Social Indicators Research Series

Volume 73

This series aims to provide a public forum for single treatises and collections of papers on social indicators research that are too long to be published in our journal *Social Indicators Research*. Like the journal, the book series deals with statistical assessments of the quality of life from a broad perspective. It welcomes the research on a wide variety of substantive areas, including health, crime, housing, education, family life, leisure activities, transportation, mobility, economics, work, religion and environmental issues. These areas of research will focus on the impact of key issues such as health on the overall quality of life and vice versa. An international review board, consisting of Ruut Veenhoven, Joachim Vogel, Ed Diener, Torbjorn Moum, Mirjam A.G. Sprangers and Wolfgang Glatzer, will ensure the high quality of the series as a whole.

More information about this series at http://www.springer.com/series/6548

Karen Bond
Editor

Sally Gardner
Consulting Editor

Dance and the Quality of Life

Springer

Editor
Karen Bond
Department of Dance
Temple University
Philadelphia, PA, USA

ISSN 1387-6570 ISSN 2215-0099 (electronic)
Social Indicators Research Series
ISBN 978-3-319-95698-5 ISBN 978-3-319-95699-2 (eBook)
https://doi.org/10.1007/978-3-319-95699-2

Library of Congress Control Number: 2018957404

This Springer imprint is published by the registered company Springer Nature Switzerland AG
The registered company address is: Gewerbestrasse 11, 6330 Cham, Switzerland

Foreword

I entered the field of arts education in the 1960s, when it was fashionable to promote the arts as ends in themselves, rather than as a means to an end, and arts education was celebrated as an important avenue for self-expression. Fifty years later, when almost all human activity is regarded primarily for its pragmatic value, the arts are more generally prized for their contribution to the economic growth of a community and the arts in education are touted primarily for their role in increasing test scores or school attendance. Under these changing conditions, considering the arts as integral to quality of life might seem just another passing trend. The quality of life discourse, however, offers a bridge between the "art for art's sake" tradition and more pragmatic values, by demonstrating how the arts can contribute to a happier, healthier, and more meaningful life for those who participate. Karen Bond (2014) has noted that, relative to other arts, dance has been marginalized as an area of serious inquiry, and this volume is a noteworthy contribution to filling an important gap in scholarship regarding dance and quality of life.

Karen and I first met at a conference of Dance and the Child: International (daCi) in New Zealand in 1985. Attending each other's sessions, we quickly realized that we were on parallel paths in our efforts to understand how young people experience dance and to include their voices in dance research literature. We continued connecting professionally for a number of years, at conferences and meetings, and eventually became co-presenters, co-teachers, co-researchers (Bond & Stinson 2000/2001, 2007/2016) – and friends.

Over the decades, as we discussed our work and that of others, we struggled to find ways to describe what we intuitively sensed was at the center of the dance experience and what made it so meaningful in our lives and the lives of others, sometimes having hearty debates about what "it" was. In retrospect, "quality of life" was perhaps the most applicable term for what we both valued in dance, and it is clear that this book represents an important strand of Karen's scholarly trajectory.

Unlike my own, Karen's belief in the power and significance of dance has never seemed to waver. As one of many possible examples of her appreciation for the potential of dance to enhance life, her 2000 keynote address at the Dance and the Child: International conference in Saskatchewan noted that she had

> identified enduring qualities and purposes of dance that could ground a caring culture for children and youth: … its contagious socializing rhythms; its value as a mode of learning, transformation, and nonverbal communication, including performance; its role in building community. (p. 13)

Revealing an affinity with the poetics of quantum physics, she concluded by stating that "dance allows expression of both difference and unity in a web of life that connects us all" (p. 13).

To say that Karen believes in the power of dance is not meant to suggest that she is a classical idealist. In our co-authored publication, "'It feels like I'm going to take off!' Young People's Experiences of the Superordinary in Dance" (2000/2001), in which we wrote individual reflections on the research findings, she stated, "as far as I can tell, there is nothing intrinsically dangerous about dancing [but]…the ease with which any manner of sociocultural ideology is able to appropriate dance and other arts complicates the issue" (p. 78). We both referenced the example of Nazi Germany's use of dance movement rituals to create citizen solidarity, and music to drown out the screams of prisoners in its death camps.

Our second co-authored article, "'It's work, work, work, work': Young People's Experiences of Effort and Achievement in Dance" (Bond & Stinson, 2007/2016), also speaks to the theme of this book. In this study, we found that when students described high levels of engagement in dance, the boundaries between work and play often dissolved; they experienced inexhaustible curiosity, challenge seeking, commitment to self-disciplined practice, and deep emotional satisfaction – all contributors to quality of life. Our analysis also identified factors inhibiting engagement and hard work, which might also be seen as obstacles to quality in one's life, including not just lack of personal interest but also fear of failure and fear of negative peer response. We concluded that "both arguments (arts as instrumental, arts as ends in themselves) seem to leave out what matters most for young people as well as adults: the creation of a meaningful life" (p. 290).

Karen's enduring belief in the possibilities of dance coexists with a rigor in scholarly analysis that has always earned my respect. Further, our collegial relationship and friendship endured my many crises of faith, as I frequently wondered whether my career in dance education was trivial in the face of the many injustices present throughout the world. I often made it through by returning to a question stimulated by Eric Fromm's (1941) thinking about freedom: If people were free from all forms of oppression, what would they then be free to do? And somehow, I could always see the arts as part of the answer, again joining Karen in reaffirming what she never seemed to doubt.

Since retiring from higher education in 2013, I have been removed from the lived experience of dancing and teaching dance and become deeply involved in responding to national, state, and local crises as well as community social action initiatives. I have questioned even more deeply whether making my professional life in dance mattered in a world that seems so broken. For others in a similar dark place, this book will offer an antidote. Reading the work of these authors is a splendid reminder of our human vocation to live fully, to stay alive and "embodied" as long as we are breathing – and the role dancing can play in that (perhaps has "always" played, as suggested in Ellen Dissanayake's Coda in this volume). As theologian and civil rights leader Howard Thurman famously affirmed, "Don't ask what the world needs. Ask what makes you come alive, and go do it. Because what the world needs is people who have come alive" (as cited in Bailie, 1996, p. xv). In the pages of this book, dance is visible as both what the world needs and as a way of coming, and staying, alive.

A quick overview of the book's sections gives a glimpse of the overall diversity to be found in this volume, a reflection of Karen's pedagogical and scholarly commitment to dance pluralism. Philosophical, historical, empirical (both quantitative and qualitative), ethnographic, autobiographical, multi-modal, and "practice-based" are among the multitude of approaches. Geographical diversity (Australia, Brazil, Denmark, Finland, Israel, New Zealand, Norway, South Africa, Taiwan, UK, USA) is also a hallmark of the book, reflecting the many connections Karen has made through Dance and the Child: International, Congress on Research in Dance, the National Dance Education Organization (USA), and 40 years of teaching and advising graduate students at the University of Melbourne in Australia and currently at Temple University in Philadelphia. This diversity adds dimensionality for the reader and also reinforces the overall premise of the book that dance is deeply connected to the human potential for thriving.

This book also represents the kind of career Karen has lived, one built on teaching and service framed in an enduring commitment to practical phenomenological inquiry – the importance of the first-person perspective "as lived" in fathoming meanings of dance. Further, constructing an edited book including the work of new, mid-career, and highly established scholars reveals her history of quietly building relationships across disciplines as well as mentoring researchers in her role as a graduate dance faculty member. Many of her students have gone on to become (some already were) established leaders, spanning the range of dance contexts – performance, invention, education, community, therapy, administration, service, research, and combinations of these. Some are contributors to this volume.

In short, this book can be seen as a worthy capstone of Karen's long career emphasizing what matters most not just in dance but in living a fully embodied life. It is also a beacon appropriate to guide future dance researchers, whose personal and professional lives will be the richer for it. In recognition of her respect for young people's meanings of dance, I will close this foreword with an excerpt revealing a Canadian high school student's holistic understanding of the importance of dance in her life, made in response to participation in a daCi conference:

> Dance is my song, my food … It promotes you, excels you, cares for you and teaches you all so simply yet so complex. This is the first time I have not felt alone… These other children too want to live dance…change the world…by connecting our different worlds, languages and traditions… We are not alone as we teach the professors, teachers and experts what we hold inside and to love dance as we do so no one will be alone. (Bond & Stinson, 2000/2001, p. 70)

Greensboro, NC, USA
April 29, 2018

Susan W. Stinson

Bibliography

Bond, K. E. (2000). Revisioning purpose: Children, dance and the culture of caring. Keynote address. In J. E. LeDrew & H. Ritenberg (Eds.), *Proceedings – Extensions & extremities: Points of departure* (pp. 3–14). Regina, SK: University of Regina.

Bond, K. E. (2014). Dance and quality of life. In A. C. Michalos (Ed.), *Encyclopedia of quality of life and well-being research* (pp. 1419–1424). Dordrecht, Netherlands: Springer.

Bond, K. E., & Stinson, S. W. (2000/2001). "I feel like I'm going to take off!" Young people's experiences of the superordinary in dance. *Dance Research Journal, 32*(2), 52–87.

Bond, K. E., & Stinson, S. W. (2016). "It's work, work, work, work:" Young people's experiences of effort and engagement in dance. In S. W. Stinson (Ed.), *Embodied curriculum theory and research in arts education: A dance scholar's search for meaning* (pp. 269–295). Dordrecht, Netherlands: Springer (Original work published 2007).

Bailie, G. (1996). *Violence unveiled: Humanity at the crossroads*. New York: Crossroad Publishing Company.

Fromm, E. (1941). *Escape from freedom*. New York: Rinehart.

Preface

> What is good, Phaedrus, and what is not good - need we ask anyone to tell us these things? (Pirsig, *Zen and the Art of Motorcycle Maintenance: An Inquiry into Values*)

The above epigraph from Robert Pirsig's (1974/1984/2011) semi-autobiographical novel has intrigued me since reading it over 40 years ago. Described variously as a "counter-culture classic" (Chawkins, 2017) and "the worst reading of Plato and Aristotle I've ever come across" (Johnson, 2010), in the 1970s West Coast environment, I was captivated by Pirsig's opus on "Quality" (with a capital Q), as were many of my friends. Over the years, I have included the question – a variation on a line from Plato's *The Phaedrus* (c. 370 BCE) – in course syllabi and lectures on epistemology, recently citing it in a book chapter on children as phenomenologists (Bond, 2018). At no point, however, have I attempted to answer the question, sometimes offering what I call the phenomenologist's disclaimer: "I am only describing language, not explaining anything." I appropriated this from Joseph Kosuth's (1991) neon art rendering of the statement (see www.pinterest.co.uk/pin/225391156321037516/) – prior to discovering it in Ludwig Wittgenstein's (1969/1974) *Philosophical Grammar* (p. 66).

Although Pirsig wrote hundreds of pages on the subject (1974/1984/2006, 1991), he struggled to define Quality. According to biographer Dan Glover (2003), one of Pirsig's premises was that Quality is not reducible to objective science, but a "way out of the 'mess' created by subject-object thinking" (p. 25), or self-other dualism. Quality precedes subject and object and is potentially accessible to all and throughout life – like dancing. Tafoya (2000) notes that in *Zen,* however, the "nameless narrator sacrifices his job, marriage, family, and sanity in his pursuit of … Quality" (p. 52). The book is abundant with unanswered, possibly unanswerable questions (Chawkins, 2017), in spite of the author's epigraphic use of a Socratic paraphrase to suggest that Quality, or *the good*, is something that everyone knows before speaking of it.

With over five million copies sold since initial publication (Chawkins, 2017), I have not been the only reader intrigued by Pirsig's metaphysical question or by his interest in "Eastern" principles such as mindfulness of nature and problems of human delusion, ignorance, and greed. Given the likely impossibility of defining Quality, Pirsig seems to advocate compassion for our collective inability to figure it out or to generate it for a sustainable future.

The same year as the publication of *Zen*, a new academic field was recognized in the launch of an international journal, *Social Indicators Research* (Alex C. Michalos, editor), specifically devoted to research on quality of life. Just over 20 years later, the first volume of Springer's Social Indicators Research book series was published (Alex C. Michalos, senior editor), with 72 volumes preceding the present one. This volume, #73, is the first in the series devoted to dance and quality of life.

In *John Dewey, Robert Pirsig, and the Art of Living,* David Granger (2006) discusses quality of life as a poetics of everyday living where "meanings of things are never final," proposing that by living life "artfully," we can increase the ability to "liberate and expand" life's potential meanings (p. 23). Further,

> When we succeed…our experiences are apt to possess a wholistic integrity. … The enhanced sense of attunement with people and things thereby created makes the world a much less forbidding and a much more fulfilling place to live in. (p. 23)

Granger views John Dewey's notion of "cultivated naiveté" as a "hermeneutics of replenishment…open-minded, not empty-minded, interested, not indifferent" (p. 23). Such cultivation is arguably a birth right, but dharmically speaking, requires "right action" (Blum, 2016) to realize it in a life worth living. As alluded to in the Foreword with the metaphor "antidote," this volume is full of "right action," as is the series in which it is housed (to be discussed further in chapter one).

I wonder whether the many scholars who have contributed to the social indicators – quality of life research field might also relate to Pirsig's (1974/1984/2006) epigraph in *Zen,* and with the following musings:

> Quality … you know what it is, yet you don't know what it is. But that's self-contradictory. But some things *are* better than others, that is, they have more quality. But when you try to say what the quality is, apart from the things that have it, it all goes *poof!* There's nothing to talk about. But if you can't say what Quality is, how do you know what it is, or how do you know that it even exists? If no one knows what it is, then for all practical purposes it doesn't exist at all. But for all practical purposes it really *does* exist. (p. 184)

Prone to cite children as theorists, I am reminded of the following epistemological reflection on dance by a North Carolina elementary school student (Bond & Stinson, 2000/2001):

> I know I learned something in dance but I just can't say what it is. It's not like it's bad or nothin', but I just don't know how to say it… It's like you want to say it, but you know you can't... It's not like you need help sayin' it, but it's just hard to say. I don't know, it won't come out ... *Life,* just put it like that, that's the best as far as I can explain it, life…period. Boom. That's all. (p. 71)

Health writer Brian Stulberg (2017) notes that even in the academic field of healthcare, quality is an elusive concept. He quotes Avedis Donabedian, a founding figure in the study of quality healthcare, whose deathbed utterances included telling a journalist that the essence of quality, echoing Pirsig, can never be measured or defined, disclosing, "Ultimately, the secret of quality is love" (n.p.). Both a long dancing life and some decades of academic inquiry into participant meanings of dance suggest to me that, ultimately, love might well be the secret of dance as well. Dutch philosopher Gerardus van der Leeuw (1932/2006) proposes that "dance and love are indissolubly bound" (p. 20), and an adolescent dancer, again in North Carolina, reflects, "I mean, if you really don't care about dance there's no reason to be doing it" (Bond & Stinson, 2007/2016, p. 164). Another puts it more simply: "It's my heart" (Bond & Stinson, 2000/2001, p. 72). Of course, in the world at large, dance is not only about love, as I will discuss further in chapter one.

I conclude this Preface with another Pirsig formulation on quality, now from his 4-year-old daughter. In Pirsig's obituary for the *Los Angeles Times*, Steve Chawkins (2017) recounts how Nell – gleefully banging on her father's typewriter – wrote the final line of *Zen's* 1984 10th anniversary edition, which reads: "ooolo99ikl;i.,pyknulmmmmmmmmm 111." May reading this volume fill you with quality.

Mount Airy, PA, USA — Karen Bond
March 20, 2018

Bibliography

Blum, H. (Ed.) (2016). Dharma jam: A modern Buddhist dance liturgy. *Dancing with Dharma: Essays on movement and dance in Western Buddhism* (pp. 147–154). Jefferson, NC: McFarland.

Bond, K. (2014). Susan W. Stinson: Teacher, scholar, advocate. In K. Harvey (Ed.), *Focus on dance: The art and craft of teaching – Proceedings of the 2013 National Dance Education Organization conference*. Bethesda, MD: NDEO.

Bond, K. (2018). "Me, a tree": Young children as natural phenomenologists. In S. Fraleigh (Ed.), *Back to the dance itself: Phenomenologies of the body in performance* (pp. 205–232). Urbana: University of Illinois Press.

Bond, K. E., & Stinson, S. W. (2000/01). "I feel like I'm going to take off!": Young people's experiences of the superordinary in dance. *Dance Research Journal, 32*(2), 52–87.

Bond, K. E., & Stinson, S. W. (2016). "It's work, work, work, work": Young people's experiences of effort and engagement in dance. In S. W. Stinson, *Embodied curriculum research and theory in arts education: A dance scholar's search for meaning* (pp. 269–298). Dordrecht, NL: Springer. (Original work published 2007)

Chawkins, S. (2017, April 24). Robert Pirsig dies at 88; wrote counterculture classic *Zen and the Art of Motorcycle Maintenance. Los Angeles Times.* Retrieved from http://www.latimes.com/local/obituaries/la-me-robert-pirsig-obituary-20170424-story.html

Dissanayake, E. (2000). *Art and intimacy*. Seattle: University of Washington Press.

Glover, D. (2003). *Lila's child: An inquiry into Quality*. Bloomington, IN: AuthorHouse.

Granger, D. A. (2006). *John Dewey, Robert Pirsig, and the art of living: Revisioning aesthetic education*. Basingstoke, England: Palgrave Macmillan.

Jones, J. (2017, April 26). Robert Pirsig reveals the personal journey that led him to write his counterculture classic, *Zen and the art of motorcycle maintenance* (1974). Retrieved from http://www.openculture.com/2017/04/robert-pirsig-reveals-the-personal-journey-that-led-him-to-write-his-counterculture-classic-zen-and-the-art-of-motorcycle-maintenance-1974.html.

Kosuth, J. (1991). *No Number #6 (On Color, Blue), 1991* [Painting]. Permanent, Museum of Contemporary Art, Chicago.

Pirsig, R. (2011). *Zen and the art of motorcycle maintenance: An inquiry into values* (40th anniversary edition). New York: HarperCollins. (Original work published 1974)

Pirsig, R. (1991). *Lila: An inquiry into morals*. New York: Bantam.

Stulberg, B. (2017, April 26). Zen and the art of Quality. Retrieved from https://www.thecut.com/2017/04/zen-and-the-art-of-quality.html.

Tafoya, E. (2000). Empty-headed musings: The holy fool in Robert Pirsig's *Zen and the Art of Motorcycle Maintenance*. In M. T. Carroll & E. Tafoya (Eds.), *Phenomenological approaches to popular culture* (pp. 49–63). Bowling Green, OH: Bowling Green State University Popular Press.

Wittgenstein, L. (1974). *Philosophical grammar* (A. Kenny, Trans.). R. Rhees (Ed.). Oxford, England: Basel Blackwell. (Original work published 1969)

Acknowledgments

Dance and the Quality of Life took root in late 2012 when senior series editor Alex Michalos invited me to bring dance into the "geological record" of the Social Indicators Research book series. Without him, it might never have occurred to me to forge pathways between the two fields, and his interest and encouragement have been greatly appreciated. Thank you to the publishing team at Springer: Esther Otten, Naomi Portnoy, Hendrikje Tuerlings, Joseph Daniels, and Lakshmikanthan Sudantradevi.

I thank the Department of Dance and Boyer College of Music and Dance for providing a sabbatical leave and stellar graduate research assistants over the years, including Julie Johnson, Nichole Arvin, Amanda DiLodovico, Kakali Paramguru, and, in particular, Matthew Olwell, who magically assembled and guided the entire manuscript into the Springer Portal. I am grateful also to doctoral fellows Robert Bingham and Molly Shanahan, who were open to a significant amount of ear-bending about the book and became contributors. Thank you to participants in my doctoral seminar, "Experience, Engagement, Multisensory Inquiry," who extended tolerance and care as I bounded toward the final publisher's deadline, which coincided with their end of semester: Pritika Agarwal, Nichole Arvin, Ziyng Cui, Colin Murray, Emily Oleson, and Kakali Paramguru.

I thank the National Dance Education Organization and the NDEO/Temple University Center for Research in Dance Education (CRDE) for its sponsorship, especially Luke Kahlich and Tom Hagood, who founded the center at Temple and understood the importance of the "quality" topic to advancing the future of dance in education, art, and life. Luke and CRDE associate Monica Frichtel provided helpful support as proposal reviewers early in the project.

I am grateful to Sally Gardner, Deakin University, Australia, whose dancing and scholarship I have long admired, for her intensive editorial contributions during the first stage of manuscript review, and by my "special request" since then. Sally's commitment has been such that I insisted she have a formal title, and we agreed to Consulting Editor (my informal title for her has sometimes been Editorial Alter-Ego).

I acknowledge three contributing authors whose work has long influenced my questioning and understanding of dance's meanings and effects: Ellen Dissanayake, Sondra Fraleigh, and Sue Stinson – thank you so much for your collaboration. I performed a wide call for papers and was determined to include everyone who appeared with an idea and stayed to closure. To all of you who communicate your unique dance knowledge and practice within these pages, and to those who helped you gather it, I am deeply grateful.

Finally, I recognize the role of family in making *Dance and the Quality of Life* come to pass, through tears and laughter: my mother Dorothy Bond (1922–2014), daughter Deanna Bond, and grandson Jesse Lloyd-Dominik, along with my rescue family whose dancily antics bring so much joy: Lucky the Dog, and cats Mama, Spot, Tiger, Jasper, Fuzzy Wuzzy, and Bo.

Contents

Graphic Essay

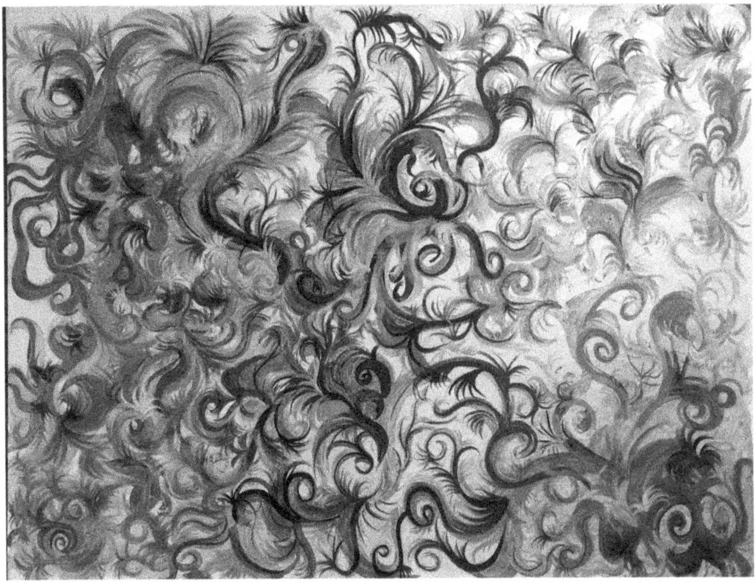

I When I agreed not to dance for six weeks (Molly Shanahan, Department of Dance, Temple University, Philadelphia, PA, USA)

Chapter 1
Introduction: At Last, Together

Karen Bond

When invited to submit an essay for Springer's *Encyclopedia of Quality of Life and Well-Being Research (EQLWR)* (Michalos, 2014), I was not familiar with the social indicators-quality of life research field. Senior editor Alex Michalos (2014) described the encyclopedia as a "fairly large" project, which turned out to be 12 volumes and 7347 pages, from "Abandonment" to "Z-values," with two further online volumes released since initial publication. In my article, I asserted that dance is underrepresented in the already-small body of literature on arts and quality of life relative to other arts (Bond, 2014). This compilation of papers on dance and the quality of life is a movement towards redressing the imbalance.

During book proposal development, I explored recent volumes in the Social Indicators Research Series online, quickly discovering Filomena Maggino's (2016) anthology, *A Life Devoted to Quality of Life: Festschrift in Honor of Alex C. Michalos*. She opens with the following tribute:

> The Festschrift celebrates his lifelong, outstanding scientific and cultural contribution to Quality of Life Research. … Taken together, the contributions from scholars around the world reflect Michalos' stance that even though there may be differences in individual scientific positions, the language in the field of quality of life has no limits and boundaries. (Preface)

Reading the festschrift, I felt drawn to this multi-disciplinary community of scholars linked by interest in understanding and bettering life on a global scale. I reflected that given the longevity of arts practice on planet Earth – at least 200,000 years – with the time arts of dance and song perhaps the earliest (see Coda), an infusion of dance perspectives into the social indicators research discourse might well aid global understanding. While the *field* of dance had not been broadly theorized within the *field* of quality of life research, I saw an analogy between the "languages" of quality of life and dance in their mutual lack of "limits and boundaries."

K. Bond (✉)
Department of Dance, Temple University, Philadelphia, PA, USA
e-mail: kbond003@temple.edu

K. Bond (ed.), *Dance and the Quality of Life*, Social Indicators Research Series 73,
https://doi.org/10.1007/978-3-319-95699-2_1

I embarked on an intensive reading program to become more familiar with the social indicators-quality of life research domain. Initial perusal of titles in *Social Indicators Research* (the journal, founded 1974) and the Social Indicators Research Series (founded 1997) evoked a similar response to that of Phillips (2016), who was "stunned by the magnitude" of the field (p. 123). Pointing to the "thousands of topics" covered in the *EQLWR* (Michalos, 2014), she deems quality of life a "somewhat mystifying area of research" that crosses boundaries readily (sounds like dance), as it "resonates deeply with many, regardless of disciplinary specialty" (Phillips, 2016, p. 124). She notes some "common views" of quality of life (QOL) studies:

> QOL embraces "the totality of human life" (Cummins, 2000); QOL has multidimensional factors measured by different life domains regardless of an emphasis on either subjective or objective aspects of life; and QOL encompasses various units of society from individual to community, to national, and to global level. (Sirgy et al., 2011, p. 128)

Michalos summarizes, "Quality of life is as varied as there are perspectives from which it can be assessed" (as cited in Weijers, 2014, p. 108). All of Sirgy et al.'s named units of society are referenced in the present volume (as cited in Phillips, 2016).

During a title scan of the book series, I noted recent expansion into qualitative research approaches. Graciela Tonon's (2015) *Qualitative Studies in Quality of Life: Methodology and Practice* aims to "show the importance of the development of qualitative studies in the field of quality of life" (Preface). An introductory chapter establishes the author's affiliation with the qualitative paradigm's emphasis on description, discovery, understanding, and articulation of diverse participant meanings in social contexts. She summarizes recent developments in two selected places: a journal – *Applied Research in Quality of Life* – and her own research group at the Universidad Nacional de Lomas de Zamora, Argentina. Most of Tonon's examples of qualitative methods are at work and play in the present volume: phenomenology, hermeneutics, grounded theory, ethnography, content analysis, thematic analysis, action research, and participative research, along with others that reach into memoir, autoethnography, multimodality, and poetics. I appreciate her perspective that qualitative research offers a theoretical outlook focused on possibilities rather than deficiencies, where a person is considered as a "subject and protagonist" endowed with human rights (p. 19).

A paper that caught my attention for its relevance to dance and quality of life is Ruut Veenhoven's (2016) "What we have Learnt about Happiness," where I discovered there is a "World Database of Happiness" (www.worlddatabaseofhappiness.eur.nl) with some 10,000 "scientific articles," the sum of which show that in terms of *outer qualities of life*, people live most happily in contexts of freedom, rule of law, economic development, and good governance (low corruption). One of Veenhoven's happiness criteria, *freedom* (in both inner and outer forms), has been closely associated with dance, ontologically and empirically (see Chaps. 10 and 20), as has the feeling state of *happiness* itself – through time and across persons, gender, age, abilities, race, class, and culture.

Dutch theologian Gerardus van der Leeuw (1932/2006) cites Molière's seventeenth century play, *Le Bourgeois Gentilhomme,* which attributes human unhappiness to the neglect of dance:

> [One] who does not dance is good for nothing. … All human unhappiness, all blows of fortune which history reports to us, all mistakes of politics, all defeats of the great commanders result solely from the fact that dance is not understood. (p. 20)

That dance and *joy* are related is an ancient idea. Plato, for example, saw dance as a fitting way to express joy, as it is impossible to remain still in the state (Davies, 1984). The human capacity for joy has also been associated with quality of life as a function of "presence" (Ventegodt, Anderson, Kromann, & Merrick, 2003):

> Somewhere deep in life exists the finest sweetness, the greatest quality in life, the pure joy of being alive that emerges when we are fully present and life is in balance. This deep joy of life is what we call experiencing the meaning of life. (p. 1183)

I dedicate this volume to my mother Dorothy Bond (1922–2014). A student of "aesthetic dance," sometimes called "free dance," in her youth, she understood my 4-year-old twirling to classical music and enrolled me in classes at a suburban ballet school north of Chicago. In retrospect, I think my mother wanted to enrich my quality of life, which dance has and hasn't done over the decades. In the next section I elaborate on dance's conundrums and paradoxes.

Dance: Conundrums and Paradoxes

As noted in the Foreword, for the most part this volume projects an "antidotal" sensibility, illuminating dance's purposes and potentials to afford a *good* quality of life. However, significant social-cultural-historical conditions have kept dance from being understood as a constituent of quality living and as a "fine art." In the West, German philosopher G. W. F. Hegel (1835/1975) relegated dance (and gardening) to the category of "imperfect art" in his early nineteenth century *Lectures on Aesthetics* (1818–1829). Due to its "inferior status," Hegel failed to give dance its own discrete place in his "system" of central, or fine arts, perhaps establishing an attitude that is alive today among philosophers of art and people-at-large. Philosopher Joshua Hall (2017) notes a continuing spillover of Hegelian thinking in the relatively low status of those associated with dancing: "women, people of color, children, and non-human animals" (p. 49).

Capitalism has compromised dance's intrinsic connections with joy and wellbeing – in its hierarchical class-ifications, exploitations, commodifications, competitions, gender binaries, and objectification of "the dancing body," particularly the female dancer. Sally Gardner notes the problem of "the gaze" (Mulvey, 1975/1999; Sartre, 1943/1992):

> The nature of the environments and structures where individuals make and experience their dancing are critical to quality of life, particularly since our bodies, and movements, can be

> subject to powerfully controlling and instrumentalising gazes and disciplinary regimes. (S. Gardner, personal communication, February 28, 2018)

Misuses of dance can often be traced to abuses of power and control, and also to the Buddha's "poisons" of ignorance mentioned in the Preface: greed, hatred, and delusion (Carter, 2010), which affect all quality of life (see Flores, 2015). Exemplifying the three poisons all at once, dancing has been forced on humans – for example, when African slaves were made to dance on ships during the 300-year Atlantic slave trade (Diedrich, Gates & Pedersen, 1999; Feelings, 2018; Sharp & Schomp, 2007) – and on nonhuman animals in captivity (Szablowski, 2014). In addition to coercion, dance has been used as punishment and humans have been punished *for* dancing (see Arcangeli, 1992, 1994).

Dance, Power, and Religion

While joy, presence, and balance might be considered inherent possibilities of dancing, van der Leeuw (1932/2006) notes that dance is capable of expressing "all the emotions…from the highest to the lowest" (p. 12). The history of world religions includes "powerful disciplinary regimes" that have suppressed or condemned dance on moral grounds (see Chaps. 7, 8, 24, and 27). Beginning with general acceptance in the Hebrew Judaic tradition as a deeply rooted mode of religious celebration, Christianity developed and changed its attitudes to dance through early anti-pagan purifications, dance epidemics, inter- and intra-denominational disagreements, formal prohibitions during the Protestant Reformation (Enge, 2017), and on to today's growing attention to religious renewal through liturgical dance (Davies, 1984; George-Graves, 2010) and the "praise dance" of the African diaspora (Daniel, 2005; Smith & Jackson, 2005). Overarching these particularities is the historical trajectory since the early Christian Middle Ages (500 CE) and the advent of Islam (610 CE), along which authorities of the world's two most populated religions have variously but consistently imposed bans on dancing.

Christians have been dissuaded through writings and sermons about the evils of dance, including threats of punishment (Arcangeli, 1992; Enge, 2017). Yet early sixteenth century Protestant reformist Martin Luther, for example, supported the role of dance in worship, especially for children (Adams & Apostolos-Cappadona, 1990; Wagner, 1997). Three centuries later, Reverend John Blake was an example of pro-dance advocacy (as cited in Kraus, Hilsendager, & Dixon, 1969/1991), observing,

> In the middle of the day…let half an hour be spent in this fascinating exercise, as a reward for good conduct as scholars, and the prediction is made with confidence, that neither boys or girls will ever be tardy. (p. 295)

Arcangeli (1992) notes an enduring paradox in Christianity's treatment of dance since the Middle Ages:

> On the one hand, dancing in this world is blamed: on the other hand, dance itself, in a different, ideal, context, is classified as one of the manifestations of joy, and as a special one, indeed: saints will not be entirely happy without it. (p. 40)

Essentially, in spite of centuries of institutionalized anti-dance bombast, children (and many adults) *will* dance spontaneously and without formal instruction, unless and until they are stopped or stop themselves. On the macro scale, however, one can't ignore the strong rhetorical thread in Christianity that equates dance with mortal sin, even when performed without "perverse" intentions (Wagner, 1997, p. 8; Chap. 8, this volume).

In Islam, rules are gender-based; women may dance in female-only settings, while for men dance is prohibited altogether (Sufi whirling dervish orders excepted). Within the third largest and widely regarded as the oldest religion, Hinduism, dance is integral to its cosmology, with beginnings in Vedic ritual around 1500 BCE (Thobani, 2017). Sitara Thobani notes that Indian dance continues to be associated with Hinduism since its twentieth century "reconstruction as classical," albeit according to contemporary understandings of Hinduism and the need to "navigate the religious/secular divide" of India's post-colonial nation state (p. 148). Globalizing the current state of religion and dance, statistics become daunting for the dance advocate. Of earth's 7.3 billion people, at least 63% (4.6 billion) possibly are or have been explicitly or implicitly discouraged from dancing on religious or moral grounds (with the exceptions of Hinduism and Judaism). Further, I estimate that in the world today, 30% of Christians are forbidden to dance (over 600 million people possibly forego this human capability). (www.pewforum.org/2012/12/18/global-religious-landscape-exec/).

Cultural theorist Jane Desmond (2001) suggests that in the West, anti-dance religious proscriptions were strengthened by modernity's "racist and colonialist cultural assumptions of an intrinsic connection between dance and sex" (p. 201). Such corruptions of indigenous courtship and fertility rituals have been used to exploit women (see Chap. 24) and children in particular. A current example of the latter is in Afghanistan, where females are not allowed to dance in public, but *bacha bazi* (under-18 "dancing boys") dressed as girls may be forced to perform for security forces, militia, and other sorts of powerful males, sometimes resulting in sexual abuse and rape (Bezhan, 2017).

Dance and Economic Wellbeing

Dancers earn well below the median hourly wage for American workers in the category of 'arts, design, entertainment, sports, and media' occupations (www.statisticbrain.com/entertainment-occupation-salary-statistics/), and dance majors in American higher education face the dilemma of whether or not to do a double major or some other kind of training that can offer financial stability if a career in dance fails to eventuate. An important question, therefore, is whether dance, especially dance performance, can be a viable career – a source of economic sustainability. In

"The Poorest Art: Dance and Money," poet and dancer Lightsey Darst (2012) writes, "Just how poor is dance? There are far too many ways to answer this question," also asserting, "I've come to a conclusion about dance and money: if dancers did not sometimes sleep with rich people, American dance as we know it would cease to exist" (n.p.). This association has a documented history in "concert art dance," for example, in the sexual abuse of dancers in the nineteenth century Paris Opera Ballet (Coons, 2014; McCarren, 1998). The article's actual "conclusion" has a more metaphysical tone, connecting with subjective quality of life: the act of dancing has intrinsic value (Darst, 2012).

> If we thought of dancers as tax-paying adults, if we took them seriously, then we'd have to take seriously the message common across practically all dance: that the life of the body matters. The moment matters: it matters how you feel, what you do to your body and to other bodies. This is what dance, unforgivably, says: the flesh is good. (n.p.)

I find myself thinking of Pirsig's (1974/2011) epigraph, "Need we ask anyone to tell us these things?" Apparently, yes.

The Economics Department at Macquarie University, Australia, has been surveying artists about career conditions since the 1980s, identifying an entrenched cultural attitude towards those who make art for a living: "Why should people be paid to do what others do for fun?" (Throsby & Petetskaya, 2017, n.p.). Similar to Darst, Throsby and Petetskaya cite non-pecuniary values, the "psychic income" afforded by the practice of dance and other arts. Close to four decades of survey data indicate that "the inner drive to make art is what encourages artists to continue… passion, self-motivation, self-belief" (n.p.).

Back to economics, it appears that dance artists working in the "fine art" concert dance realm are a particularly poorly remunerated cohort, a situation confounded by gendered pay differences. Globally, men tend to earn proportionately more than women for similar work as dancers, choreographers, and teachers (Coulangeon, Ravet, & Roharik, 2005; Throsby & Petetskaya, 2017; Van Dyke, 1992). Darst (2012) interviewed a career ballerina who informed that in the U. S. earnings begin at around $500 per week for a season of 30–40 weeks, and a former researcher for Dance/USA reported from survey data that:

> At most 6 percent of serious dance makers (including companies and independent choreographers) are offered salaries…most…make less than $25,000 a year from dancing. … Many make less, and many make their primary living outside dance. (n.p.)

He indicates further that fewer than ten American dance companies offer 1-year contracts with paid vacation, and no more than 100 dancers in the U. S. make over $100,000 a year. In contrast, market research by Ibis World (2017) reported U. S. strip club revenue at $7 billion, with an average annual income per dancer of $125,000 (www.ibisworld.com/industry-trends/specialized-market-research-reports).

Conclusion

Problems of anti-dance religious prohibitions, gender power imbalances, sexual exploitation, racism, and lack of economic stability intersect with the oppressive practices of ageism, ableism, and the "aesthetic of the thin" (Jawole Willa Jo Zollar, as cited in Kreemer, 2008, p. 34). These social fabrications can inhibit dancing or push its expression into extremes that do not support its capacity to afford a good quality of life across the human lifespan (Bolwell, 2018; Kelly, 2012; Kreemer, 2008; Lansley & Early, 2011; Nahvi, 2015; Schwaiger, 2011). Then there is the enduring myth (even among practitioners) that dancers can't learn without physical pain and emotional abuse (Lakes, 2005). In recent years, this notion was popularized through mass media on the American TV docuseries, *Dance Moms,* where in 2013, the show's inventor and outrageously aggressive dance competition coach, Abby Lee Miller, was charged by a student with assault; in its first 2 years, the show charted close to 200 million viewers (Zar, 2012), approximately half of them adults.

Sondra Fraleigh observes that dance "can offer a chance for engagement and self-knowledge or can punish and deny the body" (as cited in Bond, 2014, p. 1421). Examples of the latter phenomena abound in professional performance contexts. Upon reaching 110 pounds (50 kilos), prima ballerina Anastasia Volochkova was fired from the Bolshoi Ballet; in 2009, the injury rate for professional dancers in the UK was 80% (www.telegraph.co.uk/culture/theatre/dance/5686620/Ballet-by-numbers.html). Dancer and choreographer Molly Shanahan's series of drawings dispersed through this volume, titled "Getting to Blackbird: Early Drawings Toward a Reimagined Body," portray a living process of dance – affected and sometimes driven by bodily hatred, while seeking transformation into self-acceptance.

This section on conundrums and paradoxes of dance has considered obstacles to dance's sustainability and ability to thrive in a world of religious extremism, gender power imbalances, economic realities, and more. On these grounds, a naïve reader might think it impossible to show an intrinsic connection between dance, dancing, and quality of life. In the next section I introduce 31 chapters and a Coda that for the most part suggest otherwise, individually and collectively.

Dance and the Quality of Life

Like quality of life research itself (according to Phillips, 2016 cited earlier), dance can be described as a "mystifying area" of inquiry (p. 124) – difficult to define, understand, and justify as an element of quality of life. For my *EQLWR* article (Bond, 2014) I practiced the phenomenological epoché as I sought to affiliate dance and quality of life without falling into personal biases and "theories du jour." Asked to include a definition (a prospect that sent my epistemologist's hands fluttering with uncertainty), I offered the following:

> Dance is nonverbal behavior composed of movements that convey a heightened, aesthetic sense of body, rhythm, and space. Human dance can hold individual, social, cultural and/or spiritual meanings for both participants and observers. In its longevity and multiplicity of forms and functions, dance eludes definition. (p. 1419)

In the 1960s, a decade when dance educators, anthropologists, philosophers, and historians in the United States were attempting to cohere into a 'field' of dance research, dancer and doctoral candidate in anthropology Joann Kealiinohomoku (as cited in Bond, 2014) noted an "amazing divergence of opinions" about the origin of dance:

> We are able to read that the origin of dance was in play and…not in play, that it was for magical and religious purposes, and…not for those things; that it was for courtship and… not for courtship; that it was the first form of communication and that communication did not enter into dance until it became an "art." In addition, we can read that it was serious and purposeful and at the same time…an outgrowth of exuberance…totally spontaneous, and originated in the spirit of fun. Moreover, we can read that it was only a group activity for tribal solidarity and that it was strictly for the pleasure and self-expression of the one dancing. (p. 1419)

Given these polarities in dance's creation myths, dance might indeed be as difficult to define as quality of life.

Michalos (2014) identifies two distinct while overlapping quality of life research categories developed since the 1960s. One has a "fairly narrow focus on health-related issues" and the other a "quite broad focus" (p. 1). I recognize similitude in the distinct, overlapping categories of dance research that emerged in the United States in the 1960s, representing health (American Dance Therapy Association, founded 1966) and breadth (Congress on Research in Dance, founded 1964) of research interests.

While Kealiinohomoku highlighted wide-ranging theories of dance's beginnings, she did not identify health as an originative purpose, even though the modern profession of dance therapy was positing dance's early functions in health, healing, and "integration of the individual" (https://adta.org/faqs/), a proposition that has a ring of common sense. To date, most research on dance and quality of life comes from dance/movement therapy and allied health fields (Chaiklin & Wengrower, 2009; Hanna, 2006). Accordingly, I emphasized these areas in the *EQLWR* essay (Bond, 2014), as does the recently published *Oxford Handbook of Dance and Wellbeing* (Karkou, Oliver, & Lycouris, 2017), where the writers of its two forewords come from music therapy and dance therapy.

Further, over 60% of Karkou et al.'s 49 chapters include one or more authors trained in dance/movement therapy or dance/movement psychotherapy, and 12 chapters involve collaborations with research scientists, mostly from psychology and neuroscience. Perusing chapter titles in each of the handbook's five major sections – body, performance, education, community, and health – they appear overall to project an orientation to the "psycho-therapeutic," an impression confirmed by Karkou & Oliver (2017) in the book's Conclusion, where they state: "There is a vein of dance movement psychotherapy running through…another unifying agent among the disparate sections…" (p. 926).

In contrast, *Dance and the Quality of Life* fits the category Michalos (2014) refers to as "quite broad." As mentioned in the Foreword, the volume contains contributions from 11 countries (Australia, Brazil, Denmark, Finland, Israel, New Zealand, Norway, South Africa, Taiwan, the United States, and the United Kingdom), and an author pool of dance artists, teachers, researchers, scholars, philosophers, advocates, culture workers, health professionals, and combinations of these. A range of methodological perspectives are presented, and unlike the quality of life-social indicators field historically, these are mostly qualitative, including a strong measure of first-person studies encompassing memoir, life writing, personal narrative, autoethnography, and various phenomenological approaches.

For me, the book offers a complex assemblage of people caring about and doing similar kinds of things, while often describing or naming their "doings" with different languages, depending on discipline and other affiliations. This makes the task of chapter sequencing – compiling a categorized, logically-ordered table of contents – arduous (more dramatically, I would say "impossible"), pointing to another core value of this "bricolage": the holistic nature of dance as human behavior – multi-sensory, meta-cognitive, fundamentally improvisational, and present in every known human society (Dissanayake, 2000, 2017, Coda), perhaps in all sentient beings. If I were asked to name the top four methodological influences and themes of the volume as a whole, however, I would nominate first person methodologies, hermeneutic phenomenology (in particular, Max van Manen, 1990/1997, 2014), participatory action research, and grounded theory. At the same time, I would be prompted to paraphrase Renata Tesch's (1990) *Qualitative Research: Analysis Types and Software Tools,* the first textbook I read in the newly named field. Similar to Michalos's comment on "quality of life" quoted earlier (as cited in Weijers, 2014, p. 108), Tesch suggests there are as many definitions of "qualitative research" as there are individuals doing it.

A feature of the volume is the authors' collective interest in practice, their own and others', as evidenced in the 24 of 31 chapters (close to 80%) that highlight direct participation in or observation of live dancing, or both. In essence, the book, including the solely theoretical chapters, presents a cohort of advocates speaking to dance's possibilities when associated with subjective quality of life, possibilities that point also to potential "objective" connections, or what Michalos calls "elements of the dependent variable" (p. 108). Dancing is, of course, not only subjective experience, but also inter-subjective. Sally Gardner notes, "Dancing takes place in the world amongst others; the other's/another's body, oneself as another, is always more or less implied" (S. Gardner, personal communication, February 28, 2018). This perspective is reflected widely in the volume, where first person methods are often integrated with social epistemologies, as well as contemporary multi-modal hybrids and bricolage approaches (Denzin & Lincoln, 1994/2017; Kincheloe, McLaren, & Steinberg, 2011; Rogers, 2012; Chap. 23, this volume).

Dance and the Quality of Life also reflects the post-modern burgeoning of interest in narrative inquiry across disciplines from science and mathematics to art and education. A methodology that can be traced to oral and nonverbal narrative traditions of many cultures, van Manen (1997) emphasizes that narrative – or put simply, stories – can be a research tool for understanding particular phenomena through people's experiences and the sense they make of them. Collecting and telling stories might be particularly important where researchers and participants are concerned about personal, social, and political change (Razack, 1993), all of which are needed to improve quality of life on a global scale. Importantly, stories can reveal how social injustices and inequities are experienced and perpetuated, both individually and collectively, and also uncover resistance to such conditions (Horsfall & Titchen, 2007).

Geography and Topography: Quality and Dance

The book's main body contains eight sections followed by Ellen Dissanayake's Coda, which highlights a topic that seems crucial to understanding dance and the quality of life – the biological basis of dance and the arts. Each section holds three to five chapters, many of which could be placed in two or more sections. Such seems the nature of dance and the quality of life's plural construction – its "diversity of synchronizing rhythms" and "fluctuant motility" (Feldstein, 1979, p. 41). The opening section, "Dancing Ecology, Sustaining Earth," and the culminating "Coda" together offer perspectives of dance with, on, and for earth, a curatorial decision based on both fields' growing attention to sustainability and co-existence. The remainder of this chapter offers brief introductions to each section along with snapshots of individual chapters.

Dancing Ecology, Sustaining Earth

In this opening section three artist narratives describe embodied, aesthetic explorations of self and environment, persons and places. Each author encourages us to see ourselves as active, creative beings who exist in complex worlds that affect us as we affect them (see Berleant, 2016). Here are stories of canyons and caves, water and wind, trees and spiders, human and other-than-human. Each narrative, through words and images, offers entry points to new ways of thinking about quality of life on earth.

In "Canyon Consciousness" Sondra Fraleigh blends personal narrative, poetry, and phenomenological reflection on her practice of "intrinsic dance" in the canyons of southern Utah. She describes how dancing in nature can be a form of personal healing and spiritual practice throughout life.

Don Asker's "Dancing the Landscape" recounts his experience living and dancing on the south coast of New South Wales, Australia. Considering landscape to include both geological and human constructions, he invites us to consider the responsibilities, ethics, and relationships that are ongoing between humans and places.

"In the Shadow of Crisis: Dance and Meaning in the Anthropocene" by Robert Bingham describes the author's year of daily walking, dance improvisation, and collecting trash in Wissahickon Park, Philadelphia, USA. He asks how dance can respond to ecological crisis, theorizing that dance directly accesses quality of life.

Spirituality

While a number of chapters, such as those in the previous section, touch on holistic meanings and values of dance that reference or allude to the spiritual, this section includes ethnographic and historical studies – two of each, that foreground dance and spirituality. Ethnographic research by Adrienne Sansom, and by Ojeya Cruz Banks and Jeanette "Adama Jewel" Jackson, examine dance in relation to Māori and West African spiritual values, respectively. The two chapters by Kimerer LaMothe and Jessica Van Oort apply comparative-historical lenses to examine ecstatic dance phenomena across cultures and times. In their emphasis on "dancing nature," the first three chapters in the section continue the ecological thread begun in "Dancing Ecology, Sustaining Earth."

Adrienne Sansom's "Dance as a *Taonga* from Children to the World" documents children's expressive play and dancing during walks from their early childhood center to a nearby *maunga,* or volcanic mountain, a revered spiritual landmark. Her interest is in whether and how dance can contribute to young children's sense of identity and culture, especially when connected with place. Qualitative research findings are discussed in relation to *Te Whāriki*, Aotearoa New Zealand's early childhood curriculum based on Māori values.

In "West African Dance and Spiritual Well-Being for African Americans," Ojeya Cruz Banks and Jeanette "Adama Jewel" Jackson consider how West African dance and drum can ameliorate the effects of racism in the United States. Through autobiographical writing along with ethnographic observations and interviews, the co-authors highlight Jackson's life experience and educational activism, addressing the possibilities and challenges of cultivating an African American selfhood based on West African dance as a practice of spiritual wellbeing.

Kimerer LaMothe, in "Dancing on Earth: The Healing Dance of Kalahari Bushmen and the Native American Ghost Dance Religion," examines two traditions where ecstatic dance has prevailed in the face of Christian colonialism. She details how both dance forms assert cultural identity and cultivate relationships with nature, concluding that dancing allows people to affirm their humanity in the face of forces that would otherwise deny it.

Jessica Van Oort also presents two cases of ecstatic dance in "The Spirit Moves: Christian Trance Dance in Late Medieval Europe and Early Nineteenth-Century America." Despite condemnation by church authorities and moralists, dance was an important part of Christian practice during these times. The chapter sheds light on the complicated relationship between dance and Christianity, especially for women.

Philosophical Perspectives

In one of our editorial exchanges, Sally Gardner commented,

> In *Feeling and Form,* the American philosopher Susanne Langer (1953) argues that dance is not a product or tool of mental imagining but occurs when imagination arises from the material of movement—from bodies. Langer's notion of the dancing experience as one where bodies are agents of imagination seems crucial for the place of dance in quality of life, a premise addressed directly or alluded to in numerous places in this volume. (S. Gardner, personal communication, February 28, 2018)

In Gardner's "How *Seudati* Put Me in Touch with Birds," she alludes to the importance of bodily imagination in experienced quality of life. Recalling her study of the Acehnese dance *seudati* in northern Sumatra, she relates how the dance evoked a sense of becoming bird-like, but without mimesis. She suggests that learning *seudati* expanded her susceptibility and sensibility to another species, stating: "I feel that I possess to some extent a new quality of life in which a relation to birds is part of my being and comes through my sensing, perceiving body."

In "*Pause. Listen.* Visibility and Freedom in Choreographic Practice," dance maker Simon Ellis grapples with language – how terms like "choreographer" or "dancer" can both block and enable processes of imagination. Considering his 2014 work *Pause. Listen.,* including reflective responses of commissioned viewers, he discusses how dance-making can evoke a utopian, fluid space of imagination shared between choreographer and dancer, as well as a critical space of difference and discontinuity.

Aili Bresnahan and Michael Deckard's chapter, "Beauty in Disability: An Aesthetics for Dance and for Life," counterposes the mathematical concepts of proportion and symmetry defining beauty in the Enlightenment with eighteenth century Irish philosopher Edmund Burke's counter-imaginary of "beauty-in-experience." The authors propose a resignification of beauty in light of the dancing of so-called "disabled" bodies, as exemplified in selected mixed ability dance companies in Brazil, United Kingdom, and the United States.

Dancing Gender, Dancing Family

The three chapters in this section address two under-represented research areas: males in dance and family dance. The first two offer qualitative studies of dance programs for fathers and sons, a particularly obscure topic in dance literature. A third chapter focuses on men's constructions of gender identity in a contemporary African dance company that the author describes as "familial."

In "Just Me and Daddy," Byron Richard examines the experiences of a group of fathers and sons in a weekly dance program facilitated by the author. Drawing on multiple sources of qualitative data (video, interviews with participants and their family members, and reflective drawings), Richard describes how fathers and sons supported and mediated each other's individual movement styles and dispositions to create an "aesthetic community."

Isto Turpeinen (Finland) and Ralph Buck (New Zealand) collaborate on "Fathers, Sons and Encounters in Dance." Their chapter reveals how dance fostered relationships in Turpeinen's work with fathers and sons in Finland based on his teaching methodology, *raw-board-working*. Authors reflect on how the love that underpins a father and son relationship can be affirmed through dancing and performing together.

In "Friction: Male Identity and Representation in Umfundalai," C. Kemal Nance articulates a complex relation between the history of Umfundalai, an African diasporic dance form, and values of African American masculinity and male identity. Drawing on interviews with male Umfundalai dancers and his own experience of long-term engagement with the dance form as performer and teacher, the author proposes that Umfundalai provides a familial-spiritual environment for African-descended males in dance.

Wellbeing, Ability, Health

In spite of a wide call, we received only one chapter proposal from self-identified health professionals, this from community health nurse Uzo Nwankpa and perinatal nurse Stephanie Bevill. In addition to their chapter, this section contains two further articles that address dance and quality of life questions through mixed-methods research: a group of community dancers with Parkinson's (London), and student dancers volunteering with at-risk populations (Philadelphia). These are the only chapters in the volume based on quantitative-qualitative approaches to assess effects of dancing or facilitating dance outside of "mainstream" dance environments, all of them in "community dance" settings.

All three chapters address difficulties of applying quantitative instrumentation to validate dance in "quality" terms. Perhaps this circumstance is implicated in the relative lack of attention to the arts in the more statistically-oriented, global mission of the social indicators-quality of life research field. In any case, I value researchers who perform the "art-science duet" (Bond, 1994, 2008). The fourth chapter in this section offers holistic theorization of "somatic movement dance education" as a philosophical, cognitive, feminist, and spiritual realm of pedagogical practice that can enhance dancers' wellbeing and cognitive-creative abilities.

In "The Impact of Community Engagement through Dance on Teen and Young Adult Dancers," Miriam Giguere investigates self-esteem, empathy, artistic understanding, and career aspirations of 17 youth dancers (ages 16–21) volunteering in two community dance settings: low-income teens in an urban community center, and a wheelchair dance class for young people with cerebral palsy. Research methods included quantitative measures triangulated with qualitative data from pre- and post-engagement interviews with dancers.

Sara Houston and Ashley McGill's chapter, "Understanding Quality of Life through the Experiences of Dancers with Parkinson's," focuses on a group of dancers in their 30s and 40s with early onset Parkinson's who participated in a Popping class. This mixed-methods study suggests that for people living with Parkinson's, quality of life is not solely dependent on physical and mental functioning and can improve, despite progression of symptom severity.

In "Dance and Well-Being: Honoring Caroline Plummer," Uzo Nwankpa and Stephanie Bevill explore influences of community dance on the well-being of new mothers and their babies. Data for this mixed-methods inquiry were sourced during an 8-week program based on Nwankpa's RICHER Model of community dance. Study results are placed in dialogue with New Zealand's health model, which emphasizes Māori Hauora (well-being), western integrative medicine, and community nursing process.

Rebecca Weber's review of literature, "Somatic Movement Dance Education: A Feminist, Cognitive, Phenomenological Methodology for Creativity in Dance," situates SMDE in the broader body-mind integration field of Somatics, as well as in feminism, existential phenomenology, and theories of cognition. Along with its documented effects on wellbeing, Weber proposes that SMDE can support dancers cognitively, increasing creativity in movement generation for dance choreography.

Quality of Educational Life

Much has been written about the role of education in affording quality of life (particularly economic wellbeing). In a world where more than 159 million 3-to-6 year olds, as well as 120 million primary-age children and adolescents – over half of them girls, lack access to basic education (www.unicef.org/education/bege_61667.html), this is a vital discourse. While access to education is an objective indicator, quality of life *within* education, for students and teachers, has received minimal attention. If this were not the case, dance might by now be core curriculum in schools around the globe. Researchers in Denmark and Finland, urban USA, Taiwan, South Africa, and Brazil investigate quality of educational life in practice and theory for students, teachers, or both.

According to the World Economic Forum (2016), of the 10 countries shown to have the highest quality of life, five of them are the Nordic nations of Denmark, Finland, Iceland, Norway, and Sweden (https://www.weforum.org/agenda/2018/01/how-s-life-where-you-are/). This section begins with "Dance and the Quality of Life at Schools: A Nordic Affiliation" by Eeva Anttila and Charlotte Svendler Nielsen. Based primarily on qualitative interviews with students and teachers, the study yields comparative insights from dance research in two public schools – one in Finland and another in Denmark. The authors connect research findings to theories of embodied learning and introduce Martha Nussbaum and Amartya Sen's Capability Approach, a quality of life assessment framework, into dance education research.

The remaining four chapters focus on dance in higher education. In "Discovering Freedom in Dance Education," Monica Frichtel draws on descriptive data from students across multiple sections of a general education dance pluralism course at Temple University, Philadelphia, to ground a theoretical discussion of dance as freedom. The author proposes that the "freedom pedagogies," phenomenological and critical practices oriented towards personal change and social justice, are uniquely positioned to frame pursuits of freedom in dance education.

Yi-Jung Wu's chapter, "University Dance Students in Taiwan Step out of their 'Bubble' of Elite Dance Training," concentrates on 41 professionally-trained dance students as they confront the challenge of teaching creative dance for children during a 1-year "Dance Teaching Practicum." Wu's analysis of interns' written assignments and teaching films shows that the course supported dance majors to reconsider the meaning of dance as a holistic experience that could enhance the quality of their own dancing lives.

"'A little kind of community': South African Students Dance for Self, Other and Society," by Marelize Marx, bears a historical connection to the first volume of the Social Indicators Research book series (Møller, 1997), which provided "a frank report" on South Africa's challenges post-apartheid (p. 1). Two decades later Marx explores whether dance education can promote "social cohesion" in post-Apartheid South Africa. Her study found that 76 participants from across South Africa's multi-cultural population benefited from working together as student teachers in dance. Marx discusses research findings in relation to contemporary South African socio-political ideology and the African philosophy of *Ubuntu*.

Alba Vieira presents "Quality of Working Life for Higher Education Dance Teachers: Embodiment, Complexity, Transformation," stating that "quality of life is intimately connected to quality of working life." She supports this premise with 35 dance educators' written stories about their teaching, both "good" and "bad," submitted by email from six countries. Vieira's hermeneutic phenomenological analysis illuminates "the complex and infinite possibilities of…dance teachers' quality of life as embodied transformation."

Identity, Embodied Change, and Restoration

In this section researchers explore questions of dance and quality of life in conditions of unstable social or political dynamics outside of formal education settings. Authors examine influences and possibilities of a variety of dance forms in relation to wider cultural frames that affect their transmission and reception. Dance forms include belly dance, inclusive contemporary dance, hip hop, creative movement, and two settings of Australian Indigenous dance.

Ephrat Huss and I collaborate on "Women Span Personal to Political in an Israeli Belly Dance Setting," a phenomenological-political analysis based on participant experiences in a 6-week workshop sponsored by the Women's Forum at Ben Gurion University. The authors identify meanings of belly dancing for a multi-generational, inter-ethnic group of 22 women citizens of Israel (ages 25–60), situating the study in current literature on belly dance as a mode of empowerment, denigration, metamorphosis, or cultural appropriation, depending on context, for all genders.

Tone Pernille Østern, Elen, Øyen, and Philip Channells present "Life-Changing Life Journeys through Artistic and Educational Inclusive Contemporary Dance Contexts." Dance artists Øyen and Channells document their experiences of change through long-term engagement in dance communities composed of "differently bodied dancers with and without disabilities." Østern's "life story analysis" of her colleagues' written life reflections identified individual "nodal points" and shared themes, which are discussed in relation to theories of aesthetic transformation and learning within a wider frame of dance and quality of life.

In "Young People's Experiences in Hip Hop Participation," Jacinda Richards and Sally Gardner present a qualitative study with migrant or newly arrived youth in Melbourne, Australia. Fifteen young females and males from diverse geographic and family backgrounds and wide-ranging experiences of dislocation participated in hip hop dance classes and a dance crew. Through focus groups and individual interviews, the authors sought to understand participants' reasons for joining hip hop and what benefits, if any, they perceived.

Erica Rose Jeffrey and Leslie Pruitt, in "Dancing it out: Building Positive Peace," are circumspect about claims that might be made about the role of dance in "peace building" in situations of social difficulty or conflict. With this qualification, they present a "Typology of Dancing for Peace" that outlines six extant approaches to peacebuilding in relation to quality of life. The chapter includes also a qualitative empirical component, examining the practice of dance for peace in one particular context facilitated by a dancer trained in peacebuilding.

This section ends with Kim Dunphy and Vicki Ware's "Dance and Quality of Life for Indigenous Communities in Australia." The researchers discuss two examples of Indigenous cultural practices focused on dance: the Junba dance-song tradition of Western Australia and the Milpirri Festival of the Northern Territory, identifying factors that might enable improved quality of life. They propose that dance practices of Indigenous Australians can strengthen participant access to quality of life and wellbeing as described in Indigenous epistemology.

Dancing the Lifespan

The final section of the book presents a lifespan perspective on dance as a way of life, a potential that exists for all human beings. Two "elder tales" (one individual and one collective) are followed by a chapter highlighting a poetics of infant dance.

Elder Dance First, Teresa Benzwie's "Memoir of a Dancing Life" offers selected recollections of "a life in which dance has supported happiness, enabling a philosophy of being." Chronologically, she describes a love of dance from a young age that grew into a career-long mission to support its inclusion in early childhood education. Themes of persistence and following one's dream weave through the story, including a recent success story of her creative movement based environmental unit being taken up by an entire New Jersey school district.

Nicholas Rowe, David McMicken, and Tim Newth collaborate on the chapter, "Dancing in the Setting Sun: Performance, Self-actualization and the Elderly" a qualitative study of the Grey Panthers performing group in Darwin, Australia. The study expands the discourse on dance and the aged into the relatively unmapped territory of performance. Based on semi-structured interviews with 12 dancers and grounded theory analysis, the research elucidates Grey Panthers' motivations for dancing and performing through humanistic psychologist Abraham Maslow's hierarchy of human needs.

Infant Dance Kirsten Kaschock and I collaborate to create "Babies and Dance: Questions of Origin – A Chapter in Two Parts." In Part I, I outline my long-standing interest in university dance students' perceptions of "baby dance." Then, based on questions prompted by Part I and from student papers on the subject of babies and dance (1985–2011), Part II presents dancer, poet, and novelist Kirsten Kaschock's "Questions of Origin," a layered, poetic reflection that leaves the question of origin open, as it must be for now.

Coda

Completing this bricolage construction of dance and the quality of life, Ellen Dissanayake discusses the relationship between what she calls "making special" or "artification," and the evolution of human arts. She locates dance's evolutionary origins in the ritualized behaviors of birds, early hominin mothers and infants, and the human propensity for ceremonial ritual behavior, offering neurophysiological evidence for the quality of life indicators of entrainment, movement synchrony, euphoria, and feelings of transformation that can be experienced and observed in dance. She makes a powerful case for the arts as modes of social interaction and community cohesion, and importantly, as a biological imperative for which humans are uniquely predisposed. She concludes the Coda and the book, stating, "In the most fundamental sense, dancing is intrinsic to the vitality and quality of life."

References

Adams, D., & Apostolos-Cappadona, D. (1990). *Dance as religious studies*. New York: Crossroads.

Arcangeli, A. (1992). Dance and punishment. *Dance Research, 10*(2), 30–42.

Arcangeli, A. (1994). Dance under trial: The moral debate 1200–1600. *Dance Research, 12*(2), 127–155.

Berleant, A. (2016). The art in knowing a landscape. In *Aesthetics beyond the arts* (pp. 67–80). New York: Routledge.

Bezhan, F. (2017, August 1). *U.S. watchdog: Afghan forces still "complicit" in child sexual exploitation*. Radio Free Europe/Radio Liberty. Retrieved from www.rferl.org/a/afghanistan-dancing-boys-sexual-exploitation-officials-complicit/28653116.html
Bolwell, J. (2018). Wellbeing and the aging dancer. In V. Karkou, S. Oliver, & S. Lycouras (Eds.), *The Oxford handbook of dance and wellbeing* (pp. 311–328). Oxford, UK: Oxford University Press.
Bond, K. E. (1994). Personal style as a mediator of engagement in dance: Watching Terpsichore rise. *Dance Research Journal, 26*(1), 15–26.
Bond, K. E. (2008). The human nature of dance: Towards a theory of aesthetic community. In S. Malloch & C. Trevarthan (Eds.), *Communicative musicality: Exploring the basis of human companionship* (pp. 401–422). Oxford, UK: Oxford University Press.
Bond, K. E. (2014). Dance and quality of life. In A. Michalos (Ed.), *Encyclopedia of quality of life and well-being research* (pp. 1419–1424). Dordrecht, The Netherlands: Springer.
Carter, J. R. (Ed.). (2010). *On living life well: Echoes of the words of the Buddha from the Theravada tradition*. Onalaska, WA: Pariyatti.
Chaiklin, S., & Wengrower, H. (Eds.). (2009). *The art and science of dance/movement therapy: Life is dance* (pp. 299–316). New York: Routledge.
Coons, L. (2014). Artiste or coquette? Les petits rats of the Paris Opera ballet. *French Cultural Studies, 25*(2), 140–164.
Coulangeon, P., Ravet, H., & Roharik, I. (2005). Gender differentiated effect of time in performing arts professions: Musicians, actors, and dancers in contemporary France. *Poetics, 33*, 369–387.
Cummins, R. A. (2000). Objective and subjective quality of life: An interactive model. *Social Indicators Research, 52*(1), 55–72.
Daniel, Y. (2005). *Dancing wisdom: Embodied knowledge in Haitian Vodou, Cuban Yoruba, and Bahian Candomblé*. Urbana, IL: University of Illinois Press.
Darst, L. (2012, August 1). The poorest art: Dance and money. *Huffington Post*. Retrieved from www.huffingtonpost.com/lightsey-darst/dancer-income-wages-lifestyle-_b_1556794.html
Davies, J. G. (1984). *Liturgical dance: An historical, theological, and practical handbook*. London: SCM.
Denzin, N. K., & Lincoln, Y. S. (Eds.). (2017). *The Sage handbook of qualitative research* (5th ed.). Thousand Oaks, CA: Sage. (Original work published 1994).
Desmond, J. (2001). *Dancing desires: Choreographing sexualities on and off the stage*. Madison, WI: University of Wisconsin Press.
Diedrich, M., Gates, H., Jr., & Pedersen, C. (Eds.). (1999). *Black imagination and the middle passage*. Oxford, UK: Oxford University Press.
Dissanayake, E. (2000). *Art and intimacy*. Seattle, WA: University of Washington Press.
Dissanayake, E. (2017). Ethology, interpersonal neurobiology, and play: Insights into the evolutionary origin of the arts. *American Journal of Play, 9*(2), 143–168.
Enge, N. (2017). Anti-dance treatises. *Library of dance*. Retrieved from http://www.libraryofdance.org/manuals/antidance/
Feelings, T. (2018). *The middle passage: White ships/black cargo*. New York: Random House.
Feldstein, L. (1979). *The dance of being: Man's labyrinthine rhythms*. New York: Fordham University Press.
Flores, R. (2015). Making sense of suffering: Insights from Buddhism and critical social science. In R. Anderson (Ed.), *World suffering and quality of life, Social indicators research series* (Vol. 56, pp. 65–72). Dordrecht, The Netherlands: Springer.
George-Graves, N. (2010). *Urban Bush Women: Twenty years of African American dance theater, community engagement, and working it out*. Madison, WI: University of Wisconsin Press.
Hall, J. M. (2017). St. Vitus's women of color: Dancing with Hegel. *Comparative and Continental Philosophy, 9*(1), 43–61.
Hanna, J. (2006). *Dancing for health: Conquering and preventing stress*. Lanham, MD: AltaMira Press.
Hegel, G. W. F. (1975). *Hegel's aesthetics: Lectures on fine arts* (T. M. Knox, Trans.). Oxford, UK: Oxford University Press. (Original work published 1835).

Horsfall, D., & Titchen, A. (2007). Telling participants' stories. In J. Higgs, A. Titchen, D. Horsfall, & H. Armstrong (Eds.), *Being critical and creative in qualitative research* (pp. 88–96). Sydney, Australia: Hampden Press.
Karkou, V., & Oliver, S. (2017). Conclusion. In *Oxford handbook of dance and wellbeing* (pp. 925–928). Oxford, UK: Oxford University Press.
Karkou, V., Oliver, S., & Lycouris, S. (Eds.). (2017). *Oxford handbook of dance and wellbeing*. Oxford, UK: Oxford University Press.
Kelly, D. (2012). *Ballerina: Sex, scandal and suffering behind the symbol of perfection*. Vancouver, Canada: Greystone Books.
Kincheloe, J. L., McLaren, P., & Steinberg, S. (2011). Critical pedagogy and qualitative research: Moving to the bricolage. In N. K. Denzin & Y. S. Lincoln (Eds.), *The SAGE handbook of qualitative research* (4th ed., pp. 163–178). Thousand Oaks, CA: Sage.
Kraus, R. G., Hilsendager, S. C., & Dixon, B. (1991). *History of dance in art and education*. Englewood Cliffs, NJ: Prentice-Hall. (Original work published 1969).
Kreemer, C. (Ed.). (2008). *Further steps 2: Fourteen choreographers on what's the RAGE in modern dance*. New York: Routledge.
Lakes, R. (2005). The messages behind the methods: The authoritarian pedagogical legacy in Western concert dance technique training and rehearsals. *Arts Education Policy Review, 106*(5), 3–18.
Lansley, J., & Early, F. (2011). *The wise body: Conversations with experienced dancers*. Bristol, UK: Intellect.
Maggino, F. (Ed.). (2016). *A life devoted to quality of life: Festschrift in honor of Alex C. Michalos, Social indicators research series* (Vol. 60). Cham, UK: Springer International.
McCarren, F. (1998). *Dance pathologies: Performance, poetics, medicine*. Stanford, CA: Stanford University Press.
Michalos, M. (Ed.). (2014). *Encyclopedia of quality of life and well-being research*. Dordrecht, The Netherlands: Springer.
Møller, V. (Ed.). (1997). *Quality of life in South Africa, Social indicators research series* (Vol. 1). Dordrecht, The Netherlands: Springer.
Mulvey, L. (1999). Visual pleasure and narrative cinema. In L. Braudy & M. Cohen (Eds.), *Film theory and criticism: Introductory readings* (pp. 833–844). New York: Oxford University Press. (Original work published 1975).
Nahvi, S. (2015). *The truth about dance*. Bloomington, IN: Abbott Press.
Phillips, R. (2016). An essay in honors of Alex Michalos: Finding community in quality of life. In F. Maggino (Ed.), *A life devoted to quality of life, Social indicators research series* (Vol. 60, pp. 123–130). Dordrecht, The Netherlands: Springer.
Pirsig, R. (2011). *Zen and the art of motorcycle maintenance: An inquiry into values* (40th anniversary ed.). New York, NY: HarperCollins (Original work published 1974).
Razack, S. (1993). Story-telling for social change. *Gender and Education, 5*(1), 55–70.
Rogers, M. (2012). Contextualizing theories and practices of bricolage research. *The Qualitative Report, 17*(48), 1–17 Retrieved from http://nsuworks.nova.edu/tqr/vol17/iss48/3.
Sartre, J. P. (1992). *Being and nothingness*. New York: Simon & Schuster. (Original work published 1943).
Schwaiger, E. (2011). *Aging, gender, embodiment and dance: Finding a balance*. New York: Palgrave Macmillan.
Sharp, S. P., & Schomp, V. (2007). *The slave trade and the middle passage*. Tarrytown, NY: Marshall Cavendish.
Sirgy, J., Phillips, R., & Rahtz, D. (2011). *Community quality-of-life indicators: Best cases V*. Dordrecht, The Netherlands: Springer.
Smith, E., & Jackson, P. (2005). *The hip-hop church: Connecting with the movement shaping our culture*. Downers Grove, IL: Intervarsity.
Szablowski, W. (2014). *Dancing bears: True stories of people nostalgic for life under tyranny*. New York: Penguin.

Tesch, R. (1990). *Qualitative research: Analysis types and software tools*. London: Routledge.
Thobani, S. (2017). *Indian classical dance and the making of postcolonial national identities: Dancing on empire's stage*. London: Routledge.
Throsby, D., & Petetskaya, K. (2017, November 12). *The gender pay gap is wider in the arts than in other industries*. The Conversation, Macquarie University, Sydney. Retrieved from www.theconversation.com/the-gender-pay-gap-is-wider-in-the-arts-than-in-other-industries-87080
Tonon, G. (2015). Relevance of the use of qualitative methods in the study of quality of life. In G. Tonon (Ed.), *Qualitative studies in quality of life: Methodology and practice, Social indicators research series* (Vol. 55, pp. 3–21). Dordrecht, The Netherlands: Springer.
van der Leeuw, G. (2006). In D. Apostolos-Cappadona (Ed.), *Sacred and profane beauty: The holy in art* (D. E. Green,Trans.). Oxford, UK: Oxford University Press. (Original work published 1932).
Van Dyke, J. (1992). *Modern dance in a post-modern world: An analysis of federal arts funding and its impact on the field of modern dance*. Reston, VA: National Dance Association.
van Manen, M. (1997). *Researching lived experience: Human science for an action sensitive pedagogy*. London, ON: Althouse Press (Original work published 1990).
van Manen, M. (2014). *Phenomenology of practice: Meaning-giving methods in phenomenological research and writing*. Walnut Creek, CA: Leftcoast Press.
Veenhoven, R. (2016). What we have learnt about happiness. In F. Maggino (Ed.), *A life devoted to quality of life: Festschrift in honor of Alex C. Michalos, Social indicators research series* (Vol. 60, pp. 151–170). Cham, UK: Springer International.
Ventegodt, S., Anderson, N., Kromann, M., & Merrick, J. (2003). Quality of life philosophy II: What is a human being? *The Scientific World Journal, 3*, 1176–1185.
Wagner, A. L. (1997). *Adversaries of dance: From the puritans to the present*. Urbana, IL: University of Illinois Press.
Weijers, D. (2014). An interview with Alex C. Michalos. *International Journal of Wellbeing, 4*(1), 106–110.
Zar, R. (2012, October). Sorting the reality from the reality TV: Abby Lee Miller. *Dance Teacher*, pp. 56–62.

Part I
Dancing Ecology, Sustaining Earth

Chapter 2
Canyon Consciousness

Sondra Fraleigh

Lingering
with a question,
Why do canyons sing?
They work for nothing under the desert sun.
Outcropping, never bitching or grumbling,
Sagebrush, cactus, meandering cliffs
mid trouble of not crumbling.
Washes and weatherings pass and shift
in process, revolve in a look and stumble—
Suddenly, dreaming and falling—.
Everywhere off,
Tumbling—dancing all ways—
with eagle feathers.

Everything has a nature, even you and me. Canyons also have a nature. By nature, they have mouths or openings, cracks and fissures, flat surfaces and careening walls, somewhat like the inside of a skull. They resemble human complexities, or else I'm anthropomorphizing. Rather do we find more of our individual uniqueness and common humanness inside the skulls of canyons. And we can dance there in concert with the flows of time. We can become more of who we are when we pay attention, moving consciously without talk, making friends with canyon life and others in the dance.

I am drawn to gorges and make "place dance" videos with music from my impressions (Fraleigh, 2015a, 2015b). Gorges are cavernous, unpredictable, winding, and so sublimely deep. They give meaning to the word gorgeous. Gorges are magnificent valleys, ravines, and canyon chasms. Such are the canyons in Southwest Utah: Zion, Bryce, and Snow Canyon. Further away near Moab are the gentle greens, warm corals, and ashes of Arches National Monument, with Grand Canyon

S. Fraleigh (✉)
SUNY Brockport; Eastwest Somatics Institute, Saint George, Utah, USA

K. Bond (ed.), *Dance and the Quality of Life*, Social Indicators Research Series 73,
https://doi.org/10.1007/978-3-319-95699-2_2

on the horizon. Canyons might have streams, but can also be desolate places, hot and untenable, even foreboding and alien.

In canyons, my consciousness moves through change and morphology. I morph freely when I dance there. I often feel my body become calm and receptive, sometimes shapeless. In such states, I can dance from emptiness, and feel better. Letting go of stagnant history, I can change in the flowing present. I can heal and re-gather form. I think of this mode of being present to nature as "canyon consciousness." In touch with canyons, consciously undertaken movement and dance can expand into a state of gratitude. The valley depths of canyons invite my arms to reach out spontaneously from my heart. When I dance in canyons I have no pain or worry. Rather, I drift and linger. Healing, I believe, is a daily, always renewed, occurrence. It isn't a permanent one-time happening.

Attentiveness to valleys and alluvial plains is a moral imperative. We need to be past ignoring our relationship to nature, wasting water and forests. Appreciative attention to the natural environment can enhance quality of life. This is my commitment, and the reason I take students in my somatics program in Utah to dance in Snow Canyon, to Zion and the red cliffs above Saint George. The key word here is *attention*. We can ignore nature and its exploitation, or partner with it in a transformational dance. Attention is not all that is needed, but it is a good beginning.

I'm not speaking of dancing for an audience, but of moving intuitively in tune with the physical world, embracing the rocks, not pushing away the wind or the rain. I follow in the lineage of philosophers Simone Weil (1952/2002, 1970/2015) and Iris Murdoch (1993) who understood attention as a moral virtue. According to Weil's biographer E. O. Springsted (1986/2010), she was one of few spiritual thinkers who saw suffering as part of life and a way to overcome self-centeredness. Cultivating attention can make a difference to the world and our place in it. Paying attention to earth and the more-than-human-world, I experience myself moving toward health and wholeness, not just for myself, but for the planet. Weil (1970/2015) held that "humility is above all one of the qualities of attention" (p. 351). She understood how through attention in the arts, we unite with the world: "A true painter through paying attention becomes what he looks at. And while he is in this state his hand moves, with the brush attached" (p. 361).

We are not in this life alone: ultimately we are not separate from each other, and neither are we separate from non-human nature. Science and phenomenology both teach me this, as I will take up soon. How do we find balance in relationships with nature, understanding that despite our human cultural life, we are also natural creatures? I have a friend who is considering living in a cave. He knows someone who survives quite well there. People know where the cave dweller is, and they bring him food. Cave living is a radical idea to me; I know I couldn't manage. In any case, most of us live in society and also relate to natural phenomena within and outside of ourselves. We live in what we blithely and without thinking call "the world," which means many things: for one – vast networks of societies, and the world of the Internet. The concept of "world" often refers to nature in ordinary discourse, but it also connotes international paths of decision and intrigue that seem as unresolved as deserts and oceans. The world has complexities that we call "politics." Nature is political too, or at least suffers the impact of politics. Our human nature, what can be studied and known as natural or given in life, is in as much danger as non-human nature.

Nature is conceived and studied by the natural sciences from both physical and psychological standpoints. I acknowledge these views, but veer toward art and philosophy. Nature doesn't exist on a chart. Physical nature is alive, renewing and changing always. Phenomenology, a school of philosophy founded by Edmund Husserl early in the twentieth century, holds that nature manifests in experience, a perspective that continues to unfold in this chapter. Beginning with Husserl's *Ideas II* – a work first published in 1925 and translated into English in 1989 – phenomenology references the encompassing physical world of which humans are part as "lifeworld" (*lebenswelt*). Lifeworld is an inclusive concept that characterizes experiences of the everyday communicative personal world and the normalized world, as well as the natural environing world, the intuitive world, and the affective aesthetic world of sense and culture Husserl (1925/1989, pp. 383–390). The natural environing world includes earth as elemental nature and the world as foundational. Human subjectivity grasps nature intuitively, according to Husserl (1988/1995), "but alters nothing of the unity of nature as core in its own ontological form" (p. 189). Plants and animals, insects, microbes, and human life are part of the natural and environing world, even when nature is manipulated, and even as we change through time.

Does nature make decisions? According to Charles Darwin (1859) it does: nature makes decisions about life according to "natural selection." It is selective in its efforts to maximize life (Caldwell, 1999). We humans as eco-systems also enhance life possibilities through selectivity. Or else we are self-destructive. Our choices in the foods we eat make a difference, for instance. I propose that playful movement in tune with the natural world can make a difference in nurturing quality of life. In this chapter, I celebrate dance as playful and explorative intuitive art – a way to attend and be in tune with nature.

Humans have a nature, a human nature and first nature, one that has a basis in biology and ecology. Humans are ecosystems of a specific kind. But humans change and are affected by how they live through their circumstances and choices. In terms of movement and response, we commonly call the resulting changes of our actions a second nature, one that depends on the first. In his phenomenology of movement, *Freedom and Nature: The Voluntary and the Involuntary,* Paul Ricœur (1966) traces how what we call "second nature" develops and sediments in the body. It can develop into habits or skills. Skills, as in dance, are consciously learned and revisited, while habits, as I have studied them in phenomenology and the Feldenkrais Method®, are forgotten places in memory and movement that elude attention. They are hidden in bodily awareness. That's why we call them "habits."

People have inclinations through a first nature that are further defined in a second. These sediment in character as settled dispositions toward the world: grumpy, vicious, gentle, happy, cynical, and I could go on. Inclinations become naturalized in our life choices as characteristic patterns of movement and personality that encompass habit and sediment through repetitive direction of intentionality; what was once voluntary choice becomes embedded in the responses of the involuntary systems of the body. Fortunately, habitual responses can be brought to attention, and they can change for the better. I study this matter and teach it in somatic movement arts. In my actions, I can cultivate violence toward the earth and others, or seek to reverse the damage in process. In taking responsibility for myself, I can protect and care for life, especially attuning to nature in my dances (Fig. 2.1).

For now, I will settle on "givens" as helpful in delineating nature, and "inclinations" as naturalized predispositions that sediment in the body through repetition. These can become habits. Skills also naturalize as learned movement, consciously undertaken. At some point what was difficult now seems natural (easy as belonging

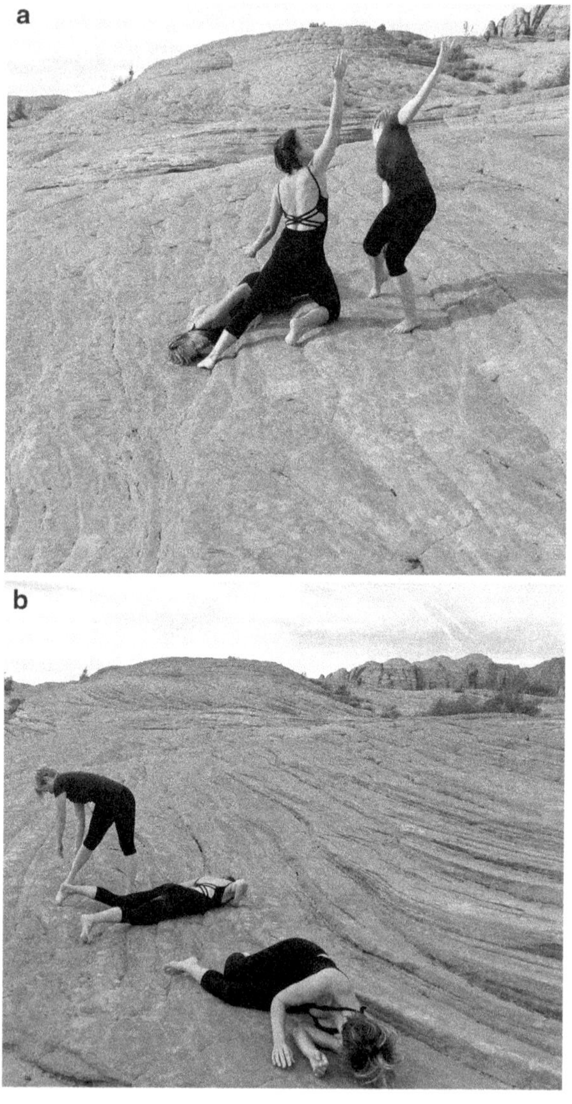

Fig. 2.1 (**a**, **b**) *Soma and Blue Muffins in Snow Canyon*, a dance improvisation structured by Sondra Fraleigh for Denise Purvis, Megan Brunsvold, and Sarah Gallo. (Photograph by Tom Gallo. © 2016)

to a person's life and movement). Skills also take on the mantle of habit, but we can renew and refine skills through attention. Here is this word "attention" again. I trust that this beginning consideration of nature and what seems natural will continue to unfold in my writing.

If I envision not what is *close* to me at first glance, but what is *closed off* from my glance, I sense that something vast, both seen and unseen, continues beyond local instances of life and work. The earth, the land and water, carries everything on its surface and in its drill holes – buildings, ships, and airplanes, impinged upon by wind and air – the sky above at sunrise – spreading its endless canopy. What is a canyon without a sky? *Nature is widely given to us,* sometimes through touch, sometimes overhead, and often more implied than seen. The word "nature" has developed several meanings. I point its meaning toward innate potential and concrete aspects of the physical universe. As given, nature is beyond total understanding or manipulation, even as it is in every respect fragile, just as human life is part of nature's fragility. As participants in the natural world, humans also influence it, and not always for the better. Ecological studies of climate change and ensuing crises are cited in the news almost daily.

Humanity is an actor in nature's morphology and needs to play its part well. Today, dancing moves close to science concerning the fragility of nature. Every living thing is subject to change; I am involved in the dance of life together with all other life. I dance in this belief, which is informed by the philosophy of Maurice Merleau-Ponty (1962), whose phenomenology describes a "primal awareness" of the world, one that does not separate humans as observers (pp. 3–5, 35, 53, 67–68). Reasons to dance in concert with the earth, and not in exploitation of nature seen merely as resource, are increasingly apparent. It is in our best interest to take care of nature, including the nature of our own bodies. What we call "self" is not separate from body and world. Rather, body and world are great teachers. I suggest that human beings need to develop greater faith in the body, and learn how to listen to it in tune with the world. This faith is cultivated in dancing, for example, through experiencing our bodies in love with the beauty of the world, while also admitting its suffering. Butoh, a *form of protest dance that began in post WWII Japan,* explores suffering as part of its aesthetic and ethos. Similarly, suffering also etches Zen Buddhism, which teaches that beauty and suffering both deepen spirit.

In my work, I aim to write through wisdom traditions and the lens of phenomenology as a philosophy. I began this journey with a book on existential phenomenology, *Dance and the lived body: a descriptive aesthetics* (1987), expanding on this in *Dancing Identity: metaphysics in motion* (2004). The latter is a syncretic work of dance theory involving phenomenology, ecology, feminism, life stories, and poetry. In *BUTOH: Metamorphic dance and global alchemy* (2010), I write about butoh's history and aesthetics, including many artists and works. Throughout its changing terrain, this unusual form of dance continues a focus on nature and suffering, as I say recently in "Butoh translations and the suffering of nature" (2016). For this present chapter I draw on heuristic phenomenology as a method of discovery that admits the descriptive power of experience, autobiography, and poetry. This method is indebted to research methods of Clark Moustakas (1990) (Fig. 2.2).

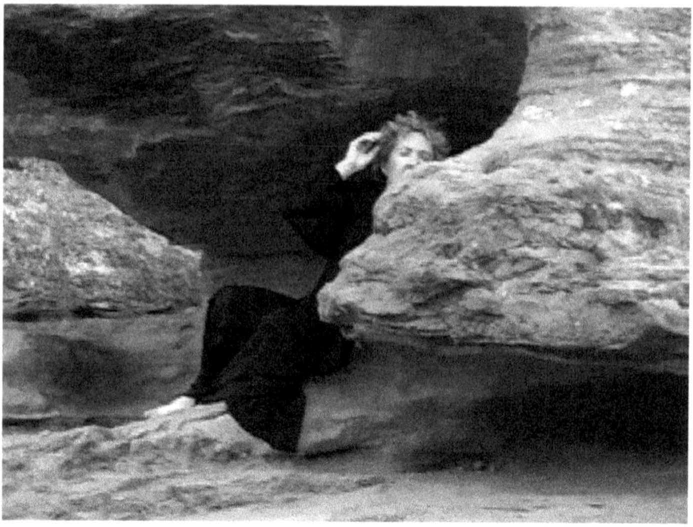

Fig. 2.2 Sondra Fraleigh in *Red Cliffs Butoh – above* Saint George, Utah. (Photograph by Mark Howe. © 2010)

As in heuristics, I use photographs and videos. Technology is not necessarily the enemy of nature. It can befriend the arts, as I write about in "Enacting Embodiment and Blue Muffins" (2015a). We humans exploit and waste, but we can use clean technologies to help restore balance with the environment, using visual technologies in thankful recognition. I suspect that the canyons I photograph are smiling – they know I'm paying attention to their beauty and suffering. Ultimately, phenomenology, for me, is a spiritual practice that gives me a way to pay attention to what is taken for granted, and this is what connects phenomenology to somatics and dance.

With its concern for cultivating consciousness, phenomenology is groundwork for an ecological philosophy. A world friendly consciousness is found in dance when it is in tune with nature. Such consciousness can give rise to love, but this does not mean it denies what is painful or messy. Heartfelt dance can swallow grief, celebrate life in its myriad forms, and doesn't deny pain. I grieve for this home we call Earth, which needs to be tended compassionately. Dancing is an aesthetic way of doing this. When I dance in Zion Canyon – *Mukuntuweap* – place, earth, home – especially at Weeping Rock, I embrace its dripping complexity and, in winter, its shards of ice. I also sense its boundless glory – as homeland of my body and the Ancestral Puebloans. We know this canyon was inhabited by a variety of villagers for at least 8000 years in the past, and the last Native Americans, the Parrusits left about 800 years ago. One of my students, Roman Morris (2016) made a video impression of his winter dance at Weeping Rock, "Exploring grief and climate change," which I include here (https://youtu.be/ehxPjrt_pJY).

Sunrise

It dawns on *Mukuntuweap, sacred ground* of the ancients,
And I wonder what music would please you.
Not one canyon, but many
Of unrelenting scratched-sandstone walls.
I have given up trying to scale your immensities,
Your ancient bodies surging through leaves of
Gold. Falling clouds, moment by moment, reflect
Glimmers, while morning grazes your massive
Landings—majesties swirling—
Chiseled by erosion over eons.
Stark uplifting monoliths of worship.

Let's play a Bach Organ Toccata, droning and soaring,
Conjure Native American Drumming,
Invoke Choirs of Angels,
For you.
And don't forget Puccini's arias.
Any music to tear the world asunder,
And your heart to pieces.

Deserts are vast places. They are natural as given, even as they evolve through time. They are also vulnerable – to radio active fall-out, for instance. Deserts can suffer along with people. I wrote about being harmed by the nuclear fall-out from the Nevada test site in the 1940s and 1950s (Fraleigh, 2004). The desert holds eternity in its sediments and substance. It isn't dead; its rocks are alive, as are its wildflowers, hawks and hummingbirds. I can sense time from geological prehistory to now in the desert. Listening and dancing with desert energies I can imagine time as eternal and space as endless. Desert canyons are part of nature's progress through time. I sense them spatially as biospheres in my body that I can dance with intuitively (Fig. 2.3).

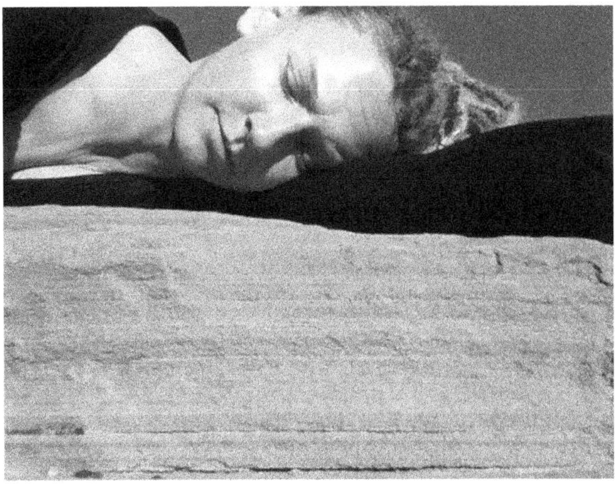

Fig. 2.3 Karen Barbour at rest, dancing in *Mukuntuweap,* the ancestral and Native American name for Zion Canyon. (Photograph by "Selfie," Karen Barbour. © 2012)

Already

My feet are sounding the earth, dancing
in gorges of vast harmonies, of vivid colors and unpredictable forms
too sublime to breathe-in; sensing delicate
and torrential waters, dizzying records of wind,
destruction through volcanoes and earthquakes,
shaking my nervous system.
The desert holds tsunami wreckages of burn
that make me shrivel.

I fear looking down over the remote distance of Snow Canyon when shadows are long and ominous early in the morning. But when I take time to relax into the canyon consciously, I breathe more freely.

At Dusk

My cells don't seem so squeezed,
When I make friends with desert elements,
Embody them as elemental in my being:
Through belly breathing, I lounge like a lazy lizard.
In standing, my chilly feet warm with
Desert sands at sunset.

At Night

The canyon stars and silky moon
Perform above a fading precipice.

Elemental nature is inspirational, even in thunder and hail. We are not separate from nature's elements; rather, they dwell within, fluid as water and murky. Nature is not simply in surroundings. *Nature is in us*. Phenomenology, especially in the thought of Husserl, holds that we are embedded in the world, and in turn, the world is in us. From him, I gain a profound appreciation of the world as being larger than scientific observations can reveal or normal everyday attention can grasp. Further: this is an awareness shared "with every mundane real thing, and all mundane truths;" in Husserl's expansive view, "Human life is *we-life*" (Fink & Husserl, 1995, pp. 167, 192). In other words, we can become aware of what we share with others, with deserts and canyons, with lakes and oceans. Shared life (we-life) can be brought forward consciously in dance and other arts (Fig. 2.4).

Site-specific somatic dance presents opportunities for *experiences of belonging*. The word "somatics" qualifies this kind of dance – where the focus is on connecting with elemental phenomena like falling water, for instance, or driftwood wedged between black volcanic rocks. Mountains of leaves shimmering in hues of honey and silver invite transformational dance through letting go of self, not in imitation of the leaves, but in touch with them in the unseen "implicate order" of nature (Bohm, 1980).

Not all site-specific dance is aligned with "green" nature. Some sites are chosen for their manufactured nature; construction sites interest me in this regard. There I can dance alone or with others to experience architectural process, as built by hand with machines and tools. Experiences of building-up, or falling apart, are special in their own ways and also lifelike, but to attend to life-in-the-making is a somatic way of paying attention to our own changing nature. When my dance attunes to the life

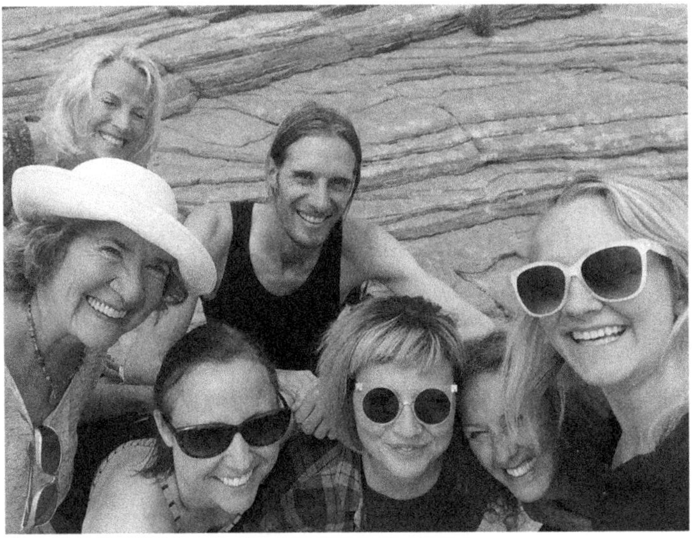

Fig. 2.4 Group photograph during dance explorations in Snow Canyon

around me, both human and other life, I am sometimes taken over by a feeling that comes from deep inside, and I weep. It is possible that I sense the child I once was when I ran and played all day in the fields of Circleville, Utah, where I was born. Perhaps I mourn the loss of innocent connection to my surroundings. I suspect I dance in nature to recover this, to belong once more without question.

My first choreographic ambition at the University of Utah in Joan Woodbury's composition class was to create a dance to Ferde Grofé's (1931) *Grand Canyon Suite*. "Sondra," Joan said, "you can't choreograph the whole Grand Canyon. Think about a more modest goal to begin with. In any case, it isn't a good idea to use overwhelming music." Now I understand a lot more about what she meant, and I don't try to choreograph the whole canyon. Instead, I go to the canyon, move out in the open to improvise a mode of "canyon consciousness." This is most simply a felt bond with the flowing life of the canyon. In eco-dances of belonging, I let nature be my guide, I don't try to harness it, or pin it down with choreography. The challenge is how to keep inspiration alive in the dance, spontaneously; and for choreographers – how to translate this more formally.

Nature is not a resource; it is medicine and teacher. Nature heals. I am content to be surrounded and permeated by nature's *atmospheres*. When I am conscious of the canyon atmosphere early in the morning, it becomes round and spherical, entering my cells and atoms. My dance emerges easily in touch with the sun beyond the rim; at dusk, I reach past the fading light.

From desert, river, and forest, I reach the sky. Skies invite upward gazes and outward reaching dances – whirling, eternally drifting and wandering. In formal sestina poetry (below), I welcome these moving states. Sestina is formed in six stanzas with an envoi of three lines at the end. The last words of the first stanza

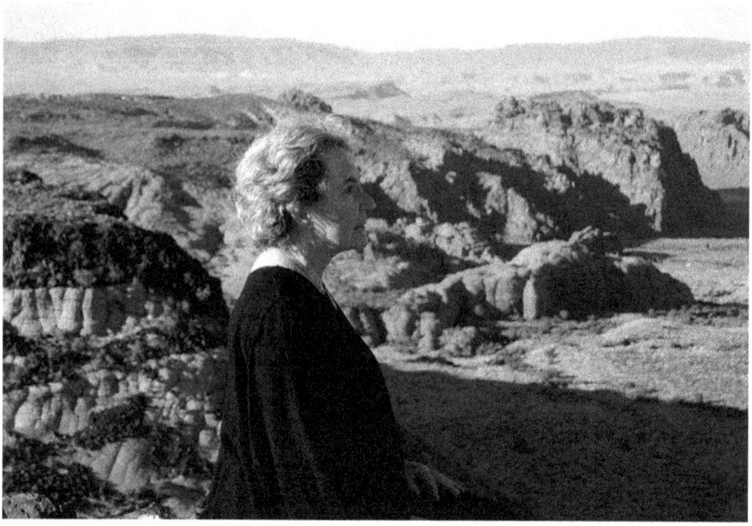

Fig. 2.5 Sondra overlooking Snow Canyon in the early morning. (Photograph by Mark Howe. © 2010)

repeat in a pattern of alternating jumps at the end of all other lines. This isn't easy, but it is satisfying over time (Fig. 2.5).

Loquitur: You need to like these words,
because they keep coming back,
stirring up strife.
Eccovi: Home at last.
in unnatural form.
The Scene: your jewel-like death
with *jongleur*, acrobat, musician, reciting…

Sky Mind

I
Worlds in this to be
I see through blue
beyond,
To what beauty bound
the heavens?
Let me lie undisturbed,

II
In summer undisturbed,
this day of floating mind. Be
whither I wander the heavens.
Up, and above blue?
And below blue? Bound
and passing through beyond.

III
Gated-paradise, beyond
count. Restored, undisturbed
remembered mind, ether bound
Abyss. Be
unruffled blue
floating gate, and first heaven.

IV
Daemonic, second heaven,
recognized in ripples and windstorms beyond
the blue.
Still, be still and drop down. Undisturbed
the roiling bodies be—
not guarded, not feared or bound.

V
Not to be bound
to any atom in heaven,
or heavens to be.
Lift past trouble, and sing beyond
the dropping dew, undisturbed
arising, with sparrows in the blue.

VI
Court no sorrow, no hope—cerulean blue
—deep violet and green. Bound.
to tear the pulsing world apart. Undisturbed,
remember my suffering, dancing heaven.
Breathe out of the blue beyond,
a calm aura, another gate to be.

VII
Where the canyon's blue heaven?
The summit crests bound hollows beyond?
Undisturbed, need bodies always be?

Ecological embodied consciousness can also be developed in the studio. Nature is there too, bounding off marley floors and windowless walls. Ecology, as interaction between organisms, is in the air and in dancing bodies. In the studio, I teach attunement to the ecological body through guiding somatic awareness of earthly elements within the body – the fluidity of water, for instance – the multi-textural cellular qualities of soil and porous bone. There is always a way to get to nature, especially through the flowing life of the human body; always a way of getting from concrete mazes of cities to places where trees and streams are singing. Dancers with imagination can travel through mindful vistas and felt sensations, and sometimes can venture out to encounter the natural world beyond studio and stage. The goodness of water is everywhere and can be transported. I have brought bowls of water to dance classes and scattered flowers on windowsills and floors, also spreading vividly colored desert rocks in circles and meanders. Enhancing the environment changes everything. Consciousness rearranges itself.

Bodies are miracles. This is what I have learned through dancing, though not all dance brings this to me – only when I sense its vibrant source. If there is a dancing way that signals a conscious path and makes use of choice, this dance offers new freedoms in charting possibilities and can also manifest as the choice to do nothing, or slow down. Dancing with nature, I can slow down. Canyons are not ambitious. They know how to meditate.

To the ancient Hawaiians and the native people of Hawaii, water was and is holy. To the native peoples of America, the land is considered holy. "Our bodies share the earth's chemistry," Santee/Cree Doris Seale (2000) explains, elaborating, "We will all experience the same fate as the earth; we know this. Mother earth is not just a metaphor, and technology will not save us." Indeed, the dominant societies, East and West, need to rediscover their rural roots and listen to what native people can teach about connection to nature – that the earth is holy and that living bodies are sacred ground.

Sticky Morphology

Morph attractors.
That's what they are.
Humid and hot, sticky visitors
In crystal waters flowing over me,
As I bend to them.

Massive slabs of old battles
And massacres emerging.
Tread carefully here in the gorge.
Fluttering cries compel my dance
Falling flat, just in time and trembling.

Fearful energies show their faces this way,
Serene in the hands that work on dreams,
Appearing's against the breadth of canyon
Backgrounds, not artificial in the damage.

Earlier modernist views of nature and dance were about domination of the natural world through human instinct. In his *The Book of Exultation*, A. K. Volinsky (1925/1983) lectures on the vertical, which he calls "the fundamental principle of classic dance" (p. 255). Noting that, "In ballet, ballerinas commonly dance on their toes," he suggests, "To understand so important an aspect of ballet, one must investigate the nature and meaning of the vertical in human life" (p. 255). Reflecting a Darwinian perspective, he posits that "man" once lived in the trees as apes do now and that after a developmental process of thousands of years, came down and stood upright, freeing arms for battle with the environment. Moreover,

> This was the moment of the greatest bloodless revolution in the history of mankind (sic). Man ceased to be horizontal and became vertical. From this time on he is identified as a man, not an ape or a primate resembling man. At the same time he acquires dominion over nature and becomes its master. This lordship is the result of the fact that man becomes conscious of his liberated arms and hands, he engages them usefully, and perfects his means

> of battle…. With the vertical begins the history of human culture and the gradual conquest of heaven and earth. (p. 256)

Contemporary scholars, however, are conceptualizing evolution in more friendly terms (Augros & Stanciu, 1988; Margulis, 1998; Margulis & Sagan, 1986). Lynn Margulis and Dorion Sagan (1986) assert,

> The view of evolution as chronic bloody competition among individuals and species, a popular distortion of Darwin's notion of "survival of the fittest," dissolves before a new view of continual cooperation, strong interaction, and mutual dependence among life forms. Life did not take over the globe by combat, but by networking. (pp. 14–15)

Robert Augros and George Stanciu (1988) also illuminate harmony in nature: "Life works with the environment, not against it. … Every living thing is beautifully attuned to its environment. Effort is … minimal because each animal and plant is so well designed" (pp. 138–139).

Harmony and freedom lie in actions we perform in concert with nature. Such actions become second nature to us; they are integral actions, emanating from an adaptable center of gravity, and have the potential to bring us into harmony with others and our surroundings. They are affined with surrender, are not control and domination. The full and easy length of my breath knows this place in body consciousness. Movements proceed naturally, aware of their environment. An easy quality of awareness is sensitive to others and fully present in the moment (Fig. 2.6).

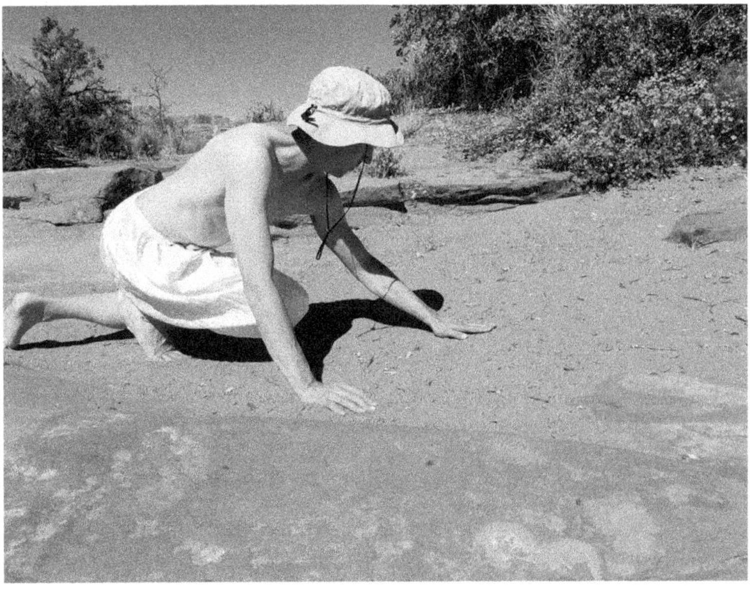

Fig. 2.6 Robert Bingham in a play of canyon consciousness. (Photograph in Snow Canyon by Sondra Fraleigh. © 2015)

Our dance seems automatic,
Confident in its emergence, not apologetic.
It radiates from a still center and
Supportive ground. When I dance from my own center And not in
imitation of others, I move freely.

I learn more about freedom arising in the nature of body from Ricœur's (1966) study of the relationship between freedom and nature in movement. His work shows how movement and knowledge are bound together in voluntary effort, as the mental and physical bring about "an undecipherable unity, beyond effort" (p. 249). When movement that once required effort ceases to be an effort, bodily spontaneity and freedom can appear. When learning a skill, for instance, I no longer need to exert myself beyond the desired effort for the movement I am learning, I can move without undue effort. I match my dance, and become one with my world and myself. I could say the dance has become second nature, or a part of me. The dance is natural to me now; there is nothing left to remember. My dance is somatic knowledge acquired through the development of skillful movement, attained through adaptations and attunements of my personal body that can be revisited consciously and with ease.

Habits, on the other hand, escape attention. Habits are hazy, embedded in automatic behaviors. I can, however, become aware of my habits and transform them. Dancing playfully, improvisationally, is one way of transforming habits, by entering processes that present new movement potentials or new ideas. Improvising in natural environments sharpens attention and requires me to apply myself in novel ways. The objects or material affordances of nature (as landscape, water, rock…) dissolve in consciousness through embodied renewal. They become part of the dance and the dancer. When I experience new movement, encounter a new idea, or change an attitude, the object of renewal – that to which I apply myself – becomes part of my consciousness and sediments in my nervous system. It becomes part of me.

I gain courage.
I loosen my neck.
My feet find a new path.
I move easily.
And dance without stress.

Paying attention in processes of learning and change is part of what dance improvisation, somatic dance, and somatic bodywork is all about. In acquiring skill and learning new movements we can experience freedom in action.

I know how to do something I couldn't do before.
My body knows the dance (acquired as skill).
Or I have experienced myself in a new environment,
And have met new challenges and freedoms there.

Moreover, my knowledge and experience has a somatic basis that arises phenomenologically in the moment – as lived. When we dance, we become the shapes of our dance – embodiment reinforces itself. What we do in turn becomes who we are. Embodied connectivity is a potential in any kind of movement, composed or improvised, but we can also feel awry. Feelings of integrative wholeness, strength, and grace are not guaranteed in dancing, but can be brought forward consciously in attuning to a malleable human nature. People sometimes feel awkward in dance; this awkwardness can be experienced as strength. Let it be, and let it change. Nature is a great teacher in this regard, as is improvisation. When I learn how to listen to my movement emerging in the moment, I don't deny who and how I am, learning how to receive and how to bend, naturally.

Dancing in continuity with nature, I discover my abilities to attune to my surroundings. I might also call surroundings my immediate environment or "place-world," after Edward Casey (2003), who says that "place-world's" local connection to the environment is more defined than "the environment" in general (p. 194). Environments are surroundings and also habitats that vary from place to place. Canyons are place-worlds of a particular kind, and the canyons near my home are still more special to me. Why? Most simply because I dance there. I feel the surfaces of the Butterfly Dune in Snow Canyon with my bare feet, and every time I visit I find a new place – to me, an entire world to explore. I pay attention to myself in relation to place, and I value both the place and my experience. Both are rooted in positive perceptions that have consequences in my perceptions of my possible-self. Suddenly, my world expands. I see, experience, and realize more.

As introduced earlier, Iris Murdoch (1993), after Simone Weil (1952/2002), describes the development of attention as "moral training." She views morality as a virtue in "looking carefully at something and *holding* it before the mind" (p. 3). Citing Weil, Murdoch elaborates that "moral change comes from an *attention* to the world whose natural result is a decrease in egoism through an increased sense of the reality of…other people, but also other things" (p. 52). I would add that attention can also be focused in different ways, and especially through performance. I see dancing as not primarily visual in focus, but as an artful and prayerful way of paying attention with my whole being. Selfless attention to nature through dance is a moral way of relating to a sense of place.

If attention is a moral virtue, then it is an aesthetic qualification as well, the same in the artist as in the scientist or teacher. Attention is a virtue not only because it contributes to well-being, but because it regards difference, allowing the other to disclose more of its nature. In his phenomenology, Heidegger (1927/1962) wrote similarly of *seinlassen*, letting beings be what they are as entities in their own right (p. 117).

Paying attention to nature I let nature be, not interfering and not manipulating. One might wonder if the canyon cares to be attended to. I imagine it does. In being appreciated in our dances, the canyon, the mountain, and the lake are revealed in their natures, perhaps in their many natures, according to the dance and the moment in time. We can attend to many kinds of nature as they are, and in the time of the dance, we are earthlings together. Dancing in continuity with the nature of canyon life creates conditions for sentient expansiveness. This is not to say that we can grasp canyons whole or that we own their wild beauty. We don't – their beauty is not ours. Canyons differ from us as specific non-human habitats. And is this not why they are able to attract and fulfill us? For myself, I will never know enough of canyons, at least not in my bones. I understand canyon beauty as a gift from nature.

Deserts are also gifts of nature. Philosophers and poets (and no doubt others) have interpreted deserts as places of desolation, devastation, and loss of meaning. Kelly Oliver explores how Hanna Arendt (2005) uses the desert as a metaphor for inhospitable regions of political geography, and Heidegger (1973) speaks of the "unworlding of the world" as the world's "desertification," when like the desert all will become diminished, without creativity or meaning (Oliver, 2015, p. 33). The beauty and biodiversity of deserts is often misrepresented. I live in the desert, surrounded by multicolored, majestic sandstone cliffs. In the evening, the transforming atmosphere and dropping clouds create incredible sunsets. I pay attention to them when I walk at dusk, or look out through my windows toward eternity.

Just above my desert home looms Pine Valley Mountain, its blue and purple peaks setting off the coral desert hues below. After rain, great arcs of double rainbows appear, the thorny cactus catching their glow. Like many, I am strongly affected by the environments in which I live. Heidegger and Arendt lived in Germany, green and lush in its forests, and so the desert for them must have seemed dry and remote in imagination. The world is not just one; it is multicolored, and there are many worlds in our one world. I would like to pay attention to the whole world, even if I can't. Earth is home to me as much as the desert. Writing about desert beauty and earth as home is a way of paying attention to my home. Dancing homewards carries my attention and writing into contemplative awe.

How I attend, and through what actions, affects me, if not immediately, inevitably. I build habits of attending, and eventually these become ethical signposts. I like to wander as a way of *not paying attention*, to diffuse my gaze, and ask my conscience to speak. Perhaps some light will appear around a flower or a tree or a shadow will suddenly look back at me. I discover ethics this way, asking into the good, into what I should do in a troublesome time or interpersonal exchange. Simply stated, I want to do the right thing. How should I act in a complex situation that involves several people? How can I act with love? I figure such things out dancing in nature, or rather the answers just come to me improvisationally. I also look wide at the landscape, the beautiful face of the canyon. It speaks to me during those times when I become humble enough to listen. In natural landscapes I have more of a chance to listen and to release my controlling mind than I do in cityscapes. Wandering in nature, I can be taught.

Improvising in the canyon, I am reminded that there are endangered places in the world; they suffer and are in need of attention. Zion Canyon, near my home, is "protected land." But it has already been dusted with poison from the testing of nuclear bombs at the Nevada Test Site for several years in the 1950s. What circulates in the water and the air reaches all, including protected canyons. Over time green and growing things are covered up with concrete, and our oceans suffocate under miles of plastic garbage. There is a danger that naturalness may disappear into social constructs, even our bodies. My ethics is to pay attention, to listen with intensity, and to dance in continuity with nature. What I attend to and how I pay attention influences the ethical positions I take. Human and non-human life are in a dance together. As we partner the world, it dances, or else it falters and falls apart. In the widest sense, we inherit the way we treat all life. Planetary transformation begins with personal transformation.

Somatic Attunement in Dance

When I dance without calculation,
I can be present with attention,
Just as I am. In tune with my nature,
I practice listening with composure,
Improvising in the studio or in nature's surroundings.

For me, paying attention in dancing is more than listening; it involves the heart. When I dance, I can listen to my feelings and connect to others without judging. Not judging is the first principle I teach in Depth-Movement Dance, a form I have evolved from nonjudgment in phenomenology as well as Buddhist teachings, and influenced by a therapeutic mode practiced generally as "Authentic Movement" (Adler, 2002). The latter is preceded by a bodily form of depth psychology pioneered in the 1950s by the late Mary Starks Whitehouse at UCLA.

When I dance, I follow the felt path of my breath until I release all need to grieve the past. I can be present in the ongoing flow of time without regret. When I am truly present in the nature of my being, I practice self-forgiveness, and thus, am not trapped in negativity. My heart is unburdened, and I can more easily respond to the heartfelt truth of others. Then I can clear away my own stories to hear the story of another. I can listen to the earth as it sings to my feet. Similarly,

I release the confusing waters of expectation.
As in yoga, I let go and get ready for surprise.

When I dance by myself in the canyon, I open the doors of sensation and invite the breeze to teach me. But I don't need to go to the cliffs or sit in the rain. I can achieve silence at home, working at my computer and living amiably there with my faults. Because I know what dancing teaches about being in the flow of time, I can let go of my inner victim and critic, not getting stuck in self-destructive narratives. Once, not long ago, when I was being witnessed in depth-movement-dance, I ended my

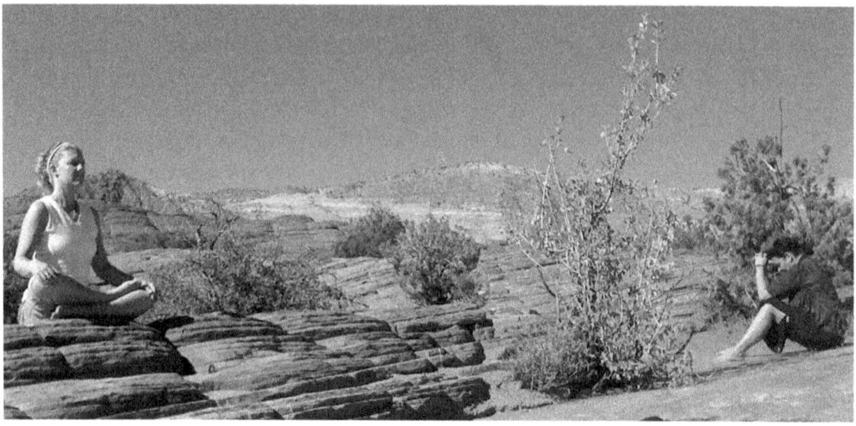

Fig. 2.7 Angela Graff and Amy Bush – Dance Meditations in Snow Canyon. (Photograph by Sondra Fraleigh. © 2013)

improvisation facing a chair. I opened my eyes, waited and watched in silence for a while, suddenly recognizing that no one was sitting there. Then I knew what the empty chair was saying. I turned to look at my witness and told him that, "for a change, and forever more, no one would judge me, at least in my mind. My inner victim was gone." Here is my poem of June 15, 2015, the day of this life-changing event (Fig. 2.7):

The Empty Chair

The chair is lonely now.
No phantom limbs or body parts
assembling there.
No one to share shattering heaviness with.
No dread.
No terrorizing or disapproving
people in the chair.

I have ached, running in buzzing loops—to
know in this naked sense,
to strike a chord in the morning or broken afternoon,
and hear the emptiness echo back.

To be suddenly awakened
to one's empty chair, and
to bury the ghosts of one's imagining
is a bright gift.

Isolated, painful, and thrilling to know
one is truly alone and happy.

Ready to weep.
Ready to shout out
the silvery freedom of absence.

No filtering to a respectable
level of "speak" ever again.
Emptiness holds reverence
for each precious, breathing moment.

When I dance freely in the moment, I can trust a deeper source than I can conjure consciously. I give up the quest for answers through intuitive dance or in gentle yoga, letting my body be the teacher. Somehow, my mind follows, or was there all along. Entering a responsive state, I wait without answers, trusting that they will arrive quite naturally if they are meant to. In depth-movement dance improvisations, I can respond to a chain of nonverbal cues, waiting for the next impulse, then the next, until I am carried past my habits of bodily thinking. I learn that my happiness is mine to seize; I can live it if I can fathom it. In living phenomenology and entering a clear mind, I give up expectations and absolutes, and as a dancer, I shine the moment.

When I dance for witnesses, I am happy for their impressions, especially when they tell me what my dance brings them – an insight, or perhaps a feeling. Dance is a way of sharing, a form of moving or nonverbal poetry. I like dancing with others when, sandwiched together in the wordless space of a canyon crevice, we feel our common humanity. For me, dance is now like meditation: I give up all intentions and purify my thoughts in movement. If thoughts stick around, I watch them pass by on the river of my imagination. What I learn through dance is something my habitual thoughts seem to stem. I learn that my happiness and suffering is not unique, nor am I. Dancing connects me to others and the world. When I was young, I lived in fear of making the wrong move. Much later I learned how to dance without judging – laterally improving – improvising where there are no wrong moves.

I enjoy helping others find their "inner dancer." All human beings have the capacity to dance, but this can become submerged in many of us at a young age. My challenge is to help people use simple improvisational methods of movement and expression to recover vitality and wholeness. For me, the body is nondual: physical, spirited and full of mind. All of this is one. The physical is never just physical. My body is primordial memory, and I can heal without words through intrinsic, intuitive dance. Sometimes the most significant dances I do are in stillness. Dance is both noun and verb; it is about moving for fun and fancy, and sometimes for show. Most fundamentally, I propose, dancing is for pleasure. I like to coax out the pleasure principle in dance, and there is nothing as pleasurable as dancing in nature's splendor, that place in consciousness, out there and in here, where there are no words (Fig. 2.8).

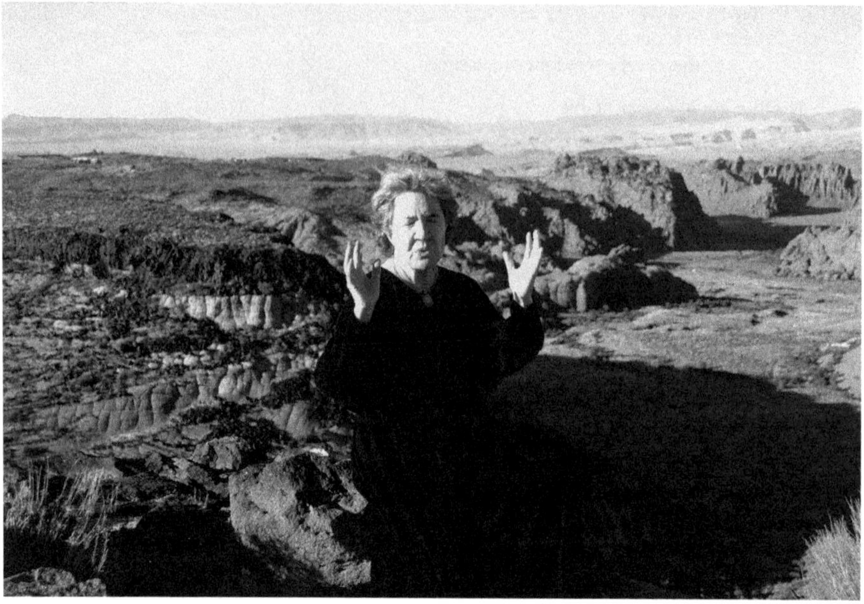

Fig. 2.8 Sondra Fraleigh looking out over Snow Canyon. (Photograph by Mark Howe. © 2010)

Primordial Memory

Remember us before language began,
We, who sought much of what we still do today.
Think back.

Remember how, without speaking about them, we possessed emotions like disgust, fear, anger, and rapture. How we later bonded in communal groups, sharing feelings of trust, contempt, and shame.

Is it likely we would have wondered about our place
in the cosmos, would have developed rules and laws,
injunctions against those who harm?

Remember that even before language
We would chant dirges,
Calls of mourning,
Shouts of greeting,
And warnings of danger.
How we would hum
Or sing, or drum—blow
Reed flutes, smoothly—
Shake rattles made of gourds—
And wearing necklaces of shells,
Whirl bullroarers.

Suppose we find new landscapes to walk,
The joy of water and vegetation,
Most likely evolve dramas that become

A privileged way of communicating,
Paint walls as a way to keep records,
And make art as way to impress
The hearts of others—

Art as social, and a way to attract mates,
Art as therapy, as sacred medicine—
Dance for war and survival,
Dance for peace.
With dancing feet,
And eyes busy watching,
Second-nature echoes through us,
Into the subconscious
Involuntary systems of tomorrow.

References

Adler, J. (2002). *Offering from the conscious body: The discipline of authentic movement.* Rochester, VT: Inner Traditions.

Arendt, H. (2005). In J. Kohn (Ed.), *The promise of politics*. New York: Schocken.

Augros, R., & Stanciu, G. (1988). *The new biology: Discovering the wisdom in nature*. Boston: Shambala.

Bohm, D. (1980). *Wholeness and the implicate order*. New York: Routledge & Kegan Paul.

Caldwell, C. (1999). A biologist's contribution to the field of somatic psychology. *Somatics: Magazine-Journal of the Mind/Body Arts and Sciences, 12*(2), 4–8.

Casey, E. S. (2003). Taking a glance at the environment: Preliminary thoughts. In C. S. Brown & T. Toadvine (Eds.), *Eco-phenomenology: Back to the earth itself* (pp. 187–210). Albany, NY: State University of New York Press.

Darwin, C. (1859). *The origin of species*. London: John Murray.

Fraleigh, S. (2004). *Dancing identity: Metaphysics in motion*. Pittsburgh, PA: University of Pittsburgh Press.

Fraleigh, S. (2015a). Enacting embodiment and blue muffins. *Choreographic Practices, 6*(2), 161–178.

Fraleigh, S. (2015b). *Blue muffins*. Retrieved from https://youtu.be/PREImPoEhqE

Heidegger, M. (1962). *Being and time* (trans: Macquarrie, J. & Robinson, E.). New York: Harper & Row. (Original work published 1927).

Heidegger, M. (1973). Overcoming metaphysics. In J. Stambaugh (Ed.), *The end of philosophy* (pp. 84–111). New York: Harper & Row.

Husserl, E. (1989). *Ideas pertaining to a pure phenomenology and to a phenomenological philosophy,* Book 2 (Ideas II) (trans: Rojcewicz, R. & Schuwer, A.). Boston: Kluwer Academic Publishers. (Original work published 1925).

Husserl, E. (1995). Appendices. In E. Fink & E. Husserl, *Sixth Cartesian meditation: The idea of a transcendental theory of method* (pp. 167, 192, trans: Bruzina, R.). Bloomington, IN: Indiana University Press. (Original work published 1988).

Margulis, L. (1998). *Symbiotic planet: A new look at evolution*. New York: Basic Books.

Margulis, L., & Sagan, D. (1986). *Microcosmos: Four billion years of microbial evolution.* New York: Summit Books.

Merleau-Ponty, M. (1962). *The phenomenology of perception* (trans: Smith, C.). New York: Routledge.

Morris, R. (2016). *Exploring grief and climate change. Weeping Rock: Selected choreography.* Retrieved from https://youtu.be/ehxPjrt_pJY

Moustakas, C. (1990). *Heuristic research: Design, method, and applications*. Newbury Park, CA: Sage.
Murdoch, I. (1993). *Metaphysics as a guide to morals*. London: Penguin.
Oliver, K. (2015). *Earth and world: Philosophy after the Apollo missions*. New York: Columbia University Press.
Ricœur, P. (1966). *Freedom and nature: The voluntary and the involuntary* (trans: Kohak, E. V.). Evanson, IL: Northwestern University Press.
Seale, D. (2000, October). *Invited lecture*. State University of New York, College at Brockport.
Springsted, E. O. (1986). *Simone Weil and the suffering of love*. Eugene, OR: Wipf & Stock.
Volinsky, A. K. (1983). The vertical: The fundamental principle of classic dance. In R. Copeland & M. Cohen (Eds.), *What is dance? Readings in theory and criticism* (pp. 255–257). New York: Oxford University Press. (Original work published 1925).
Weil, S. (2002). *Gravity and grace* (trans: Crawford, E. & von der Ruhr, M.). London: Routledge. (Original work published 1952).
Weil, S. (2015). *First and last notebooks: Supernatural knowledge* (trans: Rees, R.). Eugene, OR: Wipf & Stock. (Original work published 1970).

Chapter 3
Dancing the Landscape

Don Asker

The experience of being in a landscape reflects the relationship between person and immediate environment. This can be considered from many perspectives: how a body is active in its setting, how it physically interacts with the environment, the codependency and effect of one on the other. I understand this as a reflexive situation where person and place are mutually impacting.

Emotional responses accompany the physical interaction. For example, we might experience a landscape as relaxing, therapeutic, inspirational, or frightening. The romantic poet William Wordsworth spent considerable time walking in the Lake District of England. His wanderings provoked musings and poetics quite different from the perspectives of contemporary Lake district farmers like James Rebanks (2015) whose lives are enfolded in the sometimes life testing seasonal transformations of the same landscape. Landscape may have connotations of "country" as in indigenous culture, where topographical features are inextricably bound to a metaphysical construction of the universe and to existential wellbeing (Koori Mail, 2011, p. 35). A landscape can be so interpreted and respected that it becomes instructional, a framework guiding perception, decision-making, values and beliefs; for many, landscape arouses spiritual responses. Clearly, there is a cultural component to landscape; regions and places have characteristics that not only reflect the geophysical structures, but the living organisms including humans who inhabit them (see Ness, 2016).

This writing is autobiographical and reflective with descriptive accounts of experience – my own and those of collaborators. The dancing that I describe remains but a remembered trace. The challenge is to articulate this transcience, to outline the ongoing resonances and possible further implications for creative practice and a life well lived. I address core words that need definition as they arise. My focus is on dancing the locality I live on the south coast of New South Wales, Australia – parts I have become familiar with and other areas that remain less well known, or where I have never ventured (Fig. 3.1).

D. Asker (✉)
Victorian College of the Arts, University of Melbourne, Melbourne, VIC, Australia

K. Bond (ed.), *Dance and the Quality of Life*, Social Indicators Research Series 73,
https://doi.org/10.1007/978-3-319-95699-2_3

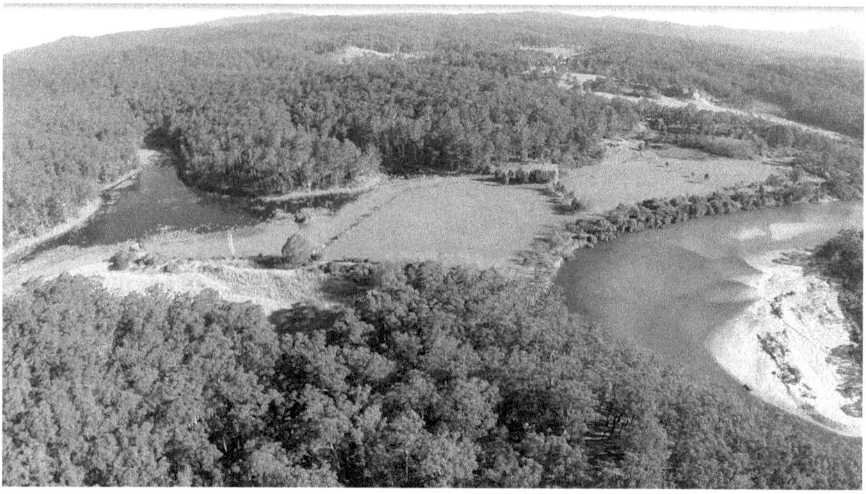

Fig. 3.1 Aerial view of site with flood-plain of the Towamba River, wetlands and neighbouring woodlands. (Photograph by Peter Whiter)

The combination of spaciousness, access to a river, and relative isolation makes the area attractive to many creatures, including humans. Tree-lined hills and ridges with valleys or gullies fold into flat expansive flood plains and wetlands before dropping into creeks and a river. One can see far across the river valley and marshlands, in contrast with some of the densely-vegetated hills where it is more difficult to move or see more than a few metres. Small clearings and rock pools dot the network of seasonal watercourses in the hills. With space or a sense of spaciousness comes a sense of freedom. As Yi-Fu Tuan (1977) put it, "Freedom implies space; it means having the power and enough room in which to act" (p. 53).

Having enough room for dancing is a subjective determination, inevitably reflecting the context and purpose of the dancer. In the past decade, I have shared the experience of dancing in the Kiah landscape (a word of the Yuin people for "the beautiful place") with others including Helen Herbertson, Ivan Sikic, Jane Mortiss, Paul Roberts, Cobie Orger, Lee Pemberton, Natalie Cursio, Janette Hoe, Kevin Jeynes, Greg Dyson, Andrew Morrish, and Ros Crisp. What follows are my accounts of some of these experiences accompanied by brief outlines of issues and insights they have precipitated. I endeavor to clarify terminology as I go (Fig. 3.2).

Sharing Landscapes

Choreographer Natalie Cursio recognised the idiosyncrasies of individual connection with place and explored this in a collaborative project with videographer Daniel Crook and me over two visits in the summers of 2013 and 2014 (Cursio & Crooks, 2015). How the human figure is perceived within landscape found a poetic realisation

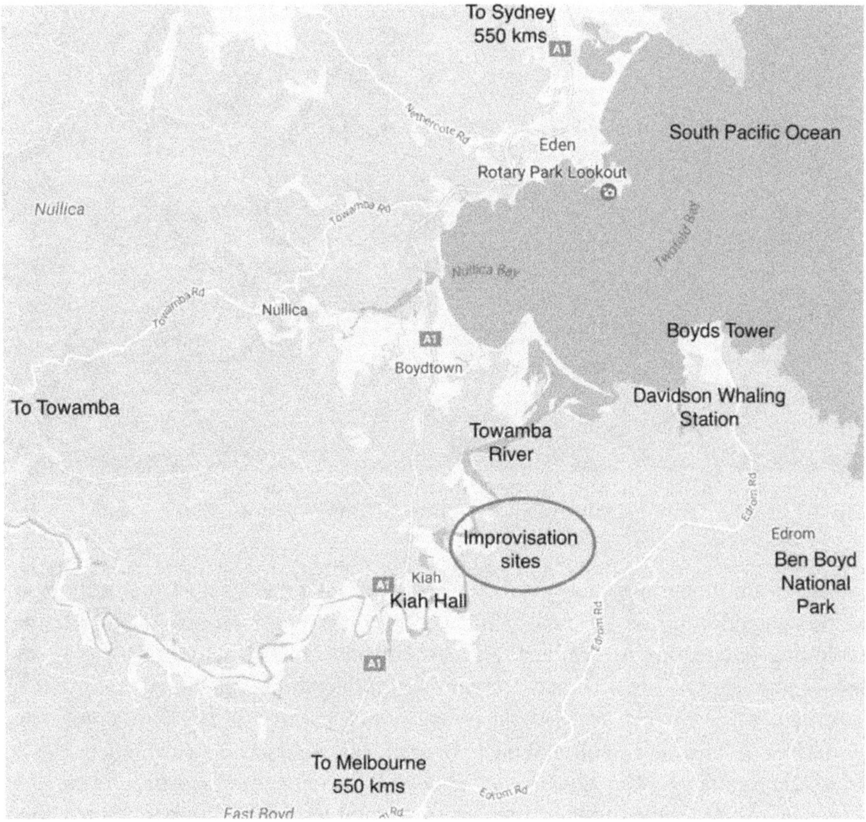

Fig. 3.2 Map showing far south coast of New South Wales, Australia with sites of dancing and other improvisations indicated

in digital media. The scoping eye of camera and director negotiated my body as subject in the landscape and also sought to explore the imaginative and interpretive aspect of that ocular perspective. Through our process, a sense of human non-fixity and impermanence emerged alongside awareness of the dynamism or flux of the landscape (Fig. 3.3).

Landscape presents its own history that we might learn, infer or uncover – a past stretching back through millennia of geological upheavals, climatic changes and seasonal weathering. It is a history we can construct from the landscape's physical surfaces, structures, and habitation. On the meanders of the south coastal New South Wales Towamba river, the landscape bears evidence of the most recent waves of human colonization: clearing for farming, timber production, fisheries. The growing attraction of eastern coastal districts as a holiday destination and place to live is reflected in the proliferation of tiny settlements. I use the term history as an accumulation of known details about the landscape and its past. In many respects, this invites all manner of perspectives and understandings.

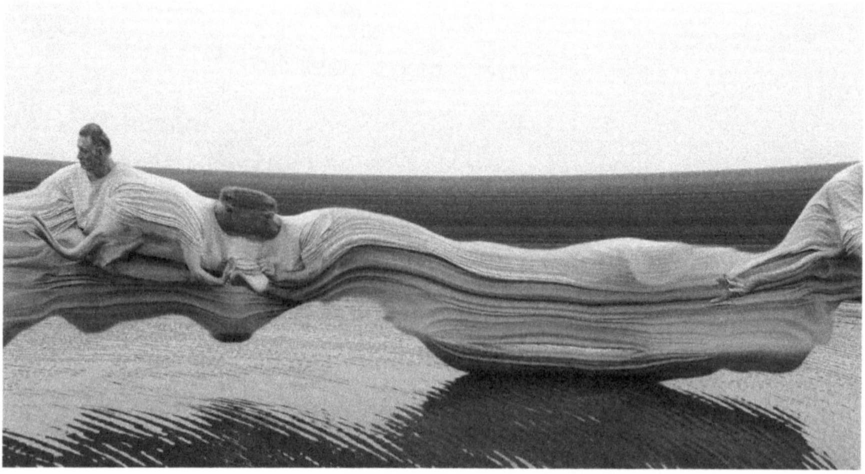

Fig. 3.3 Natalie Cursio and Daniel Crooks' *at least for a while anyway,* 2015

There are many histories of this place. Some take the form of oral tellings or stories shared with me by local people. They represent a variety of perspectives including indigenous Australians and descendants of early settlers. Explorer and settler journals provide firsthand accounts that reflect the acquisitional ambitions of the time, while more recent scholarly endeavors attempt to reconcile conflicting narratives of Australia's colonial past (Blainey, 2015; Clark, 2006; Hughes, 1987). Mark McKenna's (2002) *Looking for Blackfella's Point: An Australian History of Place,* re-examines the literature covering white settlement of this region, providing a disturbing account of indigenous displacement and genocide.

Early photographic documents of the area where I now dance show some of the wetlands cultivated for corn, dairy, and sheep and other parts supporting pig farming. The farm house in the picture below was built in 1904 replacing one swept away in a flood. It remains to this day. In a later picture from 1926, a woman stands on the cleared slope near the farmhouse, watching her child, Anna, according to the name written on the back of the photo, who holds a very large dead red bellied black snake (Fig. 3.4).

Correspondence by settler families of the time provides descriptive stories of everyday life. From a descendant of one of the first families, Monica McMahon, I have a copy of a handwritten letter describing the internment of a local settler at the small nearby Irish Catholic cemetery. The deceased was laid out at a farmhouse across the river, then ferried over and carried half a kilometer by six men to the graveside. Another letter details accounts by white settlers of indigenous corroborees and burials on a promontory of the nearby river flats. These materials contribute to my understanding of this part of the country's past, further shaping my own perspectives and informing my interactions with the place called Kiah.

There is a well in a gully through which a creek runs. It's thought that Oswald Brierly (1817–1894), acting on instructions from early entrepreneur and developer

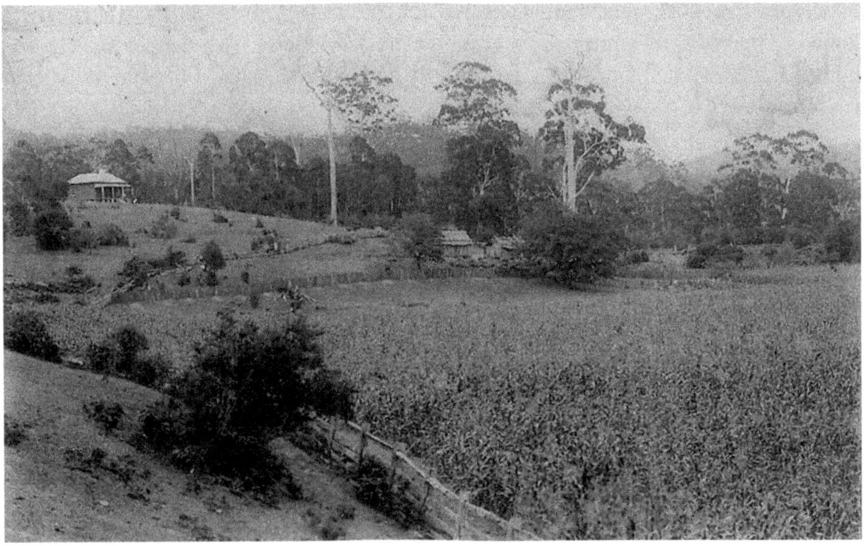

Fig. 3.4 Farm house circa 1900 above corn fields on flood plain of the Towamba River, Kiah. (Photograph courtesy of Monica McMahon)

Ben Boyd, cut reeds here to take as fodder for his horses on an explorative mission inland towards the high plains country to the west known as the Monaro – a word with Aboriginal origins. Brierly, a British marine water colorist and keen observer, left a precious record of first European contact with indigenous peoples. The aforementioned well has square sides about one and a half metres long and several corner posts and timber lining boards remain holding the well's shape and integrity. The aging of the extremely hard eucalyptus bosistoana and the post and rail handiwork dates back at least a century. The first European title of this particular part of the country dated 1887 has the name Whitaker given to a portion of land said to belong to a Granny Whitaker. Remains of horse drawn machinery, pieces of pottery, and a stone hearth dot the slopes. Flints of the dispossessed Yuin people are less conspicuous but according to BJ Cruz, an indigenous elder who walked with me here a decade ago, this is a place where food and water must have been in abundance. The well and surrounding densely forested hills is crisscrossed with human tracks. When I visit the well – the somatic experience – is interwoven with my recollections of these stories, documents and pictures.

Several years ago, on a day when a group of improvising artists and art therapists decided to choose places to dance or present ourselves, I took Kevin Jeynes as my witness to the well. I don't remember clearly the nature of my dancing, but my sense of the place and conversation with Kevin has endured. The physical effort expended by early settlers here had impressed me. Bringing water from a well – a hole in the ground requiring a bucket and rope to draw water, and navigating the steep track back up to the house, a simple dwelling vulnerable to fire and far from the nearest neighbor, meant enduring a level of isolation and self-reliance that I find hard to imagine today.

Knowledge of the place engaged my imagination. I felt intensely present here, knowing that over a century ago a group of predominantly Irish people had cleared melaleucas and eucalyptus elata in this gully and worked this soil in a bid to live and survive.

I walked near the remains of a wooden post and rail fence erected around the well. Other fence posts disappearing up the slope seemed to suggest stock once grazed in these hills. Voices would have echoed in the valley. On the day of my improvisation, Kevin and I talked in muted voices, as if we did not want to interfere with the sonic mix of wind in the leaves of trees and reeds and the voices of small birds. Waterfowl could be heard though rarely seen. I left with a feeling of connection to a colonial past; an embodied, sense of how it might have been to live a century or two ago emanated from being in the place itself.

In this writing, I use the term landscape to point to places in the Kiah region where human colonization or occupation sits in a topography that is not yet overwhelmed and totally reconstructed by humans' developmental and resource driven needs. I acknowledge the term "nature" is problematic. I don't intend to suggest a pure state free of human influence – that would sit humans outside of nature. Human complicity in the changes occurring on our planet makes it important to see the world in dynamic and evolving terms, and as much as we might think it useful to detach and find objective distance, we cannot escape our interdependence (Dorman, 2000; Ness, 2016).

So, it is for me that my dancing inevitably reflects its context, and if for a moment I don't sense human impact or presence, it is more about my attention being elsewhere and preoccupied with other things. On a day when the ash of coal fired energy generators drifts across the hills and valleys of Gippsland in the state of Victoria or dust blows off freshly felled logging coups of New South Wales state forests to find its way into my lungs, even as I stand on the banks of the sparkling Kiah River listening to the bell miner birds and helmeted honey eaters, it would seem there is no such thing as a "natural" place on earth.

My dancing in local landscapes parallels Paul Carter's literary forays, particularly his exploration of the Mallee region of Victoria, Australia, in *Ground Truthing* (2010). Carter found story lines that he could "follow up in the field" and began to sense the Mallee as a creative region, "an underlay of unedited anecdote, a fine capillary system of interconnected words, places, memories and sensations" (p. 3). Carter tried to exclude what "everybody knows" and focus on what he had "come across for myself" (p. 3). He wanted to escape the tendency to generalize and was aware that interpreting the experiences of others might infect their accounts with his own theories. To escape he had to immerse himself in the region.

Many people have experienced dancing the Kiah landscape and each has particular experiences that reflect their drives or interests. I have tended to be drawn to the voices of those whose practice is to do the dancing and for whom there is a conscious relationship to landscape. Our conversations and shared practices contribute to my understanding. With that in mind, my experience could be said to occur in a community with overlapping values.

Chilean installation and performance artist Ivan Sikic walked into the long grass and rushes of a wetland at Kiah and seemed immediately enveloped in the landscape. I saw him sporadically gesture, semaphore-like, and after a while he began to disappear only to reappear elsewhere. His initial deliberate explorative traversing became mysterious and uncertain. I realized he was divesting himself of his clothes and in some ways becoming part of the wetland wilderness, something that requires caution and alertness in those snake rich parts, especially when it is warm. After about 20 min, he retraced his steps gathering his clothes as he went (Fig. 3.5).

Clarifying some terms or values attached to my process of engagement in the Kiah landscape seems in order. The biases and values intrinsic to my work provide insight not only into my experience, but into the lenses or perspectives I have taken or perhaps adopt without conscious awareness. Dance for me is rather amorphous these days, and seems elusive to definition in any case (Bond, 2014). Although knowledgeable of the body's potentials in shape making and movement forming and the many canons influencing cultural modes of dance, I am aware also of micro movements and gestures like the softening of one's throat and the releasing of one's torso into a soft supporting chair – and how these might be experienced as dance. Clearly, though, a person's dancing, whatever that may be, reflects underlying *physical* attributes. Movement skills, aesthetic sensibilities, and patterns acquired through life, and those myriad personal contextual details shape a person's mood and disposition at any point in time. In a sense, we perform the present-ness of our dancing knowledge acquired through our past experiences and our feelings and attitudes towards dancing.

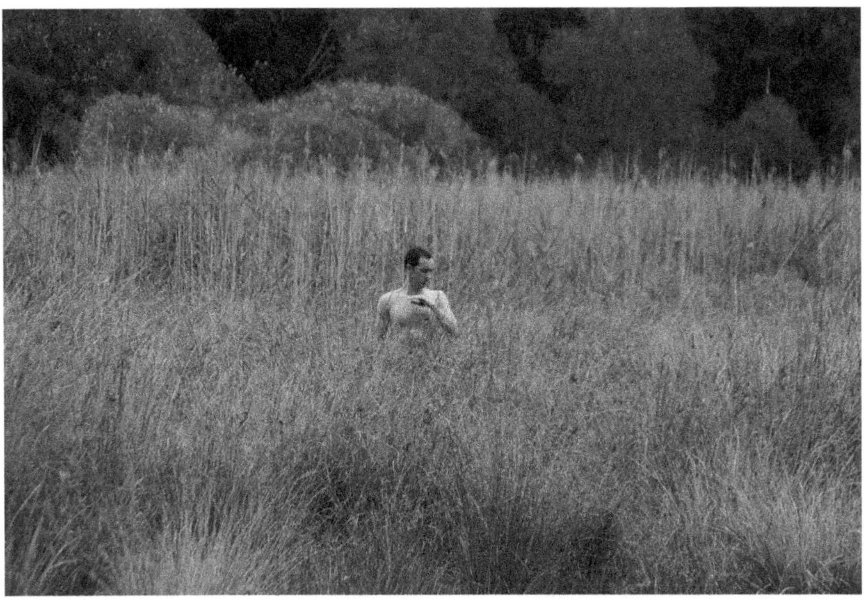

Fig. 3.5 Ivan Sikic in the wetlands adjoining Cochranes Creek, Kiah (Summer). (Photograph by Don Asker)

In the 1960s and 1970s, such aspects of everyday life were remarked upon refreshingly by the likes of dancers Yvonne Rainer (1965) and Steve Paxton. Many others including Jerome Bel further challenged conventions of dance movement vocabulary, broadening the basis of dance to incorporate other disciplinary forms. Interest in minimal movement, the provocations and initiation of gestural action is found in many movement based practices today; see, for example, Sandra Parker's (2016) performance work *Small Details* (https://vimeo.com/169191362). These "small dances" (Paxton, 1986) give access to dimensions of movement that are less spectacular than is found in traditional dance forms and have been described by phenomenologist Elizabeth Bhenke (1997) as "ghost gestures."

I tend to be consciously attentive to my possible physical articulations and sensate alertness. I notice options and select or choose, or become overwhelmed and swept away by a rush of action that could be many things from involuntary repetition of familiar action, to interaction with things that seem to be outside of pre-meditated or rationalised behaviour. Dance – my dance – can leave me refreshed, knowing differently and perhaps knowing more about others, my situation, and me. My dance isn't separate from my everyday duties, my writing, my collecting and arranging of things, my farm work, my caring for and mentoring of others. My dance doesn't really stop and simply needs me to ground my attention and thoughts in my body for it to "be."

Such self-consciousness involves capacity for self-imaging, awareness of skeleton, muscles and organs, and directing and focusing attention in the body itself, the sort of attention that Lulu Sweigard (1974) and others (Bernard, Steinmuller & Stricker, 2006; Dowd, 1995) came to call ideokinesis (see http://www.ideokinesis.com/index.htm). Susan Foster (2011) traces some of the historical features of human interest in movement and movement perception and the evolution of conceptions of kinesthesia and emotional experience (see also Sheets-Johnstone 1999/2011). Appreciation of the particularities and subjectivity of lived experience is reflected in the growing interest in the felt sense of moving that has arisen in contemporary dance (Ehrenberg, 2015).

Dancing the landscape is my means of locating myself more consciously in my place or particular placement at a moment in time. I dance the landscape to renew my contract with the rest of the world – to make connections and find myself in responsible relationship with what is around me. Apart from the personal wellness that comes with the activity – a sense of aerobic fitness, and the imaginative stimulation and deep sense of association that being in these places stimulates – there is a quality of unfolding and developing community. This latter kind of wellness is accounted for, at least in part, by the ongoing dialogues and embodied empathy that dancing for and with one another in the landscape brings. For me, the experience of dancing for Kevin Jeynes at the well described earlier had some of those social and empathic qualities.

The ever-changing landscape presents itself in all manner of ways – waterlogged, flooded, in vibrant bloom, exploited and drought affected – and provides all manner of stimulation. In 2009, I watched as Helen Herbertson walked out onto the wetland, her feet sinking into the vegetation mat that lapwings, purple swamp hens, and dotterils negotiate with ease. In this same period, Jane Mortiss stood, ran, fell, and slowly stalked heron-like, creating shadows in the waterlogged pastures (Figs. 3.6 and 3.7).

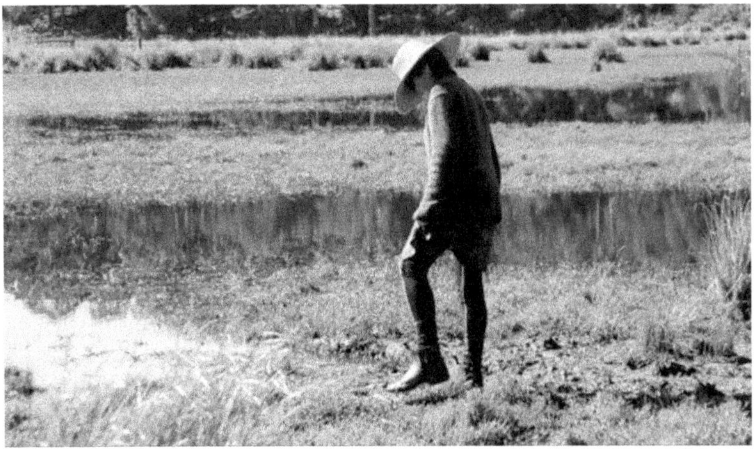

Fig. 3.6 Helen Herbertson – Autumn, Kiah wetlands. (Photograph by Don Asker)

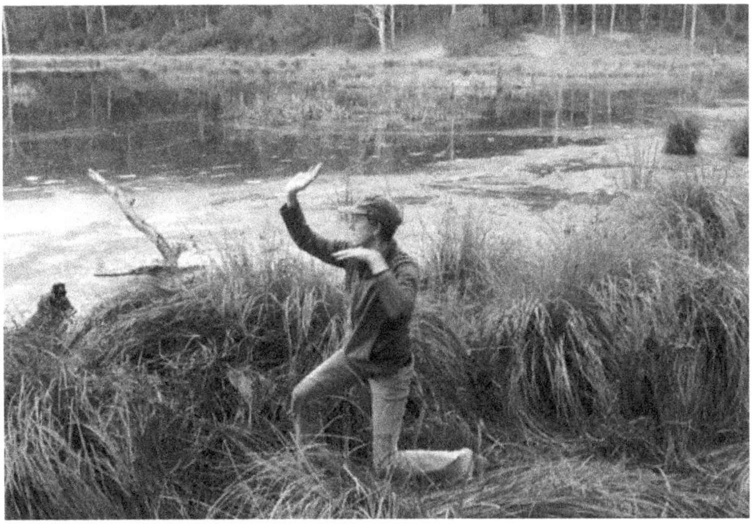

Fig. 3.7 Jane Mortiss – Autumn, flanked by phragmites reeds on the edge of Kiah wetlands. (Photograph by Don Asker)

Helen mused:

She falls to the ground covered in mud and soggy grass,
The water seeping through to her underwear,
Delicious,
The sensation of going down is what she likes,
The moment before she lands,
The softness of her body,
Easing into the ground,

Softening and easing,
Relaxing into it,
Dropping further down,
Am I lying in a cowpat?

The dialogue between dancing Jane and witnessing Helen saw physical action, conversation and poetic responses intertwining over the course of days and continue to resonate years later. The experience of dancing in the diverse environments of Kiah percolated over time. In fact, 4 years later we combined to articulate our sense of an embodied creative practice, and this hovered around a number of nodes: our bodily sense-making, the capacity for intention to arise slowly to awareness, and the interlacing of perception, imaginative process, and ideation, all grounded within the medium of our bodies and in the places and relations of our lives. Our journal article "Latitudinal Conversations" (2013) was indeed the manifestation of bearing witness to each other. Therein lies another interesting tension – between the internalizing and reflective, intra-subjective-process and the conjoining of people through conversational or respectful witnessing. Essentially, dancing the landscape feels differently enriching when it involves sharing the experience.

Reflecting on her dancing experiences at Kiah over more than a decade, Jane Mortiss mused:

> My improvising usually comes with a sense of joy and playfulness. I notice my response to trees, and to changes in the landscape. I am watchful. The dogs dance in the landscape; I relate to their rolling in the grass burning off energy, I feel a sense of freedom and exhilaration. I enjoy running round the paddock but not as I once did. There is a sense of risk and danger in a rural environment – there are snakes, holes, sticks and cow poo. (Mortiss, personal communication, January 13, 2017)

Jane describes her alertness of sight, smell, sound, touch, and kinaesthetic awareness. She is conscious of the energy and motion of her dancing and how this sensibility enables her to notice irregularities in the environment. She detects and differentiates kangaroos, deer, pollens and decomposing organic matter by smell and identifies birds as much by their call as their appearance. She talks about the environment cuing her imagination:

> My imagination works. I don't try to fly but am aware of the sensation of wind on my arms. Falling leaves sprinkle through space. The sense of colour comes more apparent with the changing of seasons. The grass goes from green to brown, the river from dark to clear. As a child, I laid on the ground watching clouds move across the sky. I still do and I see the clouds as other things. It's like being in the old farmhouse looking up at the ceiling boards and the knots in the wood grain resemble people, faces, and animals. I don't see contemporary images, but much older ones from a bygone time—the woman with the skirt has a bustle. (Mortiss, personal communication, January 13, 2017)

This partially colonised landscape – the Kiah wetlands and surrounds – attracts for its vestiges of peace and quiet, as if this country escapes the sonic violence of busy cities. Relatively speaking, there is less noise – until one sits on a tractor or happens upon a colony of noisy Bell miner birds, or territorial Wonga pigeons. But can one ever be peaceful? Is this a pointless question? Perhaps there are simply degrees of quietness, a relativity of one sound to the next, and in the space of relative quiet we might appreciate difference. I know this quietness as I dance or contemplate dancing. It is a sensory openness, a momentary emptiness before the perception of possibilities, before thought arises and I make meaning of my situation.

Being thought-full is a possibility – but when the space of my habitation demands my attention, I am less inclined to muse and reflect, but rather to be immediately responsive to my environment. As Rachel Kaplan (2003) reminds herself, "There is only this moment, this action. And then the next" (p. 226). I find myself sensorially alert as I negotiate the long grass of the wetlands, listening for sounds, looking for snakes in the next tussock, wary of the sharp blades of long leaved Garnia that can slice bare skin like razor blades, and following my impulses.

Solo improviser Janette Hoe (2017) is a Melbourne-based dancer whose performance practice has a somatic base, drawing on her body's capacity for knowing and remembering. Interested in processes of transformation and in the notion of being "medium," she describes trying to empty herself of all thought, which invites inundation from outside, from her environment, from the world in which she stands in the next moment. Switching off or letting go of obsessive or potentially fixated modes of being offers the chance of unbending from particular stances or attitudes. Let me stay with this a little longer by outlining an ongoing concern of mine, one that you might share or see its sense.

I have become entangled in the struggle to preserve parts of the natural world. This runs against conventional agri-practices and current community and corporate business commitments. Like many others, I want to see more of our forests preserved from what is now a heavily state-subsidized wood chipping for paper industry, and hope that agribusinesses will support a more responsible and sustainable use of the land. Introduced deer have adapted so well to Australian conditions that they have become pests, doing considerable damage in National Parks and farming areas. Deer hunters pay license fees providing government with important revenue and in the process, give hunters a voice in what stays.

Every action on the land has implications. The presence of cows contributes methane into the atmosphere, and their hard hooves and large body mass compact the ground. By comparison, kangaroos are lighter on the environment and also booming in numbers. They thrive in open grassy ground as indigenous peoples well knew and is reflected in their careful clearing of small areas to entice the animals within spearing range. So why, I ask, are we still farming cows when there are other options? And why are we still logging our remnant forests?

It goes on: my thoughts are often conflicted and spill out into my dancing. The personal values that guide my action in the world afford my dancing a certain agency when I let these convictions rise to the surface. There might be a common good in this, providing me a sense of purpose and fulfillment. Further, the dance that is witnessed or companioned might be the starting point of a dialogue in which dancer viewpoint becomes pluralised and then problematized as the witness responds. What might otherwise have remained an abstract thought becomes shared, and through its articulation and embodiment in dance, is grounded in the flesh and can resonate with others.

Ros Crisp, an Australian dancer and choreographer based in Paris, has visited logged sites, standing in the dust amongst the debris of discarded branches and crushed undergrowth. These are places of destruction and desolation where erosion occurs and species are obliterated or progressively selected, creating monocultures. They are difficult places to be for those concerned about the survival of fragile ecosystems. Somehow Ros has continued to bear witness to the vulnerable and exploited parts of our environment. Her dance appears to come from sensations that arise as aftershocks – where feeling, kinaesthesia, and imagination join to express bodily exclamations and impulses. She finds pleasure in publication through her dancing performance, in commitment to her own projects of natural regeneration on parts of her family's property, and in networking with other communities. There is no apparent narrative in her dancing other than her existence as one who embodies the traces of many journeys, a kind of accumulation of affect. Observing her improvise within the walls of the Kiah studio during a visit in 2016, I had a sense she was remembering paths through many different landscapes.

The landscape here has been exploited yet continues to be productive. It offers many possibilities. There is spaciousness in the sense of distance between me and the next hill, or the fringe of trees at the river or to the reeds and marshes flanking swampy areas. And this is where dancing in the landscape can come in. I can luxuriate in that state of *me* with the landscape as *respected other.* Extending theologian Martin Buber's (1923/1970) concept of human relationality, it is an "I/thou" relationship in which I am in relation with, not separate from or superior to the landscape as "other."

In 2015 Paul Roberts, joined Andrew Morrish, Jane Mortiss and me for a week-long sharing of our practices. One day Paul improvised in the open space to one side of natural wetlands, part of a flood plain area, now denuded of reeds and shrubs and partly grazed by cattle since colonial settlement in the 1850s. With a saxophonist colleague, Cobie Orger, accompanying him he danced late into the afternoon, when long shadows and still air lent a sense of peacefulness to the landscape. It was good to be there.

The grass was green and soft and with this spongy mattress underfoot we drifted with Cobie and Paul. Paul loped across the flats; he seemed to have a lot of energy, but abruptly switched to all fours, as one of the farm dogs joined him briefly. He was back on his feet and arching his back, tumbling, balancing, and seemed to forget we were with him. He circled slowly, and we adjusted our positions and walked to keep in touch with them both. Landscapes can be inviting. That day, the sun and clouds moved slowly, and frog and bird calls echoed off the hills, mixing with Cobie's sparse sounds and Paul's breathy aspirations. For me it was a dense multi-sensory experience into which thought barely trickled. Paul wrote later:

> The experience of moving and applying choreographic interests to that movement while being in a pasture made boggy by a natural watercourse, and surrounded by forest, made me feel like my very being was art and all that was required was a calling up of attentiveness. I felt held by the place, able to be courageous and big-minded about what I was doing, and the importance of my tiny place and role in the midst of so much creation and dissolution. Cobie's soundings, the attention of others, all served to locate me within dance, whilst the

> land and the sky and the sense of attendance of others—non-human others, located me in meaningfulness. (Roberts, personal communication, July 6, 2015)

In the bush, we sometimes draw mud maps to help guide strangers to particular places, including rough estimates of distances or walking time between places. Some places have names associated with what might be found there, duck ponds for example, or the names of people who perhaps established the track, like Simpsons trail. These often-simple maps can be embellished with details of what one might see or pass as one travels.

To get to where Paul and Cobie improvised we had to walk past a billabong teeming with water birds and crisscrossed with posts from a century old pig fence, and then along what we call the "corridor," a narrow paddock that serves as a route to move cattle along, and then out into an area fringed by creeks and wetlands. The wetlands are fecund places; marsh gases waft in summer and wildlife come and go. They support large populations of frogs and red-bellied black snakes and water birds. Indigenous peoples point to the bountiful resources, evidenced by flints lying on surrounding slopes. Being at the edge of these wetlands, as were Paul and Cobie, is like being close to something wild and uncivilized (Fig. 3.8).

Musing about mapping and cartographically based storytelling projects with indigenous peoples of the Tanami desert, Kim Mahoud (2016) noticed "something about the cognitive territory that maps occupy which links place to memory and emotion, short circuiting language and taking us to realms of abstraction and metaphor" (p. 194). Mappings hold a felt sense of connection of being and place, of past and present, and in abstract and poetic visual and literary forms on canvas, affirma-

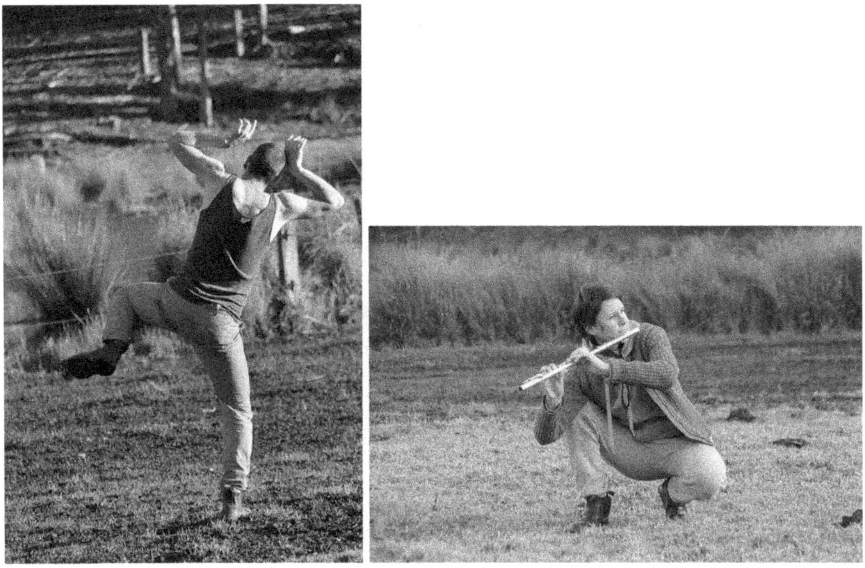

Fig. 3.8 Paul Roberts (top) and Cobie Orger improvising together at Kiah. (Photographs by Don Asker)

tion of our belonging in a place. A similar weaving can occur in dancing the landscape. The dance, ephemeral though it is, can bring to conscious awareness perceptions of who we are in this moment and how we relate corporeally, emotionally and perhaps metaphysically to the surrounding world. The emotional and sensual layers of Helen's commentary on Jane's dancing underline the capacity of dance to evoke strong resonances in others and provide in Jane's case an insight into how her seemingly minimalist gestures in the shallow waters of a flooded paddock could be experienced.

The dance can be more than its material corporeal forming and the dancer may find many cognitive processes in train, fed by the stimuli of the immediate environment and triggered memories. It seemed that at the well Kevin and I connected with the mythos or popular narratives of the place. Even more personal associations can be kindled as occurred for me in rolling, wrestling and tumbling down a hillside that I describe later. In the course of all our dancing we inevitably add new events or episodes to memory, adding to the data if I can call it that, from which we might further our practical knowing and self-understanding.

In *Locating: Place and the Moving Body,* Gretel Taylor (2009) was cognizant of the tendency to objectivise and thereby master the site. She determines to explore her relationships to place and investigate the experience of being in and with rather than detached from and superior to her environment: "My dance process and performances have engaged with places in an immersed inter-relation, valuing insights that emerged from the involvement with, or participation in, the differentiating particularities of a site" (p. 4).

Being aware of one's attitude has seemed important in my dancing. In a sense, it is a very subjective thing and worth more discussion and review over time. Nowadays I find myself putting myself in the place of the other, the patch of country or the building and asking the question, "How are you 'seeing' me?" (see Elkins, 1996). It allows the potential reciprocity between myself and other to at least be recognised. Taken to its extreme, I give imagined voice to the landscape. In fact, I am simply heightening my sensory awareness or level of alertness. This has implications for respectful relationship with what might be called the landscape, a place, or in Gretel Taylor's project, the "site."

Sometimes the dancing, as I intimated earlier, takes me by surprise, to borrow a phrase from Foster (2003). It can occur in places where one least expects dancing to happen. It underscores the dilemma of controlling dancing to particular sites, landscapes or places. The following, drawn from my journal of a day's farm work, illustrates this.

> Jane pushes open the large farm gate, kicks back her left leg in a sort of step I have seen a cow deliver at one of the kelpies when it got a little too close; then, this dancing demon arched her back, splayed her arms wide and flapped her wrists. She seems to break into these spasmodic dances, yes, I'll risk the word "dance," in the midst of doing farm work. I sit on the tractor waiting. She holds the gate open though it still vibrates with the energy of her pushing. Her face is flushed and she shuffles a few centimeters back as the large tractor tyres edge past. (Asker, journal, 2016)

Jane has given a name to this sort of "wild" dancing that differs so greatly from the modern and post-modern forms of which she was once agent and maker. She calls it "divergent dancing." The angular, breathy, impulsive, convulsive forms of this dancing seem to have distant relatives in Matts Eck's *Giselle* or Australian choreographer Phillip Adams' rapid fire classical convolutions. It happens mostly on the dirt tracks that follow the contours of the hills, where fence lines intersect at gates and barns, and the residual agribusiness of colonial times corrals us into lines and corners with fences.

I notice that when I am outdoors repairing a fence, hand feeding cattle in winter, or restoring the native vegetation along the river verges, I am sometimes prompted to stop. A sensation, sound, smell or sight catches my attention. Rather than thinking, I allow myself to listen to what is around me. I feel the articulation of my chest as I breathe or the cooling action of the wind on my face. As I relax, perhaps curving forward, letting go of the held practical body of the working me, I notice the residual tensions or possible extensions of that doing. Sometimes I bring breath and bodily shape and articulation together. I allow my attention to wander restlessly or steadily in my body, and it is interesting how quickly I am connected in awareness to the ground, to the slope and texture of the underfoot (Fig. 3.9).

When she is out in the cracked dried clay pan of the vast wetland baked in a seemingly endless summer, Jane's dance takes different forms. Sometimes I see echoes of Irish dancing – energetic prancing, toe tapping and bouncing, but this can give way

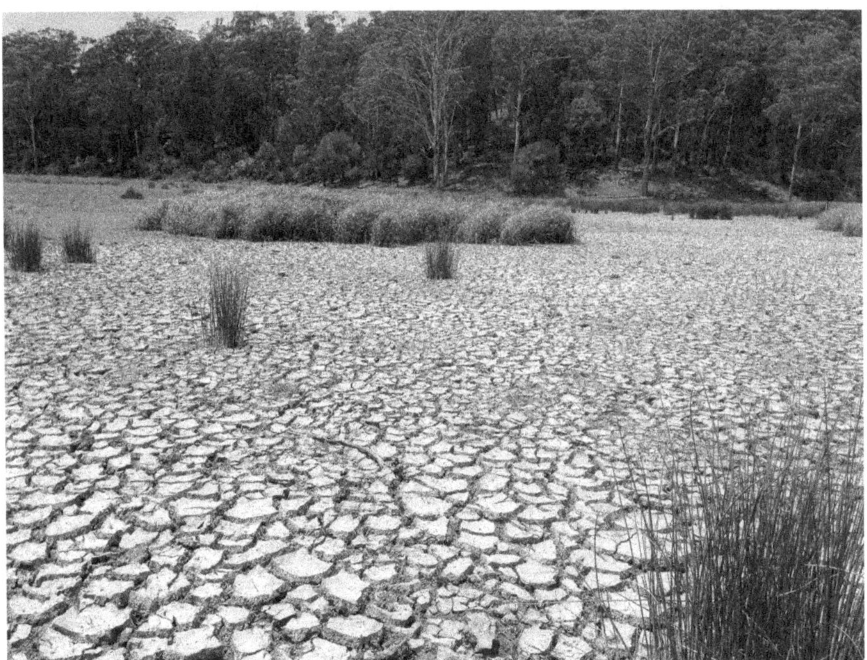

Fig. 3.9 Kiah wetlands in drought. (Photograph by Don Asker)

to wide slashing arms and leg swings, or in the blink of an eye she drops to crouch motionless like the swamp wallaby or the patient stalking egret. The wetland's grey blue fringe of melaleucas marks the boundary with the tall grey box-covered hills, and the heat causes the air to shimmer and the horizon to warp and wave. Remnant pockets of rush and reed provide cover and shelter, and late in the afternoon frogs croak, perhaps singing for rain and mate. The dance in Jane's case is never formally announced; it lurks and then asserts itself. I feel as if it is never finished.

Jane's interests have parallels with those of movement practitioner and researcher Victoria Hunter (2015), who notes a shift in her site-specific interest from urban environments to "landscape based work." The nature of her work has also changed from realizing site specific "events" to processes of "phenomenologically informed exploration and improvised performance" (p. 194) – an approach that is environmentally responsive and "focused on the exploration of improvised, organic movement responses" (p. 195). The dancer is connected to the environment and dances within and with it, rather than seeking to explain, make a story, or represent the environment. Hunter notes, "This approach is facilitated by a mobile process of dwelling in which both body and site are co-perceived by the performer, as they move along with the natural rhythms, contours, vistas and directions of the site" (p. 195).

On one occasion improviser Andrew Morrish returned to the small catholic cemetery located on the ridge above the floodplain. Descendants of families buried there continue to visit – Pendergasts, Ryans, McMahons, Whelans, Powers, McMasters, and many more as generations have married and left the district. A sense of ancestry and the uncertainty and brevity of life is often with me as I visit this place. Andrew and I had had some conversations around Irish writers and poets including Samuel Beckett and William Butler Yates. Andrew's fragmented monologue and inclusive gestures that day made Jane and me welcome attendees to something that was unusually solemn from Andrew, and sobering, if that can ever be said about an Irish cemetery. The shadows of figures from the past seemed a little more distinct as if gaps in our understanding can be filled by our imagination if we have that creative opportunity or need.

My body senses and feels. Sensory experience is constantly reattenuated as my purpose in the landscape changes. Tufnell and Crickmay (2004) suggest that as we experience our environment something within us is touched. Imagination is active. We recollect and might remember past experiences, recalling events or images of things. These are facets of the complex ways sensory perception can provide cues for association, thought, and reflection.

I startled a large lace monitor on the dusty track between mostly Cyclocarpa eucalypts and Acacia cognate – part of the track that runs on a low ridge. The 1.5 m lizard tried to climb the nearest tree but the loose bark pulled away and the creature fell backwards. After several rather frenetic attempts it turned and ambled away down the slope and into the forest. Something about the big heavily muscled creature's writhing reminded me of a wrestler. My grandfather did quite a lot of that and the wrestler's ease of moving from standing to rolling, along with my vivid memory of the startled lace monitor, stayed with me and prompted me to explore that physical capacity later that day.

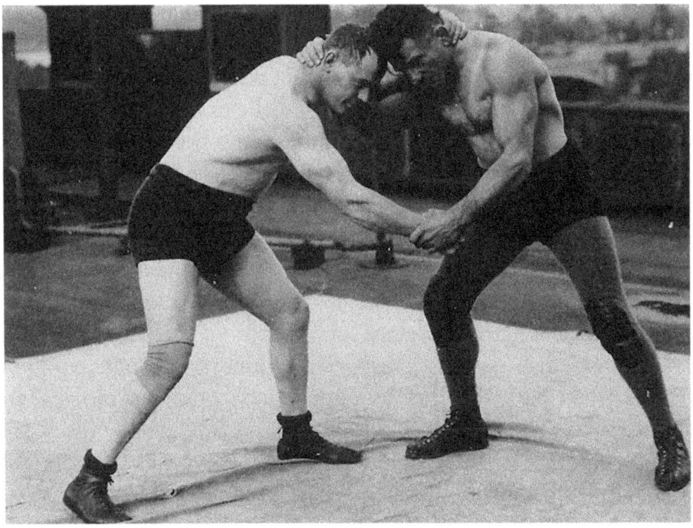

Fig. 3.10 Grandfather Albert Asker (left) and American wrestler Ad Santell, 1927. (Photograph from family archives)

I found my weight and the momentum that came with falling and rolling. This enabled me to alternately hinge and stretch legs, arms, and torso as I worked my way down a slope over the fallen logs of grey box, past anchoring rocks, and from seated postures to standing. The South African kikuyu grass gave a soft cushion while the logs needed more circumspection, as red bellied black snakes find them both good shelter for warming up and hunting grounds for their diet of crickets and frogs.

Grandfather's bouts with American wrestler Ad Santell probably led to the men becoming familiar – they would know one another's physical capacities and wrestling holds and strategies well. In a not dissimilar way, my close encounters with the side of the hill left me somehow softly massaged, aware of the odors of rotting wood, crushed grass, the prickled sensation of tussock and reedy grasses, and the passage through damp and warmth. I noticed where kangaroos had established tracks across the contours of the slope and saw their dung and their dust baths. I became hot, and my skin took on some scratch marks and blotchily responded to some of its contact with the vegetation (Fig. 3.10).

Concluding Thoughts

Through many years of dancing, I have adopted, discovered, and evolved ways of moving that "sit" in my body and support my embodied conversation and exploration of the world. In my less formal engagement today, and especially those dancing experiences in landscapes, conversation with others is central. In shared practices, there is a kinesthetic conversation or resonance and as I have suggested, even when I am the only human, the place or my environment provides the grounding for infinite interaction and reflection. In processes of empathetic exchange, sharing or reflecting back, come opportunities for mutual recognition and deeper understanding. I can sense the efficacy of gesture as inter-corporeal connection. Awareness of the particular sense of one's gestures enables differentiation and change (see Noland, 2009).

Dancing takes many forms in the landscape. It can be "conversational" in the sense that dancer and landscape are interactive. It can reflect purpose. The dancer has agency and all those witness to the event are implicated, attendance inviting response – for instance, concordance or disapproval of underlying concerns. Inevitably, dancers and witnesses experience kinesthetic and emotional resonances. These might have therapeutic, ethical, aesthetic or ecological roots, as I felt, for example, in sharing practice with Ros Crisp, and inspire discussion that is useful in clarifying perspectives. My dancing can involve a phenomenological attitude, an openness and sensory alertness – an immersion that fosters connectivity and empathy (Asker, 2018). It is situational as my episode with the goanna suggests, and has the capacity to be evocative at the same time, as memories are triggered. This creates a tension as staying somatically alert to the moment competes with the unfolding panoply of associations in thought, reflection, and remembering (Fig. 3.11).

The dancer and landscape relationship is complex, reflecting attitudes and values, emotions, physiology and bearing, and gestures of our bodies. It is accumula-

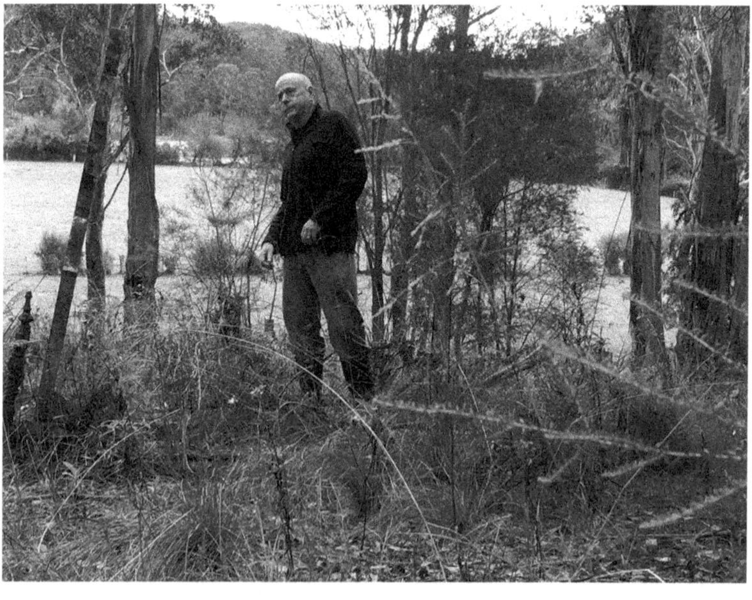

Fig. 3.11 Andrew Morrish at the Kiah cemetery. (Photograph by Don Asker)

tive in the dancer's body, which remembers or continues to be affected by particular environments long after one removes from the physical space. It was the case as Helen and I recollected dancing on the spongy wetlands years after the event. Where dancing the landscape is through a less structured or more improvised form, it is a situated real time revelation and embodiment of "values" informing the dancer's life. In this dancing, there is an intersection of practical ways of knowing – firsthand knowledge of our body's capacities and skills, experienced previously or found in the present moment – and other forms of knowing acquired through stories, perspectives, and histories of others and places. It was present in the way I experienced dancing at the well with Kevin Jeynes. Local knowledge, histories and mythology along with my particular practical skills and imaginative and creative capacities were in play that day. The everyday poetic or abstract forms of my gestures left echoes and sensations that touched emotional and thoughtful chords in me and my witness Kevin.

Choices made in dancing can be more or less conscious to the dancer, and patterns of dancing can be overturned or interrupted as the dancer finds self-critical awareness and searches for other options. Less familiar environments can heighten sensory activity and alertness; they might draw on strength, articulation, and balance, and develop physical fitness. Unfamiliarity can also arouse interest and curiosity in the environment, stimulating imagination, memories, and creative responses that reflect one's self. With increasing knowledge of the landscape and its past comes the possibility of making links and associations to one's own experiences and life narrative. The unfolding of Jane's "divergent dancing" has presented her with more choices about how she might be in this place at least. As Ivan Sikic became more and more vulnerable in the reedy, sun drenched wetlands, I recalled explorative figures like the Spaniard Cortez and the developmental pressures imposed upon indigenous cultures, subjects, and themes that Ivan's performative works have continued to explore around the world.

Experience underscores my perception of connectivity with places, and this relational aspect can raise consciousness of personal accountability and responsibility for one's actions. Shared and companioned "dancing the landscape" means embodied participation, conversation, interactivity, witnessing, and the potential for reflection and response. There is a social aspect, and rather than being individual in the world, one becomes one of many interconnected individuals. We are valuing intercorporeality in and through this dancing. The growing sense of a community of dancers at Kiah is partly that. But it also reflects the value we might place on communicating and contributing in ways that support a common good.

Particular individual and group interests can inflect dancing the landscape. Interconnections of dancer/s and landscape/s can cultivate reflection, heightened perception, and deeper understandings of one's own qualities and capacities, including strengths, endurance, and the ability to differentiate and interact with the unfamiliar.

References

Asker, D. (2016). *One day next Tuesday: A journal of life on a farm*. (Unpublished).

Asker, D. (2018). *The art of awareness*. London: Austin Macauley.

Asker, D., & Herbertson, H. (2013). Latitudinal conversations. *Journal of Artistic Research, 4*. Retrieved from https://www.researchcatalogue.net/view/29773/32861

Behnke, E. (1997). Ghost gestures: Phenomenological investigations of bodily micromovements and their intercorporeal implications. *Human Studies, 20*, 181. https://doi.org/10.1023/A:1005372501258.

Bernard, A., Steinmuller, W., & Stricker, U. (2006). *Ideokinesis: A creative approach to human movement & body alignment*. Berkeley, CA: North Atlantic Books.

Blainey, G. (2015). *The story of Australia's people, vol. 1: The rise and fall of ancient Australia*. Hawthorn, VIC: Penguin Books Australia.

Bond, K. (2014). Dance and quality of life. In A. Michalos (Ed.), *Encyclopedia of quality of life and wellbeing research* (pp. 1419–1425). Dordrecht, The Netherlands: Springer.

Buber, M. (1970). *I and thou* (W. Kaufmann, Trans.). New York: Charles Scribner's. (Original work published 1923).

Carter, P. (2010). *Ground truthing: Explorations in a creative region*. Crawley, UK: University of Western Australia Publishing.

Clark, M. (2006). *A short history of Australia*. Hawthorn, VIC: Penguin Books Australia.

Cursio, N., & Crooks, D. (2015). *At least for a while anyway*. Commissioned by Carriageworks for 24 Frames Per Second. (Single channel video). Retrieved from http://www.natcursio.com/project/at-least-for-a-while-anyway

Dorman, R. L. (2000). *A word for nature: Four pioneering environmental advocates, 1845–1913*. Charlotte, NC: University of North Carolina Press.

Dowd, I. (1995). *Taking root to fly: Ten articles on functional anatomy* (3rd ed.). New York: Irene Dowd and Contact Collaborations.

Ehrenberg, S. (2015). A kinesthetic mode of attention in contemporary dance practice. *Dance Research Journal, 47*(2), 43–61.

Elkins, J. (1996). *The object stares back: On the nature of seeing*. New York: Houghton Mifflin Harcourt.

Foster, S. L. (2003). Taken by surprise: Improvisation in dance and mind. In A. C. Albright & D. Gere (Eds.), *Taken by surprise: A dance improvisation reader* (pp. 3–10). Middletown, CN: Wesleyan University Press.

Foster, S. L. (2011). *Choreographing empathy: Kinesthesia in performance*. London: Routledge.

Hoe, J. (2017). *Performer as medium: Connecting past and present in improvisation*. MFA thesis, University of Melbourne, Australia.

Hughes, R. (1987). *The fatal shore: A history of the transportation of convicts to Australia*. London: Collins Harvill.

Hunter, V. (2015). Dancing – Worlding the beach: Connections through phenomenological movement inquiry. In C. Berberich, N. Campbell, & R. Hudson (Eds.), *Affective landscapes in literature, art and everyday life: Memory place and the senses* (pp. 189–206). Surrey, UK: Ashgate.

Kaplan, R. (2003). Some traveler's tales. In A. C. Albright & D. Gere (Eds.), *Taken by surprise: A dance improvisation reader* (pp. 215–228). Middletown, CT: Wesleyan University Press.

Koori Mail. (2011, April 20). Land is linked to well-being. *496*, 35.

Mahood, K. (2016). *Position doubtful: Mapping landscapes and memories*. Melbourne, VIC: Scribe.

McKenna, M. (2002). *Looking for blackfella's point: An Australian history of place*. Sydney, NSW: University of New South Wales Press.

Ness, S. A. (2016). *Choreographies of landscape. Signs of performance in Yosemite National Park*. New York: Berghahn.

Noland, C. (2009). *Agency and embodiment: Performing gestures/producing culture*. Durham, NC: Duke University Press.

Parker, S. (2016). *Small Details* (Video). Retrieved from http://vimeo.com/169191362

Paxton, S. (1986). The small dance. The stand. *Contact Quarterly, 11*(1), 48–50.

Rainer, Y. (1965). NO manifesto. *Tulane Drama Review, 10*, 2.

Rebanks, J. (2015). *The shepherd's life: Modern dispatches from an ancient landscape*. New York: Flatiron.

Sheets-Johnstone, M. (2011). *The primacy of movement*, Amsterdam: John Benjamins. (Original work published 1999).

Sweigard, L. (1974). *Human movement potential: Its ideokinetic facilitation*. New York: Harper & Row.

Taylor, G. (2009). *Locating: Place and the moving body*. (Doctoral thesis). Victoria University, Melbourne, Australia.

Tuan, Y. (1977). *Space and place: The perspective of experience*. Minneapolis, MN: University of Minnesota Press.

Tufnell, M., & Crickmay, C. (2004). *A widening field: Journeys in body and imagination*. Hampshire, UK: Dance Books.

Chapter 4
In the Shadow of Crisis: Dance and Meaning in the Anthropocene

Robert Bingham

> Sometimes it is not…only about the human. (Eiko Otake as cited in Yokobosky, 2000, p. 27)

From spring 2015 to 2016 I engaged in a daily practice of dancing in the Wissahickon Park, a woodland that stretches for several miles through northwest Philadelphia. I was researching ways that dance might serve as a foundation for understanding and responding to environmental crisis through its capacity to help me explore the relationship of human and nonhuman nature. My background in dance, particularly improvisation, butoh, and site specific choreography, offered guidance in structuring movement experiences outside of dance studios and theaters. Wissahickon Park was an ideal laboratory for this experiential research. Having moved to a neighborhood abutting the park 3 years earlier, I had already developed an aesthetic interest in the woods through regular walks (which increased greatly when I adopted a dog), and through dancing in and with the park as a student in Merián Soto's dance improvisation classes and as a performer in her *Branch Dances: The Practice of Peace* (2015), a sculptural work in which dancers pushed, dragged and balanced large, curving branches harvested from the park.

By 2015 my body's "entanglement" (see Barad, 2007) with the woods was well established, and I sensed that the forest lifeworld would be a fertile site for querying my embodied relationship to a planet in crisis. In March, I learned of a local writer, Bradley Maule, who had collected trash in the Wissahickon daily for 1 year and created an installation with it called *One Man's Trash* (2015). Maule's commitment to a year-long, daily practice inspired and helped clarify the structure for my research. Every day I was in town, I danced, photographed, and removed trash from the park. These three activities both deepened and recorded my evolving relationship with this particular stretch of nature. At the same time, I researched environmental crisis through publications in the sciences (for example, *Anthropocene Review, Scientific*

R. Bingham (✉)
Temple University, Philadelphia, PA, USA
e-mail: tue79791@temple.edu

K. Bond (ed.), *Dance and the Quality of Life*, Social Indicators Research Series 73,
https://doi.org/10.1007/978-3-319-95699-2_4

American, Climate Central), humanities (Bennett, 2010; Kimmerer, 2014; Scranton, 2015), arts (Davis & Turpin, 2015), and news media. Informed by these perspectives, my physical practice became the ground for aesthetic reflection on the relationship between human bodies and the earth in the context of crisis.

"In the Shadow of Crisis" is a phenomenological study. According to philosopher Maxine Sheets-Johnstone (2011), the practice of phenomenology "makes the familiar strange" in order to illuminate deeper meaning within the everyday (p. 124). Related to Husserl's (2001/1900) concept of "natural attitude," this idea stems from the notion that everyday taken-for-granted phenomena can become opaque when senses and attitudes towards them sediment into habit. Phenomenology's role, enacted through "bracketing" or suspending preconceptions, is to stir the sediment in order to refresh and deepen sensory knowing within the landscape of the ordinary. As a dance practitioner familiar with approaching habit and exploring possibilities for change somatically, I wondered how I might be changed by extending my practices of perceptual attunement beyond the frame of dance studios and art making. Through a long-term commitment to moving in the woods, I opened myself up to being moved.

Welcome to the Anthropocene

In an interview, poet and scholar Leath Tonino (2015) states that unless people "weave consciousness into the world," they are unlikely to care about its ecological plight (p. 11). Like other contemporary theorists (Abram, 1996; Brown & Toadvine, 2003; Vakoch & Castrillón, 2014), he warns of an epistemological gap separating intellectual knowledge *about* and sensuous engagement *with* the world beyond the human, and that such a gap may be a hindrance to cultivating a more ecologically sustainable planet. Intellectual representations in science are, indeed, clear and compelling, even as they are subject to debate: status quo extraction-consumption patterns are forcing the planet's climate and chemistry outside the range of natural variation, producing a net effect of what Rob Nixon (2011) calls "slow violence" including mass extinction, desertification, raging storms and tides, and forced human migration (Biggers, 2015).

While the geologic record includes many catastrophic events, such as the massive meteor that drove the dinosaurs to extinction 65 million years ago, there is no known precedent for a single species transforming itself into a geophysical force akin, in its planet-altering capacity, to large meteors and deviations in Earth's orbit (Chakrabarty, 2015). In August 2016, the International Commission on Stratigraphy overwhelmingly approved the designation "Anthropocene," first proposed by chemist Paul Crutzen in the early 2000s, for the current geologic time period so as to account for the distinct chemical "signal" human activity is inscribing into the earth's surface (Ball, 2016).

Substantial debate surrounds the term "Anthropocene." On its own, it does not account for the unequal distribution of environmental impacts within our species, nor the reality that the world's poorest citizens, who contribute least to anthropogenic climate change, tend to suffer the worst of its effects (Malm & Hornberg, 2014). Some theorists outside the sciences invoke the terms "Capitalocene" and "Eurocene" to highlight that ecological destructiveness is more directly tied to unequal patterns of consumption and exploitation of resources than to the human as ontological being per se. Scientific data bear this out, clearly demonstrating, for instance, a correlation between economic activity and CO_2 levels in the atmosphere (Klein, 2012; Steffen, Crutzen, & McNeill, 2007).

Other debates surrounding Anthropocene are temporal, focusing on what date should be designated as the beginning of the geologic "Age of Humans" (Robin, 2016). Should it be the Industrial Revolution, when humans first began in earnest to shift from renewable energy harvested from the planet's surface – plants, water, wind, muscle – to *previously* renewable energy buried underground for millions of years? Among its many "triumphs" (Klein, 2012, p. 173), the technology of the coal-fired steam engine allowed industry to untether itself from natural earth surface patterns of weather, health, seasons, decay, and regeneration, etc. Might the start of the Anthropocene be better attributed to "Trinity," the first atomic blast, which occurred in 1945 in New Mexico's Jornada del Muerto desert, ushering in the nuclear era? Radioactive fallout from thousands of bombs tested subsequently and used in war now blankets the globe, inscribing fissile debris into the earth's geologic record. Should the Age of Humans be pegged to the Great Acceleration following World War II? Graphs of population, carbon emissions, and economic activity all show a sharp increase at this time (Steffen et al., 2007). Today, we continue to live the Great Acceleration, with population growing by a billion every 12–13 years, and economic activity growing even faster, albeit highly unequally. Cumulative effects of just the last few decades will extend their reach into geologic time (Berwyn, 2016).

Graphs, pie charts, statistics, and scientific papers describe the status quo with great specificity, but how effective are they on their own in igniting change? For Nixon (2011), the ontological crisis represented by anthropogenic forcing is accompanied by a crisis of storytelling. In today's media-saturated world, which encourages an ongoing state of "partial attention" (p. 13), the pace of slow violence creates a narrative dilemma (Fig. 4.1):

> Different kinds of disaster possess unequal heft. Falling bodies, burning towers, exploding heads, avalanches, volcanoes, and tsunamis have a visceral, eye catching and page-turning power that tales of slow violence…cannot match. Stories of toxic buildup, massing greenhouse gases, and accelerated species loss due to ravaged habitats are all cataclysmic, but they are scientifically convoluted cataclysms in which casualties are postponed, often for generations. … How can we convert into image and narrative the disasters that are slow moving and long in the making, disasters that are anonymous and star nobody? (p. 20)

For some contemporary philosophers and dance artists, storytelling in the Anthropocene, whether or not it references specific disasters, centers on age-old questions about what it means to be human. These include the relationship of humans with nature, wilderness, animals, things, and the more-than-human world (Abram, 2011; Galanter, 2009; Kloetzal, 2011; LaMothe, 2015; Lepecki, 2016;

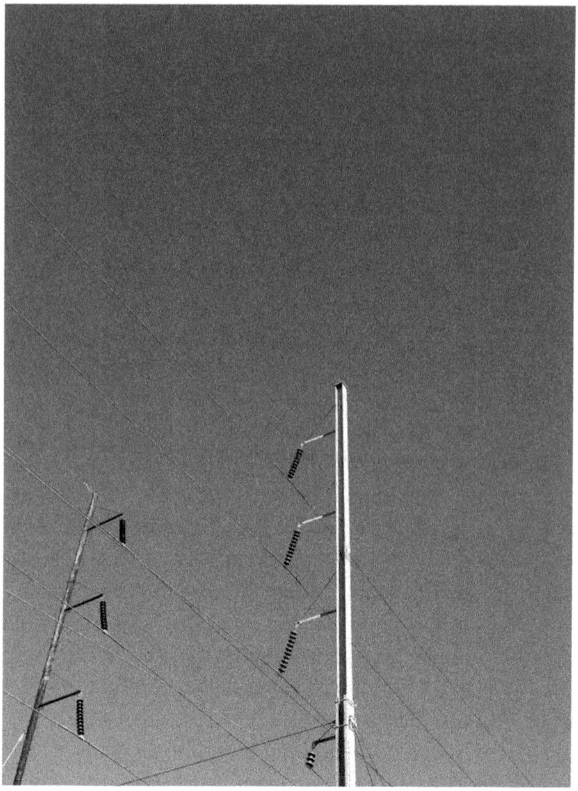

Fig. 4.1 Wissahickon Park (Summer). (Photo by Robert Bingham)

Monson, 2016; Olsen, 2002; Takenouchi, 2016). Philosopher Roy Scranton (2015) interrogates philosophy itself, concluding that the ancient practice of reflecting on the nature of reality exists precisely to offer guidance during critical times such as the current dawning of the Age of Humans. Philosophy is learning how to die, he asserts, referencing French Renaissance philosopher Michel de Montaigne. In a dying world, philosophy can guide us towards dying gracefully.

Sondra Fraleigh (2016) notes that the human body is always already a philosopher, and dancing is a way for body to reflect on world through conscious participation in movement. Somatic attention to self as evolving body in evolving world offers a means of relating to the world's dying presence, as she describes in an account of dancing in the Utah desert:

> In dance of many kinds we learn how to pay attention, how to fall, how to get up, and how to stroll and stride…Now in advanced age, I take what I've learned into the fields and tall grasses, kneeling down, lying down, and breathing. Through this dance, I feel what happens in and around me. … I become present to the canyon, to others and myself, and I think about change and age. Doesn't the mountain die at last, the lake, and do not the canyons also morph? (p. 71)

As she continues this reflection, Fraleigh alludes to the violent history of Cold War nuclear testing that took place 65 miles to the west, raining toxic debris throughout the region. The dancing she describes does not resist those memories living in the red rock, but allows them, instead, to participate in a moment of transformation: "[Here] I lie…in the suffering, consenting to have nothing but love in my life" (p. 71).

For choreographer and teacher Arawana Hayashi (as cited in Galanter, 2009), consciously embodying one's relationship to a context of environmental destruction can facilitate personal transformation towards action. Rather than casting blame on others, which she considers a form of disengagement, she proposes dancing as a tool for owning one's role in a long and continuous history of crisis and directing this somatic knowledge towards change:

> I am part of a collective creation. This is the product, this mess we are in…I can, with friends who are also creating this system, make some changes…[T]hat brings enormous power once you engage with that. (p. 25)

For Hayashi, inquiring into personal responsibility is a tool for connecting more fully with one's embodied agency in making change.

Woodland Phenomenology

Novelist Kevin Kling's statement that storytelling is asking questions in front of other people (as cited in Tippett, 2016, n.p.) suggests that a good story asks good questions. When I began my forays into the woods in spring 2015, I hoped that the questions I posed, for myself and for dance, would have impact by increasing dance artists' and scholars' engagement with environmental crisis. At the time, I was aware of only a few dance scholars, notably LaMothe (2015) and Olsen (2002), who were addressing meanings that emerge when dance studies is framed in the context of environmental crisis. I was asking questions I hoped others were asking, such as how dance practices support responding and adapting to crisis and how dancing can help develop and nourish an ecological ethics for the Anthropocene. My working theory was that the spatio-temporal structure I established – 1 year of deep engagement with a particular stretch of earth – would lead me towards deeper insight, if not to solid conclusions (van Manen, 1997).

By framing the study in relation to a problematic, what I had come to think of as the "shadow of crisis," my intention was not to assume the stance of a "presuppositionless beginning" as proposed by Husserl's (2001/1900) transcendental phenomenology. Nor was I attempting to make a determination about whether or not a crisis existed. Rather, I was seeking greater insight into a crisis I already believed existed, drawing upon my feelings about the circumstance to help me stay committed to paying attention over the course of a year. Phenomenology is *per se* a practice of close attention to experience, including its affective qualities, and illuminating its meanings through reflection. By engaging the phenomenological method somatically, as an improvising dancer, I accepted my bodily-affective entanglement with the world while at the same time endeavoring to maintain an open center and allow predeterminations to fall away. I entered the woods each day with an intention to create space for the world-as-represented in the Anthropocene literature to give way to an immediate experience of world-in-itself. Ultimately, I sought to integrate knowledge received in the woods with knowledge received from the page.

For the first several months, my practice centered on walking. I pushed myself to travel ever-farther afield, beyond the network of familiar trails near home, and to walk for longer than I wished. This was a conscious effort to part from habitual patterns of walking that had already been established within my everyday life. Very quickly, I became aware of a kind of invisible fence bordering these familiar patterns. As I pressed beyond the border, whether spatially or temporally, anxious thoughts began to kick in:

> I'm far from home and getting thirsty, and I forgot to bring water. I'm hungry, and it could be hours before I eat. What a waste of time! I should be reading more theory. How will what I'm doing ever be taken seriously as scholarship?

When such thoughts arose, I continued walking, recalling Buddhist nun Pema Chödrön's (1994) advice to connect with the "feeling beneath the storyline" and remain present to the possibility of emergent, fresh awareness (p. 28).

Sometimes, along a distant stretch of park, the banality of walking with mental restlessness transformed, and I found myself sensing, in-depth, the rise and fall of the paths, the vertiginous drops towards the creek, the sounds of breathing, footfall, and trickling water. I had entered a flow and, within this flow, I might pause to listen more intently, lifting my head from the tops of my ears and seeing with clear eyes unshrouded by thinking. One morning, I recalled the words "doe eyes," something Joan Skinner said during an improvisation class 20 years back. In that moment, my eyes softened outward towards my temples, while the sounds of the woods entered my limbs and spine. In a flash, I was animal, fully alive in my senses and with the ground and trees. When I continued walking a few minutes later, I felt gratitude for the gift of memory and its mysterious life within the flesh.

Several months into the practice, I described what I was doing to a neighborhood friend, a sociology professor, explaining that this was a choreographic improvisation centered on patterns of walking, photographing, and removing trash. "That's interesting," she said. "But I don't understand how it is dance." I began describing the influence of my past training, including postmodern walking dances, before thinking to myself, 'This is too abstruse. I am not dancing in any conventional sense, nor am I presenting choreography for an audience. I will have difficulty communicating what I am doing as dance research.' I decided that from that day on, I would encourage, within the practice, "superordinary" movements such as stamping, jumping, rolling, falling, melting, balancing, shape-shifting, and stillness.

The shift in my experience of the practice was immediate, initiating reflection on the difference between dancing and walking relative to perception:

> It seems that the lifeworld of the woods becomes more vivid when I dance, in part, because there is a relationship between my habits of perception and my habits of movement. When I am in everyday walking mode—forward, frontal focus—that vividness tends to be obscured, as thoughts buzz around like flies. But something as simple as pausing and

> rotating to sense the space behind my body, or going upside-down, or balancing on one foot, or lying down on a rock to see the sky, changes my entire perceptual system, which re-orients itself, and I see and feel things afresh. (Bingham, 2015)

When I only walked, it might take 45 min or longer for my everyday consciousness to transform into a consciousness fully attuned with the sensuous depths of the woods. When I danced, however, the shift was often instantaneous. Over time, I began to comprehend habit in a new way, not simply as a matter of movement but one of perception, and this led me to reflect on two decades of prior training and experience of dance.

As a student of contemporary western theatrical dance techniques, how many hundreds of hours had I spent dropping my weight into gravity, sensing the support of the floor, opening out into the constructed spaces of dance studios and theaters whose architecture separated and marked them as special places for dancing? I was grateful to those open spaces and sprung-wood floors that were the sites of my artistic training and yet, now, I felt cheated by them, as their partitioning obscured deeper somatic meanings of gravity, earth, and space, in particular the fact that other, nonhuman beings experience these phenomena, too. I was habituated to thinking of dancing as something that humans do with and for other humans. Gradually, however, this assumption melted away as my dancing in the woods evolved into a form of witness to how nonhumans within the "living ambiance" (Nagatomo, 1992, p. xxv) expressed movement, silence, sound and stillness. The lifeworld itself was becoming a dance (Fig. 4.2).

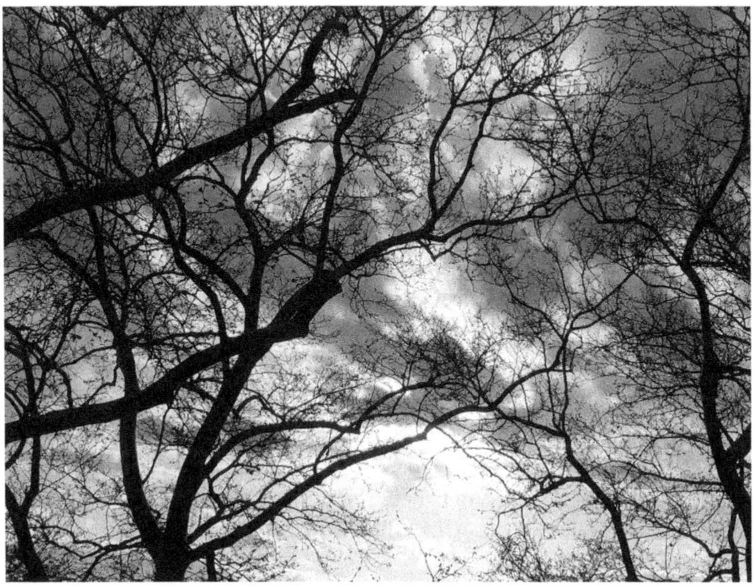

Fig. 4.2 Wissahickon Park (Fall). (Photo by Robert Bingham)

Over time, dancing in the woods cohered into a practice of attunement through body (Nagatomo, 1992) oriented to deepening the meaning of my connection, as body, to the materiality of earth. Often, I struggled to remain present to my dancing, particularly given the lack of accountability to any human witness or audience, save an occasional passerby. Even without an audience, I was witness to myself, and my inner critics sprang to life readily. When they did, I attempted to settle into the somatic qualities of self-criticism and allow these to move me, reminding myself that the goal was attunement through my body, not artistically-satisfying choreography. More often, however, it was something in the woods – a pattern of movement, a shift of sound or light – that brought me back to my senses and to specific, ever-changing qualities of body and ambiance. One morning, a lackluster sequence of dancing vivified into a tiny duet with a fly:

> I'm back in the woods. I go to my regular spot with large trees spaced twenty yards apart. There is a patch of sunlight, which I enter and assume a wide stance. Immediately, my right arm begins to rise, and with it the thought comes: "There it is again: always initiating movement with that arm." But the dance has begun, and so I follow its course. My arm continues towards the familiar high-diagonal stretch but then reaches a little further, pulling my center with it. I begin pouring awareness into the left side of my body, while thinking "left nervous system." Left body-half now starts tugging away from right arm, creating a whole-body morphing rotation that drags my focus across the spongy forest floor until it arrives at a broad tree, just three feet away. The grey trunk is lit up brilliantly, and my eyes crawl upwards along its scaly body. Suddenly, there's a buzzing: a fat, blue fly spirals around before landing directly in my line of vision. My right arm, unhappily removed from the action, floats over to hover, fingers slightly extended, an inch from the tree. I wait. Then I have a thought: can I touch the tree with such gentleness that the fly will remain? I make contact. The fly buzzes away. Within seconds, though, it is back. I contact again. The fly is gone, then returns again. This is a game we repeat three more times, before I have had enough and continue my rotating. Feet rooting, spine spiraling, I turn back to where I began and dissolve the dance and continue with my day. (Bingham, 2015)

Over the course of the year, these kinds of kinesthetic interactions with animals, trees, rocks and waterways accrued towards an encompassing sense of sensual and emotional entanglement with the woods. Walking home one morning after dancing in the area surrounding a fallen tree (Fig. 4.3), which I had visited daily for over a month, I imagined how I might feel if these woods were torn down in order to extract minerals, coal or oil to multiply corporate wealth. What if this lifeworld, which I had come to love and respect, were transformed, for the sake of profit, into a landscape of ravaged ground and poisoned water?

The sense of violation was a visceral blow sending a sticky cocktail of dread and helplessness through my veins, even as this was only an exercise in thinking likely triggered by accounts I had recently read of corporate incursions into the Amazon and American Southwest. I continued walking as thoughts boiled over and then simmered back down, eventually melting into the steady rhythms of footfall, breathing, a dog barking somewhere in the distance. Just come back to earth, the rhythms said, trust earth to do what it will do. Allow the healing movements of change to unfold through time. Allow time.

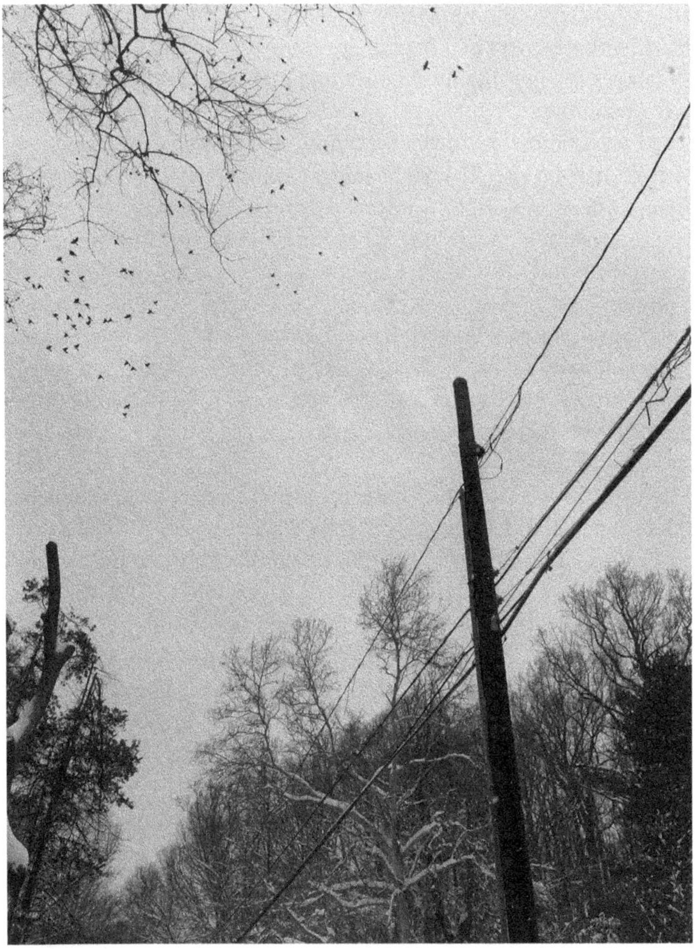

Fig. 4.3 Wissahickon Park (Winter). (Photo by Robert Bingham)

Flow

The role of consciousness is choice. (Deborah Hay, 1994, p. 3)

"Making the familiar strange" (Sheets-Johnstone, 2011, p. 124) is aided by slipping around familiar patterns of thought and perception. It is a task to which dance, as "conscious participation in the rhythms of bodily becoming" (LaMothe, 2015, p. 7), is well suited. When I participate somatically in bodily becoming, I can guide my movement past grooves of habit towards lesser-known terrain, where seeds of new movements and perceptions await, ready to stir to life. With dedicated attention, my senses are born anew, bringing fresh awareness to the vibrant materiality (Bennett, 2010) of the environment in which I dwell. At times, the inter-resonance of my self and the living ambiance (Nagatomo, 1992), and by extension world, becomes unmistakable, and in a fleeting moment I grasp that bodies and their environments "intra-actively bring forth new worlds" (Barad, 2007, p. 170) in an ensemble dance of becoming.

Consciously participating in the unfolding patterns of movement – perceiving them growing, dissolving and transforming – plants seeds of comprehension that the general patterns of my living – my food and trash, my speaking and breathing – are never only mine, and never only what I think they are. Rather, they are woven within the vast, patterned movement of the "worlding" world (Heidegger, 1927/2010, 1971) – a process, not a thing – and the pathways of my living are like phrases spinning into and out of a never-ending dance. I am part of the earth's dance and of the universe's dance, even as the restless winds of thinking make me forget. When I dance, I bring myself back to the patterns here and now – these vibrant trees, this vibrant ground, this vital body – and for a moment I remember what is forever slipping towards the forgotten.

David Bohm (1980), elaborating upon the discoveries of quantum physics, writes that the universe and all phenomena contained therein are movement. Cities, oceans, mountain ranges, and thoughts are patterns emerging from and dissolving back into what he calls "undivided wholeness in flowing movement" (p. 14), which for me echoes Husserl's "flowing live present" (as cited in Bruzina, 2004, p. 30). Flow appears to characterize all being yet is irreducible to a determinate substance and unavailable, according to Bohm, to final analysis. Still, flow patterns emerge in dancing, just as they do in mountains of trash – the detritus of American consumption – as vividly displayed in Robert Sullivan's (1998/2012) description of garbage mounds tucked out of sight of New York City's skyline:

> The…garbage hills are alive…billions of microscopic organisms thriving underground in the dark, oxygen free…after having ingested the tiniest portion of leftover New Jersey or New York, these cells exhale huge underground plumes of carbon dioxide and warm moist methane, giant stillborn tropical winds that seep through the ground to feed the meadowlands fires, or creep up into the atmosphere, where they will eat away at the…ozone… I walked along the edge of a garbage hill, a 40-foot drumlin of compacted trash…. There had been rain the night before, so it wasn't long before I found a leachate seep [that] was pure pollution, a pristine stew of oil and grease, of cyanide and arsenic, of cadmium, chromium, copper, lead, nickel, silver, mercury, and zinc. I touched this fluid – my fingertip was a bluish caramel color…warm and fresh. A few yards away, where the stream collected into a benzene scented pool, a mallard swam alone. (p. 97)

How might understandings of consumption – someone's or everyone's – change if viewed not dualistically as consuming subjects and consumed objects, but holistically as movements, more or less harmonious, within the ancient life-enabling patterns of the earth system? As I look around me, I can imagine the objects I see as movements in earth's dance.

"Everything around you comes from Mother Earth," boomed a woman with a bullhorn at a recent rally protesting the North Dakota Access Pipeline. Quantum theories suggest that every "thing" interweaves or "entangles" with all other things as they pass through shared planetary and cosmic histories. When I dance, my perceptions awaken to vibrant matter-energy – the vibrancy of this body changing with the changing environment – evoking at times an image of the world as dancing

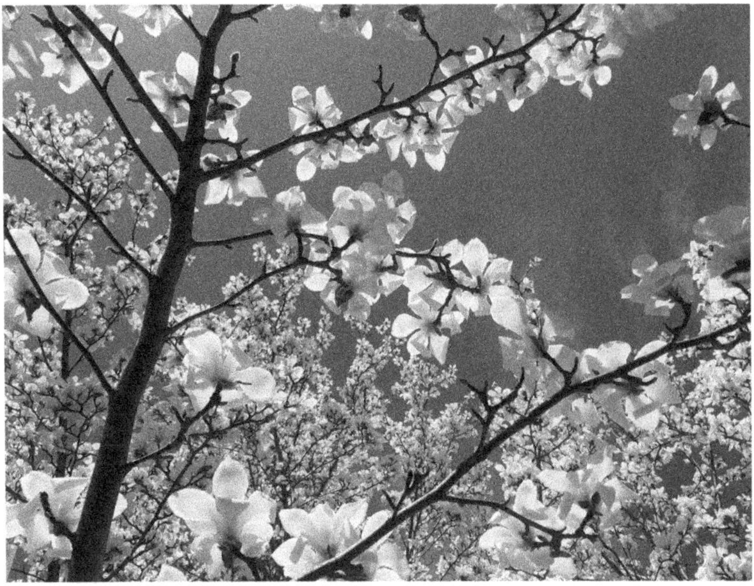

Fig. 4.4 Wissahickon Park (Spring). (Photo by Robert Bingham)

(Bingham, 2017). This image orients me as I try to locate my place in an injured world, and I sense in an immediate way that this and every moment of the world's becoming creates the conditions of possibility for future moments.

What seeds, I wonder, might I plant today? Joanna Macy (2014) offers a reminder that decisions made today "under pressure for profit…will affect whether beings thousands of generations from now will be able to be born sound of mind and body" (n.p.). I search for a felt connection to those faraway beings, and to those beings presently on earth with whom I am entangled but will never meet. In a world stressed by pressures for profit and growth, which force dangerous new rhythms into the planetary dance, this search feels like an ecological necessity (Fig. 4.4).

Showing Up

A full year has passed and I am ready to review the photographs I took every day, documenting my visits to the woods. There are hundreds. Looking through, I notice that I have aimed the lens towards contrasts, favoring patterns of light, shadow and color that play off each other in striking ways: autumn leaves curling in on themselves; spider webs heavy, yet intact, after rainfall; trees 80 feet tall spreading across the sky like branching veins; a single ladybug radiant on a spring leaf; the crumbling, charred remains of a nineteenth century stone cottage, the word "LUST" splashed across one of its remaining walls. I go back to the beginning and scroll again, quickly this time, and see a blur of color marking the year's passage through familiar seasons: grey turning to green, green to dark green, dark green to rust, rust to grey, and then, suddenly, white – the day of the blizzard, when I hurled myself again and again into soft, thick pillows of untrammeled snow.

I reflect on this year of listening through the medium of movement to the life-world of the woods. Thoughts bloom in quick succession: these woods matter; matter matters; matter and meaning are entangled (Barad, 2007). Through my attention I can choose to find new meaning in the taken-for-granted, as I understand that their origins and futures are earth's. Reflecting on the stubborn persistence of violence against the earth's life systems, Macy (2014) states that, "the biggest gift you can give is to be absolutely present," adding, "The main thing is you're showing up, that you're here and finding the capacity to love the world. That is what's going to unleash our solidarity for the healing of the world" (n.p.).

After a few minutes my thoughts change direction, towards food. Food is, unquestionably, matter that matters, yet 40% of what is grown in this country ends up in landfill (Modi, 2016). During this year of eco-phenomenological inquiry, I paid closer attention to my patterns of consuming and throwing away food asking, as somatic movement techniques have taught me, if there were other ways to move. Through the movements of questioning, my pathways changed as I sought out new possibilities. I was moved to begin learning the ropes of growing food, volunteering at an urban farm and joining a community garden, where new rhythms – squatting, digging, pulling, squeezing – cohered into a practice that, like dance, demanded skill, patience and perhaps most importantly, open senses.

I discovered that, again like dance, this practice enhanced quality of life, affording a sense of living into the world, participating robustly in its animacy (Abram, 1996). Its reward was renewable curiosity and fresh understandings gleaned from casual exchanges with people I met amidst crops: plants communicate; soil needs to rest; Philadelphia is, as one activist told me, "where it's at" for sustainable urban farming and food justice activism in the United States. The bio-web of species, from bipeds to composting microbes, is sustained through dynamic balance held by reciprocal exchanges of energy. In the Age of Humans, this balance is in peril, as noted by another veteran gardener who quipped: "When one species dominates, you get global warming and stinky compost."

I move on from the photographs and begin to pore through field notes. Page after page I see rambles and rants: descriptions of dances in the woods, moments of sentimentality, and flashes of clarity – sticky compost feeding a story I wish to tell. My eyes land on a pile on my desk, a jumble of hand-written notes and unfiled bills. I pick out a wrinkled, partially crossed-out page. It is barely legible, the words written in a hurry.

> I am patterns of movement
> When I pay attention, I can change them
> When I pay attention, I discover they are already changing
> I do not know how I know this
> The world that I think about is not the world I perceive
> The first appears solid
> The second is dancing

I lean back, take a deep breath, and vow that I will never forget to dance.

References

Abram, D. (1996). *Spell of the sensuous: Perception and language in a more-than-human world*. New York: Vintage.

Abram, D. (2011). *Becoming animal*. New York: Vintage.

Ball, D. (2016, September 14). *The new Anthropocene epoch has dawned, and it's "very worrisome"*. Retrieved from http://www.metronews.ca/news/vancouver/2016/09/14/new-anthropocene-epoch-has-already-dawned-warn-researchers.html

Barad, K. (2007). *Meeting the universe halfway: Quantum physics and the entanglement of matter and meaning*. Durham, NC: Duke University Press.

Bennett, J. (2010). *Vibrant matter: A political ecology of things*. Durham, NC: Duke University Press.

Berwyn, B. (2016, September 5). Far from turning a corner, global CO_2 emissions still accelerating. *InsideClimate News*. Retrieved from https://insideclimatenews.org/news/19052016/global-co2-emissions-still-accelerating-noaa-greenhouse-gas-index

Biggers, J. (2015, August 28). *Call it what it is: A global migration shift from climate, not a migrant or refugee crisis*. Retrieved from http://www.huffingtonpost.com/jeff-biggers/call-it-what-it-is-a-glob_b_8056186.html

Bingham, R. (2015, December). *In the shadow of crisis: Dance and meaning in the Anthropocene*. Paper presented at the annual Eastwest Somatics Network Conference, Springdale, UT.

Bingham, R. (2017). *Improvising meaning in the age of humans*. Doctoral dissertation, Temple University, Philadelphia.

Bohm, D. (1980). *Wholeness and the implicate order*. London: Routledge.

Brown, C., & Toadvine, T. (Eds.). (2003). *Eco-phenomenology: Back to the earth itself*. Albany, NY: SUNY Press.

Bruzina, R. (2004). *Edmund Husserl and Eugen Fink*. New Haven, CT: Yale University Press.

Chakrabarty, D. (2015, December). *The geophysical agency of humans and climate change*. Retrieved from http://globalenergyinitiative.org/insights/161-climate-change-and-the-geophysical-agency-of-humans.html

Chödrön, P. (1994). *Start where you are*. Boston: Shambhala.

Davis, H., & Turpin, E. (Eds.). (2015). *Art in the Anthropocene*. London: Open Humanities Press.

Fraleigh, S. (2016). Butoh translations and the suffering of nature. *Performance Research, 21*(4), 61–71.

Galanter, M. (2009). Dance, ecology, and the deep world. An interview with Arawana Hayashi and Jennifer Monson at SEEDS. *Contact Quarterly, 34*(2), 20–25.

Hay, D. (1994). *Lamb at the altar: The story of a dance*. Durham, NC: Duke University Press.

Heidegger, M. (1971). The origin of the work of art. *Poetry, language, and thought* (A. Hofstadter, Trans.). New York: Harper & Row.

Heidegger, M. (2010). Being and time (J. Stambaugh, Trans.). Albany: SUNY Press. (Original work published 1927).

Husserl, E. G. (2001). *Logical investigations* (D. Moran Ed.). London: Routledge. (Original work published 1900/1901).

Kimmerer, R. W. (2014). Returning the gift. *Minding Nature, 7*(2), 18–24.

Klein, N. (2012). *This changes everything: Capitalism vs. the climate*. New York: Simon & Schuster.

Kloetzal, M. (2011). *Site dance*. Gainesville, FL: University Press of Florida.

LaMothe, K. (2015). *Why we dance: A philosophy of bodily becoming*. New York: Columbia University Press.

Lepecki, A. (2016). *Singularities: Dance in the age of performance*. New York: Routledge.

Macy, J. (2014, November 6). *A wild love for the world* [Interview]. Retrieved from www.onbeing.org/program/joanna-macy-a-wild-love-for-the-world/

Malm, A., & Hornberg, A. (2014). The geology of mankind? A critique of the Anthropocene narrative. *The Anthropocene Review, 1*(1), 62–69.

Modi, P. (2016). *Exclusive interview with the director of Harvard's Food Law and Policy Clinic*. Retrieved from www.change.org

Monson, J. (2016). Artist statement. *iLand*. Retrieved from http://www.ilandart.org/artist-biography/

Moran, D. (2000). *Introduction to phenomenology*. New York: Routledge.

Nagatomo, S. (1992). *Attunement through the body*. Albany, NY: SUNY Press.

Nixon, R. (2011). *Slow violence and the environmentalism of the poor*. Cambridge, MA: Harvard University Press.

Olsen, A. (2002). *Body and earth*. Middlebury, CT: Middlebury Bicentennial Series.

Robin, L. (2016). How do people live in the Anthropocene? *Geophysical Research Abstracts, 18*. Retrieved from http://meetingorganizer.copernicus.org/EGU2016/EGU2016-3339.pdf

Scranton, R. (2015). *Learning to die in the Anthropocene*. San Francisco: City Lights.

Sheets-Johnstone, M. (2011). *The primacy of movement* (2nd ed.). Amsterdam: John Benjamins.

Steffen, W., Crutzen, P. J., & McNeill, J. R. (2007). The Anthropocene: Are humans now overwhelming the great forces of nature? *Ambio: A Journal of the Human Environment, 36*(8), 614–621.

Sullivan, R. (2012). *The meadowlands: Wilderness adventures at the edge of a city*. New York: Scribner. (Original work published 1998).

Takenouchi, A. (2016). *What is Jinen?* Retrieved from http://www.jinen-butoh.com/top_e.html

Tippett, B. K. (Host). (2016, May 19). Kevin Kling: The losses and laughter we grow into. In B. K. Tippett (Producer), *On being with Krista Tippett*. Minneapolis, MN: KTPP.

Tonino, L. (2015). David Hinton on the wisdom of ancient Chinese poets. *The Sun, 469*, 4–12.

Vakoch, D. A., & Castrillón, F. (2014). *Ecopsychology, phenomenology, and the environment: The experience of nature*. New York: Springer.

van Manen, M. (1997). *Researching lived experience: Human science for an action sensitive pedagogy*. New Palz, NY: SUNY Press.

Yokobosky, M. (2000). Movement as installation: Eiko & Koma in conversation with Matthew Yokobosky. *Performing Arts Journal, 64*, 26–35.

Part II
Spirituality

Chapter 5
Dance as a Taonga from Children to the World: A Perspective from Aotearoa New Zealand

Adrienne Sansom

Introduction

This chapter highlights the presence and role of dance in the early years of learning within a specific community. The setting is Aotearoa New Zealand where early education is underpinned by New Zealand's early childhood curriculum, *Te Whāriki: He Whāriki Matauranga mō ngā Mokopuna o Aotearoa* (Ministry of Education [MoE], 1996) and the *Treaty of Waitangi* (*Te Tiriti o Waitangi,* 1840), Aotearoa New Zealand's founding document. The treaty is both a political treatise for the everyday functioning and future aspirations of Aotearoa New Zealand as a bicultural and, consequently, multicultural nation, and a reminder of a nation's ethical and moral obligation to *all* children and their education. *Te Whāriki* is based on a set of principles that reflect Māori or indigenous ways of knowing.

Te Tiriti o Waitangi was a pivotal development in the history of Aotearoa New Zealand, as it was written as a contract between the Māori people and the British Crown, which in return for New Zealand sovereignty guaranteed specific rights for Māori (Hill & Sansom, 2010; see also Nwankpa & Bevill, Chap. 17, this volume). Māori rights include acknowledgement and appreciation of their cultural epistemologies, or ways of knowing, and ontology, or ways of being (Ritchie, 2001). A significant contribution to honoring Māori indigenous epistemologies is found in *Te Whāriki*, the first codified bicultural and bilingual curriculum in Aotearoa New Zealand. *Te Whāriki* is viewed as a curriculum that plays a politicized role in upholding the rights of all children in Aotearoa New Zealand, especially pertaining to their individual uniqueness and ethnicity (May, 2009).

The chapter centers on a case study in a Kaupapa Māori-medium early childhood center where the focus is on all things Māori but without full immersion in *te reo* Māori (Māori language), thus differing from *kōhanga reo*, or full immersion Māori

A. Sansom (✉)
University of Auckland, Auckland, New Zealand
e-mail: a.sansom@auckland.ac.nz

K. Bond (ed.), *Dance and the Quality of Life*, Social Indicators Research Series 73,
https://doi.org/10.1007/978-3-319-95699-2_5

language early childhood centers. Kaupapa Māori is related to *mana tangata,* or the ability to stand confidently in both worlds, that is, the Māori world and the colonized or Pākehā world. The overarching question for the study was: *How can dance, especially when connected with place, contribute to young children's sense of identity and culture?* I address this question in dialogue with *Te Whāriki*'s Māori principles and practices, and with the Māori philosophy of the early childhood center where the study took place (to be discussed later).

A further aim of the study is to extend the literature on evidence-based advocacy for children's right to make meaning of their lives through dance experiences. The aesthetic experience called dance arises from children's multi-sensory, bodily engagement, when it allows expression of feelings and thoughts, and supports imagination and sociality (Bond, 2000, 2008, 2018; Bond & Deans, 1997; Bond & Stinson, 2000/2001; Greene, 1995; Stinson, 1988). Empowering young children as both creators and appreciators can release emerging agency (Anttila, 2007), a premise that correlates with the aspirations of *Te Whāriki* principles of *kotahitanga* (the holistic way children learn and grow) and *whakamana* (empowerment), as well as with the Kaupapa Māori philosophy of the early childhood center.

For purposes of this article and research setting, I define dance for these young children as bodily aesthetic engagement that grows or emerges out of the opportunity to move and play in open environments. I see these early movement explorations as sources of kin-aesthetic awareness, enabling young children to discover what they can do with their bodies and experience what it is like to dance just for the sake of dancing. While some anthropological definitions might not consider young children's spontaneous emotional kinetic expression as dance (e.g. Hanna, 1988, 2006), I agree with Karen Bond (1991) that, "there is a fine line between spontaneity and intentionality in young children; and the ability to employ aesthesia and rhythm in the service of nonverbal communication is clearly present from infancy" (p. 12) (see Dissanayake, Coda, this volume). Indeed, on quality of life grounds, children's moments of impromptu bodily-affective expression can be acknowledged and extended to foster optimal development. Further, through a phenomenological hermeneutic lens (van Manen, 1997), the young child's ubiquitous "free expression" can be understood as a form of "early dance," rather than as "dance-like" or "pre-dance" behavior (Bond, 2018). According to Sue Stinson (1988), dance is "making movement *itself* significant" (p. 2), a human capability in which young children can excel (Bond, 2000, 2018; Sansom, 2013; Stinson, 2002).

Dance as a Taonga

Some years ago, I wrote an article titled "Mindful Pedagogy in Dance: Honoring the Life of the Child" (Sansom, 2009). My intention was to address the privilege that can be experienced in everyday encounters with young children, that is, the gifts they present, in this case the *taonga* (gift) of dance. The premise of the article came from a keynote address, "Revisioning Purpose: Children, Dance and the Culture of Caring," presented by Karen Bond at the 8th Dance and the Child International Conference in Canada (2000), and her reference to "receiving the dance of the child" (p. 4), a mode of pedagogy she first articulated two decades earlier (Bond, 1978). This notion of receivership was poignant as it aligns with the tenets on which the early childhood curriculum in Aotearoa New Zealand was founded. These tenets include noticing, recognizing and responding to the interests and cultural experiences of the child (MoE, 1996). As a lecturer in teacher education with a background in early childhood, my pedagogical philosophy upholds these tenets, which link to the *Treaty of Waitangi* (1840) and honor indigenous ways of knowing.

Early Childhood Education in Aotearoa New Zealand

Māori values and beliefs that underpin *Te Whāriki* include the principles of *kotahitanga* (holistic development), *whakamana* (empowerment), *whānau tangata* (relationships), and *ngā hononga* (family and community). These principles interweave with the strands of *mana atua* (well-being), *mana whenua* (belonging), *mana tangata* (contribution), *mana reo* (communication), and *mana aotūroa* (exploration) (MoE, 1996). The word *mana* signifies sources of strength or status and represents domains of the *atua* (spiritual), *whenua* (land or place), *reo* (language), the world of *aotūroa* (light and nature), and *tangata* (people). The concept of *mana* evokes a positive image of the child as one who is empowered to learn and develop. *Mana* relates to the principle of *whakamana* (empowerment), which holds notions of identity and agency (Lee, Carr, Soutar, & Mitchell, 2013).

Te Whāriki is viewed as an open curriculum that offers a wide range of possible interpretations appropriate for the distinctive setting of each early childhood center. This value resonates with the curriculum's sociocultural underpinnings and the importance of linking to people, places and things that are part of the child's life (May, 2009; Pohio, Sansom, & Liley, 2015). A chief focus in *Te Whāriki* is "equity and respect for children's rights" (Lee et al., 2013):

> The curriculum looks ahead to citizens who can make responsible and informed choices, respect the ideas and beliefs of others, include diversity in their world-view and have an understanding of both major cultures and languages of the country. (p. 3)

The formulation of *Te Whāriki* reflects significant educational developments in Aotearoa New Zealand that recognize Māori culture, tradition, and customs (*tikanga* Māori) and the revitalization of the Māori language (*te reo* Māori), for example, success of the Kōhanga Reo movement, which was open to both Māori and non-Māori children, provided the incentive to conceive an early childhood curriculum based on Māori values and beliefs for all children in Aotearoa New Zealand. A strong aspect of *Te Whāriki* is that it highlights ways of teaching and learning founded on Māori cultural epistemologies and ways of being while also upholding promises found in the *Treaty of Waitangi*: "All children should be given the opportunity to develop knowledge and an understanding of the cultural heritage of both partners to *Te Tiriti o Waitangi*" (MoE, 1996, p. 9). A curriculum that is inclusive as well as holistic honors the rights of the child and views the child as competent and confident (MoE, 1996).

From a Māori perspective, concepts such as *tino rangatiratanga* (self-determination or governance), together with underlying principles such as *manaakitanga* (caring) and *kaitiatikanga* (stewardship) (Ritchie, 2010), provide a sound basis for ecological understandings of the natural world, thereby supporting sustainability, social justice and democratic citizenship. The corollary is that pedagogical practice embedded in the principles of *Te Whāriki* "considers the perspectives, hopes, rights, and voices of children, their families, and their communities" (Pacini-Ketchabaw, Nxumalo, Kocher, Elliot, & Sanchez, 2015, p. 119). These principles echo the sentiments that inspired me when listening to Bond's (2000) keynote address, contributing to my ongoing commitment to cherish life in all its forms in whatever pedagogical ventures I may undertake. As a result, I have become more and more cognizant of the myriad ways children offer their *taonga* – their gifts – and thus their understandings of the world in which they live.

As noted by Mackey (2014), Māori principles of *manaakitanga* (caring) and *kaitiatikanga* (stewardship) encourage young children to "interact with the natural world and, as a consequence, better understand how to be caring and be appreciative of others in their lives" (p. 188). Caring about others and the world can help to develop a heightened understanding of the environment as well as their agency as active citizens to care unconditionally for all things (Noddings, 2003). Such a "culture of caring" (Bond, 2000, 2014) must surely contribute to quality of life for humans and other species in the world we share.

As a bodily aesthetic practice, dance can be considered a form of *manaakitanga* and *kaitiatikanga* that can help to establish reciprocal and possibly empathetic relationships with others and with the environment.

Kaupapa Māori: All Things Māori

As noted, the heart of this chapter is a study with children, teachers, and *whānau* (family members) from a Māori-medium early childhood center in Auckland (Tamaki Makaurau), Aotearoa New Zealand. The center espouses a philosophy based on Kaupapa Māori, which promotes all things Māori. Kaupapa Māori aims to teach *tamariki/mokopuna* (young children) to become enthusiastic and engaged learners using *te reo* and *tikanga* Māori (Māori language, protocols and customs). These include the observance of "*whānaungatanga* (responsibility and reciprocal obligations towards others), *manaaki* (respectful relationships), *tuakana/teina* (to look after each other), and *mana tangata* (to be able to stand confidently in both worlds)" (Pohio et al., 2015, p. 105).

Guided by *Te Whāriki* and by association the *Treaty of Waitangi*, my interest as a researcher was in indigenous ways of knowing, in particular the significance of the environment or land. I chose this particular center as a research site for its regular visits to a nearby volcanic mountain, a revered local landmark. The mountain overlooks the center, which nestles in a valley just below. For the center's teachers, children and families, the mountain is a guardian. To Māori, *whenua* (the land) and all that it includes – such as *maunga* (the mountains), *ngahere*, (forests and trees), *moana* (the oceans), *awa* (rivers), and *roto* (lakes) – is endowed with *wairua* (spiritual meaning), or *ihi* (energy) and *ora* (life) or *mauri* (life force), which cannot be separated from those who live on and with the land and all those who have gone before (Pohio et al., 2015). Ritchie, Duhn, Rau, and Craw (2010) explain:

> Papatuanuku (Earth Mother) and Ranginui (Sky Father) look after all of us. The sun, wind, rain and air look after the plants that look after us. …In caring for our natural environment, the *tamariki* [children] are developing respectful relationships with nature while nurturing their health, wellbeing and *wairua* [spirituality/soul] within. (p. 78)

The *maunga* is such a site.

A Dancing Center I also chose this center for its well-developed dance program. Children at the center are involved in dance in multiple ways as part of the curriculum and therefore know dance as a word and as a practice. Some of the dancing reflects the Kaupapa Māori philosophy of the center, as evident in teacher Shelly's description:

> One boy really loved the *haka* and although we hadn't done it before, he spontaneously started doing it. We drew on his passion and decided that whenever we had a *powhiri* [welcome ceremony] or a *mihi* [tribute] or we had a visitor, we would ask him "do you want to lead the *haka*?" Because we were doing it more, the *tamariki* [children] knew it and the young boy became the *kaea* [leader] of the dance. When we were learning the dance, he was connecting to everyone…it is a special feeling to have people you know standing next to you and you are all doing the same quite vigorous and energetic *haka* or *waiata* [song, chant]. That was *manaakitanga* [respect, hospitality, kindness], and that's the *kaupapa* [program] right there.

Other center dance experiences evolve from the children's specific culture and dances learned from family members. Shelly describes:

> We play different types of music so that children are able to express themselves in different ways. We have a Nigerian girl who loves to dance and she's quite expressive in that way. She's only eighteen months and not yet verbal. Another example is a young boy who is Niuean/Cook Island and he loves drumming. For his grandmother's birthday, he and his cousins had learned to dance, so he was doing the dance at the center. One of my colleagues is Niuean and she got into the dance… the young boy was shining. You can see that a young child recognizes when their culture is being expressed and when they're being recognized for what they can do. He was quite shy at the beginning, but once he saw that we were enjoying watching his dance and the other children were joining in, he could see himself as a beautiful being in his own culture.

The Research Design

The qualitative study I undertook at the center employs an interpretive phenomenological perspective to examine how, in terms of *Te Whāriki,* dance can play a meaningful role in young children's lives. Data were gathered from observations of children and teacher interviews (to be described in more detail below). The study was approved by The University of Auckland Human Participants Ethics Committee (UAHPEC).

Having been influenced by Max van Manen's (1997) hermeneutic phenomenology, I was conscious that my initial observations needed to be attentive and reflective, rather than guided by assumptions about children's meanings of dance. As a participant observer, my aim was to be unobtrusive, while at the same time being responsive to children if they engaged me in their dancing, for example, inviting me to skip with them through the long grass. I really wanted to capture the quality of children's lived experiences of "dancing the mountain." In dialogue with my knowledge as an early childhood educator and dance specialist, I analysed the data for examples of dance experiences and related these to the principles and goals of *Te Whāriki* and the Kaupapa Māori, philosophy of the center. Ultimately, this chapter illuminates dance as a dynamic source of meaningful engagement and agency in young children's lives, that is, as a fundamental area of learning during the early years of education. Moreover, the chapter highlights the potential of dance to connect children with identity, cultural heritage, and place.

Since the project involved only one early childhood education and care center as the research site, I chose a case study approach. Case study provided the opportunity to describe what was happening in the actual context as part of everyday experience. This approach allowed me to apply descriptive and interpretive lenses without a concern for generalization to a population. As stated by early childhood researchers Rolfe and MacNaughton (2010), "Case study research may seek to create change or understand a particular aspect of a specific setting. In this research, validating arises through the way in which the research is conducted and analyzed rather than through its replicability and generalizability" (p. 8).

The Research Process

Twenty children (12 males and 8 females) aged three to 5 years participated in the study. The majority had Māori ancestry, with a small number of European descendants. Four teachers accompanied the children on fortnightly excursions to the volcanic mountain landmark, together with parents and grandparents. Qualitative data were collected through observation and interviewing. I carried out five 2-h observations (four during mountain excursions and one in the center) over 6 months, employing written field notes, photography and video, finding photography the most flexible. I looked for opportunities to photograph when children were exploring the environment bodily, particularly trails and pathways, embankments and grassy areas, the trees they encountered, the flat open area toward the top that overlooked the skyline, and, of course, when children spontaneously danced with each other. I videoed incidents where I perceived the possibility of a movement emphasis, but found videoing difficult to sustain as a participating observer. When not photographing, I took field notes, and sometimes joined in the children's activities.

I also conducted a one-hour semi-structured individual interview with each of two teachers (at their convenience). My purpose in interviewing was to gain teachers' perspectives on how dance might contribute to children's understanding of their identity and cultural heritage, especially when connected to place. In addition, I was interested to hear how both the children's and the teachers' understandings were being incorporated into the overall program of the center. The five observations took place at times agreed to by the center. Self-selected pseudonyms are employed for the teachers.

Hermeneutic, or interpretive, phenomenological inquiry focuses on examining lived experience as the basis of human meanings (van Manen, 1990/1997). This approach framed my analysis of observational data, while narrative inquiry informed analysis of interviews (Clandinin & Connelly, 2004), where my aim was to pay attention to teachers' *maunga* stories and what meanings they hold for them. As explained above, *Te Whāriki* and the *Treaty of Waitangi*, together with the Kaupapa Māori philosophy of the center, provided the interpretive framework for analysis. I first created textual descriptions (discrete episodes and composites) of children's responses to the local landmark, drawing on photographs, video footage and field notes. Then, with the aid of teacher interviews, I analyzed how these anecdotes illustrate important Māori concepts and indigenous epistemologies. The following section presents findings of the study, offering multi-sensory descriptions of children's dancing and reflections on how the *taonga* of their dancing can be translated through principles and concepts of *Te Whāriki* together with Kaupapa Māori beliefs.

Dancing on and with the Mountain

Dancing on and with the mountain developed over time as children made their fortnightly visits. Each visit enabled them to become more familiar with the *maunga* and what it had to offer. Mountain offerings included climatic conditions, which changed from hot, sunny days when the grasses were wispy and crisp with dryness, to times when wind or rain provided wet, muddy terrain underfoot and long damp grass to wade through. Teacher Aroha described how children responded to the wind on the mountain, where they would put their arms out wide and experience the elements of the weather with their bodies. She explains:

> There's nothing like feeling that different kind of wind and we're always talking about the different types of wind; what type of wind will come from this side and how it will be different from the other side and at times they've felt and moved like the different winds.

On warmer days, we could go with the flow of trails around the mountain and take time to rest and observe the scenery. On days when the weather was tempestuous with rain or strong winds, children braced their bodies against its intensity while moving along the mountain's edges or standing on exposed ridges. They navigated steep inclines and stony meandering pathways as they traveled up and down the mountain. They explored hollows full of native bush located down steep embankments, a legacy of early Māori settlements where the craters afforded protection from weather and large trees to climb, balance on, and shelter beneath. Climatic and environmental variants found on the mountain became the genesis for many dance experiences as children discovered ways to engage through expressive bodily responses to the landscape.

Bodily-Affective Engagement

Dancing the mountain was largely initiated by children, occurring spontaneously in their physical encounters with the environment. Over the 6 months of my observation visits, I noticed increasing adeptness as children revisited special places and established ritualistic or repetitive engagement with the space, for example, following regular pathways in a zigzag pattern from one side to the other, or creating labyrinths or mazes through the grasses. Shelly describes how children were developing their visual-kinesthetic capabilities through visits to the mountain: "When we visit the maunga the children know which way to go and we follow them. And they know the places to go back to that they enjoy – the trees they like climbing, the hut they made last time." She also reflected on children's overall attraction to the mountain:

> If I try to imagine how the children see their connection to the maunga, I notice that they get excited about going there, like visiting a friend. It is a form of friendship, that connection… they're excited to see if the leaves are still the same color or is the treasure I buried still here? So the connection is emotional, physical, spiritual and familial. It's definitely a relationship of appreciation: it's a different kind of day going there and I can see the tamariki developing in different ways. I mean they just wouldn't use their bodies in the same way if they couldn't climb the trees and roll down the hills, and run through the long grass.

Physical creativity became more apparent as children's developing familiarity with the environment supported their freedom to explore space with full bodily engagement: running, twirling, skipping, leaping, galloping, tumbling, rolling, jumping, and "flying." Moreover, children's bodily expressions appeared to become progressively more spontaneous with each mountain excursion I observed. For example, one young boy had a distinctive full-bodied style of dance in which he appeared to delight in the sensations of loose pebbles beneath his feet. He displayed hints of Māori *haka*-like movements in his *takahia* (stamping actions) as he practiced his unique dance each visit, taking command of his expression on the mountain. I noticed that the girls often engaged in partner dances that developed in scope over time, for example, skipping through the long grass side by side to skipping holding hands to facing dances with side to side arm swings (Fig. 5.1).

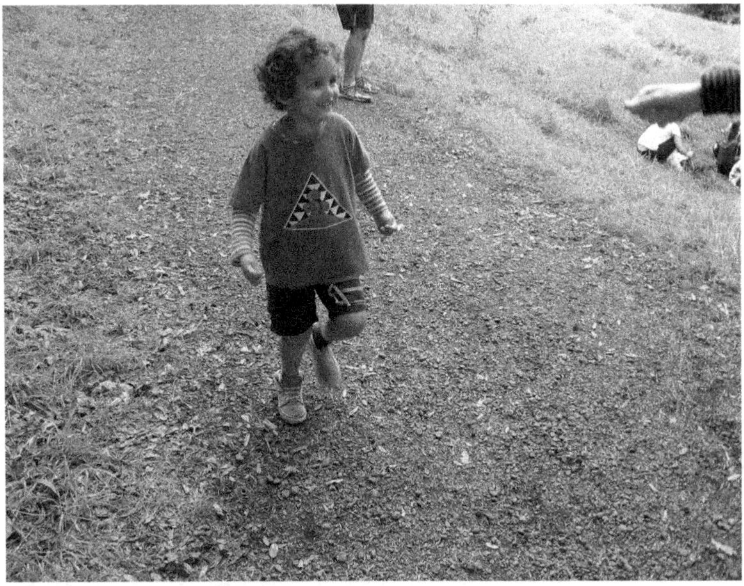

Fig. 5.1 *Haka*. (Photo by Adrienne Sansom)

The open spaces, created pathways, shapes of the terrain, and various obstacles all appeared to invite unprompted expressions of creative movement, which, as discussed earlier, I consider a form of dance. These emergent moments of dance arose from one child or a small group and varied in duration. I observed children shaping their bodies to replicate vegetation found on the mountain, such as the pointed spiky leaves of the *harakeke* (flax bush) as well as assorted visual landmarks, like the cityscape that could be seen from many vantage points. They nestled in trees, using bodies and limbs to match the shapes of branches or become part of a tree. They became immersed in tall grasses and simulated the natural movement – softly swaying or moving vigorously as they navigated their way through the grass and created visible pathways. Many of the children's dance experiences arose from play or were indeed a form of play (Lindqvist, 2001; Sheets-Johnstone, 2011; see Anttila & Nielsen, this volume), in keeping with the adventurous exuberance that can be generated in the outdoors.

As noted by Shelly, also, children seemed to particularly enjoy rolling down embankments when the grass was long and lush following the summer rains, and imitating shapes in their visual field. She commented,

> I think they enjoy the space of the maunga…they extend their play to be covering more, and they begin to move and stretch out more, exploring the different angles of the whenua so they can roll and jump in the grass. And then they climb high to this vast flat area where you can see the Sky Tower and they love to look at the view of the harbor and the whole city below them and sometimes they make shapes with their bodies to look like the Sky Tower or the harbor bridge.

On one occasion, I, too, saw children creating their own pathways and body shapes in the flat expansive spaces near the top.

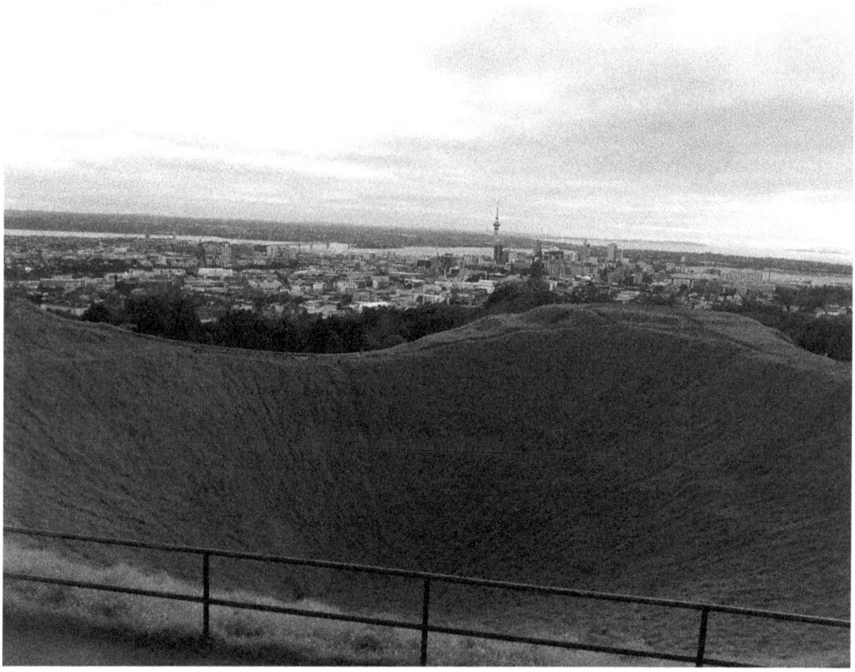

Fig. 5.2 *Maunga*. (Photo by Adrienne Sansom)

On two occasions during my observations teachers became involved as interactive partners with the children, copying their actions or following their lead as they journeyed through the mountain terrain. On one of these occasions, a teacher initiated a chant, which was quickly picked up by the children as they followed each other along a meandering path. The chant sustained the rhythmic actions of this impromptu dance – including march-like steps incorporating stamping actions (*waewae takahia*), pulsating pumping arms (*ringaringa*) moving up (*ki runga*) and down (*ki raro*) and in (*ki roto*) and out (*ki waho*), and clapping (*paki paki*) – until a particular destination was reached. Children's dancing in the ways synthesized above was combined with specific Māori dances performed on the mountain, such as the *haka*, *poi* and *taiaha*, which they learned from and shared alongside adults – both teachers and the *whānau* (family members) (Fig. 5.2).

Ecological Bodies

From a *Te Ao Māori* or Māori world view, there is interconnection between all living things – whether human or other animal, plant, or earth and sky. Everything Māori are involved in, including dance, maintains this interconnection to the life force or *mauri* of all living things past and present. From this ecological perspective, Shelley recalls a particular visit to the mountain:

> We did a haka for Standing Rock. We climbed up and faced towards the water in a line. We talked to the tamariki about why we were doing the haka for Standing Rock because in America there was another iwi who were worried about their water.

For Māori, dance has always been an expression of the *whenua* (land and people). Māori see themselves as the *kaitiaki* (guardian or caretaker) of the land, from which some Māori dance originates. Just as the children might say a *karakia* (prayer) or sing a *waiata* (song) composed for the mountain, Māori have long performed dances as offerings and as a ritual form of thank you to the *maunga*. Shelly elaborates on children's strong identification with the *maunga*:

> I am amazed at how much the tamariki connect with the maunga. When we go for a walk to another center or we're on the bus going to swimming lessons, children always see it…they will turn and say, "there's Maunga." When I started at the center I wasn't aware of that level of the skyline; I didn't know that you could see that maunga from all these different points, but the children showed me "there it is, that's our maunga." We always do a mihi to Maunga when we go there, and when we can see it from far away we also say, "kia ora, Maunga, there it is."

On visits to the mountain, children appeared to adhere consciously to certain boundaries. Shelly affirmed,

> They know the boundaries, and then I feel assured as a kaiako [teacher] that they're not going to wander away because this is their place. And I think it's really important to empower children to interact with a space but also teach them that they are an important part of looking after that space, and can be involved in the things they see happening, which links to kaitiatikanga [stewardship].

Responsibility, Reciprocity, Respect As introduced above, a sense of camaraderie seemed integral to children's mountain dancing and I understand this as *whānaungatanga* (responsibility and reciprocal obligations towards others), *manaaki* (respectful relationships), and *tuakana/teina* (to look after each other). The quality of children's mutuality demonstrated awareness, not only of their relationship with the environment, but of their connection with each other. Children would come together and help each other to achieve particular goals: to climb trees, traverse stiles, share a tire swing, balance along tree trunks, follow weaving pathways, tumble together in the long grass, or hold hands to support each other up and down the stony trails. A sense of collaboration and caring for each other was evident, for example, when a child encountered difficulty climbing the steep embankments and another showed compassion, offering a helping hand and waiting until the challenged child could rejoin the group. On each of my four visits to the mountain I observed children forming an improvised follow-the-leader pattern as they ascended and descended, copying each other's movements.

Cultural Identity and Place

Through close observation, phenomenological description, and teacher interviews, I am able to propose that children's spontaneous and cultural dance experiences in relation to the mountain support their sense of cultural identity and place, reflecting *Te Whāriki*'s goals of *mana whenua* (belonging) where children develop "knowledge about the features of the area of physical and/or spiritual significance to the local community, such as the local river or mountain" (MoE, 1996, p. 56), and *mana atua* (well-being) or *wairuatanga*, which has been described as "a source of spiritual and emotional well-being" (Ritchie, 2015a, p. 157). Through these forms of knowing, children "can participate and take risks without fear or harm," and respect others and the environment (MoE, 1996, p. 52).

During their mountain excursions children became better acquainted with their cultural roots (Davies, 2000; Golden, 2013). Familiarity with the land magnified the possibility for children to deepen their connection to their culture, especially as Māori, but for all the children as citizens of Aotearoa New Zealand. As explained by Rose Rangimarie Pere (1994), Māori view the child as precious *taonga*, a cherished gift from the *whānau* (family genealogy). At their early childhood center, children participate each morning in the daily ritual of *mihi mihi* (greeting), sharing their *pepehā* (declaration) or *whakapapa* (ancestry) – where they come from, and their *maunga* (mountain), *awa* (river), *waka* (canoe), and *marae* (gathering place) (Pohio et al., 2015). This ritual enacts a form of connectedness to *whānau*, "the principal social kinship unit in Māori society" (Lee et al., 2013, p. 34).

These links to *whānau* and to the land situate the children in a history that played out in the very place and space they explore. With this awareness, children can learn to respect the environment. I observed respect in the way children treated the surroundings, for example, by taking care to not harm any living things. They often left gifts for the *maunga*, such as an ephemeral installation made from broken twigs found on the ground. In return, the *maunga* rewards children with the gifts of Papatuanuku (Earth Mother) and Ranginui (Sky Father), which represent interconnectedness between human, nonhuman and more-than-human, reflecting Māori concepts of *manaakitanga* (caring) and *kaitiatikanga* (stewardship).

While these young Aotearoa New Zealand children might not have been fully cognizant of their unique cultural or spiritual connection with the *maunga*, evidence of embodied identification was clear. A mother commented that her daughter loves visiting the mountain, and both teachers I interviewed remarked that the children view the mountain as *theirs*. One of the children told me personally, "This is my mountain." Confirming her colleague Shelly's perspective recounted earlier, teacher Aroha elaborates:

> I know that a lot of the children think that the mountain is "my" maunga. They could be beside another mountain: "no, Maunga is my maunga." They are quite staunch saying: "it's my maunga, I have another maunga somewhere but that's my maunga."

The reason a center teacher instigated visits to the mountain was that the *maunga* has spiritual meaning to the *iwi* (group of people with common ancestors) who belong to the land on which it sits; she considered it important for the children to understand this connection beyond just seeing it as a "big hill." My own memories of childhood that remain vivid are those times I spent dancing in nature through my bodily-affective engagement. These memories are not necessarily romanticized or even nostalgic memories of place or space, but visceral associations (the rough and the smooth, the pleasures and pains of which there were many).

Cultivating a Culture of Care

According to Mackey (2014), when children understand the power of their own agency they are capable of caring for things they believe in or value, which might include the environments they occupy and their association with the culture and history of place. Through embodied participation in the local community children can begin to understand how they might contribute to sustainability of their environment, and also nurture their own emotional *mana atua* (well-being) and *mana whenua* (belonging). As reiterated by Mackey (2014), "As [children] learn to care and show empathy to improve the life of others, it is hoped that the skills learnt will be transferable between the human and nonhuman world" (p. 188).

In dialogue with the cultural perspectives of *Te Whāriki*, this chapter conceptualizes children's lives as intertwined ecologically in a world where human beings live with both human and nonhuman others. The intent of *Te Whāriki* is to enable children to engage in a world that goes beyond a "romanticized" version of nature, i.e., a view of nature that is only seen as inherently full of natural goodness and beauty, to one that is collectively, politically, and materially reconfigured (Taylor, 2014). An aspect of this reconfiguring is a moving engagement that requires a different form of appreciation in order to address real world issues. Ritchie (2016) supports this perspective, particularly given the standardized or universalized concept of quality sometimes seen in early childhood education. She argues that "such qualit*ies* need to engage a reorientation away from humanistic, individualist modes to ways of seeing, feeling and being…that recognise human inter/dependence" (p. 2), in a world where ways of life are becoming endangered through loss of threatened species and tracts of land, as well as through loss of diverse languages and cultural heritages.

For example, early childhood educators are charged with the responsibility to research and learn about the Māori creation stories of Papatuanuku and Ranginui, and to understand and use the language of "the *waiata* (songs), and *haka* (dances) for the *whenua* (land) and the *mokopuna* (children/grandchildren)" (Ritchie, 2015b, p. 46). Despite this call, however, the wisdom and values inherent in the curriculum from a Māori worldview tend to be forsaken due to Education's increasing focus on standardization and normalization, which is alleged to increase student achievement, but clearly results in narrowing the curriculum.

Ritchie (2016) goes on to say there is a need to bring in "a different sensibility – a different set of qualit*ies* that reflect our embodied beingness *with*(in) our world" (p. 2). Dance offers this opportunity to be embodied in the world, where communities come together in a form of unity for the land (*whenua*) on which they live, or as expressed by Māori, their *turangawaewae* – a place to stand. Children's fortnightly visits to the mountain ensure they have this opportunity to appreciate their bodily-affective relationship with the environment and to establish their cultural affiliation with the land – their *tino rangatiratanga.*

Conclusion

This case study set out to address the following research question: *How can dance, especially when connected with place, contribute to young children's sense of identity and culture?* This study suggests that place can be a felt, visceral experience, showing how young children's bodily-affective connection to the land can support a *kotahitanga* (holistic or spiritual) and *whakamana* (empowering) affiliation. Building consciously embodied relationships with the environment is part of *tino rangatiratanga* or children's rights, the right to know what it means to identify with the land where one lives and what this might mean from personal, social, cultural, political and historical perspectives. Conversely, the study illustrates how embodying place or memories of place can stir feelings from within, including joy and altruism – a kind of consciousness that transforms everyday movements into dance (Bond, 2000, 2018; Bond & Stinson, 2000/2001; Stinson, 1988, 2002, 2004). The case study presented in this chapter is the first phase of a larger project. The second phase is to examine the visual arts experiences associated with children's visits to the mountain together with the possibility of combining visual arts with dance (Bond & Deans, 1997; Deans & Brown, 2008; Deans & Wright, 2018). Children's graphic representations of their thoughts and feelings in relation to the mountain, together with teachers' perspectives drawn from interviews, will broaden understanding of how this relationship is manifested in the center's program. In addition, further research will be informed by Reggio Emilia pedagogy, which focuses on comprehensive documentation of children's learning (Rinaldi, 2006) and includes children's portfolios and learning stories.

As evident in these first findings, I propose that the "aesthetic embodiment" (a bodily-sensory-affective phenomenon) that characterizes early childhood spontaneous and patterned dance provides a vital medium and process for children's building of identity. Amongst the children in my study dancing erupted "naturally" in response to the *maunga,* supporting knowledge creation in place and links to cultural heritage. Through regular excursions to the mountain, children, together with their teachers and family members, became increasingly familiar with the terrain.

Over the four occasions I observed children dancing with the mountain, their physical engagement with the space became more confident. Further, Māori dances such as the *haka*, *poi* and *taiaha,* which are shared both in the center and on the mountain, create links between the center and the community and also contribute to children's sense of cultural heritage and identity. As one of the teachers commented, the children's visits to the mountain are more than "just going outdoors" – they are about connecting to culturally significant landmarks where Māori once lived (and, I would add, danced) – the very land where some of the children's ancestors lived.

On my fifth research visit, which took place at the center, I observed a group of children physically expressing the explosion of a volcano. They were jumping with extended arms and legs, and shaking their bodies to replicate the quaking earth. This was followed by their volcanic eruption and flowing like lava, expressed through sinking and rolling movements, as the lava moved down the mountainside. The children drew me into their volcano dance, telling me to be careful because the lava was coming and it was very hot. I responded by asking, "what should we do to protect ourselves?" One young girl stood directly in front of me as I was crouched low to the ground, quivering. With her arms outstretched in a large curved shape, she offered me an imaginary bowl, explaining, "the bowl will catch the lava – but it might get crumpled," as we melted down onto the floor.

I was moved by this young child's expression of empathy and concern for my welfare – the caring and altruistic way she responded to my "endangerment." I understand this as an example of *tuakana/teina* (to look after each other) and *manaakitanga* (caring). Connecting with Māori cultural heritage, the imaginary bowl is associated with the legend of Mataaoho, a giant who once lived on the *maunga*, where the *atea* (sacred crater – an open space where offerings or declarations occurred), represents the giant's food bowl. In her gesture, I saw the relationship between cultural heritage, place, and the creation of dance.

In the terms of *Te Whāriki,* the child's mana *aotūroa* (exploration) and *mana tangata* (contribution) to creating dance are enabled and valued. When a child's contribution is honored, so too is their *mana atua* (well-being), which unconditionally authenticates the child's meaningful engagement and quality of life. Correspondingly, when a child's *mana whenua* (lived experience) and thus identity and belonging become central to the creation of dance, a connection can be made to the image of the child as *whakamana* (powerful) and to education as a *kotahitanga* (holistic) endeavor that weaves together "cognitive, social, cultural, physical, emotional and spiritual dimensions" of being human (Lee et al., 2013, p. 59).

Movement is the genesis of dance. When linked to cultural identity through *ngā hononga* (relationships) with people, places and things, dancing provides potential access to *ihi* (energy), *wairua* (spirit), and *mauri* (life force), or quality of life. Adults who nurture the lives of young children have the opportunity to bear witness to these moments and to receive the *taonga* of dance that young children so generously share with the world.

References

Anttila, E. (2007). Children as agents in dance: Implications of the notion of child culture for research and practice in dance education. In L. Bresler (Ed.), *International handbook of research in arts education* (pp. 865–879). Dordrecht, The Netherlands: Springer.

Bond, K. (1978, July). *Receiving the dance of the child: An application of developmental and humanistic learning theories to teaching dance*. World Congress, International Society for Education through the Arts, Adelaide, South Australia.

Bond, K. (1991). *Dance for children with dual sensory impairments*. PhD thesis. Bundoora, Australia: La Trobe University.

Bond, K. (2000). Revisioning purpose: Children, dance, and the culture of caring. In J. LeDrew & H. Ritenberg (Eds.), *Proceedings – extensions & extremities: Points of departure* (pp. 3–14). Regina, SKN: Dance and the Child International.

Bond, K. (2008). The human nature of dance: Towards a theory of aesthetic community. In S. Malloch & C. Trevarthen (Eds.), *Communicative musicality: Exploring the basis of human companionship* (pp. 401–422). Oxford, UK: Oxford University Press.

Bond, K. (2014). Dance and the quality of life. In A. C. Michalos (Ed.), *Encyclopedia of quality of life and well-being research* (pp. 1419–1424). Dordrecht, The Netherlands: Springer.

Bond, K. (2018). "Me, a tree": Young children as natural phenomenologists. In S. Fraleigh (Ed.), *Back to the dance itself: Phenomenologies of the body in performance* (pp. 205–232). Urbana, IL: University of Illinois Press.

Bond, K., & Deans, J. (1997). Eagles, reptiles and beyond: A co-creative journey in dance. *Childhood Education, 73*(6), 366–371.

Bond, K., & Stinson, S. (2000/2001). "I feel like I'm going to take off!" Young people's experiences of the superordinary in dance. *Dance Research Journal, 32*(2), 52–87.

Clandinin, D., & Connelly, F. (2004). *Narrative inquiry: Experience and story in qualitative research*. San Francisco: Jossey-Bass.

Davies, B. (2000). Eclipsing the constitutive power of discourse: The writing of Janette turner hospital. In E. S. Pierre & W. Pillow (Eds.), *Working the ruins: Feminist poststructural theory and methods in education* (pp. 179–198). New York: Routledge.

Deans, J., & Brown, R. (2008). Reflection, renewal and relationship building: An ongoing journey in early childhood arts education. *Contemporary Issues in Early Childhood, 9*(4), 339–353.

Deans, J., & Wright, S. (2018). *Dance-play and drawing-telling as semiotic tools for young children's learning*. London: Routledge.

Golden, A. (2013). Preschool children explore the forest: The power of wild spaces in childhood. In D. Meier & S. Sisk-Hilton (Eds.), *Nature education with young children: Integrating inquiry and practice* (pp. 123–136). New York: Routledge.

Greene, M. (1995). *Releasing the imagination: Essays on education, the arts, and social change*. San Francisco: Jossey-Bass.

Hanna, J. L. (1988). *Dance and stress: Resistance, reduction, and euphoria*. New York: AMS Press.

Hanna, J. L. (2006). *Dancing for health: Conquering and preventing stress*. Lanham, MD: AltaMira Press.

Hill, D., & Sansom, A. (2010). Indigenous knowledges and pedagogy: A bicultural approach to curriculum. In D. Chapman (Ed.), *Examining social theory: Crossing borders/reflecting back* (pp. 259–270). New York: Peter Lang.

Lee, W., Carr, M., Soutar, B., & Mitchell, L. (2013). *Understanding the te whāriki approach: Early years education in practice*. Oxon, UK: Routledge.

Lindqvist, G. (2001). The relationship between dance and play. *Research in Dance Education, 2*(1), 41–52.

Mackey, G. (2014). Valuing agency in young children: Teachers rising to the challenge of sustainability in the Aotearoa New Zealand early childhood context. In J. Davis & S. Elliott (Eds.),

Research in early childhood education for sustainability: International perspectives and provocations (pp. 180–193). New York: Routledge.
May, H. (2009). *Politics in the playground: The world of early childhood in New Zealand* (Rev. ed.). Dunedin, New Zealand: Otago University Press.
Ministry of Education. (1996). *Te whāriki: He whāriki mātauranga mō ngā mokopuna o Aotearoa: Early childhood curriculum*. Wellington, New Zealand: Learning Media.
Noddings, N. (2003). *Caring: A feminine approach to ethics and moral education* (2nd ed.). Berkeley, CA: University of California Press.
Pacini-Ketchabaw, V., Nxumalo, F., Kocher, L., Elliot, E., & Sanchez, A. (2015). *Journeys: Reconceptualizing early childhood practices through pedagogical narration*. Toronto, ON: University of Toronto Press.
Pere, R. (1994). *Ako: Concepts and learning in the Māori tradition*. Wellington, New Zealand: Te Kohanga Reo National Trust Board.
Pohio, L., Sansom, A., & Liley, K. (2015). My past is my present is my future: A bi-cultural approach to early years education in Aotearoa, New Zealand. In L. Kroll & D. Meier (Eds.), *Crossing borders of reflection: Educational change in international early childhood contexts* (pp. 103–122). New York: Routledge.
Rinaldi, C. (2006). *In dialogue with Reggio Emilia: Listening, researching and learning*. New York: Routledge.
Ritchie, J. (2001). Reflections on collectivism in early childhood teaching in Aotearoa/New Zealand. In S. Grieshaber & G. Cannella (Eds.), *Embracing identities in early childhood education: Diversity and possibilities* (pp. 133–147). New York: Teachers College Press.
Ritchie, J. (2010). Fostering communities for ecological sustainability within early childhood education. *Early Education, 47*, 10–14.
Ritchie, J. (2015a). Disentangling? Re-entanglement? Tackling the pervasiveness of colonialism in early childhood (teacher) education in Aotearoa. In V. Pacini-Ketchabaw & A. Taylor (Eds.), *Unsettling the colonial places and spaces of early childhood education* (pp. 147–161). New York: Routledge.
Ritchie, J. (2015b). Social, cultural and ecological justice in the age of the Anthropocene: A New Zealand early childhood care and education perspective. *Journal of Pedagogy, 6*(2), 41–56.
Ritchie, J. (2016). Qualities for early childhood care and education in an age of increasing superdiversity and decreasing biodiversity. *Contemporary Issues in Early Childhood, 17*(1), 78–91.
Ritchie, J., Duhn, I., Rau, C., & Craw, J. (2010). *Titiro whakamuri, hoki wakamua: We are the future, the present and the past: Caring for self, others and the environment in early years' teaching and learning*. Final Report for the Teaching and Learning Research Initiative. Wellington, New Zealand: NZCER.
Rolfe, S., & MacNaughton, G. (2010). Research as a tool. In G. Mac Naughton, S. Rolfe, & I. Siraj-Blatchford (Eds.), *Doing early childhood research: International perspectives on theory and practice* (2nd ed., pp. 3–34). Crows Nest, Australia: Allen & Unwin.
Sansom, A. (2009). Mindful pedagogy in dance: Honoring the life of the child. *Research in Dance Education, 10*(3), 161–176.
Sansom, A. (2013). Dance with connections to moving and playing in the early years. In B. Clark, A. Grey, & L. Terreni (Eds.), *Kia tipu te wairua toi – Fostering the creative spirit* (pp. 100–112). Auckland, New Zealand: Pearson.
Sheets-Johnstone, M. (2011). *The primacy of movement* (2nd expanded ed.). Amsterdam: John Benjamins. (Original work published 1999).
Stinson, S. (1988). *Dance for young children: Finding the magic in movement*. Reston, VA: AAHPERD.
Stinson, S. (2002). What we teach is who we are: The stories of our lives. In L. Bresler & C. M. Thompson (Eds.), *The arts in children's lives: Context, culture, and curriculum* (pp. 157–168). Dordrecht, The Netherlands: Kluwer Academic.

Stinson, S. (2004). My body/myself: Lessons from dance education. In L. Bresler (Ed.), *Knowing bodies, moving minds: Towards embodied teaching and learning* (pp. 153–167). Boston: Kluwer.

Taylor, A. (2014). Situated and entangled childhoods: Imagining and materializing children's common world relations. In M. Bloch, B. Swadener, & G. Cannella (Eds.), *Reconceptualizing early childhood care and education: Critical questions, new imaginaries and social activism* (pp. 121–130). New York: Peter Lang.

van Manen, M. (1997). *Researching lived experience: Human science for an action sensitive pedagogy* (2nd ed.). Albany, NY: State University of New York Press. (Original work published 1990).

Chapter 6
West African Dance and Spiritual Well-Being for African Americans

Ojeya Cruz Banks and Jeanette "Adama Jewel" Jackson

> Why should we be enslaved to bad thoughts, bad education, poverty, lack of opportunity, lack of ambition, lack of greatness. We are created to be great, and this culture creates a platform by which our babies can begin to see themselves as great…it all starts with them hearing, and feeling, the beat of the drum. (A. Jewel, personal communication, January 11, 2016)

Many African Americans have found a lifeline through igniting a relationship to the percussive tradition of the *djembe,* a West African hand-drum originally from Mali. Synching up heart and body to its sonic vibration and rhythms can declutter and purge negative thought patterns and recalibrate the somatic experience of a dancer with joy and self-assurance (Dunham, 1969, 1989; Primus, as cited in Schwartz & Schwartz, 2011), while carrying out community rituals of "respect for ancestors and elders" (Monteiro & Wall, 2011, p. 245).

We propose that when African American dancers synchronize their movements to the drum, this constitutes a recovery of cultural transmission interrupted when African people were kidnapped and sold during the Atlantic Slave Trade (c. 1500–1850 CE). Regaining cultural fluency in West African dance can be a critical part of cultural, emotional and spiritual restoration. We view dance retrieval as a sign of recuperation that enables African Americans to tap into an African worldview and to heal from traumatic events of forced migration, cultural dislocation, and racism.

To explore how West African dance is an important practice for African American spiritual well-being, this paper provides a glimpse into the life, pedagogy, and cultural activism of West African dance educator, Jeanette "Sista Adama Jewel" Jackson. In 1998, Jewel founded African Soul International (ASI), a non-profit organization based in Los Angeles, articulating the following mission:

O. Cruz Banks (✉)
Denison University, Granville, OH, USA

J. Jackson
African Soul International and University of La Verne, La Verne, CA, USA

K. Bond (ed.), *Dance and the Quality of Life*, Social Indicators Research Series 73,
https://doi.org/10.1007/978-3-319-95699-2_6

> To preserve and present the best of African Culture through the dances, songs, rhythms and stories of the African/African-American experience. ASI uses the arts to keep youth off the streets, bring community together and build bridges of joy and compassion through positive artistic experiences. (www.africansoulinternational.org/)

The chapter highlights Jewel's journey toward becoming an avid West African dance educator. Reflecting on her life and educational work provides a springboard for discussing the psychological consequences of racism and miseducation, as well as insights into the significance of West African dance for cultivating spiritual well-being.

Gabriel Fara Tolno, a former member of Les Ballets Merveilles of Guinea and well known *djembe* and dance teacher, said that in a ritual dance circle, the musicians' job is to "give the light" (Tolno, personal communication, August 3, 2014). Tolno explained that the art of *djembe* is designed to support and uplift dancers. Tuning into the beat of the drum is to plug into rhythms whose primary function is to elicit oral history as well as a heightened sense of a spiritual and community consciousness (Billemeir & Keita, 1999; Price, 2013). Jewel notes that the dance and drum connection can induce and exude joy, peace, and harmony, stating, "This is why the dances of Africa resonate with people from all backgrounds and are essential for Africa's descendants. They hold the DNA of generations of triumph, resilience and culture" (A. Jewel, personal communication, August 9, 2016).

West African dance has been fundamental to strengthening and mobilizing African American identities and communities in the United States. Recent studies have illuminated West African dance as a vehicle for political movement and spiritual capital, a remedy for Eurocentric American education and curricula, and a tool to (re)construct understanding of Africanity and develop Diaspora networks (Cruz Banks, 2009, 2010, 2014; Gittens, 2012; Nur Amin, 2016; Watson, 2008; Welsh Asante, 1993; Zabriskie, 2013). The late dancer-scholar, Pearl Primus, who was one of the first to bring dance from Liberia, Nigeria, Ghana, Zaire and other locations on the African continent to the US, wrote:

> Dance is my medicine. It is the scream which eases for awhile the terrible frustration common to all human beings who because of race, creed, or color are invisible. … Instead of growing twisted like a gnarled tree inside myself, I am able to dance out my anger and fears. (as cited in Schwartz & Schwartz, 2011, n.p.)

Since antiquity, dance has been a bedrock of indigenous health and education on the African continent (Diallo & Hall, 1989; Monteiro & Wall, 2011). This philosophy of well-being through dance survived the Atlantic Slave Trade in the Americas where dance was suppressed on the plantations by legal restrictions and Christian dogma that deemed it paganist and uncivilized (Daniels, 2005; Hazzard-Gordon, 1996; Stuckey, 2002, 2013). Despite attempts to erase Africa from the bodies of African-Americans, the movements, songs and rhythms persisted in embodied memories of the people. Before there were opportunities to travel back to Africa and link movement to origins, Africa seeped from the creative bones of her children; take for instance, the ring shout, the jook, and the juba dance (Hazzard-Gordon, 1985, 1996).

In addition to African American dance pioneers Katherine Dunham and Pearl Primus, other living treasures carrying the mantle forward include Baba Chuck Davis, Amaniyea Payne, Kariamu Welsh, Baba Robert Crowder, Dorothy Wilkie, and Wilhelmina Taylor. Numerous others, less widely known, have also expanded the reach of African dance to communities across the US, including Najwa I, Denise Bey, Barbea Williams, Donald Eno Washington, Aminisha Cunningham, Ferne Yangeti Bronson, and Linda Thomas-Jones, to name a few. These teachers have been inspired by the work of master artists from West Africa such as Ladji Camara, Assane Konte, Marie Basse-Wiles, Raymond Sylla, Zak and Naomi Diouff, Kemoko Sano, and others. Several generations in the diaspora and from the continent have revitalized the transmission and evolution of African dance through advocacy, research, performance and teaching. To further explore the significance of West African dance, this chapter tells the story of Adama Jewel and the importance of her *djembe* worldview and culture for enhancing spiritual well-being.

Theoretical Context

Carter G. Woodson's (1933) influential book, *The Miseducation of the Negro,* argued that schooling institutionalized the disgracing of African Americans by disseminating histories and ideas that ensured a sense of racial inferiority. He asserted that nourishing the Black mind is not the project of Eurocentric American education. This historical backdrop is what Gloria Ladson-Billings (2006) calls the outstanding educational debt, the unequal distribution of educational resources that is arguably responsible for racial achievement gaps in US schools. Cornel West (1993) noted that while racism is a socio-economic tool, how it influences human desires, values, and self-concepts is just as important. Madison (2011) might call what Woodson, Ladson-Billings and West are describing as the "hidden circling of race" (p. 87).

We argue that these ambiguous social constructions of self and social alienation can be remedied through experiencing the "healing wisdom of Africa" (Dillard, 2008, Dillard & Okpalaoka, 2011). Cynthia Dillard (2008) suggests that rituals of fellowship grounded in African cosmologies can have tangible effects on our souls; and that spiritual praxis is an imperative action for divesting race and colonial internalizations and habits. This could explain why worldwide, oppressed dance traditions are being revived in the interest of centering ancestral knowledge and accessing "spiritual capital" (Cruz Banks, 2009, 2014). Spiritual capital references the (re) generation of intellectual, spiritual and cultural knowledge in the wake of colonialism, racism and post-slavery trauma – enlivening alternative realms, transcendence, and freedom that increase one's sense of spiritual well-being. For instance, Jewel explains that her West African dance pedagogy is about nourishing self-efficacy and communities that "hold ourselves to an ethic of care and love so we can attract positivity and demand it as well. No one can mandate that another person respect you, but when you respect yourself, it changes the dynamics" (A. Jewel, personal communication, August 9, 2016).

This study is situated in existing scholarship examining the prominence of African Diaspora dance in the United States as a critical pedagogy and a disseminator of epistemologies of rhythm, somatic grounded(ness), body power, communion, and spiritual capital (Cruz Banks, 2010; DeFrantz, 2001, 2002, 2004; Gottschild, 2003, 2005; Nur Amin, 2016). For African Americans, dance has been an important tool of self-affirmation and resistance – a way to "strike back" at racism (Hazzard-Gordon, 1996, p. 221). Thomas DeFrantz (2001) agrees that dance is a practice where racial identity can be contested, and comments that the drum is a tangible hallmark of African retentions: its "insistent rhythmicity," "individualism within a community dynamic," "temporal presence," and "ubiquitous spirituality" (p. 15). Some scholars suggest that African dance aesthetics enhance a sense of identity, body image and educational experiences (Cruz Banks, 2010, 2012, 2014; Gittens, 2012; Kerr-Berry, 1994; Monteiro & Wall, 2011).

This study adds to the conversation a teacher's life story of how West African dance loosened and released racial chokeholds while boosting ancestral literacy of *djembe* rhythms. Describing *djembe* culture, Jewel notes:

> The 'marriage' between the dancer and drummer is an intimate connection, symbolic of our relationship with life itself. Sometimes the drummer leads, sometimes the dancer does. The most critical thing is that they both listen to and connect with each other. (A. Jewel, personal communication, August 9, 2016)

The practice can usher in what DeFrantz (2004) calls the "sacred dimensions" (p. 72). Like Dunham's decolonizing dance pedagogy, West African dance is vital in the diaspora for boosting self-optimism, sense of roots, and spiritual alertness for African Americans (Cruz Banks, 2009, 2014; Gittens, 2012; Price, 2013). Cruz Banks (2012, 2014) also found spiritual well-being benefits of West African drum and dance for culturally diverse youth. In spite of the positive indicators, West African diaspora dance continues to be absent or fall low on the priority list for public school and university curriculums in the US (Kerr-Berry, 2012). Monroe (2011) found that some University students undervalue West African dance because they don't perceive it as a helpful movement technique. Addressing this issue, Nur Amin (2016) argues for a "reimagining of curricula" that destabilizes the privileging of Western movement approaches (p. 15).

A half-century after passing of the *US Civil Rights Act of 1964*, there is still a lack of positive portrayals of Africa and African Americans in American mass media, both as places and as people, as well as in the ambiguously inconsistent and contested historical narrative of African American peoples disseminated in American schools (McCarthy, Crichlow, Dimitriadis, & Dolby, 2005). Civil rights lawyer and writer Michelle Alexander (2010) asserts that a new Jim Crow era is emerging in the United States in the form of a racial caste system. Police brutality statistics and excessive incarceration rates of African American males, for example, continue to take a toll on African Americans' lives: "African-Americans are more likely than other racial and ethnic groups, including Asians, Hispanics and Whites, to be exposed to traumatic events" (Alim et al., as cited in Walker, 2015, p. 1). Created in 2012 as a political intervention to address these issues, the now well-established Black Lives Matter movement is evidence that the U.S. is not a "post-racial" society (www.blacklivesmatter.com).

A premise of this study is that West African dance educational experiences are a force for healing from the arrows of racial ideologies – both inferiority and supremacy. For African Americans, this is accomplished by Jewel and others through gifting the trajectories and experiences of African culture that are not tainted in the media by over-representations of poverty, war, disease and strife.

Research Methodology

Our research methodology blends autobiographical reflection with an "ethnographic eye," integrating Jewel's first person perspective with Cruz Banks' ethnographic observation and analysis. Memoirs emphasizing excerpts of the life story written by Jewel – her personal theories and verbatim quotations – are focal points (Fetterman, 2010; Madison, 2011). Tuning into Jewel's articulation enabled an opportunity for active listening and learning (Ladson-Billings & Donnor, 2008) in order to understand the importance of her involvement in West African dance. This is compatible with critical ethnography, which strives to centralize the voice of people and their efforts toward social justice (Madison, 2011).

This is not a classical ethnography that assumes a concentrated participant-observation time of 6–12 months (Fetterman, 2010) in the field. Instead, the study includes observations of Jewel's teaching at Camp Fareta, a weeklong intensive West African dance and drum camp held annually in the southern Sierra Mountains at Dunlap, California, during 2014 and 2015. Intensive fieldwork weeks were followed up with two informal conversations and ongoing email interviews and correspondence. Camp Fareta is where we, the authors, met, and participation at this event inspired conversations that led to this collaboration. The above-listed materials were collated and analyzed to understand how West African dance has contributed to Jewel's personal well-being and in turn inspired a passionate pedagogy.

The study is grounded also in Cruz Banks' practitioner-researcher experience over 15 years of studying West African dance in Africa and the United States, and by Jewel's wellspring of knowledge about the social history of African American and West African dance forms. We both intend for the paper to be meaningful to West African dance communities in the USA and to wider academic stakeholders, but more importantly to portray optimistic social change efforts. As co-authors, we collaborate to integrate our shared insights as African American women, dance educators, scholars and long-time practitioners of West African dance. Ethical approval for this research was granted by Academic Committees at the University of Otago.

The Beat of the Drum

The upcoming personal narrative reveals how West African dance opened up a new world to Jewel, and that her journey towards becoming a cultural educator-advocate was not without hurdles. It chronicles her navigation of socio-economic limitations, family alienation, and demoralization from racism. The sting of racism throbbed less when she was introduced to positive African and African American history and scholars that helped her to realize the unfortunate miseducation she received in school. The critique of white supremacy and racism gained from African Studies equipped her with a meaningful worldview and stimulated an educational mission. Jewel wanted to shine a positive light on African heritage and, particularly, to pursue a mission to promote emotional and spiritual resilience and well-being. She felt empowered through Dance, which helped her to divest the wounds of racism from the psychological foreground of her identity.

Jewel's introduction to the *djembe* through master teachers from Guinea and Senegal living in the US was a turning point in her life. Inspirational teachers and dance class experiences propelled her on to a professional dance career and now she is an avid West African dance educator and community facilitator. What follows are insights into Jewel's journey – in her own words – prompted by the question: *What was the momentum that led you to establish your organization African Soul International?*

"Sista" Adama Jewel and African Soul International

January, 2015

I was born in 1972 to a teenaged mom – the second of two children by the time she was 15. Growing up in the inner city of Cleveland, Ohio, I know what it's like to not have access to the arts, or a family that prioritizes your artistic ambitions…whether because of a lack of time and resources, or because the arts are considered a tertiary aspect of life for people who are struggling to survive and maintain. I'm the only artist in my family. Nobody "got" me growing up…so I know the feeling of wanting to express your gift, but not having that outlet.

At 18, I experienced a racist incident towards the end of my high school career. A crowd had assembled outside my English class, and a friend told me I wouldn't believe what was on the board. When I finally got inside, I saw it. On the wall, someone had written, "Niggers go back to Africa." The message shook my core. This experience broke the childhood illusion of school as a "safe space." It conjured up a mix of feelings – confusion, fear, betrayal, anxiety, shame… The event invoked self-consciousness about my ancestors and my inherited DNA, but not in a positive way. I don't know why it hurt me so. I had heard the words used in rap lyrics and on the street…but this was different. A white classmate wrote it. My mind was racing with crazy questions: Do they hate all of us? Were they upset with one person? Why? What's going on? Is someone here plotting to hurt us?

As appalling as the chalk board message was, the response from the administration was far worse. They demanded that it be erased and forgotten…as if that were possible. Thereafter there was no reconciliation, no gathering around the camp fire, no Kumbaya singing and telling us that we were all one. There was just emptiness. The administration never conducted an investigation, possibly waiting for the school year to end so they could move on to summer plans in hopes this would blow over before the next year. That didn't happen. I could not understand how my principal, with his thick Irish accent, couldn't understand. Weren't the Irish fighting for their own independence, freedom, and dignity? Couldn't he see that this incident created fear in students? Didn't he care? Didn't he value his Black students and want to ensure we felt accepted at school?

In my neighborhood, when the word *nigger* was used in a derogatory manner, that was "fighting words." So, when a large student group including myself gathered to demand action, school administrators ran out after us. The principal assured me he'd take care of it. I trusted him. I went back to class and when the girl who admitted to being the writer of the racist slur gave me a smirk. I seethed inside. But I chose to drop it and let the situation go.

However, she approached me after school by my bus stop. I felt threatened and feared she was going to assault me.

We ended up fighting and the principal came out to break it up. When he asked us who hit first, I told the truth. That truth cost me: I was expelled from school and not allowed to attend my prom or any other activities associated with graduation. The pain of this incident made me realize how little I knew about life. I felt that I would be judged as an African-American woman when I left the familiarity of school. After all the years of education, I felt I had no self-concept. I didn't know who I was or how to go out into the world as an African-American woman and be successful.

Things started to change for me when I joined an African study group and began to learn about Molefi Asante, Yosef Ben-Jochannan, Asa Hilliard, Leonard Jeffries, Ashra Kwesi, Maulana Karenga, Frances Cress Welsing, Neely Fuller, and many others who exposed me to a world that *I never knew existed!* What a way to come into adulthood! It hurt, though, that I had *never* through my K-12 experience heard of *any* of it. I wanted to do something about that. I wanted to teach young people how beautiful they were, before the streets or this society could tell them otherwise.

Dance was a highlight of my childhood – I had an immense love of movement. I danced at parties, family gatherings, or just all over the house. I think if someone assessed me as a child, I might have been labeled ADHD because I was ALWAYS moving. Dancing was part of my personality, which I think must have inspired leadership qualities. A cousin recently told me that I made them all learn choreography when they came over to visit. I started my first hip-hop group at 16. My best friend and I were called Jewel and Jetta, and we rapped, danced and sang. We used to go to the weekly talent show at the skating rink, win $50, and invest it in new clothes for the show the next week. Those were the days. But the icing on my cake was when I started learning African dance after meeting Linda Thomas-Jones, founder of the Imani dancers in Cleveland, at a party. I pretty much bear hugged her when she told me who she was and what she did. The next day I rode my bike across town to be at her 9:00 a.m. class. I was hooked!

From that group I was able to get on a national tour with Omowale, a group from Detroit directed by Sundiata Keita. This experience changed my life. It was the first time I had met Africans – proud, powerful, gentle, confident Africans: I was home. The tour took us to Washington, DC for the Kankouran West African Dance Conference with Assane Konte. Imagine being 18 and seeing Assane, Mama Kadiatou Conte, Youssouf Koumbassa, Marie Basse, and the chorus of beautiful, Black, powerful drummers. Where else was I to GO!? I was HOME!!

I worked with Wonde, a children's company in Columbus, Ohio directed by Kaikpai Paasewe of Liberia. The group rehearsed in a city recreation center in the projects, and the kids literally walked past drug dealers, liquor stores and everything you can imagine to get there. Opportunities to perform were the bright spots in these kids' lives. They told me how they stopped "hanging" with certain people, stopped being friends with little boys, and made sure they finished their homework because they didn't want to mess up their chances to perform. Seeing children perform on college campuses when no one in their families had gone past high school was so rewarding. I knew this was what I wanted to do. In 1998, at age 26, I wrote my first grant proposal. I'd had a son and was in a job training program, learning to type and use Microsoft Office. My teacher said we should each have a project that we wanted to learn these skills for, so my project was to get a grant from the Ohio Arts Council and offer free classes for the children in my community. I received the grant, graduated from the program, and the rest is history.

Cruz Banks Above, Jewel has narrated "the good and bad" of her life that inspired her to found African Soul International (ASI), grounded in her love of dance since childhood. She now facilitates weekly youth and adult Guinea, Mali and Senegalese dance classes, provides master classes for several universities, and runs dance residencies at local schools. Jewel holds an annual intensive dance and drum conference featuring West African dance teachers from Guinea, Senegal, and Mali, and has established her own dance company in Los Angeles. Over 100 students attend her dance immersion program. She also hosts and organizes special workshops and residencies for well-known master artists such as Djeneba Sako (Mali), Youssou Koumbassa (Guinea) and the late Abdoulaye Sylla (Guinea). As a veteran of the West African (USA) dance circuit, I can say that Jewel has a reputation as an extremely knowledgeable dancer with impressive precision and charisma. Her many influential teachers have been role models for Jewel's teaching philosophy and cultural activism. Following is her response to the question: *Who are your influential dance teachers and what made them influential?*

Jewel Papa Assane Konte, Mama Naomi and Dr. Zak Diouf, Youssouf Koumbassa, Moustapha Bangoura, Djeneba Sako, Mouminatou and Marietou Camara, Mareme and Marie Basse are like legends to me. They exhibit so much grace and knowledge. More than anything, their commitment to spreading this art to the community has been so influential. The story of how West African dance circulated throughout the US is one of resilience, cultural preservation, and love. These artists came here and lived *in* the community, teaching in schools, churches and community centers, building and repairing communities, families and children. It's a legacy that I hope to continue through my work.

August, 2016

Cruz Banks Later in our collaboration I asked Jewel to elaborate on how West African dance and drum have contributed to her well-being.

Jewel The dance and drum scene was amazing to me, as I had never functioned outside of the hegemonic narrative of Black, inner city life. Here were these Black folks that were FREE!!! It was like growing up on the plantation, with the illusion of freedom, because you're free within boundaries. But once you ask for your humanity to be valued, you're reminded that you're not that special. I can liken it to the feeling I imagine people had when they left the south for Harlem. Seeing Black folks, free, living, happy – you just realize… where was I and why didn't anyone tell me this was an option? It's funny now, but that's how I felt. I couldn't understand how they were all free, but I didn't know that freedom (that is, value) was available. Since I realized it, I've never turned back. The opinion of others is irrelevant to me – I have my tribe, and that's where my value lies. I dance it, I drum it, I live it…I am Africa. It's the freedom to commune with artists, to dance, to experience the atmosphere, to live.

Camp Fareta

In 2014 Jewel offered to teach at Camp Fareta, and Youssouff Koumbassa welcomed the idea. Serendipitously, Koumbassa was one of the dance teachers who made Jewel's heart sing at 18 and inspired her career path (A. Jewel, personal communication, July 20, 2014). Since then, Koumbassa has come to work with ASI many times. Jewel directed the children's dance program for Camp Fareta, and her youth company performed as part of the event's talent show. On the evening of July 9, 2014, an ensemble of eight African American youth dancers accompanied Jewel along with a musical section that included two skilled young male drummers who played with special guests – master drummers Mbembe Bangoura and Mangue Sylla from Guinea. They performed a dance called *Coucou*, a rhythm from the Bela people of Guinea, choreographed by Jewel.

The camp cafeteria was transformed into a theatre. When the percussion began, the crowd roared. The group danced through the lanes between the tables all the way to the front where the drummers stood. The choreography was fluid, dynamic, and athletic; synergy with the drumming was strong. The lead drummer mapped the rhythmic topography of the choreography. I found the playful interchange between youth and master percussionists extremely touching – I wept through most of the performance. I was so deeply proud and happy to see ownership of djembe culture displayed by young African Americans during this opportunity to play with legendary musicians. Their self-assurance and skill was not far from virtuosic. In general, the youth empowerment embodied in this performance was, for me, remarkable. Six months later, I asked Jewel via email: *What have been your most rewarding moments as a teacher?* She responded,

> My greatest rewards are with my kids, of course! To see young people who come from dysfunctional homes, yet they shine brilliantly on stages in union theaters, and begin to envision themselves as a vital part of the world is a feeling that goes beyond words. To see young people who have grown up come back and ask that *their* children be a part of my program, or to go to McDonald's and an employee says, "Hey Mama Jewel, do you remember when you taught me this?" and just busts out dancing at their job…I mean, young people let you know they appreciate the life and gift that you saw in them. They let you know when you have taught them to see themselves differently. That's the reward. I wish I could track them all – I could read *their* stories and how THEY felt about the work. (A. Jewel, personal communication, January 10, 2015)

On July 9, 2015, I observed Jewel teaching a children's dance class at Camp Fareta. She wears an embellished bright pink, fitted t-shirt with bling letters that says: *Dance It, Dream It, Live It.* A year later I asked her about the meaning of this mantra, and she wrote that the words encourage us to live out Africa in each step, rhythm and song…to show our solidarity with Africa, our love of Africa, our connection to Africa, beyond the dance and drum space. She went on to say it is about "LIVING it, not exercise, but the culture…we live it" (A. Jewel, personal communication, August 8, 2016)! Following are my field notes from the class observation:

> Jewel is teaching a rhythm and dance called *Sinte*, a rite of passage dance for young girls from the Boke region of Guinea, which is indigenous to the Baga and Landouma people. When I arrive, she is breaking down the musical composition of the *dunduns* – the *dundunba, sangba,* and *kenkeni.* These three drums played with sticks accompany the *djembe* and set the tempo of the music and the dance. She is playing the rhythm while explaining to a young boy how to switch from the chorus (a repetitive beat) to the breakdown.
>
> Two skilled teenage male *djembe* players are accompanying the class and while Jewel is organizing the music and assisting the less experienced drum student, the dance students mingle around the *djembe* players – jumping, doing cartwheels, even juggling to the beat of the drums. The dance portion of the class begins and Jewel has a group of about eight engaged children, including her youngest daughter, standing behind her. They all face the drummers, listening to the music and striving to synchronize their actions to the beats. Jewel sings and counts the rhythm to help them match their moves to the pocket of the music. I observe collective energy and mutual support through participants' commitment to the rhythmic groove.
>
> Jewel now has them marching to the tempo now; once they have it, she adds movement embellishments. The dancers dip their bodies to one side and perform triplet hops that match the musical break. Jewel presents as a joyful and enthusiastic teacher, smiling a lot

> and vocalizing affirmations such as "Come on everybody," "Good," "Yes, keep going," and the kids pick it up. She counts the steps out for them, too, turning around frequently. She makes regular eye contact with the student dancers and drummers. I see a fostering of musicality and an ability to match students' moves to the drumbeats.

Jewel's pedagogy in this workshop was about strengthening students' connections to rhythm, rather than how to move their bodies per se; so, she did not fuss about the shapes or steps their bodies were performing, but focused on how they were moving in relation to the beats. She did an exercise about becoming familiar with the "breaks" in the music. Breaks are the drummers' way of communicating to the dancer and signal when they start or change or stop dancing. This can be tricky, as sometimes students get caught up in the various polyrhythms and can't hear the break, therefore missing important cues that keep the entire ensemble together.

When asked to elaborate on her teaching objective, she explains that "when the cadence of the break is played, each student has to stop and clap the break at the appropriate time. This practice assists the students with hearing the music in order to learn to converse with "drum talk," a fundamental of African dance" (A. Jewel, personal communication, August 9, 2016). Since Guinea dance is rhythmically constituted, Jewel assists the children to attune their bodies to the music through movement repetition. While *djembe* rhythm comprehension can take many years, learning to hear the music and move to the textures of the groove is an important process for transmitting West African heritage and promoting cultural values (Billmeier & Keita, 1999; Price, 2013).

In an early email interview, Jewel stated that her overall teaching ambition is "to develop a healthy African concept," elaborating:

> As we learn the truth about Africa, and how her wealth and children have fed the world, we see ourselves as productive, vital and necessary. As we see Mama Africa's innovation, we know that we too can produce. As we see her humanity, we realize the humanity in ourselves and develop a deeper spiritual sense of who we are. In essence, when we dance Africa and we drum Africa, we begin to LIVE Africa, and that's a beautiful place to live. Living Africa is a direct opposition to the life that we were bred or forced to live here. Our defiant return to our traditions here are synonymous with revisiting the "Door of No Return," our obstinate way of saying that when you told us we couldn't, we decided that we could. The connection that you cut and told us to cut, we will reestablish and grow. (A. Jewel, personal communication, January 25, 2015)

Reflection

Jewel's life narrative and Cruz Banks' ethnographic observations highlight someone for whom West African dance (practice & theory) made a life-changing difference. Jewel's first-person account of a racist incident in high school illustrates how such experience can trigger a mentality challenged by distrust, fear, anxiety, antagonism, internal turmoil, and lack of confidence; however, it also fueled important questions about equality, human respect and kindness, and cultural difference, planting the seeds for founding African Soul International. Jewel's story reveals a distressed psychological state prompted by a racist slur being disentangled through empowering studies of Africa and Africa-America. Her paradigm shift was reinforced rhythmically by *djembe* drum and dance culture, affording mental and spiritual uplift. Jewel believes this helped her to see beyond the "hegemonic narrative of Black life" that can be perpetuated in institutions such as schools.

Jewel's journey towards becoming a cultural practitioner and teacher of West African dance represents the human possibility of self-renaissance and cultural reclamation. Her coming of age memoir demonstrates how dance participation immersed her within empowering communities and historical narratives of Africa that fed her spiritually. Her story signposts the steady momentum of African dance in the US for endowing African-Americans with cultural literacy, emancipatory articulations, and miseducation repair vital to healthy identities, reflecting an-going Afro optimism and the positive steps taken towards healing from the traumas of slavery, racism, and geographical dislocation. For the heirloom *djembe* beats and moves were designed to keep heritage alive and embodied, and to ensure psychological, emotional and spiritual well-being.

Across cultures and centuries dance has been a vehicle for youth initiation rituals and preparation for adulthood (Billmeier & Keita, 1999; Charry, 2000). Jewel gained cultural pride and a liberating trajectory when she discovered West African dance. Inspired and equipped with cultural knowledge, she assists African American youth in acquiring self and cultural understandings that promote their spiritual well-being through rhythm knowledge. In Camp Fareta, during observations of Jewel's performance pedagogy, Cruz Banks observed a youth ensemble activating DeFrantz's (2004) sacred dimensions of rhythm, electrifying the cafeteria with Guinea drum and dance. In the teaching session, I noticed how her focal point was about cultivating attention to the rhythm protocols of dance to develop what Jewel calls drum talk competency. The music became an anchor of group connection and a methodology for Jewel to immerse young people in an African world. Placing Jewel's dance pedagogy in the context of her racist high school, I see her educational efforts clearly divesting racist attitudes and negative associations with Africa. Her organization, African Soul International, invests in preserving and presenting "the best of African Culture" (www.africansoulinternational.org/). Jewel's teaching emphasizes community togetherness, compassion, and joy.

Benefits of music and dance are receiving increasing attention from Western science, pointing to the progressive nature of indigenous West African dance epistemologies. Hanna (2016) and Lovatt (2011, 2013) report studies showing that dance might spark new brain cells, change self-perception, improve memory, reduce stress, release empowering hormones, and promote physical well-being. The 2009 World Science Festival in New York hosted a dialogue between neuroscientists of music and singer Bobby McFerrin to discuss the relationship between music, neurons and the central nervous system. One panelist proposed that a primordial function of music is to line up people's brain waves to enable social cohesion and community. Others discussed music as a central nervous system experience and how music and dance can evoke both negative and positive emotions (Schaefer, McFerrin, Levitin, Bharucha, & Parsons, 2009/2014).

Djembe drumming and dance specifically have been found to enhance social and emotional well-being and to treat depression, a global health concern (Anderson, 2010; Locke & Clark, 2009). Since ancient times, African societies throughout the continent and the diaspora have viewed music and dance as mediums of social medicine (Daniels, 2005; Monteiro & Wall, 2011). Dance is a medium for socializing and nurturing African spiritualties and healthy people (Billmeier & Keita, 1999; Charry, 2000; Diallo & Hall, 1989; Monteiro & Wall, 2011).

Conclusion

For Jewel, teaching West African dance is about "intervening in the life trajectory of our future generations…that's powerful in and of itself" (A. Jewel, personal communication, January 10, 2016). Her autobiographical narrative illustrates that for one person West African dance was a (re)educative process, transforming a skewed self-orientation with optimism and ancestral heritage. Dance can help address the educational debts and gaps that many African Americans have endured as a consequence of slavery, racism and continuing adverse legacies. Dance touched Jewel and roused the prophetic philosophy: "Dance it, Dream it, Live it." Hers is a quintessential story of how the reverberation of the drum can change cognitive patterns and even ameliorate the effects of racism for African Americans. Her testimony illustrates how dance amplified a sense of cultural integrity and spiritually transformed her quality of her life.

This chapter has attempted to capture a salient story of resilience and cultural work by a West African dance practitioner, a perspective that could easily escape the dance studies radar. There is a need for further autobiographical accounts of dance educators like Jewel, specifically, qualitative research that explores whether others have experienced the same transformational qualities, for example, in relation to how African dance might counter the negative influences of racism on African American youth in the United States. Research that examines dance educators' influence on the lives of youth at-risk or young people with extraordinary untapped potential would be useful as well. While the spiritual benefits of West African drum and dance on youth self-esteem have been described (Cruz Banks, 2009, 2014), this study adds an intergenerational counterpoint – how West African dance enhanced an educator's life, resulting in an aspirational pedagogy. In conclusion, this story is about the invigoration of an African American identity, self-worth and sense of place and history through West African dance. For Jewel, tapping into the ancestral wisdom and rhythms of West African dance gifts her with a sense of agency and a direction in life that energizes spiritual well-being.

References

Alexander, M. (2010). *The new Jim Crow: Mass incarceration in the age of colorblindness*. New York: The New Press.

Amin, T. N. (2016). Beyond hierarchy: Reimagining African diaspora dance in higher education curricula. *The Black Scholar: Journal of Black Studies and Research, 46*(1), 15–26.

Anderson, J. D. (2010). *Moving to the beat of djembe drums: African dance and reported feelings of depression*. Senior thesis, Claremont McKenna College, Claremont, CA.

Billmeier, U., & Keita, M. (1999). *Mamady Keita: Life of the Jembe tradition & rhythms of the Malinke*. Brussels, UK: Arun.

Charry, E. (2000). *Mande music: Traditional and modern music of the Maninka and Mandinka of Western Africa*. Chicago: University of Chicago Press.

Cruz Banks, O. (2009). Critical postcolonial dance recovery and pedagogy: An international literature review. *Pedagogy, Culture & Society, 17*(3), 355–367.

Cruz Banks, O. (2010). Critical postcolonial dance pedagogy: The relevance of West African dance education in the United States. *Anthropology & Education Quarterly, 41*(1), 8–34.

Cruz Banks, O. (2012). Katherine Dunham: Decolonizing anthropology through African American dance pedagogy. *Transforming Anthropology, 20*(2), 159–168.

Cruz Banks, O. (2014). West African dance education as spiritual capital: A perspective from the United States. *Journal of Dance, Movement & Spiritualities, 1*(1), 163–179.

Daniel, Y. (2005). *Dancing wisdom: Embodied knowledge in Haitian vodou, Cuban yoruba, and Bahian candomblé*. Urbana, IL: University of Illinois Press.

DeFrantz, T. F. (2001). Foreword. In D. Fisher-Hornung & A. D. Goeller (Eds.), *Embodying liberation: The black body in American dance* (pp. 11–16). New Brunswick, NJ: Transaction.

DeFrantz, T. F. (2002). *Dancing many drums: Excavations in African American dance*. Madison, WI: University of Wisconsin Press.

DeFrantz, T. F. (2004). The black beat made visible: Hip hop dance and body power. In A. Lepecki (Ed.), *Of the presence of the body: Essays on dance and performance theory* (pp. 64–81). Middletown, CT: Wesleyan University Press.

Diallo, Y., & Hall, M. (1989). *The healing drum: African wisdom teachings*. Rochester, VT: Inner Traditions/Bear.

Dillard, C. B. (2008). When the ground is black, the ground is fertile: Exploring endarkened feminist epistemology and healing methodologies in the spirit. In Y. S. Lincoln, N. K. Denzin, & L. T. Smith (Eds.), *Handbook of critical and indigenous methodologies* (pp. 277–292). Singapore, Singapore: Sage.

Dillard, C. B., & Okpalaoka, C. (2011). The sacred and spiritual nature of endarkened transnational feminist praxis in qualitative research. In N. K. Denzin & Y. S. Lincoln (Eds.), *The Sage handbook of qualitative research* (pp. 147–162). Thousand Oaks, CA: Sage.

Dunham, K. (1969). *Island possessed*. Chicago: University of Chicago Press.

Dunham, K. (1989). Katherine Dunham. In B. Lanker & B. Summers (Eds.), *I dream a world* (pp. 28–29). New York: Stewart, Tabori, Chang.

Fetterman, D. M. (Ed.). (2010). *Ethnography: Step-by-step* (Vol. 17). Thousand Oaks, CA: Sage.

Gittens, A. F. (2012). Black dance and the fight for flight: Sabar and the transformation and cultural significance of dance from West Africa to black America (1960–2010). *Journal of Black Studies, 43*(1), 49–71.

Gottschild, B. D. (2003). *The black dancing body: A geography from coon to cool*. New York: Palgrave Macmillan.

Gottschild, B. D. (2005). Crossroads, continuities, and contradictions: The Afro-Euro-Caribbean triangle. In S. Sloat (Ed.), *Caribbean dance from Abakua to Zouk: How movement shapes identity* (pp. 3–10). Gainesville, FL: University Press of Florida.

Hanna, J. L. (2016). *Dance: Neuroplasticity and brain fitness*. Retrieved from http://sharpbrains.com/blog/2016/01/22/what-educators-and-parents-should-know-about-neuroplasticity-learning-and-dance/

Hazzard-Gordon, K. (1985). African-American vernacular dance: Core culture and meaning operatives. *Journal of Black Studies, 15*(4), 427–445.

Hazzard-Gordon, K. (1996). Dancing under the lash: Sociocultural disruption, continuity, and synthesis. In K. Welsh Asante (Ed.), *African dance: An artistic, historical and philosophical inquiry* (pp. 101–130). Trenton, NJ: Africa World Press.

Kerr-Berry, J. A. (1994). African dance: Enhancing the curriculum. *Journal of Physical Education, Recreation & Dance, 65*(5), 25–47.

Kerr-Berry, J. A. (2012). Dance education in an era of racial backlash: Moving forward as we step backwards. *Journal of Dance Education, 12*(2), 48–53.

Ladson-Billings, G. (2006). From the achievement gap to the education debt: Understanding achievement in U. S. Schools. *Educational Researcher, 35*(7), 3–12.

Ladson-Billings, G., & Donnor, J. K. (2008). Waiting for the call: The moral activist role of critical race theory scholarship. In Y. S. Lincoln, N. K. Denzin, & L. T. Smith (Eds.), *Handbook of critical indigenous methodologies* (pp. 61–84). Singapore, Singapore: Sage.

Locke, K., & Clark, D. (2009). Can African drumming impact the social/emotional development of young children. *Canadian Children, 34*(2), 10–15.

Lovatt, P. (2011). Dance confidence, age and gender. *Personality & Individual Differences, 50*(5), 668–672.

Lovatt, P. (2013). Dance psychology: The power of dance across behavior and thinking. *Psychology Review, 19*(1), 18–21.

Madison, D. S. (2011). *Critical ethnography: Method, ethics, and performance*. Thousand Oaks, CA: Sage.

McCarthy, C., Crichlow, W., Dimitriadis, G., & Dolby, N. (Eds.). (2005). *Race, identity, and representation in education* (2nd ed.). New York: Routledge.

Monroe, R. (2011). "I don't want to do African… What about my technique?": Transforming dancing places into spaces in the academy. *The Journal of Pan African Studies, 4*(6), 38–55.

Monteiro, N. M., & Wall, D. J. (2011). African dance as healing modality throughout the diaspora: The use of ritual and movement to work through trauma. *Journal of Pan African Studies, 4*(6), 234–252.

Price, T. Y. (2013). Rhythms of culture: Djembe and African memory in African-American cultural traditions. *Black Music Research Journal, 33*(2), 227–247.

Schaefer, J., McFerrin, B., Levitin, D., Bharucha, J., & Parsons, L. (2009, June 12). *Notes and neurons: In search of the common chorus*. Panel, World Science Festival, John Jay College, New York. Retrieved from https://www.youtube.com/watch?v=S0kCUss0g9Q

Schwartz, P., & Schwartz, M. (2011). *The dance claimed me: A biography of Pearl Primus*. New Haven, CT: Yale University Press.

Stuckey, S. (2002). Christian conversion and challenge of dance. In T. F. Defrantz (Ed.), *Dancing to many drums: Excavations of African American dance* (pp. 39–58). Madison, WI: University of Wisconsin Press.

Stuckey, S. (2013). *Slave culture: Nationalist theory and the foundations of black America*. Oxford, UK: Oxford University Press.

Walker, L. (2015). *Trauma, environmental stressors, and the African-American college student: Research, practice, and HBCUs*. Philadelphia, PA: Penn Center for Minority Serving Institutions. Retrieved from http://www2.gse.upenn.edu/cmsi/content/reports

Watson, A. (2008). Guinea. In R. M. Juang & N. A. Morrisette (Eds.), *Africa and the Americas: Culture, politics, and history: A multidisciplinary encyclopedia* (Vol. 1, pp. 535–540). Santa Barbara, CA: ABC CLIO.

Welsh Asante, K. (1993). African American dance in curricula: Modes of inclusion. *Journal of Physical Education, Recreation, and Dance, 64*(2), 48–52.

West, C. (1993). *Race matters*. New York: Vintage.

Zabriskie, Q. M. (2013). *Reconstructing Africanity: Constructed knowledge, diasporic networks, and cultural power in Chicago's African dance and drum communities* (Doctoral dissertation). Northwestern University, Evanston, IL.

Chapter 7
Dancing on Earth: The Healing Dance of Kalahari Bushmen and the Native American Ghost Dance Religion

Kimerer L. LaMothe

From the sixteenth to the nineteenth centuries, forms of ecstatic or transformative dance around the world suffered from concerted attempts on the part of western European empires to establish religious, military, economic, intellectual and cultural domination over indigenous ways of life. Forms of dancing that elicited intense sensory experiences through music and movement, and that claimed access to prophetic insight, healing power, ancestors, or other spiritual entities proved particularly volatile points of contention. Where western Europeans and then Americans fought to suppress these dances, indigenous peoples often refused to relinquish them.

Arguments levied by largely Christian imperialists against ecstatic dancing sounded out similar themes. Dancing was a sign of resistance to western, Christian beliefs, values, and practices; it represented allegiance to pagan gods and ways of life. Dancing took time and energy away from productive work, while encouraging laziness, lust, and even outright rebellion. US agents on the Pine Ridge Reservation in South Dakota went so far as to blame dancing for making people sick, as the native dancers would sweat in the snow (Holler, 1995, p. 118). Instead of dancing, colonialists insisted, people should be reading and writing, learning from books how to assume western Christian ways of believing, worshiping, thinking, and acting. In the US, government laws forbidding Native Americans to dance were on the books well into the twentieth century (Holler, 1995; Wenger, 2009). Yet, officials' vociferousness in targeting indigenous dancing tacitly acknowledged a power of dancing that went beyond diversion or consolation and rivaled Christianity on its own turf. Against devastating odds, forms of ecstatic dance found ways to survive colonial oppression and even thrive anew in the so-called post-colonial period.

In seeking to explain the resilience and resurgence of these dances, scholars trained in modern western forms of knowledge have offered a range of explanations

K. L. LaMothe (✉)
Independent Scholar, Granville, NY, USA
e-mail: klamothe@post.harvard.edu

K. Bond (ed.), *Dance and the Quality of Life*, Social Indicators Research Series 73,
https://doi.org/10.1007/978-3-319-95699-2_7

focusing on political and social concerns. Sometimes, as in the case of Indian classical arts, the revitalization of dance traditions occurred under the auspices of a new national government seeking to institutionalize folk and religious forms into effective signs of national integrity (Foster, 2009, p. 120). Sometimes, as in the case of the Native American powwow, tribal peoples found in revived dance traditions an effective expression of ethnic identity (Krystal, 2012). Sometimes canny business people, in search of tourist dollars, catalyzed the recovery, as with the Pueblo dances of the American southwest (Sweet, 1985). In other cases, artists of a particular lineage, taking responsibility for being living carriers of the dance, began teaching a new generation of students and creating work for a concert stage (Shea Murphy, 2007).

Indigenous peoples, however, often counter such explanations with the language of religion, asserting that their dancing is spiritual or religious (Keeney, 2010; Wenger, 2009). The implication is that their choice of dancing as a medium of resistance to coloniality is neither accidental nor symbolic. Dancing is fundamental to who they are and what they know: a human cannot live a good life, a purposeful life, a holy life without it. There is no equivalent. Nevertheless, by adopting religious language, indigenous people run the risk of being misunderstood. It is easy for readers trained in the modern west to hear the terms "religious" and "spiritual" as referring to intellectual, emotional, and inward states concerned with belief, meaning, and their textual expressions (LaMothe, 2004, 2008). Such understandings of religion, coextensive with the rise of both the modern west and the field of religious studies, have served to justify colonial repression of ecstatic dancing in the first place. *How then are scholars to understand indigenous claims for religious significance in ways that take seriously the value and agency of dancing action?*

This chapter examines two cases in which practices of ecstatic dance, though caught in the crosshairs of Christianity and capitalism, refused to die: the healing dance of the Kalahari Bushmen and the Native American Ghost Dance. Both are circle dances, involving a whole community, female and male, young and old, singing and stepping together, so as to propel some of their members to access prophetic, visionary and/or healing abilities for the benefit of all. This chapter begins with the premise that I, as a modern western scholar of religion and dance, have something to learn from these cultures about what "religion" and "dance" are, what they do, and how they matter.

For the Bushmen living in the Kalahari Desert, driven from South Africa by Dutch then British forces, and now restricted by the governments of Botswana and Namibia to a fraction of their former nomadic range, all-night, communal healing dances remain a living, central element of culture. Their dances are so important that over the past 20 years Bushmen elders have asked a number of western scholars – whom they call paper people – to write about their dancing (Guenther, 1999; Katz, Biesele, & St. Denis, 1997; Keeney, 2010). In addition, a group of elders have given their own account of their healing dances in a book edited by Bradford Keeney and Hillary Keeney (2016): *Way of the Bushman as Told by the Tribal Elders*. In this book, Bushmen elders assert that the time has come to share their spiritual knowledge with the world.

For Native Americans across the western regions of the United States, the Ghost Dance Religion emerged in the late nineteenth century in response to cultural and environmental devastation wrought by white Europeans and Americans. The Ghost Dance gained notoriety among white Americans for its purported role in provoking US soldiers to massacre over 300 Sioux at Wounded Knee Creek in 1889. Commentators at the time predicted that the Ghost Dance would die along with the slain Native Americans. However, more recent writers have revisited this incident and the attitudes towards dancing that emerged in its wake, arguing that the Ghost Dance did not die, and continues to carry forward distinctive, constitutive elements of native religious traditions (Eppes, 1956; Holler, 1995; Kehoe, 2006; Neihardt, 1932; Smoak, 2006).

In relation to each of these dances, I find in practitioners' appeals to religious significance a challenge to western assumptions about what religion is. For people in these two traditions, dancing is essential for quality of life; and it is so for the ways in which dancing cultivates sensory awareness of human participation in the ongoing life of what the dancing enables them to perceive as the natural world. For people in these cultures, the practice of ecstatic dancing is not simply a mark of ethnic or cultural or even religious identity. It is a means for ensuring that their thoughts and actions, their values and ideals, their quality of life, "remain faithful to the earth" (Nietzsche, 1954, p. 125).

In what follows, I introduce an ecokinetic approach to guide my study of these two cases. For each case, I then examine primary and secondary sources, focusing on the language of religion as it appears in modern western interpretations and indigenous responses. In a careful analysis of each dance, I mobilize an ecokinetic approach to reveal how indigenous uses of religion language attest to the agency of dancing in promoting an earth-friendly quality of life.

An Ecokinetic Approach

As first articulated in "Transformation: An Ecokinetic Approach to Ritual Dance" (LaMothe, 2014), an ecokinetic approach to the study of ecstatic dance is rooted in a philosophy of bodily becoming. A philosophy of bodily becoming affirms the centrality of bodily movement to all aspects of human life; it presumes that humans *are* an ongoing rhythm of creating and becoming patterns of sensation and response. It holds that culture consists of these bodily movements – of movement patterns that have been discovered, remembered, and passed on for their ability to help humans cultivate life-enabling relationships with sources of sustenance present in their natural and social environments (LaMothe, 2015a).

While this philosophy owes its shape to many sources, it is most deeply indebted to the American modern dancers (especially Isadora Duncan and Martha Graham); to phenomenologists of religion (especially Dutch philosopher Gerardus van der Leeuw); to Friedrich Nietzsche, feminist philosophy, and my own practical study of dance traditions including African, Haitian, Sufi, classical Indian, ballet, and American modern. In privileging movement, this philosophy also aligns with recent research across fields, including neuroscience, developmental psychology, anthropology, and evolutionary biology in which bodily action plays an integral role in human evolution and development (LaMothe, 2015b).

Notably, from the perspective of bodily becoming, "religion" appears as a collection of movement patterns in the form of symbols, practices, or beliefs whose primary function is to teach people how to participate consciously in the rhythms of bodily becoming. Said otherwise, the movement patterns comprising religion are those proven to awaken *kinetic creativity* – the ability to find ways to move in relation to others, including the natural world, that sustain life-enabling relationships (LaMothe, 2015a, 2015b).

An ecokinetic approach to the study of ecstatic dance mobilizes this concept of religion to understand indigenous claims for the religiosity of their dancing activity. As "kinetic" it attends to the bodily movements participants make. It acknowledges that each movement is a *relationship* that *educates the senses* to certain possibilities of thought, feeling, and action. As "eco" it attends to the matrix of these relationships – the world or "whole" or "earth," which the action of making the movements *makes real and believable* for those who participate (LaMothe, 2014, 2015b). It identifies the ways in which the practice and play with movement patterns helps people cultivate connection with sources of sustenance.

An ecokinetic approach proceeds in four steps. After studying firsthand accounts of these dances in order to discern their movement patterns, I first imaginatively recreate the sensory education that making these movements affords (LaMothe, 2008). I assess the ways in which this sensory education orients dancers' perceptual range and triggers their kinetic creativity. I correlate this sensory education with the kinds of religious claims made by participants for the dance. Finally, I evaluate how the action of dancing these dances contributes to what participants perceive and value as an earth-friendly quality of life in the wake of colonial persecution and its lingering legacy.

The Ju|'hoansi or Bushmen of the African Kalahari

Although Bushmen people (a name they now choose) have been studied intensively since the late nineteenth century (Keeney and Keeney, 2012), only recently have scholars acknowledged their all-night communal dances as a central, constitutive element of their culture. This shift began with the research of Harvard anthropologist Richard Katz. His book, *Boiling Energy* (1982), sparked debate over how integral the dancing is to the longstanding psychological, physical, and spiritual health of the people. In Katz's account, dance is not a way to consume excess calories, as surmised by at least one researcher before him (see Lee, 1979). Rather, dance delivers modes of healing that sustain the specific needs of Bushmen in living their nomadic life: sharing resources, cooperating in hunting and child rearing, and releasing tensions that arise among individuals (Katz, 1982, p. 3). In a later work, *Healing Makes Our Hearts Happy*, Katz et al. (1997) suggest that the all-night healing dances might even provide Bushmen with a medium for discerning workable strategies in their efforts to resist attempts by western organizations and their own national governments to impose modern forms of education, medicine, and dwelling onto their nomadic culture.

While Katz's (1982) work garnered attention for the dance as a cultural and political resource, the Bushmen take issue with his interpretations of the dance as evoking fear, requiring battle with evil spirits, feeling like death, and most of all, involving "trance." Where Guenther (1999), for example, follows Katz's lead, asserting that "the objective of the curing dance is to achieve the state of trance… and thereby transcend ordinary life and reality" (p. 182), the elders disagree. They insist: "Anyone who says we go into 'trance' and have a 'trance dance' is mistaken" (Keeney and Keeney, 2016, p. 16).

In searching for alternative words to describe the transformative efficacy of their dance, the Bushmen turn to the language of "love," "God," and "Creation." According to the elders, the shaking, seeing, pulling, and healing of the dance happen as a direct reception of "God's love, the source of the universal life force or what we call n|om" (p. 4). For them, a healer's shaking and stomping is a spontaneous, full bodily experience of being moved by love. While Katz (1982) did identify an "open heart" as key to the ritual's efficacy (p. 130), the Bushmen push further. The dance is what it is because of love – because of human love for God, and God's love for humans, where God is a Sky God who can take many forms, including male, female, and plural.

For the Bushmen, the fact that their dancing evokes and expresses God's love is what renders it powerful within their communities and relevant for the world – not its ability to promote political action or anchor ethnic identity. As they aver, their dance embodies a "spiritual knowledge" that Bushmen have kept alive since the beginning of time – a knowledge that the rest of the world has forgotten (Keeney, 2010; Keeney and Keeney, 2016). With such statements, the elders call attention to what they believe most western scholars have not grasped: *they dance in order to dance*. The practice of dancing itself is essential for the survival of humans on earth.

While Bushmen's appeals to God, love, and creation make sense as responses to materialist explanations of their dancing, they also carry risks. The word "love," for example, does not necessarily mean the same thing to a Bushman as it does to a reader educated within the context of modern western scholarship. As an ecokinetic approach helps clarify below, the love the Bushmen describe is one defined by the *experience of doing the dance*. As Keeney and Keeney (2016), both anthropologists and recognized shamans within the Bushmen communities, aver, "We are speaking about an awakened and energized love that inspires us to spontaneously tremble and shake in ecstatic bliss" (p. 4). For the Bushmen, love is (and is not) an emotion or idea. Love is a sensory awareness of vibratory, relational movement connecting humans, ancestors, and all moments of the natural world.

A Healing Dance

While the Bushmen have several kinds of dances, and no two are alike, a dance generally progresses through four stages (LaMothe, 2015a) whose duration, intensity, and reach vary depending upon the participants and the dynamic they create together. I lay out these four stages, recreating in relation to each: the movement patterns required; the sensory education they afford; and the perceptions of God, love, creation, and nature they make possible. The details are culled from the work of Katz (1982), Katz et al. (1997), Keeney and Keeney (2012, 2013, 2016) and Bushman elders (Keeney and Keeney, 2016).

Warm Up A dance begins with a group of women who sit on the ground around a fire and start singing, clapping out their own musical accompaniment. As community members gather, children practice their dance moves while adults chat and tell jokes. In these initial moments of the dance, the patterns of song and movement invite everyone to come together into a group. The songs awaken aural spaces and pace breathing; they pull forth visceral, sensory memories of past dances. The sharp clapping grabs people's focus, hooking them under the ribs, stirring them to join in.

People start paying attention to one other. They experience being moved by one another's movements. Their own stepping and stamping awakens in them a sensory awareness of what they are feeling, of the ground, and of their connection to it. Stepping and stamping together educates the senses of participants to movements in them and around them, joining them.

Practice The singing intensifies. Children drop out of the dance. The circle of dancers, mostly men, tightens in a ring around the singers. The dancing gathers strength and precision. The stepping and stamping are more pronounced. Participants prepare for the rise of *n|om*. As the elders tell, "We dance and sing in order to heat n|om" (Keeney and Keeney, 2016, p. 10).

Though sometimes interpreted by anthropologists as a "spiritual" power (Katz, 1982), n|om is not opposed to a power that is physical or material. For the Bushmen, n|om refers to the energy of any life form and of the endless web of ropes that connects and sustains all momentary bursts of itself. To heat n|om is to open to feel the sensation of this pulsing web, to welcome that sensation, and to coax it into fuller form, so that this stronger sensory awareness of relational movement becomes a doorway, a threshold, and a compass for further thoughts, feelings, and actions.

Play When n|om heats and rises to a certain point, the Bushmen say that it "boils." At that moment, one or more dancers *kia* – or awaken – to a new level of feeling. The movement of the dancers who kia changes. It becomes spontaneous and freeform. It rises and ruptures into sudden bursts of action or sound. The dancers tremble and shake. This shaking is "a sign that they are waking up;" they are shifting into a n|om-centered, n|om-enabled experience where their perception of themselves and the world changes (Keeney and Keeney, 2016, p. 39).

What those who shake see is "sickness" in others. They not only see it, they are impelled to move toward it, to lay hands on a person, and to pull that sickness out. The shaking is critical for healing. "This is when our dancing turns into the stomping movement of an awakened healer. The movement helps us not fall over as n|om gets stronger and each stomp on the ground sends more vibrations into the body" (p. 22). The vibrations coursing through the body, rooted in the ground, train the senses of those present to perceive their own bodily selves and the bodily selves of others as sites where movements are emerging, coming forth, and becoming real – where healing is happening.

According to the Bushmen, this heightened emotion that manifests as shaking is "love." The intensification of all feelings and any feeling resolves itself in this shaking love. In this way, the progression of the Bushman dance prepares people not only to sense impulses to move arising in themselves, but to seek out those that appear in the shape of heart-felt compassion for people in their community. The experience of shaking educates people to feel both a desire to help and faith in one's ability to do so. The experience of shaking thus offers all present a chance to perceive their own bodily-movement-making as actively participating in endless currents of creation. As described by Keeney and Keeney (2016), "For ecstatic shamans…it's the arousal of intense feelings that lead to song, movement, and synesthetic experience that marks the authenticity of a spiritual voyage" (p. 97).

Cool Down After the healers pull out the sickness they have seen, the level of energy fades, and the dancing and singing quiet down. Dancers and singers rest, absorbing the impact of the waves of sensory awareness that have just coursed through them.

Throughout the night, a dance runs through these phases of practice, play, and cool down several times. The singing and dancing heat to a pitch of intensity; individual dancers kia, shake, and pull sickness from others; and the activity slows and fades before building again. At dawn, as the sun rises, the dance reaches a climax before entering its final arc. The singing subsides. The dancing stills.

People break off into small groups, talking and sharing. In the final moments of the dance, the movements-made settle into the bodily selves of those who made them. Participants not only carry with them memories of what happened, they have become the patterns of sensing and responding that they have been practicing and playing with throughout the night – the feelings of openness, compassion, and connection that they know as love.

Shaking as God's Love

An ecokinetic approach reveals the play in the Bushmen's use of religious language. While the terms may sound familiar to western ears, the way in which the words mean is different. Shaking itself, as the Bushmen practice it, is a culturally specific medium of sensory perception. As Keeney and Keeney (2010, 2012) insist, the shaking movement is not "dance" in the western sense of a planned and rehearsed movement sequence. Nor is it an "improvisation" in the sense of some intentional exercise in inventing movement patterns. It is not "religious" in the sense that it expresses beliefs concerning sacred or divine powers that are codified in textual or visual forms.

The Bushmen case redefines these terms. Their dancing *is* dance in the sense that the stepping, circling, and shaking represent bodily patterns that participants are creating and becoming. It is dance in the sense that it occurs as a letting-happen of movement patterns that people in that culture have learned to value as beneficial for their well-being. Moreover, it is religion in the sense that the action of dancing and shaking educates the senses of those present to possibilities of life-giving, life-enabling experiences that they may not access otherwise, namely, what they call "love."

The lived experience of shaking provides a sensory awareness of all reality – including and especially the natural world – not only as connected with one another but as generative of one another, as n|om, as God's love. Shaking, a person creates and becomes the movement of exchange – a vibratory connection – that can catalyze a healing that is always already at work; she thus strengthens the "ropes," the reciprocal relationships, that enable and sustain all life. As the elders affirm, "When we make our ropes stronger, it helps strengthen all the ropes in nature" (Keeney and Keeney, 2016, p. 30).

First and Second Creation

When describing how shaking heals, the Bushmen use terminology that again must be understood in terms of the sensory education that shaking provides: "First Creation" and "Second Creation." In First Creation, the Bushmen explain, not only are there no distinctions among separate things, but every unit is itself changing forms – humans into animals and animals into one another. In First Creation there is no suffering or pain. Second Creation, by contrast, refers to the world of everyday life. In Second Creation, every animal has a name that fixes its identity and limits its being so that it becomes a site of illness and death. For Bushmen, then, the antidote to any form of injury or hurt is to enter First Creation (Keeney and Keeney, 2013).

Nevertheless, neither "creation" is a fixed place. Both are better understood as modes of experience. According to the Bushmen, First Creation refers to the mode of experience in which people know viscerally that everything that exists is movement – everything is change. First Creation exists as the quickened sensory awareness of movement that the effort of stepping and stamping and circling with others requires. By dancing and shaking, then, humans *heal* – in any and all senses of that word, by tapping into a visceral experience of endlessly explosive, dynamic movement as more real than what otherwise appears as finite and painful. As the Keeneys affirm, "Anything can be transformed as it is embraced by the energy of change that underlies primary creation" (Keeney and Keeney, 2016, p. 61).

In assessing the mechanism of this transformation, it is again tempting to think of it as psychological. Yet, the Bushmen reject such interpretations. The Keeneys write: "With a Bushman dance, changing one's relationship with present experience sets in motion self-correcting means for altering whatever has been stuck, maladaptive, or non-resourceful in one's life" (p. 59). This "self-correcting means" can be elaborated through the notion of *kinetic creativity*. From the perspective of bodily becoming, all humans *are* a capacity to sense and respond to pain by receiving impulses to move differently. It is a capacity that humans must exercise from birth (if not before) in order to learn how to connect with the sources of life-enabling nourishment (LaMothe, 2015a). Healing is always happening; and while this kinetic creativity operates at all levels – physical, emotional, intellectual, spiritual – the fundamental form and prime catalyst is bodily movement.

From an ecokinetic approach, then, the Bushman dance represents patterns of bodily movement discovered and passed down over centuries based on their ability to catalyze, orient, and ground people's kinetic creativity. As an elder confirms: "Rather than crying, we shake. In this way, we change the sadness of suffering into the reenergizing presence of n|om. We cook our suffering. When it boils, we experience joy in being spiritually wealthy with n|om" (Keeney and Keeney, 2016, p. 2). The movement patterns of stepping, singing, and shaking wake up a sensory awareness of impulses to heal that are always already emerging at every point in the pulsing web of life.

Although they call it love or entering First Creation, Bushmen are clear that names are just names – agents of Second Creation that arrest and kill the truth. What matters is the experience: "When we are in *thara* [shaking], we are awake and living inside the world of creation" (p. 57). What matters is the shaking. This dance is a knowledge, the Bushmen affirm, that human quality of life on earth requires. "The world needs to have teachers and healers who sing, dance, and tremble as God's love flows through their hearts" (p. 32; see also Widlock, 2001).

Native American Ghost Dance Religion

The Ghost Dance began with a Paiute man, Wovoka, living in land now part of Nevada (see Kehoe, 2006; Mooney, 1973). During the solar eclipse of 1889 Wovoka received a vision containing a twofold instruction for all native tribes in North America: dance and live cleanly. Wovoka predicted that a new era was coming: within a year, the buffalo would return, the earth would regenerate, and the white people would disappear. All the Indians needed to do, according to Wovoka's vision, was to dance regularly, three to five times a week, and live a moral and honest life free from alcohol and other white vices. While the dance Wovoka taught was called different names by different tribes (Kehoe, 2006), and while practices varied from tribe to tribe, in every case the organizing purpose of the dancing was to receive visions that corroborated and nuanced Wovoka's original vision. Dancing in this way would align the people's attention and efforts with the imminent regeneration of the earth and its natural bounty.

Within a year the Ghost Dance spread widely. Though not every community introduced to the dance chose to practice it, the Ghost Dance reached multiple tribes across a wide swath of western states, including Idaho, Utah, Wyoming, Colorado, Missouri, Iowa, and Oklahoma (Mooney, 1973, p. 902). The Ghost Dance was never taken up by southern tribes, including Apache and Pueblos (p. 805). Rich Plains tribes who traded profitably with the Whites, like the Navajo and Hopi, laughed at the message (pp. 809–810, 813). Nevertheless, those who chose to dance embraced it fervently, believing that if they danced, the Great Spirit would restore their quality of life.

Interpreting the Ghost Dance

The Ghost Dance Religion has been subject to a fraught history of interpretations, in large part due to its disputed involvement in the massacre noted above of unarmed Sioux women and children at Wounded Knee Creek, South Dakota. In 1890 the US Government commissioned the first study of this event, sending anthropologist James S. Mooney to determine whether the Ghost Dance had in fact incited the Sioux to revolt against the US military presence on the Pine Ridge Reservation. *Was dancing to blame*?

Mooney's (1896) massive 1000-page analysis concludes that the Ghost Dance religion did not foment resistance to the Pine Ridge agents and their military reinforcements. To the contrary: "The Ghost dance itself, in the form which it assumed among the Sioux, was only a symptom and expression of the real causes of dissatisfaction…not the cause of the outbreak" (p. 828). In making his case, Mooney argues that the Ghost Dance is "a religion" (p. 928ff). He defends his claim by documenting instances of ecstatic dance not only among Native Americans, but in religious contexts around the world. As part of his case, Mooney establishes that dancing is and can be religion, even within the history of Christianity (as addressed by Jessica Van Oort in the next chapter, a study of ecstatic dance during two periods of Christianity).

Nevertheless, the notion of "religion" that Mooney mobilizes to defend the dancing is one indebted to traditions of modern western scholarship. As a result, Mooney predicts that the Ghost Dance is on the verge of dying out (p. 927). Assuming that religion is primarily a matter of belief, and dancing is only viable as a mode of expressing belief, Mooney concludes that the Ghost Dance religion would end once its Indian practitioners realized that its predictions were not going to happen. As Holler (1995) confirms,

> The assumption that the Ghost Dance withered away or collapsed under the weight of its own absurdity persists probably because its tenets are completely implausible from a scientific point of view that misconstrues religious discourse as propositional. (p. 218)

The Ghost Dance, however, did not die. Recent scholarship is revisiting the question of why not. As a handful of authors have established, not only are there a few places where the Ghost Dance is actively practiced, but, even more significantly, the Ghost Dance remains a constellation of movement patterns that comprise a potent fund for ongoing attempts to revive native cultures (Eagle, 2000; Holler, 1995; Kehoe, 2006; Neihardt, 1932; Smoak, 2006). It was never just about the beliefs.

Several of these interpretations focus on the ethnic, cultural, and political import of the dance. For Smoak, the Ghost Dance has been an invaluable tool for "identity formation" in the face of Euro-Americans' refusal "to understand and accept aboriginal conceptions of identity and social relations" (p. 8); it has given Native Americans "a vehicle for the expression of ethnic and racial identities" (p. 202). Alternately, for Holler, the Ghost Dance secures the longevity of cultural forms. He writes: "the idea of rejuvenating traditional culture through ritual dance is precisely the essence of the Ghost Dance" (pp. 150–151). Yet, as Alice Kehoe notes, the reasons Native Americans give for continuing to dance the Ghost Dance, even as a vehicle for expressing ethnic identity or rejuvenating culture, are resolutely religious. Describing the Sioux Wahpeton Reserve's New Tidings community, a contemporary example of the Ghost Dance Religion, she affirms that, "The religion stimulated creative pruning of unobtainable or anachronistic elements, such as emphasis on bison, while incorporating effective new symbols" (p. 50). Here "the religion" has agency in generating and shaping itself.

Black Elk Nowhere are claims for the religious import of the dance stronger than in the legacy of Black Elk. Black Elk participated in the Ghost Dance as a young man and was present at Wounded Knee. At the turn of the century, Black Elk converted to Catholicism. Then, after another 30 years, he delivered a rousing affirmation of Native American dance in two dictated accounts, published as *Black Elk Speaks* (DeMaille, 1984; Neihardt, 1932) and *The Sacred Pipe* (Brown, 1953). In these narratives, Black Elk locates the practice of ecstatic dancing securely at the center of native life as site and source of their distinctive earth-honoring religion.

Black Elk's use of the terms "religion" and "spiritual" marks his response to Mooney and those who agreed with Mooney. For even though he had honored the Ghost Dance as "a religion," Mooney explained its transformative efficacy by claiming that the Native Americans had learned to manipulate capacities latent in the human physiology; without knowing it, they were practicing what Europeans call "hypnotism." As Mooney writes: "It can not be said that Indian priests understand the phenomenon, for they ascribe to it a supernatural cause, but they know how to produce the effect, as I have witnessed hundreds of times" (p. 922). Modern commentators have followed suit. Kehoe (2006), for example, describes the dance as a "trance" (p. 8).

Black Elk, by contrast, consistently describes dancing as a source of spiritual power – and one that cannot be substituted by any other means. As he affirms, a vision alone is not enough: "A man who has a vision is not able to use the power of it until after he has performed the vision on earth for the people to see" (DeMaille, 1984, p. 238; Neihardt, 1932, p. 204). A vision often contains a ritual that a person must "perform" in and as a dance.

In relation to his own vision, received at age nine, that predicted his power to heal others, Black Elk describes the transformation that the dances he made accomplished:

> Of course it was not I who cured. It was the power from the outer world, and the visions and ceremonies had only made me like a hole through which the power could come to the two-leggeds. If I thought I was doing it myself, the hole would close up and no power could come through. (Neihardt, 1932, pp. 204–205)

For Black Elk, at least as described by Neihardt, dance opens the "hole," the circle, through which a power that extends through but beyond him – a spiritual power, healing power, the power of the Great Spirit – flows.

Performing a Vision

From an ecokinetic perspective, the question to pose in the face of these claims is not whether such a power is real, or whether a "supernatural" exists. Rather, the relevant question to ask is: *How does the dancing educate the senses of participants so that they are able to perceive as real what they conceive as spiritual or sacred?*

When viewed through an ecokinetic lens, the Ghost Dance, like the Bushman dance, appears as a progression of movement patterns that educates dancers' sensory awareness to ranges of perception and action that are otherwise unavailable to them. The dancing makes possible experiences that transform their current situation; it does so by granting participants a visceral sense of a living, moving, generative matrix of which their movements, the natural world, and their ancestors and gods are all a part. The following rendering of the dance is culled from first person reports of nineteenth century dances chronicled by James Mooney (1896/1973), Black Elk (DeMaille, 1984; Neihardt, 1932), and Alice Kehoe (2006).

Warm Up Before the dance begins, tribal members often engage in extensive preparation, making special shirts painted with images and symbols from Wovoka's vision, setting up a central pole, and rehearsing songs. The dance itself begins when one or more singers or leaders of the dance gather at a designated center, sometimes marked with a cedar pole, and sing songs that signal community members to join them. Those who respond take one another's hands. Alternating male and female, they interlace fingers, and join in the singing.

Ecokinetically, the act of coming together, drawing near, circling up, in a round that includes everyone regardless of gender or age, cultivates in those who make these movements a sensory awareness of the group in relation to themselves, and of themselves in relation to the group (Kehoe, 2006, pp. 7–8). This sensory awareness travels through clasped hands, as each member holds onto two others, and is gripped in return. A Ghost Dance circle could be small or expand to include over 300 people.

Practice As the singing intensifies, members of the dancing circle move together clockwise around the circle, tracing the path of the sun, with a series of shuffles and a stomp. These repetitive, punctuated movements draw dancers' attention down through their legs, to the soles of the feet, where they make contact with the earth, sounding out its support. As they stamp their feet, guided by songs, tribal members awaken and enhance the knowledge that they are dancing on earth, for the wellbeing of the earth and all earth's creatures. Their stamping and singing are visible and audible to others in the circle. Any one person may feel the presence of the group as waves of sound and movement, pulsing together with him or her, lifting, supporting, and amplifying his or her own individual patterns.

Play As the dancing and singing grow in volume and intensity, certain individuals, often women first, begin to tremble and shake. The change in movement patterns signals to those present that the person is entering another dimension of experience. After some shaking and trembling, the dancer falls down on the ground and lies still as the rest of the community continues to dance and sing around the circuit. When the fallen person is ready, he or she wakes up. The dance pauses, and the one who fell shares stories of what he or she has seen.

These visions often contain symbols and images that are familiar to all. Visions frequently involve passage to places where people who had died recently go about ordinary tasks, hunting and playing. The visions may contain songs and rituals, offering guidance for future dances. The Ghost Dance shirt, for example, was such an innovation, received in a vision by Black Elk himself (Neihardt, 1932, p. 243). After the sharing, the dance would continue, beginning another cycle, inviting, receiving, and attending to another round of visions.

Cool Down After several cycles, depending on time and place, and on leaders and participants, the dancing and singing wind down, and participants toss their blankets or shawls into the air in a final gesture of release.

In what sense are the movements of this dance essential for accessing, directing, and conceiving what Black Elk means by spiritual power? As with the Bushmen, indications point to *kinetic creativity*. In the Ghost Dance, the bodily movements in and around the circle, hands clasped all together, train the senses of those present not only about *what* to think, feel, and see, but *how* to see, where to look, and what to expect. The dance provides them with a time and space where they are encouraged both to feel the pain and suffering of their current situation and to receive some impulse to move that may transform it.

The Ghost Dance itself originated in a vision. When dancing, participants expect visions. They expect to be moved by what they see, hear, and feel. Such impulses to move, while sharing a common pattern of hope and encouragement, are also distinctive. They emerge in the moment, for the moment, in a particular individual for a given community as an expression of and a response to the movement of the gathered crowd. The dance educates the senses of those present to the creative potency of their own movement-making.

In performing the Ghost Dance, then, Native participants are not just preserving tradition or asserting racial or ethnic identity. They are not even practicing a religion per se in the sense of following a set of beliefs. Rather, they are exercising the most effective medium they have discovered for participating in the ongoing creation of the world as they know it. They are accessing a proven means of discerning how to move in ways that cultivate relationships of reciprocity with life-enabling powers of the earth itself. As evident from Wovoka's very first vision, dancing is the ongoing practice of sensory education that ensures that whatever cultural evolution occurs – whatever thoughts and actions and intentions Native Americans have – remain faithful not just to "tradition" as a fixed set of artifacts in the abstract, but to their ongoing ability to know and cultivate a visceral connection with a life-giving, earthbound whole.

The Ghost Dance keeps alive in participants the will and the ability to participate humanly in their unfolding future, step by step, day by day, in small and large ways. The agency unleashed by the dance is not an agency of individuals or of the tribe, per se, but the agency of something like life-force itself manifesting in the movements of kinetically creative bodily selves, seeking a way to flow fully and swiftly in line with the good health of the whole human-earth matrix that the dancing enables those bodily selves to perceive.

Dancing for the Earth

In the case of the Bushman dances and the Ghost Dance Religion, ecstatic dancing appears to those who do it as an essential component of a human life. The practice of dancing is integral to the process by which bodily selves in these two cultures become fully realized humans, living in reciprocity with the natural world, able to think and feel and act in ways that sustain the ongoing lives of themselves and their communities.

As framed by an ecokinetic approach, this dance-enabled alchemical action is not a mental act of will in which a person chooses to look on the bright side. It is a thoroughly bodily phenomenon, an experiential shift that awakens the pleasure of finding and making movements at all levels – in thought, feeling, and action – that do not recreate patterns of pain (LaMothe, 2015a). Such movements may be and often are overtly political or strategic, but nowhere more so when they appear as expressions of love in a world that denies it. As Keeney (2010) writes of the Bushmen, "This kind of dancing is… pure and simple joy, the highest form of tender loving care" (p. 5).

In relation to both dance traditions, the devastation wrought by imperial powers continues. Both cultures remain in subordinate status to governments founded in the wake of colonialism. In both cases, these governments fail to recognize the rights of native peoples to the land, the livelihood, and the life that they enjoyed before colonial conquest. In both cases, native peoples are still struggling to find a voice and express it in ways that carry authority and will be heard.

It is easy to see these cultures as doomed to eventual assimilation into the cultures that press and prey upon them from every side. However, the dancing vital to each offers another perspective. Dancing provides immersion in sensory experience that can shift the reality of oppression, such that it no longer appears as an unyielding monolith of pain, but rather as an ever-evolving pattern of relationships that include the earth in which every movement made, even the smallest movements of one human bodily self, matters.

For both the Bushman and the Native American, dancing taps and mobilizes a human power – a kinetic creativity – that will not disappear as long as humans persist. This power lies at the source of attributes that native peoples value highly: compassion, love, resilience, and respect for the natural world. In light of the sensory experiences provided by these dances, "earth" is not a thing or material reality existing independently of human bodily movement. *Earth is what the dancing enables them to perceive as the generative source of their own ongoing life, as holy or divine*. Dancing thus not only provides indigenous peoples with a sensory education that counters the education thrust upon them by western scholarly conventions, but sets in motion an alternative dynamic ground for perceiving, understanding, and envisioning the future.

The Bushmen assert what they know to be true: the dance *will* be reborn. They are sure of it. For them dance has a life of its own – one that is inextricably entwined with the unique paradoxes that accompany human life as both mind and body, individual and social creature, earthly and visionary. Dance is itself a power and a player. Practitioners of the Ghost Dance hold a similar faith: the dance has its own agency as an expression of life force bent on nurturing a human connection to the earth. Dancing, for them, is the most effective practice that humans can do in order to align with this ongoing restoring and regenerating movement of earth itself that they conceive as sacred.

For representatives of these two traditions, then, the challenge is clear. They are not under the illusion that they must "preserve" a dance and teach it to others as a reminder of what has been lost. Rather, they intend to keep their experiences of dancing alive long enough that the forms they have discovered can serve as crucibles of alchemical potential – marking a site and space where others can see and recognize the power of dancing to create our bodily selves and the world as we want and need it to be. That world, in so far as it remains accountable to the ongoing practice of dancing, will evolve beyond the cultural intolerance of colonial oppression, giving rise to new paradigms of thinking, feeling, and acting that privilege *bodily movement* as the source and telos of a human's quality of life.

References

Brown, J. E. (Ed.). (1989). *The sacred pipe: Black Elk's account of the seven rites of the Oglala Sioux*. Norman, OK: University of Oklahoma Press. (Original work published 1953).

DeMaille, R. J. (Ed.). (1984). *The sixth grandfather: Black Elk's teachings given to John G. Neihardt*. Lincoln, NE: University of Nebraska Press.

Eagle, B. M. (2000). *The last ghost dance: A guide for earth mages*. New York: Ballantine.

Foster, S. L. (Ed.). (2009). *Worlding dance*. New York: Palgrave Macmillan.

Guenther, M. (1999). *Tricksters and trancers: Bushman religion and society*. Bloomington: Indiana University Press.

Holler, C. (1995). *Black Elk's religion: The sun dance and Lakota Catholicism*. Syracuse, NY: Syracuse University Press.

Katz, R. (1982). *Boiling energy: Community healing among the Kalahari Kung*. Cambridge, MA: Harvard University Press.

Katz, R., Biesele, M., & St. Denis, V. (1997). *Healing makes our hearts happy: Spirituality and cultural transformations among the Kalahari Ju|'hoansi*. Rochester, VT: Inner Traditions.

Keeney, B. (2010). *The Bushmen way of tracking God: The original spirituality of the Kalahari people*. New York: Atria Books/Beyond Words.

Keeney, B., & Keeney, H. (2012). Dancing nom. *Journal of Dance and Somatic Practices, 1*(1), 11–22.

Keeney, B., & Keeney, H. (2013). Reentry into first creation: A contextual frame for the Ju|'hoan Bushman performance of puberty rites, storytelling, and healing dance. *Journal of Anthropological Research, 69*, 65–86.

Keeney, B., & Keeney, H. (Eds.). (2016). *Way of the Bushman as told by the elders: Spiritual teachings and practices of the Kalahari Ju|hoansi*. Rochester, VT: Inner Traditions.

Kehoe, A. B. (2006). *The ghost dance: Ethnohistory and revitalization* (2nd ed.). Long Grove, IL: Waveland.

Krystal, M. (2012). *Indigenous dance and dancing Indian: Contested representation in the global era*. Boulder, CO: University Press of Colorado.

LaMothe, K. L. (2004). *Between dancing and writing: The practice of religious studies*. New York: Fordham University Press.

LaMothe, K. L. (2008). What bodies know about religion and the study of it. *Journal of the American Academy of Religion, 76*(3), 573–601.

LaMothe, K. L. (2014). Transformation: An ecokinetic approach to the study of ritual dance. *Dance, Movement, & Spiritualities, 1*(1), 57–72.

LaMothe, K. L. (2015a). *Why we dance: A philosophy of bodily becoming*. New York: Columbia University Press.

LaMothe, K. L. (2015b). Becoming a bodily self. In J. Rieger & E. Waggoner (Eds.), *Movement matters: New materialism and religious experience* (pp. 25–53). New York: Palgrave Macmillan.

Lee, R. B. (1979). *The !Kung San: Men, women, and work in a foraging society*. New York: Cambridge University Press.

Mooney, J. (1973). *The ghost dance religion and wounded knee*. New York: Dover. (Original work published 1896).

Neihardt, J. G. (Ed.). (1979). *Black Elk speaks: Being the life story of the holy man of the Oglala Sioux*. New York: William Morrow. (Original work published 1932).

Nietzsche, F. (1954). Thus spoke Zarathustra. In W. Kaufman (Ed.), *Portable Nietzsche*. New York: Penguin.

Shea Murphy, J. (2007). *The people have never stopped dancing: Native American dance histories*. Minneapolis, MN: University of Minnesota Press.

Smoak, G. E. (2006). *Ghost dances and identity: Prophetic religion and American Indian ethnogenesis in the nineteenth century*. Berkeley: University of California Press.
Sweet, J. D. (1985/2004). *Dances of the Tewa Pueblo Indians: Expressions of new life*. Santa Fe, NM: School of American Research.
Wenger, T. (2009). *We have a religion: The 1920s Pueblo Indian dance controversy and American religious freedom*. Chapel Hill, NC: University of North Carolina Press.
Widlok, T. (2001). The illusion of a future? Medicine dance rituals for the civil society of tomorrow. *African Study Monographs, 27*, 165–183.

Chapter 8
The Spirit Moves: Christian Trance Dance in Late Medieval Europe and Early Nineteenth-Century America

Jessica Van Oort

Introduction

Around the world and across time, participation in religious rituals has helped people sustain or improve their quality of life. Through such rituals, participants can gain a sense of community, healing, insight, and purpose. It is unsurprising that dance has often been a part of religious ritual, as dance itself is credited with encouraging bonding between humans, releasing tension, healing pain, forming culture, and helping people negotiate their place as individuals within a group (LaMothe, 2015; Thomas, 2008). One subset of religious dance, trance dance, has a particular capacity to create a heightened emotional state that can bring joy and well-being. Trance dancers are often empowered with a sense of meaning and purpose that bring change to their own lives and the communities around them. In Christianity, however, unlike in many other religions, dance has not had an important role. In fact, Christian moralists have often prohibited dance (Amoah, 2004; Wagner, 1997; Chaps. 1 and 7, this volume).

Have Christians, therefore, been denied important experiences and states that would add important dimensions to their lives? The answer is not as obvious as it might appear. Despite prohibitions, some Christians have engaged in religious dancing, including trance dance. Trance dance in Christianity has not often been performed by clergy or by those in positions of power, but instead by the poor and oppressed, especially women and, in antebellum America, African-Americans (Thomas, 2008; Van Oort, 2009).

This chapter presents the meanings ascribed to trance dance by those who performed and those who observed, in both thirteenth- and fourteenth-centuries Europe and early nineteenth-century America. I selected these as examples of revival and change as eras when old religious traditions were no longer fulfilling people's needs,

J. Van Oort (✉)
Independent Scholar, Pawlet, VT, USA

K. Bond (ed.), *Dance and the Quality of Life*, Social Indicators Research Series 73,
https://doi.org/10.1007/978-3-319-95699-2_8

and Christians were seeking new ways of bringing meaning and quality to their lives. As I will demonstrate, trance dance provided joy, community, and empowerment to these Christians.

Ecstatic Dance and Trance Dance

In the context of religious or spiritual practice, scholars have identified a form of dance that is healing or transformative to individuals and communities. This dance need not be associated with organized religion; in modern-day Western cultures it often appears in clubs, raves, and concerts (Becker, 2004; St. John, 2004; Sylvan, 2005). Whether it is called ecstatic dance (Thomas, 2008), the "superordinary" (Bond & Stinson, 2000/2001), or raving (St. John, 2004; Sylvan, 2005) this kind of dance enables people to feel freedom, joy, connection with others or with a higher being or state, or a greater "internal somatic experience" (Sylvan, 2005, p. 67). Performers may sense that boundaries normally dividing them from others, such as ethnicity, class, or gender, vanish as they dance (St. John, 2004).

When experienced as part of formalized religion, healing and transformative dance can provide a ceremonial path to the divine, reinforcing the beliefs of participants and increasing their sense of well-being (Thomas, 2008). A particular religious context will shape both the experiences of the dancers and the meanings they draw from their dance (Becker, 2004).

Religious trance dance is a subset of the larger category of healing and transformative dance. Becker (2004) identifies commonalities among religious trances, which include emotional arousal, loss of a sense of self, an intense ability to focus, a halting of inner thoughts, an extraordinary ability to withstand fatigue, and sometimes a loss of memory. In this research I combine Becker's commonalities with LaMothe's (2015) definition of dance as an "emergent phenomenon" (p. 7) that arises out of movement as the mover becomes consciously aware of and participates in his or her "bodily becoming" (p. 4). This definition moves beyond the binary of danced and non-danced bodily movement and permits a broad examination of trance dance within Christianity.

Christian Attitudes Toward Dance

Christianity is one of the few world religions that lacks a strong tradition of sacred dance and therefore also lacks a reliable way for worshippers to understand and make meaning of trance dance. In Hinduism, one of Shiva's many forms is Nataraja, the divine dancer and creator. In many African and other-than-Western religions, dance is essential as a way to communicate with the deities (Frembgen, 2012; van de Port, Hansen, & de Haan, 2011; Younger, 2001). By performing specific movements that reflect the characteristics of a deity, dancers invoke that deity to possess them and dance through them (Ajayi, 1994). In Christianity, on the other hand, dance has rarely been sanctioned as a form of worship, and even dance as secular entertainment has often fallen under censure. Beginning around the fourth century many church authorities, drawing on a neo-Platonic hierarchy of spirit above body, preached against dance and sometimes banned it entirely (Amoah, 2004; Maynard, 1992; McDonnell, 1969).

In medieval Christian Europe social dance was a popular form of communal celebration, especially on Sundays and feast days. Most of the authorities of the Catholic Church, which dominated Europe at this time, tolerated laypeople dancing, but a few disapproved, associating dance with sins such as gluttony, pride, and luxury (Arcangeli, 1992). Church councils were less tolerant of dancing by clergy, in churches or churchyards, or as part of the official festivities for holy days (Backman, 1952; Mews, 2009). It seems likely, however, that sacred dance went on despite official prohibitions; church councils would not have felt the need to repeatedly sanction religious dances if they had been completely stamped out.

Christian opposition to dance was even stronger in nineteenth-century America than in medieval Europe. The new evangelical Protestant denominations, the Methodists and Baptists, condemned social dance for various reasons – it was of the flesh and not the spirit, it was irrational, it aroused pleasurable feelings, it wasted money, and most importantly, it was a worldly amusement that got in the way of a relationship with God (Wagner, 1997). At the same time, some revivalists who preached against social dance encouraged religious trancing and trance dance among their congregations, though they called such performances "exercises" rather than dance (Stone, 1847).

Trance Dance in Late Medieval Europe

Medieval European Context The thirteenth and fourteenth centuries in Europe saw religious changes that, while they did not alter the hierarchy of the Catholic Church, did bring about new religious options, especially for women. During the disasters of the fourteenth century – the Black Death, numerous famines, and the Hundred Years' War between France and England – performative penitential movements such as the flagellants became more widespread (Hamilton, 2003). Even before these disasters, however, Europeans had been seeking religious change. In the twelfth through thirteenth centuries local priests and laypeople, fearing that the church had become wealthy and corrupt, challenged religious norms (McGinn, 1991; Simons, 2001). Today we would call this a "grassroots" movement, motivated from below rather than above. Men and women left their old lives behind to embrace poverty and itinerate preaching, in imitation of the apostles. New religious groups sprang up, including two monastic orders, the Franciscans and the Dominicans, as well as groups open to laypeople such as the penitents, flagellants, and beguines (Grundmann, 1935/1995; McGinn 1991). Clergy often viewed these lay religious groups with suspicion since they were outside the church's authority (McDonnell, 1969; Murk-Jansen 1998).

The beguines were a uniquely female phenomenon, women who took temporary religious vows rather than permanent ones like nuns. Most beguines lived communally and supported themselves by manual labor. Some, however, lived solitary lives, and might wander and beg for a living, or even preach, which was not acceptable for women in this era (Grundmann, 1935/1995; Kittel & Suydam, 2004; McDonnell, 1969; Simons, 2001). Two of these solitary beguines used trance dance to present Christ to the world and to claim authority for themselves as laywomen outside the hierarchy of religious power.

Christina the Astonishing and Elisabeth of Spalbeek: Two Beguines Who Danced

Christina the Astonishing (1150–1224) According to thirteenth century Dominican biographer Thomas de Cantimpré (1999), the beguine Christina the Astonishing gave violent performances in which she climbed to the tops of trees or buildings to pray, immersed herself in icy water, or leaped into hot ovens. The people of her town, Saint-Trond in Belgium, thought her mad, but Christina eventually found church approval when religious men and women who came to see her determined that she was inspired. De Cantimpré did not refer to her performances as dances, but said that Christina was physically demonstrating the horrors of purgatory in order to lead people toward salvation.

Some of Christina's performances included trance dance. While praying in a state of "spiritual inebriation" she would sometimes perform contortions in which "all her limbs were gathered together into a ball as if they were hot wax and all that could be perceived of her was a round mass" until she finished praying, whereupon "like a hedgehog her rolled up body returned to its proper shape and the limbs which had been bent formlessly were once again extended out" (p. 24). When someone in Saint-Trond died, Christina would perform. If the person's soul had been damned, she "wept and twisted herself and bent herself backwards and bent and rebent her arms and fingers as if they were pliable and not made of bones" (p. 30). If the dying person had been saved, however, "she leaped and jumped so high that it was a great marvel to see. From behavior like this, the people knew the power of her spirit and could easily mark by her joy or sorrow what would happen to the dying in the town" (p. 31). In other words, Christina's performances were prophetic.

Though not a nun, Christina often spent time at the nearby convent of Saint Catherine. While speaking with the nuns she would sometimes enter trance through performance:

> Her body would roll and whirl around like a hoop … with such extreme violence that the individual limbs of her body could not be distinguished. When she had whirled around for a long time…, it seemed as if she became weakened by the violence of the rolling and all her limbs grew quiet. (p. 36)

After finishing this dance, she would stand up and call the nuns to join her in song: "the nuns of the convent came running from all sides and greatly rejoiced in Christina's solace and she began to sing the *Te Deum laudamus* and all the convent joined in" (p. 36). Afterwards, Christina had no memory of what she had done (Fig. 8.1).

Elisabeth of Spalbeek (1246/7–1304) The beguine Elisabeth of Spalbeek lived near the city of Liège in Belgium in the late thirteenth century. Through dramatic trance dances, she portrayed Christ's Passion at each hour of the divine office, the seven daily times for prayer. Elisabeth was well known in her community for being a holy invalid and for displaying the stigmata, copies of Christ's wounds (Njus, 2011; Rodgers & Ziegler, 1999; Simons, 1994). Philip, abbot of the monastery of Clairvaux, visited Elisabeth in 1267, when she was 20. Observing her, he became convinced of her sanctity and wrote a detailed description of her performances, which he did not call dance, but rather "a wondrous mode of lively representation" (*Catalogus*, 1886, p. 363).

Elisabeth's bed was right off the chapel where she performed, and she would lie in bed before rising to dance. She always performed in a particular order, beginning in stillness and proceeding to specific poses and movements that corresponded to the scripture readings for that hour. Philip understood her stillness to be a trance state:

> Before she rises she is raptured, and for a long time she remains completely stiff in that posture in which she is raptured, without feeling or moving or breathing, like an image of

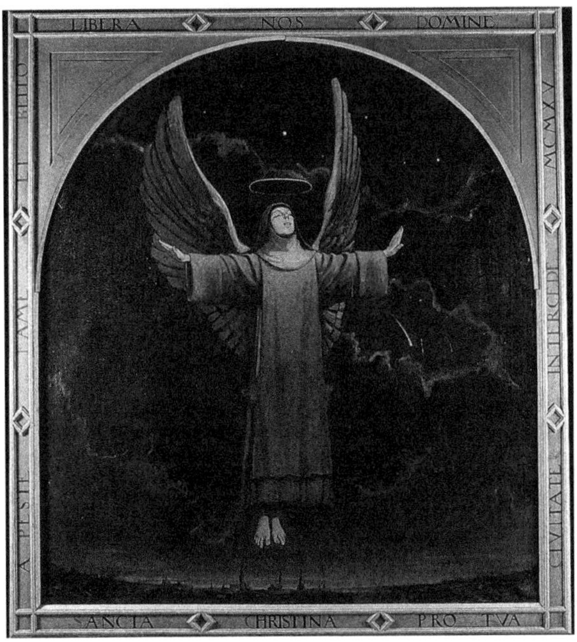
LIBERA NOS DOMINE
CIVITATE INTERCEDE MCMXV
SANCTA CHRISTINA PRO TVA

Fig. 8.1 Christina the Astonishing (1150–1224)

> wood or stone, in such a way that no part of her may be touched or moved, not even the smallest finger, without the whole structure being moved. (p. 364)

After her stillness, Elisabeth rose from her bed and walked back and forth, striking her face repeatedly with her palms, creating a sound that Philip compared to drums or cymbals. She displayed intense emotion: "Frequently she gives out, between her punishments, groans and sobbing as if she were dying" (p. 366). She then moved from striking her face to beating various parts of her body,

> …in such a strong way that other parts of her whole small body bend toward the ground from the weight of the beatings, now on the jaw, now on the back of the head, now between the shoulder blades, now on the neck. And then she strikes herself precipitously upon the previous parts, or with a marvelously curved body dashes her head toward the ground. (pp. 364–365)

Elisabeth's beatings escalated from rhythmic cheek-slapping to striking her entire body to acrobatic feats. Rodgers and Ziegler (1999) point out that striking oneself rhythmically is a method used to induce trance in various cultures throughout the world.

Besides striking herself, Elisabeth also shaped her body into various poses. In one of her most dramatic poses, she performed as Christ on the cross:

> She quickly gets out of bed and places one foot above the other and one wound above the other, standing upright, with her hands and arms stretched out in the form of the cross; … she remains immovable…, with her eyes open but seeing and sensing nothing. (*Catalogus*, 1886, p. 369)

After trancing in this posture for some time, Elisabeth lowered herself backward to the ground, beat her breast repeatedly, and then began to dance along the floor:

> Instead of walking with her feet (because she cannot walk with one foot always set atop the other) she changes position while lying down by rolling herself over her breast and back and sides, in a way that cannot be described. And then she rises quickly and stands upright upon her foot which is the only thing touching the ground, without the support of the other foot or hands. Let the reader note how miraculous this is. (p. 370)

Still in a crucifix shape, Elisabeth rolled on the ground and then rose suddenly to stand balanced on one foot. Philip expressed wonder at the difficulty of her movements and, as he often did, attributed Elisabeth's dance to divine influence (*Catalogus*, 1886).

What meanings did Elisabeth, Christina, and their audiences draw from their trance dances? Since neither woman left a written record, we have only the word of the two men, Thomas and Philip, who observed Christina and Elisabeth, respectively. Both admired the women's performances and considered them authentically holy. From their descriptions, it seems evident that the dancers experienced strong emotions while performing, including joy, sorrow, and pain. They also drew spiritual authority from their performances of trance dance. Christina prophesied through movement and visually taught Christians about the horrors of purgatory. Her trancing seems to have given her authority with the group of nuns, as her dance led them all into a performance of praise. Elisabeth, too, taught others through her performances as she shaped her body into images from scripture. Philip claimed that even illiterate people could understand the faith by watching Elisabeth dance:

> An ignorant man, just as if he were learned, is able to read, not in parchment or paper, but in the limbs and body of our girl . . . a living picture of salvation and an animated narrative of redemption. (p. 373)

Elisabeth's trance dance empowered her to take on a role reserved for male priests, that of representing Christ (Simons, 1994; Rodgers & Ziegler, 1999). Her dedication to a grueling schedule of performances suggests that she found this role fulfilling, a fulfillment that she would otherwise have been denied due to her gender. It is important to note, however, that Christina and Elisabeth's performances were individual and unique. Both used trance dance for religious purposes but were not part of a community of trancers. There was, however, a group of dancers in the fourteenth century who may have practiced trance.

The "Dance Epidemic" of 1374

In 1374, a large group of itinerant dancers appeared in Liége and other cities along the Rhine. They were clearly not from the Rhine area as they used foreign words in their songs; the locals believed they were calling out the names of devils. They had a particular form of dress, with wreaths on their heads and cloths tightly tied around their waists. In the streets and in churches, especially before altars, these dancers performed vigorous movements such as leaping, rolling, and falling to the ground. Sometimes they cried out as if in pain (Backman, 1952; Bartholomew, 2000). As they travelled from city to city, the dancers attracted a following. Church authorities, perhaps afraid of the size and popularity of this dance movement, pronounced the dancers demon-possessed and tried to exorcise them (Waller, 2009).

Many twentieth-century scholars have assumed that the dancers of 1374 were suffering from physical or mental illness, and used the terms "dance epidemic," "dance plague," and "dance mania" to describe the phenomenon (Backman, 1952; Lueger, 2015; Waller, 2009). Others, however, have suggested that the dancers were a traveling religious group (Bartholomew, 2000). It is hard to know what prompted these dancers' performances but since they displayed heightened emotion and their movements sound similar to those used by religious trance dancers in other times and places, it seems likely that they were also trancers, dancing to bring about a transformation in the quality of their lives, whether from sickness to health or from one spiritual state to another.

Trance Dance in Early Nineteenth-Century America

American Context

After the American Revolution (1765–1783), the new country experienced political and social changes including rapid territorial expansion, the growth of cities, sectionalism, and burgeoning industry (Ott & Schell, 2015). Religion was changing as well; the old Calvinist doctrines of predestination no longer meshed with the new American ideals of free will, optimism, and belief in the goodness of humanity (Evans, 2013; McLoughlin, 1978). Methodist, Presbyterian, and Baptist preachers stressed a personal, emotional experience of conversion, a heart religion rather than a head religion. These preachers were especially effective on the sparsely populated frontier. The white settlers who had begun to move into this area were strongly individualistic small farmers with little education or wealth, the structures of civilization were few and far between, and violence was common (Boles, 1972).

In this setting, around 1800 a series of religious revivals began to sweep the new American nation. Sometimes called the Second Great Awakening, these revivals brought an increased emphasis on performance, including trance and dance, and new roles for laypeople, especially women and African-Americans (Kling, 1993; Thomas, 2008).

Revivals started among the congregations of the Presbyterian minister James McGready in Logan County, Kentucky, in the latter part of 1799. By the summer of 1800, revival meetings were springing up all over Kentucky and in neighboring parts of Tennessee, and by 1805 they had spread through the entire South (Boles, 1972; Ott & Schell, 2015). Similar revivals appeared in the cities of the Midwest in the 1820s (McLoughlin, 1978) and also in New England (Kling, 1993), though it was at the outdoor revivals in the South, known as "camp meetings," that trance and dance were most common (Boles, 1972; Evans, 2013).

Attendance at camp meetings could number in the thousands. After the ordained preachers finished, non-clergy continued praying, singing, and preaching to each other long into the night – such lay preaching was known as "exhorting" (Johnson, 1955). Many people at camp meetings, especially women and children, had deeply emotional and physical conversion experiences (Boles, 1972; Thomas, 2008). These experiences transformed their lives both personally and communally. They renounced practices such as gambling, drinking, swearing, and sexual practices or acts regarded by the church as immoral; felt a strong emotional connection to the divine; and were drawn into a new, supportive religious community (Johnson, 1955; Wagner, 1997). Modern-day ravers speak of their first rave experiences in similar terms, as a conversion from a former way of life into a new, transformative community (Sylvan, 2005), albeit one that does not renounce pleasures of the senses.

Trance Dance at Revivals and Camp Meetings

Many people who attended revivals experienced states of trance. In a common pattern, repeated again and again in autobiographical accounts, people would hear preaching, enter a state of heightened emotion (often fearing God's anger), and fall to the ground. Barton Warren Stone (1847), a Presbyterian preacher during the Kentucky revivals, described how those who fell "continued for hours together in an apparently breathless and motionless state – sometimes for a few moments reviving, and exhibiting symptoms of life by a deep groan, or piercing shriek, or by a prayer for mercy most fervently uttered" (p. 34). James Finley (1853), a Methodist minister, noted that some who fell appeared lifeless, while others showed signs of consciousness:

> Some were unable to stand, and yet had the use of their hands and could converse with companions. Others were unable to speak. The pulse became weak, and they drew a difficult breath about once a minute. In many instances they became cold. Breathing, pulsation, and all signs of life forsook them for hours. (p. 367)

The person who fell and lay in trance might feel an altered sense of self; some saw or heard divine revelations. Zilpha Elaw, a free black woman who became a preacher, felt the overwhelming presence of God at a camp meeting in 1817 and fell, later reflecting:

> While I was thus prostrate on the earth, my spirit seemed to ascend up into the clear circle of the sun's disc; and, surrounded and engulphed in the glorious effulgence of his rays, I distinctly heard a voice speak unto me . . . Truly I durst not move, because God was so powerfully near to me; for the space of several hours I appeared not to be on earth, but far above all earthly things. (Andrews, 1986, pp. 66–67)

Elaw's sense of self changed, as she experienced herself lifted above the earth and swallowed up in God. This experience of changed consciousness is an indicator of trance.

After lying for some time, trancers would rise up to shout aloud, sing, clap their hands, leap, spin, or dance. Stone (1847) saw the converted shout with joy: "The gloomy cloud, which had covered their faces, seemed gradually and visibly to disappear, and hope in smiles brightened into joy – they would rise shouting deliverance" (pp. 34–35). Not only the new converts shouted; other Christians shouted as well, to express their own joy and to help others become converted. Peter Cartwright (1857), a Methodist, was preaching in Ohio in 1805 when over 30 people fell. He stopped preaching in order to pray for them, noting, "There were a few scattered members of the Church around this place, who got happy and shouted aloud for joy, and joined in and exhorted sinners" (p. 96). This sort of performance appears in multiple accounts, with converted Christians gathering in circles around fallen "sinners" or "mourners" to pray, sing, shout, or dance in order to assist them in finding salvation (Taves, 1999).

This common conversion experience of falling and rising, with its heightened affect and loss of a sense of self, shows the hallmarks of trance, as does another performance known as the "jerks" or the "jerking exercise." This was a repetitive jerking movement in a single part of the body or the whole body:

> When the head alone was affected, it would be jerked backward and forward, or from side to side, so quickly that the features of the face could not be distinguished. When the whole system was affected, I have seen the person stand in one place, and jerk backward and forward in quick succession, their head nearly touching the floor behind and before. (Stone, 1847, p. 40)

Cartwright (1857) believed that jerking was involuntary. Those affected were "seized with a compulsive jerking all over, which they could not by any possibility avoid, and the more they resisted the more they jerked" (p. 48). Lorenzo Dow, another revival preacher, agreed that the impulse to jerk was involuntary, but that "the consent of the will" was required – in other words, a person had to give in to the impulse for the jerks to take hold. Jerking could be exhausting to those who performed it, so might eventually lead to falling (Watson, 1819).

Congregations at revivals also performed movements that contemporary observers labeled as dancing. Cartwright (1857) and Dow (as cited in Watson, 1819) both saw jerking turn into dancing. Dancing, in fact, could ease the violence of the jerks: "persons taken with the jerks, to obtain relief…would rise up and dance" (Cartwright, 1857, p. 48). Stone (1847) also saw people move from jerking to dancing:

> The subject, after jerking awhile, began to dance, and then the jerks would cease. Such dancing was indeed heavenly to the spectators; there was nothing in it…calculated to excite levity in the beholders. The smile of heaven shone on the countenance of the subject… Sometimes the motion was quick and sometimes slow. Thus they continued to move forward and backward in the same track…till nature seemed exhausted, and they would fall prostrate…, unless caught by those standing by. While thus exercised, I have heard their solemn praises and prayers ascending to God. (p. 40)

This trance dance clearly brought joy to performers. Stone distinguished this sacred dancing from secular social dancing by pointing out that there was no "levity" even though the dancers smiled with joy and seemed as graceful as angels.

What did these performances mean to those who experienced and those who observed? Clergy often interpreted the performances of their congregations as a sign of God's presence, affirming their preaching. Cartwright (1857) said that when he spoke "an awful power fell on the congregation, and they instantly fell right and left, and cried aloud for mercy" (p. 86). Revival preachers wanted their congregations to experience God visibly. While they might condemn certain types of performance as wild or extravagant, they saw most performances as miraculous signs, indications that the revivals were God's work (Cartwright, 1857; Finley, 1853).

Performers often experienced a deep sense of joy. When Stone (1847) asked about the inner experiences of those who fell and jerked, they told him, "those were among the happiest seasons of their lives" (p. 40). John Fanning Watson, a Methodist who was against vigorous performances, nonetheless noted that a woman who leaped and shouted during services “found a lively sensibility of pleasure in the exercise, but dreadful deadness when quiet” (Watson, 1819, p. 19). Dow, too, learned from the performers of the jerks and dancing that “the dancing if resisted makes very great deadness of mind” (p. 158).

These reports of pleasurable emotions are unsurprising, since experiencing joy during trancing is common (Becker, 2004). Ravers today may feel a euphoric joy during the peak moments of their music- and dance-induced trancing (Sylvan, 2005). A feeling of “deadness” followed by release and joy in performance is a powerful impetus for dance, both in the nineteenth century and today (Bond & Stinson, 2000/2001; St. John, 2004). These intense moments of joy increase the performers’ senses of well-being and, when experienced communally, draw people together into a close-knit and supportive group (Thomas, 2008).

Women’s Participation in Revivals

In early America, women outnumbered men in the rolls of church membership, but during the revivals of the early nineteenth century this trend became even more pronounced. Attending revivals gave women opportunities for socialization, public speaking, and intense emotional experiences that could help them shape their identities apart from their male relatives (Kling, 1993). Women were more likely than men to perform at revivals. John Dixon Long (1857), a Methodist from Maryland, describing a prayer meeting among black converts, pointed out that the women shouted louder and more vigorously than the men (p. 383). At one of her prayer meetings, Jarena Lee noted a bench of women all falling and screaming at once (Andrew, 1986, p. 45). This abundance of female performance drew the attention and ire of preachers. Watson (1819) complained,

> Why is it that for one man who jumps or screams, there are so many women? . . . How is it that many instances of women who, while single, are conspicuous in these things desist altogether after marriage? (p. 27)

Since women, especially single women, were more likely to perform, Watson found such performances suspect.

Like Christian women of the late medieval era, American women drew spiritual authority from their performances of trance and dance. In the nineteenth century none of the major American denominations ordained women, but women still found ways to perform their faith as well as preach it. At revivals, one or two women’s performances often provided the spark that converted others. Stone (1847) observed this when two girls were “struck down under the preaching of the word.” They fell, lay motionless in trance, then sprang up and spoke of their experiences, and “their addresses made deep impressions on the congregation” (p. 36). Finley (1853) tells of Eliza Hawkins, who fell in the road on her way home from a camp meeting. She was carried, seemingly lifeless, back to the meeting spot and many people gathered around her. They sang and prayed for 32 h as she remained in trance, after which Eliza:

> …sprang instantly to her feet, and commenced singing and shouting alternately. Her face seemed lighted up with an unearthly radiance; and, as she spoke of Jesus and heaven, in strains of the most inimitable eloquence and sweetness, the whole congregation was overwhelmed, and we felt ourselves in the presence of a superior being, rather than of an artless, unsophisticated country girl. (p. 231)

Witnessing Eliza's performance invigorated the camp meeting, which went on for 10 more days, with over 100 people converted.

Zilpha Elaw had a similar influence when at a camp meeting she fell, lay in trance, and received revelations:

> When I recovered from the trance or ecstasy into which I had fallen, the first thing I observed was, that hundreds of persons were standing around me weeping . . .when the prayer meeting afterwards commenced, the Lord opened my mouth in public prayer; …it seemed as if I heard my God rustling in the tops of the mulberry trees. Oh, how precious was this day to my soul! I was after this very frequently requested to present my petitions to the throne of grace in the public meetings at the camp. (Andrews, 1986, p. 67)

Elaw's performance of falling and trance, like those of Eliza and many other unnamed women, had a powerful effect on those around her. Her trance gave her courage to speak publicly, and the visible sign of her performance showed others that she was authorized by God.

This divine authorization could give women power over those to whom they would usually be subordinate. Cartwright (1857) saw a Baptist minister's daughter become converted at a camp meeting. The young woman, after lying on the ground and praying all night, "rose and went over the camp-ground like a top." When she encountered her father, she "begged him to repent and get his soul converted. She made him kneel down, and she engaged him in mighty prayer" (p. 121). Despite her father's age and status, the minister's daughter became his teacher through her experience and performance of the divine.

When women usurped male clerical authority it could lead to a power struggle. A Methodist preacher's class meeting was disrupted when a woman "rose up to speak her state – after declaring her sense of a glorious change wrought, she began to close it with stamping, clapping her hands, and at last jumping" (Watson, 1819, p. 19). When the preacher asked her to sit down, she shouted louder, "No man shall stop me from praising God aloud! No man shall make me be still. You, Sir, are an opposer to the work of God, and I will shout his praise" (p. 19). This woman understood her leaping and shouting to be authorized by God. The preacher, however, valued orderliness above ecstasy. Taves (1999) discusses this same phenomenon where female congregation members appropriated power from preachers by disrupting meetings. Since Christian women who leaped, shouted, and danced believed that their performances were a necessary work of God that improved the lives of their communities by bringing sinners to salvation, they felt justified in disregarding preachers who tried to stop them.

African-American Participation in Revivals

African-Americans played an important role in early nineteenth century revivals and derived benefits from trance dance. Early American slave owners had cared little about sharing Christianity with their slaves (Thomas, 2008), but African-Americans began to convert in the waves of revival that swept the nation first in the 1740s and again around 1800. According to Raboteau (1978/2004), at camp meetings African-Americans experienced the same pattern of falling, trance, leaping up and shouting that white converts did, though African-Americans danced more frequently than whites, used dance to achieve trance, and had a particularly rhythmic and musical quality to their performances. Black converts felt a special connection to danced worship because of their African heritage (Thomas, 2008). For African-American Christians, singing was closely connected to dancing (Todd, 1886):

> As the leader struck the first notes..., peculiar motions, confined to no particular portion or member of the body, indicated the time in which the piece was to be rendered; and significant glances in the direction of the chief "men-singers and women-singers" brought them, one by one, into position for effective action, in a hollow circle facing inward. The space thus inclosed was devoted to penitents. (p. 180)

Creating a ring of singers around penitents or mourners was common among both whites and blacks. Taves (1999) suggests that such praying rings had both African and European influences, producing an interracial amalgam. In the above description, the uniquely African-American element is not the ring but the "peculiar motions" of the song-leader, which suggest the African aesthetics of polyrhythm and polycentrism – performing multiple different rhythms at once and using all parts of the body equally (Asante, 1994).

African-Americans often danced while singing hymns and spirituals: "With every word so sung, they have a sinking of one or other leg of the body alternately; producing an audible sound of the feet at every step" (Watson, 1819, pp. 30–31). Later in the century Payne (1888) observed African-American Christians dancing in a ring at a camp meeting near Philadelphia. As they sang, they "clapped their hands and stamped their feet" (p. 253). This rhythmic, circular song and dance later became known as the ring shout, a sacred dance form with African roots that survived into the twentieth century in the Sea Islands of Georgia and South Carolina (Raboteau, 1978/2004; Stuckey, 2002). The early nineteenth-century revivals, where trancing and performance were encouraged, seem to have been a fertile ground for the creation of new performance traditions for both whites and blacks, and an environment in which African-influenced dancing was not out of place.

For African-Americans, dance had a special association with trance. Long (1857) witnessed a dance at a prayer meeting in which, after singing and praying,

> the company will then form a circle around the singer, and jump and bawl to their heart's content . . . After a prolonged continuation of these violent evolutions, some will swoon away; their muscles will become perfectly rigid, and they will lie as motionless as though they were dead. Sand thrown in their eyes, while in this state, will not make them wink. Many persons think this condition is the result of supernatural power, and regard the subjects of it with reverence. (pp. 383–84)

While falling in a motionless trance was common to both black and white Christians, among white converts trance seems to have been induced by hearing powerful preaching and feeling a sense of one's own sin. In this all-black prayer meeting, a long period of rhythmic performance preceded falling and trance. The dancers may have been dancing with the intent to achieve trance; ritualized performance of rhythmic movement is a traditional way of entering trance and continues to be used in West African religious practices in continental Africa and the African diaspora (Ajayi, 1994; Lum, 2000; Olupona & Rey, 2008; Saraiva, 2013). As African-Americans performed trance dance they were able to improve their quality of life by experiencing feelings of joy and, at least temporarily, softening the effects of external oppression through communal bonding (Thomas, 2008).

The dances of African-American Christians likely influenced white forms of worship. Taves (1999) sees evidence for a give-and-take between black and white Christians in the development of the ring shout, observing that a prayer circle around struggling sinners had a European background and was first seen among whites, while formal movement around the mourners seems to have been more African-influenced. Other evidence for the influence of black performance on white performance includes Watson's (1891) complaints about jumping and shouting in white churches. He claims that such performances "began in Virginia, and as I have heard, among the blacks" (p. 27). Todd (1886) reports that when, at the end of an interracial camp meeting black Christians went "leaping, shuffling, and dancing" around the camp, whites would sometimes "echo back, in happy response, the jubilant shout of the rejoicing slaves" (Todd, 1886, pp. 182–83). It is common in the study of dance and music to find that performance styles beginning in African-American culture, from jazz to hip-hop, have later been appropriated by white culture (Given, 2015; Gottschild, 2003). It would not be surprising if, long before the Cakewalk or the Charleston, African-American styles of song and dance were influencing the worship of white Christians.

Like women who shouted during sermons, taking power away from the preacher, black performers also appropriated power. Todd (1886) observed that, in interracial preaching services, it was common for African-Americans to call out praise or suggestions during the sermon. These remarks could be helpful to the white preacher who paid attention: "Many a discourse, really but a moderately good exhortation, was metamorphosed into a great sermon . . . by a volley of well-timed negro shouts, poured in at a critical juncture" (p. 184). The influence of black congregation members extended beyond the preacher. When African-Americans began to shout during a service, the performance "quite frequently would be echoed back again from the more impressible and enthusiastic in front, until a general shout of victory crowned the hour, and scores of awakened souls were weeping and pleading for mercy" (p. 183). The people "in front" were white (African-Americans often sat behind the preacher in segregated camp meetings). These church services provided a situation in which African Americans in the congregation possessed an authority, denied them elsewhere, to lead the whites (from behind) toward a spiritual transformation.

Conclusion

For Christians in both late medieval Europe and early nineteenth-century America trance dance brought new, often highly enjoyable and satisfying, experiences and dimensions to their lives. Dancers frequently experienced joy and release, though joy was not the only emotion; they might also weep and cry out. Trance dances were more than emotional outlets, however: they were also transformative, empowering individuals, especially those at the bottom of oppressive, hierarchical power structures, to claim direct inspiration from God and gain spiritual authority. Trancers prophesied, received revelations, and preached, sometimes usurping power from the clergy as they did so. This spiritual authority could increase an individual's sense of purpose and fulfillment. A Christian woman in thirteenth-century Europe who believed that preaching was her life's purpose could not be ordained as a priest but she could, by preaching through dance, fulfill her calling.

Through trance dance, groups of Christians became communities. United by common belief and a common, ecstatic experience of the divine, Christian trancers reinforced their own faith identities and forged connections across race and gender divides. Trance dancers were also influential in social change. The revivals of the early nineteenth century fostered the growth of voluntary societies that focused on temperance, foreign missions, women's rights, and the abolition of slavery (Evan, 2013; McLoughlin, 1978).

Trance dance, in both religious and non-religious settings, continues to play a positive role in adding important dimensions to people's lives today. In Pentecostal churches in the United States and throughout the world, worshippers in trance fall, rise, and shout for joy (Becker, 2004). Young people seeking connection crowd onto dance floors and move together to driving electronic rhythms, transcending their individual selves in what many describe as a mystical union (St. John, 2004; Sylvan, 2005). Trance dance continues to open a path toward regions of experience that humans have always sought beyond economic survival and the mundane: ecstatic joy, empowered purpose, and immersive community.

References

Ajayi, O. S. (1994). In contest: The dynamics of African religious dances. In K. W. Asante (Ed.), *African dance: An artistic, historical and philosophical inquiry* (pp. 183–202). Trenton, NJ: Africa World.

Amoah, M. (2004). Christian musical worship and "hostility to the body". *Implicit Religion, 7*, 59–75.

Andrews, W. (Ed.). (1986). *Sisters of the spirit: Three black women's autobiographies of the nineteenth century*. Bloomington, IN: Indiana University Press.

Arcangeli, A. (1992). Dance and punishment. *Dance Research, 10*(2), 30–42.

Asante, K. (1994). The Zimbabwean dance aesthetic: Senses, canons, and characteristics. In K. W. Asante (Ed.), *African dance: An artistic, historical and philosophical inquiry* (pp. 203–220). Trenton, NJ: Africa World.

Backman, E. L. (1952). *Religious dances in the Christian church and in popular medicine*. London: George Allen & Unwin.
Bartholomew, R. E. (2000). Rethinking the dancing mania. *Skeptical Inquirer, 24*, 42–47.
Becker, J. (2004). *Deep listeners: Music, emotion, and trancing*. Bloomington, IN: Indiana University Press.
Boles, J. (1972). *The great revival 1787–1805: The origins of the southern evangelical mind*. Lexington, NC: University Press of Kentucky.
Bond, K. E., & Stinson, S. W. (2000/2001). "I feel like I'm going to take off!" Young people's experiences of the superordinary in dance. *Dance Research Journal, 32*(2), 52–87.
Cartwright, P. (1857). In W. P. Strickland (Ed.), *Autobiography of Peter Cartwright, the backwoods preacher*. New York: Carlton & Lanahan.
Catalogus codicum hagiographicorum bibliothecae Regiae Bruxellensis (1886). Vol. 1. Brussels: (n.p.).
de Cantimpré, T. (1999). *The life of Christina the Astonishing* (M. H. King, Trans.). Toronto, ON: Peregrina. (Original work published 1232).
Evans, C. H. (2013). *Histories of American Christianity: An introduction*. Waco, TX: Baylor University Press.
Finley, J. B. (1853). *Autobiography of Rev. James B. Finley, or, pioneer life in the West*. Cincinnati, OH: Cranston & Curts.
Frembgen, J. W. (2012). DHamāl and the performing body: Trance dance in the devotional Sufi practice of Pakistan. *Journal of Sufi Studies, 1*(1), 77–113.
Given, W. (2015). Lindy hop, community, and the isolation of appropriation. In N. George-Graves (Ed.), *Oxford handbook of dance and theatre* (pp. 729–752). Oxford, UK: Oxford University Press.
Gottschild, B. D. (2003). *The black dancing body: A geography from coon to cool*. London: Palgrave Macmillan.
Grundmann, H. (1995). *Religious movements of the middle ages* (S. Rowan, Trans.). Notre Dame, IN: University of Notre Dame Press. (Original work published 1935).
Hamilton, B. (2003). *Religion in the medieval west* (2nd ed.). London: Hodder Arnold.
Johnson, C. (1955). *The frontier camp meeting*. Dallas, TX: Southern Methodist University Press.
Kittel, A., & Suydam, M. (2004). *The texture of society: Medieval women in the southern low countries*. London: Palgrave.
Kling, D. (1993). *A field of divine wonders: The new divinity and village revivals in northwestern Connecticut 1792–1822*. University Park, PA: The Pennsylvania State University Press.
LaMothe, K. (2015). *Why we dance: A philosophy of bodily becoming*. New York: Columbia University Press.
Long, J. (1857). *Pictures of slavery in church and state*. Philadelphia, PA: J. Long.
Lueger, M. (2015). Dance and the plague: Epidemic choreomania and Artaud. In N. George-Graves (Ed.), *Oxford handbook of dance and theatre* (pp. 948–964). Oxford, UK: Oxford University Press.
Lum, K. A. (2000). *Praising his name in the dance: Spirit possession in the spiritual Baptist faith and Orisha work in Trinidad, West Indies*. New York: Routledge.
Maynard, S. W. (1992). *Dance in the arts of the middle ages (doctoral dissertation)*. Tallahassee, FL: Florida State University.
McDonnell, E. (1969). *The beguines and beghards in medieval culture*. New York: Octagon.
McGinn, B. (1991). *The flowering of mysticism: Men and women in the new mysticism (1200–1350)*. New York: Crossroad.
McLoughlin, W. (1978). *Revivals, awakenings, and reform: An essay on religion and social change in America, 1607–1977*. Chicago: The University of Chicago Press.
Mews, C. (2009). Liturgists and dance in the twelfth century: The witness of John Beleth and Sicard of Cremona. *Church History, 78*(3), 512–548.
Njus, J. (2011). What did it mean to act in the middle ages? Elisabeth of Spalbeek and *Imitatio Christi*. *Theatre Journal, 63*(1), 1–21.

Olupona, J. K., & Rey, T. (2008). *Òrìṣà devotion as world religion: The globalization of Yorùbá religious culture*. Madison: University of Wisconsin Press.
Ott, D., & Schell, H. (2015). *Christian thought in America: A brief history*. Minneapolis, MN: Fortress.
Payne, D. (1888). *Recollections of seventy years*. Nashville, TN: A.M.E. Sunday School Union.
Raboteau, A. (1978/2004). *Slave religion. The 'invisible institution' in the antebellum South*. Oxford, UK: Oxford University Press.
Rodgers, S., & Ziegler, J. (1999). Elisabeth of Spalbeek's trance dance of faith: A performance theory interpretation from anthropological and art historical perspectives. In M. Suydam & J. Ziegler (Eds.), *Performance and transformation: New approaches to late medieval spirituality* (pp. 299–355). New York: St. Martin's.
Saraiva, C. (2013). Pretos Velhos across the Atlantic: Afro-Brazilian religions in Portugal. In C. Rocha & M. Vasquez (Eds.), *The diaspora of Brazilian religions* (pp. 197–222). Leiden, NL: Brill.
Simons, W. (1994). Reading a saint's body: Rapture and bodily movement in the *vitae* of thirteenth-century beguines. In S. Kay & M. Rubin (Eds.), *Framing medieval bodies* (pp. 10–23). Manchester, UK: Manchester University Press.
Simons, W. (2001). *Cities of ladies: Beguine communities in the medieval low countries, 1200–1565*. Philadelphia: University of Pennsylvania Press.
St. John, G. (Ed.). (2004). *Rave culture and religion*. New York: Routledge.
Stone, B. (1847). *The biography of Eld. Barton Warren Stone, written by himself: With additions and reflections by Elder John Rogers, written in part by John Rogers*. Cincinnati, OH: (n. p.).
Stuckey, P. (2002). Christian conversion and the challenge of dance. In T. DeFrantz (Ed.), *Dancing many drums: Excavations in African American dance* (pp. 39–58). Madison: University of Wisconsin Press.
Sylvan, R. (2005). *Trance formation: The spiritual and religious dimensions of global rave culture*. New York: Routledge.
Taves, A. (1999). *Fits, trances, and visions: Experiencing religion and explaining experience from Wesley to James*. Princeton, NJ: Princeton University Press.
Thomas, K. (2008). *The religious dancing of American slaves, 1820–1865: Spiritual ecstasy at baptisms, funerals, and Sunday meetings*. Lewiston, NY: Edwin Mellen.
Todd, R. (1886). *Methodism of the peninsula*. Philadelphia, PA: Methodist Episcopal.
Van Oort, J. (2009). *Dancing in body and spirit: Dance and sacred performance in thirteenth-century beguine texts (doctoral dissertation)*. Philadelphia, PA: Temple University.
Wagner, A. (1997). *Adversaries of dance: From the puritans to the present*. Urbana, IL: University of Illinois Press.
Waller, J. (2009). *Dancing plague: The strange, true story of an extraordinary illness*. Naperville, IL: Sourcebooks.
Watson, J. F. (1819). *Methodist error: Friendly Christian advice to those Methodists who indulge in extravagant emotions and bodily exercises*. Trenton, NJ: D. & E. Fenton.
Younger, P. (2001). *Playing host to deity: Festival religion in the south Indian tradition*. Oxford, UK: Oxford University Press.

Part III
Philosophical Perspectives

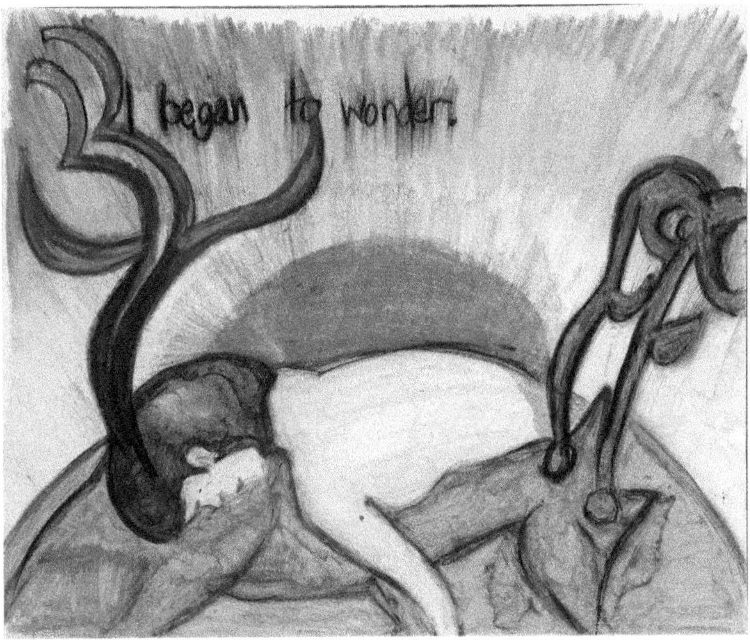

II I began to wonder (M. Shanahan)

Chapter 9
How *Seudati* Put Me in Touch with Birds

Sally Gardner

> Vitality affects give rise to forms of life that are fundamentally shared. …
> There is no reason why this nonlocal linkage cannot reach into the sky. (Massumi, 2003, pp. 7, 12)

An acquaintance from Aceh told me how in his region villagers will call to each other to come and shoo away the birds from the rice fields. As he talks I imagine the people running and calling out from different directions and the birds flying up and perhaps wheeling around before disappearing into the bright or clouded sky or, alternatively, coming to land again elsewhere, possibly lining up on a wire, or settling temporarily in a tree. This image of a kind of sport or contest between birds and people over rice – whether apt or not in local terms – comes to me strongly because I have been involved in learning *seudati*.

Since having the opportunity to learn some of the movement aspects of this Acehnese music/dance form in Aceh, Sumatra, Indonesia in 2012 I have become more aware, observant and discerning of, and interested in birds. You might say that my world is now different from what it was before I had my encounter with *seudati*. I feel that I possess to some extent a new quality of life in which a relation to birds is part of my being and comes through my sensing, perceiving body. This relation in turn gives me an imaginative investment in *seudati* that is alive and ongoing.

Previously, I would have construed dance practices as effecting a change in my body, thus isolating my bodily self from my world, even as I understand and acknowledge different dance styles and the social contexts of their practice to constitute different worlds, or different sub-cultures. I emphasize that there has been a change in my world, furthermore, because this feels different to the mere acquisition of information in a cognitive sense. This feeling could be similar to Daniel Vermonden's (2011) reflection in "Cuculano: Myths, Legends, Tales, Fables or Sedimented Tools for the Transmission of a Perception? Questioning Mind-Centred

S. Gardner (✉)
Deakin University, Geelong, VIC, Australia
e-mail: sally.gardner@deakin.edu.au

K. Bond (ed.), *Dance and the Quality of Life*, Social Indicators Research Series 73,
https://doi.org/10.1007/978-3-319-95699-2_9

Theories and Assumptions of Knowledge Transmission," where he writes of studying story forms in Buton, Indonesia, saying, "...I had rather the impression that the world was changing" (p. 41).

In this chapter, I discuss the background to this experience and try to theorise mechanisms by which it occurred. My broader aim is to use this personal, cross-cultural experience to suggest how dance practices have potential to maintain in play, and through time, heterogeneous cultural elements and perceptions. Statements made about *seudati* in this chapter are based on research in a body of material available in library collections/online databases in the English-speaking West, and my understanding of physical experiences and conversations I had with *seudati* practitioners on two visits to Banda Aceh in 2012 and with others in Melbourne in 2013. The practitioners include the late Pak Zulfikhermi, Cut Yuza Nadhira, Cut Zona Anjana, Pak Jamil Cehmin, and Bang Murtala.

Seudati: Background

There is no doubt that *seudati* contains what I will call "avian" characteristics. The written archive contains numerous, often apparently minor, references to the form's avian dimensions, including mention of bird-related costume elements, dance formations, and a relation to the cockfight (Amir, 2005, 2006; Kartomi, 2003, 2004). These references exist somewhat in the margins of discussion about *seudati*, and this could relate to the fact that foregrounding so-called "animist" values is not encouraged by various state authorities in Indonesia, nor has it been since colonial times (Geertz, 1975).

At present, *seudati* has official state recognition and promotion, and at stake is the perception of Aceh or of Indonesia as "modern," both at home and abroad. In addition, discussion or description of *seudati* by Westerners has tended to come from scholars or visitors who have not been in a position to explore the embodied dimensions of the dance directly – like Margaret Kartomi (1984), an Australian ethnomusicologist renowned for her documentation and analysis of Sumatran musical forms and practices, or like the colonial era anthropologist, Christian Hurgronje, who was a spy for the Dutch government in the late 1800s (see De Vries, 2011). Dancers, generally, can be familiar with the phenomenon whereby somatic, experiential and kinaesthetic dimensions of practices are not well recognised or discoursed in official knowledges.

Seudati is performed currently by groups of eight, usually males (musician-dancers), in addition to two "alternating solo singers" (*aneuk syahe*). In this case, it is known as *seudati agam,* whereas performed by eight women it is called *seudati inong* (Kartomi, 1999, p.12). To my knowledge, based on seeing the *seudati* practice and performances of members of *Sanggar Leumpia* in Banda Aceh, the terms *agam* and *inong* are names, as one might name a male or female child (respectively), and do not indicate different versions of the form other than in relation to the placement of the characteristic body slapping (sides of the chest for men, sides of the hips for women). There may be regional differences, however, in the form. *Seudati* denotes a combination of rhythmic body percussion, dance choreography, storytelling, and recitation of love or other poems, along with some religious pedagogy (Kayam, as cited in Raseuki, 1993, p. 2). *Seudati* comprises a number of different named sections, each quite distinct in tone and contents, some or all of which will be performed on any one occasion depending, in the present era, on time constraints and decided by the lead dancer.

Since colonial times *seudati* has been resilient in having survived falling in and out of favour with various authorities (Amir, 2006). It is currently learned and performed for both state sponsored events and occasions, and is to some extent still passed on in villages and learned in independent *sanggars* (studios or clubs) such as the *Sanggar Leumpia* in Banda Aceh which I visited twice, once with a group of university students undertaking a dance study tour. Hurgronje (1906) described and discussed *seudati* in his two volume report *The Achehnese,* noting it mainly as a vehicle for Islamic messages. Kartomi (1984) mentions it being a "former court dance" that displays the legendary martial skills of the Acehnese and the bravery of soldiers about to go into battle (p. 19). She classifies *seudati* ethnomusicologically as a standing rather than sitting "body percussion" form.

Comprising as it does movements, body percussion rhythms, song, story, and prayer, *seudati* has great capacity for a range of ironic or reflexive meanings and subtexts. At the verbal level, according to Iwan Amir (2005), it is a means to express prevailing opinions through criticism, jokes, and ribaldry, and makes room for up-to-date story-telling "tucked away in the background" (n.p.), including in the *estra* or *lanie* section when performers include contemporary songs and other material from worldwide (Kartomi, 2012, p. 305).

Even though numerous descriptions trace its origins to early Muslim saints in Aceh and focus on the religious content of the songs, according to Amir (2005) *seudati* represents a counter-point to religiosity, playing against the stereotype of Acehnese identity as "predominantly segregated and knee-deep in Islam" (n.p.). In fact, Amir (2006) writes that at the first modern Festival of Acehnese Arts in 1958, "The *ulama* vetoed *seudati* and some even declared it to be *haram*" ("forbidden" in Islam) (p. 135). This banning had a complex background in colonial and post-colonial politics and in the fact that seudati lyrics were a place for lively critique of religiosity (pp. 130–137). It may also suggest that *seudati* was, at the time, deemed irreligious and backward on account of its animistic elements. For a video of *seudati* see, for example: http://www.seputaraceh.com/read/7016/2012/04/13/seudati-aceh-tarian-gembira-penuh-heroik.

Without doubt, *seudati* has been a vehicle to spread Islamic ideas, to comment ironically or critically on them, and contains non- or pre-Islamic elements. Our teacher at *Sanggar Lempia*, Pak Hermi, said that *seudati* contained or could contain songs and movements from around the world (*seluruh dunia ada geraknya di dalam seudati*) possibly referring to the *estra* or *lanie* section mentioned above. He also said that *seudati* was *induk tari sedunia,* the "mother of all dances" or "pregnant with dances of the world." Further, it was important to learn (movements) from nature or *alam* ("world," "realm," or "nature") – for example, listening to the fall or movement of leaves in the wind, going in a boat to learn the movement of waves, or being guided by animals (*jurus binatang*). Similarly, in a presentation in Jakarta in 2006, Syeh Lah Geunta said the movements of *seudati* grew out of a closeness to nature. "You can make the motions of waves and trees," he said. The sense I obtained from Pak Hermi was of *seudati* as a vast archive or repository of memory, knowledge, perceptions and meanings.

It is worth noting that Hurgronje (1906) describes and includes a photograph of two young boys dressed in a feminine way as members of a *seudati* troupe, a practice that apparently continued to some extent up till the 1980s (p. 221). Based on comparisons with Indian examples such the *gotipua* singer-dancers of Odisha, a phenomenon associated with changes to temple dance practices during the period of the Mughal invasion (sixteenth century) and prohibition of women appearing in public (Allen, 1997; Citaristi, 2001), the presence of young boys could suggest that the form may have pre-Islamic roots and may once have been primarily a women's form. Amir (2006) notes, however, that there are many examples of cross-dressing (boys) in performance forms throughout Southeast Asia, and he considers the boys in *seudati* to have been the troupe's singers (*aneuk syahe*) rather than performing as dancers.

Learning *Seudati*

My experience with *seudati* is discussed here against the current background of a certain Islamisation and nationalisation of *seudati* and thus a potential loss (or temporary eclipse) of heterogeneity in its values and meanings and in the social/cultural memory it might carry forward. Ashis Nandy (2002) notes how both secular modernity and official religion share similar values of rationality and logic. He makes a distinction between religion as "faith" on the one hand and "ideology" on the other:

> By faith I mean religion as a way of life, a tradition which is definitionally non-monolithic and operationally plural... By ideology I mean religion as a sub-national, national or cross-national identifier of populations contesting for...non-religious usually political or socio-economic, interests... The modern state always prefers to deal with religious ideologies rather than faiths. (pp. 62–63)

In Indonesia, Islam is often viewed and valued as modern in distinction from other customs or *adat* (Abdullah, 1966), for example cockfighting (Geertz, 1975), which may be viewed as "backward," "irrational," and not befitting a modern nation (Butterworth, 2011; Feillard & Madinier, 2011). My linking *seudati* explicitly with birds, therefore, may associate it (and thus those who perform it) with the backward and superstitious.

Reticence to make explicit reference to a connection with birds or with the cockfight might also be related to a preference of senior teachers that *seudati* remain a form of secret knowledge. Writing on Javanese practices and forms, Foley (1990) says that because "principles of *ilmu gaib* (secret mystical knowledge) and *kabatinan* (spiritual practice) are involved with most traditional performance, the conversations that surround verbalizations about it are charged" (p. 77, f/n 1).

For my own part, the new attention to or knowledge of birds to which this form opened me is not of a scientific or taxonomic order, nor is it necessarily an Acehnese knowledge, as I am not claiming to have come to experience *seudati* in a more Acehnese way – not least because I assume that Acehneseness itself is heterogenous. Similarly, this discussion of *seudati* is not ethnomusicological, choreological, anthropological, ethnographic or historical, even if it draws on an archive established within those fields. It is not the result of a long period of fieldwork supported by a rigorous formation in, say, anthropological or sociological practice and observation. I want to say less what *seudati is or means,* and more instead what it *did* in my case.

Initially, I did not make a connection between the *seudati* practice that I saw and avian elements or qualities. When, as a casual visitor with a background in American modern dance, I first saw this music/dance form being rehearsed and learned at the *Sanggar Leumpia*, I appreciated it for its three dimensionality and sense of "the back." The eight young women, dressed mostly in tracksuit pants and T-shirts, who were practising under the guidance of Pak Hermi, seemed to weave around each other and turn upon themselves in surprising and unpredictable ways. Changes of speed or timing were also a feature, as was slapping the hips and clicking the fingers. I liked this form very much because of its dynamic and playfully complex arrangements and qualities (I did not understand the verbal components), and it appeared to have quite a different premise to the local dances I had become familiar with such as the *rateb meuseukat* or *ratoh duek* – both body percussion forms in which performers kneel side by side in a line, or the *ranup lampuan* where the women elegantly carry and present their betel offerings to guests.

When I was trying to learn *seudati* moves from teacher Pak Hermi and his assistants Cut Yuza and Zona Anjana, as a beginner I really struggled with the rhythm and patterns because I could no longer step with certainty or ease or with the familiar sense of feeling the counterthrust from the floor, even though I could see that for Pak Hermi and the others it made physical sense. When you shift your weight in slow or fast locomotor steps in *seudati* you have to lift your lower leg in a lightly accented way before putting it down to complete the weight transfer. The feeling of a step's completion is somewhat undercut, however, by the subsequent lightly accented lifting up of the *other* lower leg. In other words, instead of placing the weight *down,* the locomotion in *seudati* requires that you somewhat *retract* from the ground.

The most basic locomotion was confusing for me in what I would now call its avian aspects. The way of raising the arms with an impulse from the back of the shoulders and the particular way the arms folded down to slap the sides of the body (of the chest for men, hips for women) was also somewhat bird-like. The physical confusion and unsettled body state of trying to come to terms with a new way of moving is the opening Sally Ann Ness (1992) refers to, or what I would call a dislocation necessary to acquire new corporeal schemas. When I was subsequently reading and watching the dvds made by Amir and Kartomi, I did begin to see birds "in the wings" of – that is, as somewhat marginal references in these sources, and simultaneously began to open or become available to the bird world. Amir (2006) writes, "Formations can also be modelled on animals, natural or mythical, as in the *cicem po* ("flying bird") or *buroq meunari* ("dancing buraq bird") formation. This formulation emulates birds flying with the dancers flapping their arms" (p. 143).

Clearly there was something relating to birds in *seudati* even if this aspect, as I gradually began to interpret from the available literature, is not brought forward explicitly in current discourses (including in the several *sanggar,* or studios, I attended). Had I seen this performance form in Aceh but not attempted to understand it in a practical way in my own body, I might not have paid much attention to these references, or acquired an avian dimension to my world through my changed perception. As Vermonden (2011) writes of his experience of becoming literate in an initially unfamiliar local world of stars and fish, the idea of an "accumulation of content in the mind misses (the) dimension of world transformation" that can occur through embodied experiences (p. 44).

Obviously, birds exist: I could see them out and up there at any time. But now they are more present for me and I feel more alive to them when I see them. Once, since my experience with *seudati,* while taking off from Jogjakarta on a Garuda flight, I had a hallucination where I quite literally felt that I was flying on the back of a huge bird and could feel my fingers digging into the warm, feathery body. I felt completely safe.

Pointing to Birds

When French philosopher Maurice Merleau-Ponty (1964) writes that, "Through its 'sensory fields' and its whole organization the body is, so to speak, predestined to model itself on the natural aspects of the world" (p. 7), it might appear that both the human body and the "natural world" are here assumed to be basically natural, and that this discussion of *seudati* and birds could end there. But the human sensory fields are always already cultural fields: "the world which is given in perception...is the concrete, intersubjectively constituted life-world of immediate experience" an experience that is always cultural (Edie, 1964, p. xvi). Both "nature" and "body" are mutually cultural experiences. Bodily experience and the world are co-nascent – they develop together and the world is always the world for those who experience it. As John Martin (1939/1985) observed, the qualities of things are not given to consciousness as attributes of those things but are rather a function of our corporeal relationship with them: "When we pronounce the log heavy (or say that it is lying on the ground) ... we are actually describing not so much the log itself...as the motor reactions which occur in our own bodies at sight of it" (p. 45).

Merleau-Ponty (1964) was trying to concretely gain access to the structure of the perceived world – that which is "buried under the sedimentations of later knowledge" (p. 5). This later knowledge radically separates subject from world, creating an opposition between culture and nature, self and other. Merleau-Ponty (1964) believed that critical thought had "broken with the naive evidence of *things*, and when it affirms, it is because it no longer finds any means of denial" (p. 3). As part of bringing into relief what he understands to be "buried," Merleau-Ponty invokes the phenomenon of *pointing*, a gesture about which he says:

> This insertion of our factual situation as a particular case within the system of other possible situations begins as soon as we *designate* a point in space with our finger. For this pointing gesture...supposes that we are already installed in virtual space—at the end of the line prolonging our finger in a centrifugal and cultural space. This mimic usage of our body is not yet a conception, since it does not cut us off from our corporeal situation: on the contrary, it assumes all its meaning. (p. 7)

Merleau-Ponty suggests that, at its most basic, the gesture of pointing establishes that the pointer is located materially just like, and in the same space as, the thing or being pointed to. Similarly, C. S. Pierce wrote that the "index" designates its object, "because it is in dynamical (including spatial) connection, both with the individual object, on the one hand, and with the senses or memory of the person for whom it serves as a sign, on the other hand" (as cited in Clark, 2003, p. 245). Whereas language can refer to a world "in the mind," pointing retains an awareness that the subject is sharing a world with other situated objects and beings (of course, the gesture of pointing can also take on specific cultural meanings).

Pointing also leads "participants to *focus attention*" on the object being indicated (p. 246). Learning aspects of *seudati* in Aceh was for me as though it had the effect of a kind of pointing. The movements themselves, as I tried them, seemed to orient me to birds, not as concepts or representations of them, but as other objects/beings whom one might or could both pay attention to and with whom one shares a corporeal situation and a "mutual permeability" or "mutual binding." *Seudati* seemed like a form for the re-membering – the putting back together – of a specific human-bird cross-over and co-presence.

There is another, related way of thinking about the way that *seudati* connected me to the bird world. In his essay "Archive of Experience," Brian Massumi (2003) discusses an intriguing aspect of the phenomenon of movement and its perception. Quoting phenomenologist Albert Michotte he says that, "Movement has the uncanny ability ... 'to survive the removal of its object'" (p. 2). He gives the example of one billiard ball hitting another, noting that "what we perceive is the movement of the first ball *continuing* with the second." He calls this phenomenon a "perceptual feeling" (p. 2) and goes further to argue that, in our perception, movement continues across changes of object and state.

Massumi is trying to re-orient thinking away from (visual resemblances between) objects and instead to focus on relations between *events*. Relationship, he argues, is the event of movement's appearing to continue across different objects. He also draws on Daniel Stern's (1985/2010) discussion of "vitality affects," where Stern argues that the felt rhythms and qualities of events can jump, not just between situations but also between sense modes, such as when an infant can associate going to sleep with certain heard or felt rhythms without the activity producing that rhythm having to be the same every time: the mother can pat, rock, sing or hum, or dim the lighting achieving an effect for the infant that *feels* the same. Stern observes that, "Infants...appear to have an innate general capacity, which can be called *amodal perception,* to take information received in one sensory modality and somehow translate it into another sensory modality" (p. 151). He continues:

> For instance, a rhythm, such as "long short" (------ -), can be delivered in or abstracted from sight, audition, smell touch or taste. For this to occur, the rhythm must at some point exist in the mind in a form that is not inextricably bound to one particular way of perceiving it but is rather sufficiently abstract to be transportable across modalities. (p. 152)

Further, Stern states that vitality affects give rise to *forms of life* that are fundamentally *shared,* and that their "activation contour" links them together. Massumi (2003) elaborates that experiences can be "archived" and classified with other experiences according to processes and attributes other than the more dominantly recognised intellectual, visual, or verbally generated resemblances. Thus, it may have been the kinds of energetic or vitality affects that Stern (1985/2010) describes in musical terms – crescendo, decrescendo, "bursting," "drawn out," etc. (p. 54) that "continued across" from birds to dancing.

I consider that in *seudati* I had an "education to attention" *vis à vis* the realm of birds and that I have come to experience a new poetics of dwelling (Vermonden, 2011, p. 44). While I was trying to learn *seudati* movements, the dance itself (as an ambiguous kind of transcendence or repository of knowledge) was opening me to new perceptions. In my own dance background, I have placed knowledge in the figure of the choreographic artist and in the dancer, and had little time for a concept of "the dance." Now, however, I have *witnessed* that a particular idiom is much more than what any individual intends: it can harness a current of movement that flows through bodies and through time, animating them (Ness, 1992, p. 1). The dance can reveal or initiate in a transcendent way, "continuing across," mediating, and entwining different beings and different becomings that might (as in my case) have lost touch with each other.

Reflecting further on the nature/culture relation in this chapter and through the *seudati* experience, I would say that as humans we are intertwined with what we call "nature." This intertwinement, however, is obscured (by the "sedimentations" that Merleau-Ponty [1964] refers to) and often only becomes visible as ecological or other crisis. With the help of Massumi and Stern, I am arguing implicitly that it can also become felt or visible in the kinds of experiences discussed in this and other chapters. The term "ecological animalism" coined by the late Val Plumwood (2012) seems apt, suggesting a "human/animal continuity" (p. 83) that is consonant with the way Massumi (2003) is conceiving connection, and also pointing to the possibility of survival. In her homage to Plumwood, Deborah Bird Rose (2013) writes that her "philosophical animism...opens the door to a world in which we can begin to negotiate life membership of an ecological community of kindred beings" (p. 93). Bird Rose insists that for Plumwood this approach was not a doctrine "but rather a path, a way of life, a mode of encounter" (p. 93).

Lifeworld

After my encounter with *seudati* I am much more frequently aware of birdlife, and I see it in more detail. I perceive and appreciate the way groups or small flocks of birds of different kinds can wheel and bank around in the air above land or water, sometimes suddenly turning back on themselves, or suddenly dipping down or soaring higher. I also now enjoy how on a bright sunny day a group of birds might fly up and gradually disappear from vision as though *into* the sky as they get higher and higher, going back up to the stars. I also see differently the intense industry of a small group of hens sorting through a garden's leaf litter. I no longer have a general, verbal, assumed image of birds but instead they come into view for me through the movements of which they are capable and which I enjoy and feel part of.

I have always thought that birds are some of the most difficult creatures that I might try to mimic or emulate physically – (even though members of some communities and some children are completely adept at this) because of the peculiar suddenness of their ground-based movements and capacity for absolute stillness in between those light sudden moves; and, of course, because of their flight and thus particular use of their upper appendages. Now, I feel that I have had some experience, however partial, of 'becoming bird' not because I succeeded in mastering the bird-like aspects, as I came to see them, of *seudati,* as I was far from doing that, but because birds – their behaviour – themselves have become more part of my everyday world and distinctions. I feel closer to and more able to participate at a distance with birds when I see them in action. In the struggle to take on *seudati* behaviour, which at first was opaque to me in terms of any poetics or meanings, I came to perceive something in the world to which I had not previously been alive. This process or phenomenon could be thought of as my undergoing a kind of initiation. According to anthropologist Edith Turner, "the communitas that occurs during ritual...is the consequence of the connectedness by which the human world's meshing with the nonhuman world becomes possible and manifests itself" (as cited in Dubisch, 2008, p. 331).

At this point of conclusion, it might seem that I have displaced a question of cultural difference onto one of species relations but this would be only in terms of a thought that assumes the "pure" naturalness of "nature." In claiming that *seudati* has avian characteristics, I am not essentialising the *seudati* body or claiming that cross-culturally I can speak for it since, remaining in repertoire, to use a term from Diana Taylor (2003), it has an extraordinary range of resonances and meanings that come through different poetic, religious, comedic sung and spoken language, events of performance, the movements, their performers, the audiences, and in different eras and times. I do not want to suggest that *seudati* is "about birds" or is a *representation* of birds. I am more interested in the force and transporting effects of a performance form, something that seems much more difficult to find language for. *Seudati* according to this measure might be something like a counter-archive, potentially conserving worlds of felt relations across space, time and bodies.

References

Abdullah, T. (1966). Adat and Islam: An examination of conflict in Minangkabau. *Indonesia, 2*, 1–24. Retrieved from http://www.jstor.org/stable/3350753

Allen, M. H. (1997). Rewriting the script for South Indian dance. *The Drama Review: TDR, 41*(3), 63–100.

Amir, I. (2005). *Seudati: percakapan dengan seniman* (Digital video disc.). Melbourne, VIC: Monash University.

Amir, I. (2006). *Sing, adapt, persevere: Dynamics of the traditional vocal performers in the Islamic region of Aceh from the late 19th to the early 21st century.* Doctoral thesis, Faculty of Arts, Monash University, Clayton, Australia.

Bird Rose, D. (2013). Val Plumwood's philosophical animism: Attentive interactions in the sentient world. *Ecological Humanities, 3,* 93–109. Retrieved from www.environmentalhumanities.org

Butterworth, D. (2011). Ritual preparation for living. *Indonesia and the Malay World, 39*(113), 49–67.

Citaristi, I. (2001). *The making of a guru: Kelucaharn Mohapatra: His life and times.* Delhi: Manohar.

Clark, H. (2003). Pointing and placing. In S. Kito & M. Plank (Eds.), *Pointing: Where language, culture and cognition meet* (pp. 243–268). London: Psychology Press.

De Vries, I. (2011). *Christiaan Snouck Hurgronje: History of orientalist manipulation of Islam.* Retrieved from http://www.newcivilisation.com/home/1605/ideas-philosophy/christiaan-snouck-hurgronje-history-of-orientalist-manipulation-of-islam/

Dubisch, J. (2008). Challenging the boundaries of experience, performance and consciousness: Edith Turner's contribution to the Turnerian project. In G. S. John (Ed.), *Victor Turner and contemporary cultural performance* (pp. 324–337). New York: Berghahn.

Edie, J. (Ed.). (1964). Introduction. In *The primacy of perception and other essays on phenomenological psychology, the philosophy of art, history and politics* (pp. xiii–xix). Evanston, IL: Northwestern University Press.

Feillard, A., & Madinier, R. (2011). *The end of innocence? Indonesian Islam and the temptations of radicalism.* Singapore: National University of Singapore Press.

Foley, K. (1990). My bodies: The performer in West Java. *The Drama Review: TDR, 34*(2), 62–80.

Geertz, C. (1975). Deep play: Notes on the Balinese cockfight. In *The interpretation of cultures* (pp. 412–454). London: Hutchison.

Hurgronje, C. S. (1906). *The Achehnese, Volume II.* Leyden, NL/London: Late E. J. Brill/Luzac.

Kartomi, M. (1984). Music and dance in Aceh: A preliminary survey. *Indonesia Circle – School of Oriental & African Studies Newsletter, 9*(24), 15–28.

Kartomi, M. (1999). Seudati inong: The female form of the martial art genre in Meulaboh, West Aceh, Indonesia. *ISIM Newsletter*, 12.

Kartomi, M. (2003). *Seudati music and dance in Aceh.* Distinguished performance series (Digital video disc.). Melbourne, VIC: Monash University.

Kartomi, M. (2004). Some implications of local concepts of space in the dance, music and visual arts of Aceh. In *Yearbook of traditional music, 36* (pp. 1–49). Ljubljana: International Council for Traditional Music.

Kartomi, M. (2012). *Musical journeys in Sumatra.* Urbana/Champaign, IL: University of Illinois.

Martin, J. (1985). *Introduction to the dance.* New York: Dance Horizons. (Original work published 1939).

Massumi, B. (2003). The archive of experience. In J. Brouwer & A. Mulder (Eds.), *Information is alive: Art and theory on archiving and retrieving data* (pp. 142–151). Rotterdam, The Netherlands: V2 Organisatie/EU European Culture 2000 Program.

Merleau-Ponty, M. (1964). An unpublished text. In J. Edie (Ed.), *The primacy of perception and other essays on phenomenological psychology, the philosophy of art, history and politics* (pp. 3–11). Evanston, IL: Northwestern University Press.

Nandy, A. (2002). *Time warps: The insistent politics of silent and evasive pasts*. Delhi: Permanent Black.

Ness, S. A. (1992). *Body, movement, and culture: Kinesthetic and visual symbolism in a Philippine community*. Philadelphia: University of Pennsylvania Press.

Plumwood, V. (2012). *The eye of the crocodile*. (L. Shannon, Ed.). Canberra, Australia: ANU Press. Retrieved from http://press.anu.edu.au?p=208511

Raseuki, N. I. (1993). *Seudati in Acehnese tradition: A preliminary study.* Master's thesis, University of Wisconsin Press, Madison.

Stern, D. (2010). *The interpersonal world of the infant: A view from psychoanalysis and developmental psychology*. London: Basic Books. (Original work published 1985).

Taylor, D. (2003). *The archive and the repertoire: Performing cultural memory in the Americas*. Durham, NC: Duke University Press.

Vermonden, D. (2011). Cuculano. Myths, legends, tales, fables or sedimented tools for the transmission of a perception? *Indonesia & the Malay World, 39*(113), 29–47.

Chapter 10
Pause. Listen.: Visibility and Freedom in Choreographic Practice

Simon Ellis

Authority

> Inasmuch as I am at the heart of nature a simple given, nothing is mine. (de Beauvoir, 1987, p. 137)

> I am a dancer.
> I am a choreographer.
> I work with others.
> I am indebted to others.

Here is a chapter in a book about dance and the *quality of life*. The book's title presupposes that dance has some relationship to quality of life or even that it might improve the quality of our lives. But it is, I imagine, also a book implicitly about the lives, attitudes and desires of academics – each of us trying to carve out an existence through publication, based on a perceived (and sometimes even real) authority and expertise. Don't be fooled: each of us is contributing to this book – or indeed any other book – because our quality of (academic) life demands this kind of writing and scholarship. And don't be fooled again: each of us so-called authors are dependent on the lives and experiences of others. We define ourselves while defining others around us; we are made through them as we write of and about them. We are 'blinded' by ourselves (Cage, as cited in Larson, 2013, p. 187) and by our (perceived and real) authority and power.

Here is a chapter in a book in which I reflect on and write about the conditions of production and performance of a dance called *Pause. Listen.* (2014). In doing so I aim to reveal some of the ethical values in making and presenting the dance, and how these values might contribute to conversations and experiences in dance of ownership, attribution, responsibility, and status. The chapter is divided into five parts: (1) *Authority*, this current section in which I introduce and frame the writing

S. Ellis (✉)
Coventry University, Coventry, UK

K. Bond (ed.), *Dance and the Quality of Life*, Social Indicators Research Series 73,
https://doi.org/10.1007/978-3-319-95699-2_10

in relation to authorship and personal ambition; (2) *Visibility*, to discuss agency and (in)visibility for dancers and choreographers; (3) *Other Voices*, a small collection of writings by other artists in response to their experiences of *Pause. Listen.*; (4) *Freedom*, in which I draw together thinking by Simone de Beauvoir, Ilya Prigogine and Henri Bergson to consider indeterminacy and freedom in relation to novelty and an ethics of choreography; and, finally (5) *Letters*, a collection of letters I wrote to dancer Chisato Ohno at the very beginning of what would become *Pause. Listen.* Together, I hope these seemingly disparate written forms will help to imagine a new type of choreographer-as-author: the *steward*, whose role and attributes might challenge how the dance community and marketplace valorizes choreographic authorship. I should be clear that *Pause. Listen.* is not a dance *about* freedom or visibility or ethics, but that, within the dance's processes, performances, and underlying values, rests an opportunity to consider dance and the quality of life.

But whose lives, and what qualities?

Pause. Listen. is a dance by Chisato Ohno (performance), Jackie Shemesh (design), and me – Simon Ellis (choreography). The brackets around those words – performance, design, and choreography – are more than syntactical economy; they are meant to allow the artistic roles-as-words to be ghost-like, floating between uncertainty and clarity. The three of us are marked by those roles in this dance, but marks can be deceiving. *Pause. Listen.* was a small dance, for a few people. Its ambitions were – and remain – discreet. Since the three of us expressed interest in making a work by understanding and adapting performance practices and environments, it was developed only through residencies: first in the Garage Nardini space at Bassano del Grappa in Italy in October–November 2013, and then again in the Founders Studio at The Place in London in August–September 2014. This residency approach meant that each version of the amalgamated choreographic, dance and design practices would be shaped – or afforded – by time in the spaces we were working and performing. We hoped to inhabit these spaces-to-be-danced-in in order to evoke what anthropologist Tim Ingold (2000) describes as a "poetics of dwelling" (p. 26), a term he uses to describe the sensitivity and responsiveness akin to intuition, and developed through time in environments.

Pause. Listen. was also another opportunity for me to question the role, status, and ethics of the choreographer in collaborative processes (e.g. Ellis 2010, 2015) – to seek methods of practice and performance that would bring into focus the tremendous corporeal and cognitive intelligences of the dancer Chisato Ohno, while exercising humility as a choreographer. There is a paradoxical desire here in the dance and this writing: to acknowledge or recognize my role as the choreographer while attempting not to draw attention to it. Further still, the chapter is written without the direct voice or perspectives of Chisato; a problem or perhaps *friction* that produces a matrix of absence and presence between her, me, the performance and this writing.

Two overlapping questions stayed alive throughout the processes and experiments of *Pause. Listen.*: How might I invoke choreographic absence, or somehow reduce my authorial presence in the work? What is the least I need to do in order to make space for – or get out of the way of – Chisato's readiness to practice performance? For my part, a key aspect of the development and performance of *Pause. Listen.* was to heighten my sensitivity to the experience, thinking, skill and decision-making of Chisato, while finding strategies to minimize the impact of my taste, vision and general authorial presence on her dancing and the work itself.

The challenge here and now is to write, represent and reflect on this choreographic work, and the work of these people involved, that is not "replete with clichéd, ready-made (some would even say cowardly) ideas of proprietorial authorship, the book, originality, fixity, and the finished object" (Hall, 2016, p. xiv). Such a proposition demands sensitivity to ownership, privilege, power and authority. It demands that you the reader remembers that these ideas are constructed as they are written, that I am – even as I type *these words here and now,* and whether I like it or not – in the process and muddle of expressing desires: to make sense, to be clear, to acknowledge accurately the work and roles of the collaborative team, to be open and vulnerable, to ask difficult questions, to not pretend, to not seek regard, to not make absurd claims. These desires are qualities I would like to have in my professional life, and although ambitious and beyond my capacities, they are how I want to come to dancing, and they are how I attempted to approach *Pause. Listen.*

Visibility

> Man cannot escape from his own presence, nor from the singular world that his presence reveals around him; his very effort to uproot himself from the earth causes him to dig a hole for himself. (de Beauvoir, 1987, p. 138)

In *Performance as a Political Act*, dancer, sociologist, and Marxist Randy Martin (1990) applies the terms *conceiver*, *performer* and *consumer* to the production of dance. He suggests that performance is the "spatial and temporal terrain upon which the conceiver and consumer meet," and what is mediation for the choreographer and audience is "experience for the dancer" (p. 83). This claim was part of Martin's efforts to elevate the agency of dancers over the authority of the choreographer, and his agenda was born out of the anecdotal history in dance of *silent dancers*, or dancers understood as being on the receiving end of (choreographic) authority and power.

Dance scholar Sally Gardner (2007) has criticized Martin's industrializing the roles of the dancer and choreographer as not reflecting the history of modern dance (in which the choreographer was often also one of the dancers). Furthermore, Gardner expresses concern that Martin's "industrial metaphor" (p. 49), in which the "dancers are workers to the choreographer's 'capital'" (p. 47), eclipses the choreographer by a type of transfer of power from mind (choreographer) to body (dancer), whereas in historical modern dance the choreographer authored the dance through her body.

There continue to be multiple versions of the ways in which choreographers, dancers and choreographer-dancers access, devise, manage, and question their work together. Yet the agency of dancers in choreography continues to be a sore point in contemporary dance practice; sore enough for the Swedish site *Sarma* to have produced *The Dancer as Agent Collection* (Parkinson & Peeters, 2014). The site is edited by Chrysa Parkinson and Jeroen Peeters and contains a broad collection of materials (video, writing, drawing) that celebrate and foreground the work, thinking, and actions of dancers, many of whom explicitly avoid calling themselves choreographers.

Whereas Martin pulled apart the roles of choreographers and dancers in order to elevate the value and agency of the worker-dancer, Gardner's (2007) argument is that contesting the choreographer-dancer binary (a binary that doesn't survive historical analysis) makes possible more complex processes of "transmission where authority might remain with the choreographer but also belong to the dancers" (p. 50).

> What can the dancer and the choreographer know and be with respect to one another in modern dance if we do not accept that they simply fall on either side of binary divisions between art and craft, self and other, subject and object, mind and body. (p. 37).

Notwithstanding Gardner's concerns about the pertinence of Martin's Marxian framework for thinking choreographic *production*, his description of conceiver, performer and consumer provides a useful means to question who is responsible – and when – for authoring choreographic work and to what extent the terms of this responsibility are able to be disrupted or circumvented in ways that reflect Gardner's challenge to various binaries.

Martin's diachronic approach – a process of transferring authority over time – doesn't necessarily reflect more common choreographic processes that involve a synchronic *give and take* between the artists. Martin (1990) himself recognizes this synchronic transfer of roles in the work of John Cage and Merce Cunningham in which "the conceiver is located inside the performance rather than in the process of conceiving it" (p. 84). There are also many examples of choreographers looking to bend and extend rehearsal dialogues and practices between choreographers and dancers into performance.

In *Sunstruck* (Herbertson & Cobham, 2008) Melbourne choreographer Helen Herbertson sends instructions and feedback to dancers Trevor Patrick and Nick Sommerville via wireless earpieces as they perform the movement materials. Similarly, in *The Boom Project* (Crisp & Herbertson, 2015), Australian dancer-choreographer Rosalind Crisp dances while "artistic companion and provocateur" Herbertson quietly speaks responses, ideas and thoughts into the space to nourish Crisp's dancing. William Forsythe has long used live directorial strategies to explore choreographic possibilities. For example, in *Sleepers Guts 3* Forsythe (1996) directed the dancers what to say in real time (based on their text from the first act). In *Artifact* Forsythe (1984) "calls out [dancers] waiting on the side and gives drastically varying directions" (Caspersen & Steinwald, 2007). In the same interview Forsythe's long-term collaborator Dana Caspersen relates that [Forsythe] is "interested in how set structures change when a few basic instructions are altered" (2007). Perhaps his curiosity in structural and temporal complexities made directorial interventions at the moment of performance almost inevitable. Forsythe was perhaps influenced by his historical predecessor Trisha Brown in *Solo Olos* (1976), for example, in which dancer Lisa Kraus leaves the dance to call out instructions to the four other dancers.

Dances like these collapse Martin's conceiver-performer-consumer description of production. At varying stages, choreographers are performing directions, dancers are adapting and conceiving while performing dances, and the performances to a certain extent (and more than is usual in choreographies) are consumed as they are produced; they possess a quality of aliveness that is built into their construction. Nonetheless, in the examples I have described, *at some point in time* each work contains some version of a directorial presence that extends beyond the rehearsal period, and that adapts, adjusts and sets possibilities in motion for the dancer to notice, absorb, manage, create and even reject.

This relationship between director and dancer(s) holds even for Rosalind Crisp's *The Boom Project* in which, although Crisp is described as both dancer and choreographer (akin to other examples at the heart of Gardner's 2007 article), it is clear from Helen Herbertson's visible yet subtle spoken interventions-as-companion that *direction* – even in the loosest sense of the word – is being communicated (Crisp & Herbertson, 2015). These choreographic-danced scenarios are distinct from the diachronic transfer of agency in traditional choreographic practices that follows the visibility of the key participants: at a certain point in the production process the choreographer-director steps back from her role and the dancers *assume* ownership of – and visibility in – its performance, with the audience subsequently assuming its (visible) role in experiencing and reading the work.

In these examples of dances by Crisp, Herbertson, Brown, and Forsythe, agency is shared between people and through and across time. It is a form of *distributed agency* in which making (or choreography) is stretched through time into performance, and the responsibility for it overlaps as it is distributed across the dance's collaborators (dancers, choreographers, designers, etc.). These are instances of dancers who make or create while in the practice of choreographic performance. The works contain degrees of visibility in the various roles and at various times for the participants-agents, and these degrees have dramaturgical value. That is, the means by which relationships of visibility are constituted both in outcome and process influence how the performances are practiced, experienced, and apprehended.

Furthermore, when distributed agency is built into the construction and performance of work, it has the capacity to reveal an ethics of agency, power, and authorship that might disrupt, for example, long-held patterns of the dancer's body as object that is "always directed and reactive" (Gardner, 2007, p. 44). In such an ethics, we can ask who might be responsible to make and practice performance, and how and *when* might the interventions or conversations between collaborators occur?

In *Pause. Listen.* I was interested in devising a system with Chisato in which – unlike the examples above – I attempted to remove my authorial taste and presence from the performance of material while maintaining for Chisato in particular a sense of distributed agency. Chisato and I created a lexicon of choreographed movements, stimuli, and micro-scores that were randomly combined and then projected to her via three small screens hidden from the audience. The lexicon was long enough for Chisato to be unprepared for the combinations, and for her to have to build the performative, movement and creative opportunities afforded by what was displayed for her on the irregularly updating screens. The technology was not there to *command* Chisato, but to make complex propositions available in order for her to continue to question her own performance practice. As the *choreographer* during the performance I was only responsible for pressing start on each set of randomized projected stimuli.

The irony of what I understand on my part to be an ethical *desire* is that the mechanics of *Pause. Listen.* are counteracted by a much larger politics of authority. Such politics are independent of my relative (in)visibility and try as I might to step back from the performance-as-creation by Chisato Ohno in *Pause. Listen.* those ghostly brackets around my role-as-choreographer press me into high-vis visibility. Whereas Gardner and Martin are calling on histories and modes of production in relation to the politics of performance, I'm referring here to a type of popular or celebrity *culture* that lauds the choreographer-as-author and inadvertently diminishes the dancer as artist-maker. Perhaps a culture that prizes the obvious or straightforward author is an example of a conceptual framework "always at work making some things visible and sayable and obscuring others" (Gardner, 2007, p. 50; Fig. 10.1).

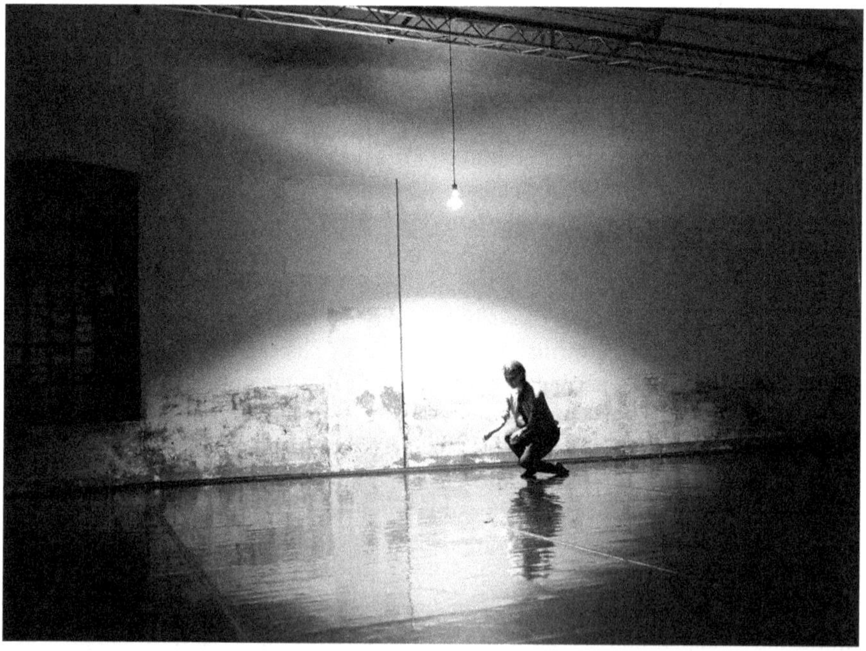

Fig. 10.1 Chisato Ohno at Centro per la Scena Contemporanea di Bassano del Grappa, October 2013. (Photograph: Simon Ellis)

Other Voices

> There is no such thing as an empty space or an empty time. There is always something to see, something to hear. In fact, try as we may to make a silence, we cannot. (Cage, 1961, p. 8)

I commissioned three artists – Charlie Ashwell, Guadalupe Núñez-Fernández and Lucy Cash – to write reflective responses to their experience of *Pause. Listen.* They are welcome interlopers in this text and their writing functions to distribute authorship of this text that speaks to and about *Pause. Listen.* They are a reminder of the extended community of people – away from the author's voice – that are involved in how performance is made and experienced. Excerpts are included below, and complete copies of the written responses, along with a video edit of *Pause. Listen.*, are online at https://www.skellis.info/work#/pauselisten/.

Different Ears: Guadalupe Núñez-Fernández (2014)

There was sound, but she was moving as if dancing to the music in her head, or with an invisible companion – not chasing her own shade but playing along with it.

I wondered what was prompting her from motion to motion, and from scene to scene, because her movement had pattern to it, punctuation, a continuum of beginnings, middles, ends, always beginning again. It felt new each time, unrehearsed, like breathing can be, each breath different than the one before – not assumed or taken for granted. Improvised somehow, though always ongoing.

To me, her dancing felt like a form of meditation, both for herself and for the audience, as she moved through the room and at once closed the windows, rolled down the blinds, made the place smaller and turned down the sound; as she walked to the edges of the space and found places, as if they hadn't existed before; and as her breathing became something we could all experience a lot more closely. Its pace and the way it seemed to go behind and along all her movement was a mirror to all our darting thoughts. It wasn't awkward, self-conscious or intimidating in any way. It was enrapturing.

I've been listening to my neighbors' music with different ears since, whether it's loud Eurotrash or Albanian folk, I've been remembering Chisato Ohno's near silent dance and meditating as I listen to the breath under the floorboards.

Time Within Time: Lucy Cash (2014)

Time lies in this dance. There is the time of the church clock striking, people speaking and the cars as they pass in the street below. There is the way time feels inside the dancer and the way her mind reveals it for us to see. The time that it takes for her body to remember these movements and the time that we have to see them. Time also lies in our thoughts as we watch. The last time we saw a head nod like this, and our anticipation of when such a nod might happen again.

There is time within time as the fragment of music arrives, extending itself into the present, reminding us of what we have already left behind.

The city lies in this dance. It is in the building that surrounds this dance; the ceiling that receives the shadow of the dancer before we can see the dancer herself. The floor that lies beneath the dancer, remaining constant. The windows that begin as open and will end as closed and that cast their shadow on the patient floor until the blind is drawn and erases the shadow … The woman pacing in front of the window in the house opposite, her cigarette smoke, the road, the street lamps, the moon – these bits of city are also in this dance.

And air lies in this dance. It comes in from the night outside. It brings the city closer. It is the current beneath the dancer's arms, and our breath as we watch her.

Solitude with: Charlie Ashwell (2014)

Philosopher Elizabeth Grosz (2005) writes of thinking as "a mode of inadequation of the real" (p. 74). I like that. How about dancing as a mode of inadequation of the real, as well? Dance as excess; as spilling-over. Dance you cannot work out; perpetually not fitting any system; altering the very terms by which we might try to measure or value or even perceive it. I believe the woman next to me is not a serial contemporary-dance-watcher, although maybe she will become one. She cheers and claps loudly and enthusiastically at the end and immediately proclaims the piece a success.

She dances. She teaches. She gifts us the dance that she does. She makes it pretty good. She wraps. HA. She raps nicely. She riffs. Bone. Black. Wood. Applause. I borrow her moves. This dance is our library, hey? Moves we've not done. She dances them, many. She dances all there is to dance. I feel digested. Accounted for. Responded to. Cared towards. There is always that moment of crisis when a dancer goes 'what am I doing with my life?' She doesn't do that here. I've been trying to think about dance as a mode of criticality and then also a mode of healing, to some extent. What, I'm not sure. Perhaps dance doesn't heal wounds but airs them; doesn't bridge gaps but occupies and exceeds them. Dance as magnet; attraction and repulsion. Dance as salt.

There is a paradoxical idea that in solitude, we engage primarily with our peripheral vision – it is softer – more open and receptive to information from others. In company, in the conscious presence of another, the gaze hardens, things form – subjects and objects – and perceptions narrow. Watching another, with others, I try to delay this moment. Solitude in and as community, perhaps. Solitude *with* (Fig. 10.2).

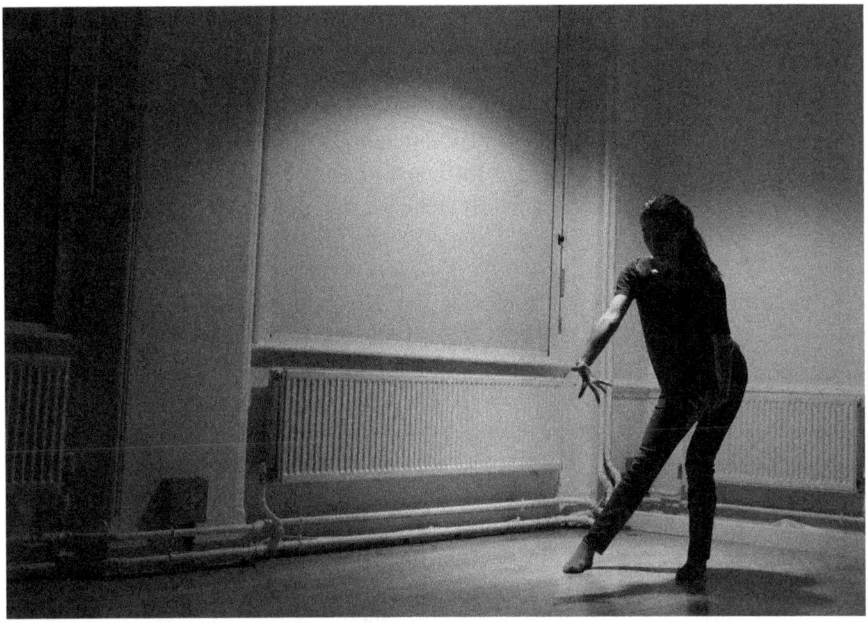

Fig. 10.2 Chisato Ohno dancing in The Founders' Studio. (Photograph: Stacie Bennett)

Freedom

Artists talk a lot about freedom. So, recalling the expression 'free as a bird,' Morton Feldman went to a park one day and spent some time watching our feathered friends. When he came back, he said, "You know? They're not free: they're fighting over bits of food." (Cage, 1961, p. 265).

In Simone de Beauvoir's (1944) first philosophical essay, "Towards a Morals of Ambiguity, According to *Pyrrhus and Cinéas,*" she asks, "under what conditions, if any, may I speak for/in the name of another?" (Bergoffen, 2004, n. p.) and queries the limits of "any human project" (de Beauvoir, 1987, p. 136).

Pause.

I need to be careful.

My appropriation of de Beauvoir's ideas here in a book about dance and the quality of life is awkward at best. *Pyrrhus and Cinéas* was first published just after the liberation of France in 1944, and in it de Beauvoir grapples with the ways in which freedom and violence are common to human experience, in which "one always works for certain men (sic) against others" (de Beauvoir, 1987, p. 139). And yet here I am ostensibly writing about choreographic practice and how it is that choreographers and dancers *are* in relation to each other. This is academic hubris at the very least, but perhaps mining de Beauvoir's war-time thinking might help afford certain ways of being between choreographers and dancers, and how these ways, approaches, and *values* might extend into the future. Aren't we all, whether we like it or not, implicated in experiences of agency, power, and freedom?

At the heart of de Beauvoir's understanding of freedom is that although we all share freedom, it is only, for example, the miserable who "can declare themselves free at the heart of misery" (p. 140). By not helping, de Beauvoir states that she is in fact the "face of that misery" (p. 140), and that in this case freedom exists only for the other and cannot be directly touched by them (Bergoffen, 2004). De Beauvoir's non-negotiable freedom is to choose whether or not to accept the other's misery.

The essay starts with a conversation between Pyrrhus and Cinéas in which Cinéas repeatedly questions Pyrrhus's desire to continue with new projects of conquest. De Beauvoir celebrates Pyrrhus's restlessness, for it is by continually finishing and starting projects that transcendence – to make a change in the world – is possible. But for these projects, we need others, and in fact we "depend upon the freedom of the other" (de Beauvoir, 1987, p. 142). In her outline of *Pyrrhus and Cinéas* philosopher Debra Bergoffen (2004) writes that in order to give our projects a future we need others and are "enjoined to appeal to their freedom" (n.p.).

Perhaps I can suggest that in *Pause. Listen.* I was appealing to Chisato's freedom – that she was not simply fighting-dancing over bits of food? Regardless, it is in the way de Beauvoir signals that freedom might make possible uncertain futures that interests me in this part of the chapter, not least because it invites a conversation that includes thinking by philosopher Henri Bergson and physical chemist Ilya Prigogine. De Beauvoir (1987) writes:

> We must assume our acts in uncertainty and risk; precisely here does the essence of freedom lie, it isn't decided in view of a salvation accorded in advance; it signs no pact with the future; if it were defined by the end it aims at, it would no longer be freedom. (p. 142)

This seems critical: although we can be clear of our aims, if we are defined by what any version of the end will be (and how we are getting there), then we are not acting freely.

In 1997 Belgian physical chemist Ilya Prigogine published *The End of Certainty*. The book is an account of Prigogine's thinking and research into nonequilibrium thermodynamics and indeterminacy. It seeks to reconcile the disparity between the feeling human beings experience or sense that time is moving forwards, with the notion in classical physics that time is reversible in that its laws hold regardless of the direction of time. He asks, "How can we conceive of human creativity or ethics in a deterministic world?" (p. 6).

The so-called "arrow of time," developed in the early twentieth century by Arthur Eddington, is analogous to irreversible (entropic) processes in the universe. According to Prigogine, such processes play a "fundamental constructive role in nature" (p. 27) and demand an understanding of the laws of nature built on "possibilities" and not "certitudes" (p. 29). The arrow of time has both unity and diversity. There is unity because the arrow is common to all parts of the universe ("your future is my future; the future of the sun is the future of any other star" (p. 56)), and diversity as we only need look around us. In a dynamic system with distinct and known initial conditions, we cannot predict the outcome, only possibilities. There are many different and unpredictable ways for this (dis)organization to occur. For Prigogine, the "universe around us is only one of a number of possible worlds" (p. 59).

Prigogine cites philosopher Henri Bergson for whom time is a "vehicle of creation and of choice" (Bergson, 2007, p. 98) and its directionality proves that there is indeterminacy. Indeed, Bergson understands time to be "indetermination itself" (p. 98), and in *The Possible and the Real*, he argues that the possible does not precede its reality until its reality has appeared. In other words, the possible is "the mirage of the present in the past" (p. 107). If we put the possible back into its proper place, evolution becomes something quite different from the realization of a program: the gates of the future open wide; freedom is offered an unlimited field (p. 110).

In the overlap between Bergson's philosophy of time, Prigogine's understanding of thermodynamics, and de Beauvoir's (1987) thinking that freedom has "no pact with the future" (p. 142), we end up with an indeterminate and irreversible "flow of unforeseeable novelty" (Bergson, 2007, p. 112).

What might all this have to do specifically with *Pause. Listen.*, and more generally choreographic processes, and dance and the quality of life?

Pause. Listen involved a delicate organization of people, space, time, environment, and action, but with many possible and unpredictable ways of being performed and experienced. It involved a single stance to developing choreography – represented by residencies in the performance and practices spaces – which made possible the system within which the time irreversible performance occurred. The performance's irreversibility was foregrounded by devising very specific conditions by which Chisato Ohno made possible the performance; she brought its trajectory – a trajectory unable to be determined by what precedes it, including the work of the choreographer – into being. I imagine that Chisato was able to author the body and the experience to make what dancer Chrysa Parkinson (2014) describes as "agential cuts in the fabric of culture," cuts in which dancers have choices to author "experience itself" (p.17).

Together, these thoughts on novelty, indeterminacy, freedom, uncertainty, and time invite an ethics of choreography that *does not know*, and under which the simplest of working conditions afford indeterminate possibilities. It is an ethics that queries the cultural status of the choreographer as author, and foregrounds the artistry, autonomy, and intelligences of the dancer; it is choreographers that begin to understand that the freedom of dancers cannot be touched, and who recognize that (after de Beauvoir) they – the choreographers – are the face of the disempowerment of dancers. It is an ethics of choreography that reconfigures our relationship to time and novelty, whereby our role as *makers* is minimized by the ongoing trajectories and incalculable possibilities of practice-as-performance.

How then might we – choreographers, dancers, and academics – continue to challenge the commonly held hegemonic status of *the choreographer*? It is a status afforded to "signature artists" (Roche, 2015) by the contemporary dance marketplace, in which the creative work of dancers is predicated on disappearance (p. 2). What kinds of violences are perpetuated by this dominant order? What violences –

"the violence that [dominant] order does to themselves and others" (Martin, 1998, p. 26) – have I committed or been privy to?

Here is a call for alternative ways for choreographers to be in the world, and to be (un)seen in the world:

> Thus, my environment is the world as it exists and takes on meaning in relation to me, and in that sense it came into existence and undergoes development with me and around me. Secondly, the environment is never complete. If environments are forged through the activities of living beings, then so long as life goes on, they are continually under construction. (Ingold, 2000, p. 20)

Anthropologist Tim Ingold writes of the environment as Ilya Prigogine writes of thermodynamics. They both experience time and nature in which novelty and ongoing construction place human endeavor in perspective. This perspective is akin to the conditions in which I understand the *choreographer-as-steward* to be working:

> A steward is someone who accepts responsibility for taking care of something that is deemed worthy of care. Stewardship implies a lightness of touch and time in which the steward—at the request of someone else, or acting on their behalf—may manage resources, frames or contexts, materials and even culture. A steward is accountable and responsible. (Ellis, 2015, p. 98)

The steward is constantly and lightly aware of being in relation to the (eco)systems of change and possibility. They are uncertain of the future and understand that along the arrow of time there are many possibilities to accept the status and work of the other. They revel in the paradox of acute responsibility for the conditions of the performance of the work, while acknowledging their role is finite as the work extends through time beyond the boundaries of its performance. The choreographer-as-steward is not the choreographer as "manager, facilitator, or director of all those involved in the collaboration" (Foster, as cited in Kolb, 2013, p. 35). Instead, they are an author that positions the intelligences and autonomy of the dancer-as-artist, "a source of knowledge and as capable of self-representation" (Roche, 2015, p. ix) – ahead of all other concerns.

For all my attempts to redirect attention away from *me me me,* it is the nature of one's *involvement* that is key. I am not apart from this world or these choreographic and performance practices. I am not a casual observer or innocent bystander. By attempting to separate myself from – or diminish my role in – the observation and stewardship of these choreographic and performance practices performed by Chisato Ohno in *Pause. Listen.*, I embody a dualism or binary that not only smooths over the edges of choreographer-dancer messiness (see Gardner, 2007), but is unethical. The ethics lie in understanding that "novelty, choice, [and] spontaneous action" (Prigogine, 1997, p. 12) are made possible by listening gently and carefully to the indeterminate potential of actions and the "reality of time and change" (p. 12) in others. As a choreographic steward I recognize that the nature of my propositions and interventions are limited and brief, and yet in their brevity lies a politics of authority that recognizes and celebrates the agency of the dancer-as-artist: their decisions, their understanding, their voice, their experience of time, and their capacity for newness; such markers of agency are qualities of living worth pursuing.

Letters

> If one is making something which is to be nothing, the one making must love and be patient with the material he chooses. Otherwise he calls attention to the material, which is precisely something, whereas it was nothing that was being made; or he calls attention to himself, whereas nothing is anonymous. (Cage, 1961, p. 114)

Following are a series of letters I wrote to Chisato Ohno during our first meetings in the studio in 2012. Even at this early stage I toyed with the desire to diminish my role in the work to the extent that I would be absent from the performances of what would become *Pause. Listen.* I planned to leave these letters for Chisato before her performances, or perhaps even suggest that she read them out to the public. In the end, I handed Chisato three of the letters on different days just prior to sitting at a small desk at the back of the Founder's Studio in London to become *Pause. Listen.*'s *operator* – an ironic gesture and title if ever there was one.

The letters are at times terribly naïve on my part. How am I able to give something to another without imagining that I *own* it in the first place? They also clearly reveal the paradox of drawing attention to one's self while hoping to deflect or diminish that attention. For Randy Martin (1998) even "to be self-reflexive about the ability to speak to others can be problematic when that particular voice of self only amplifies a privileged position" (p. 27). These letters are a dance of words to the self, disguised, at least in part, as an expression of humility; isn't this the living breathing definition of privilege – that the choreographer-man thinks or knows he is in a position to dictate the terms of the economy, relationship, or exchange? Nevertheless, I've included the letters here as a way to exit the more scholarly ideas in the chapter with a reminder that dance, like so many other human activities, assumes its most valuable qualities when we attend to the nature of relationships.

Saturday 24 November 2012: A Different Kind of Death

Dear Chisato

We've been working together for some time now, but this is my first letter to you. It is a letter from a choreographer to a dancer, and I imagine that you will read it at some stage in the future. I wonder what will have transpired in the time between now and then?

Today you danced with remarkable breadth and playfulness. I admired – as we worked – your capacity to shift from quite staccato and strong movements to dancing like quicksilver.

But this writing is not really supposed to be about what we did today. It is more to set the stage. I would like to suggest to you that I have considerable doubt about how responsible I might be for how this performance is about to look and feel.

A while ago Roland Barthes (1977) wrote an essay called "The Death of the Author" (1977). He was challenging the idea that creator and creation are related, and that "to give a text an Author is to impose a limit on that text" (p. 147).

But I would like to suggest that my absence is a different kind of death. I like to think of it as the beginning of my silence. And this is probably quite funny for those who know me because I simply talk too much. (Even my mother would agree.)

So, I wish you good dancing, and I wholeheartedly give this work to you. Tonight. Now.

With best wishes, and into the silence,
Simon

Saturday 15 December 2012: Without Me

Dear Chisato

On the first day we worked together, you said "without me it won't happen." I liked this a lot, it stripped power away from me – the *choreographer* – and placed it between us. And there it has remained, although I should admit to being tempted to pick it up, and to wear that power as a means of protecting my vulnerability and uncertainty as our dancing relationship has developed.

On the second day we worked together – this was in October 2012 – you talked about our meeting as being "Chisato meets Simon." You were clear that this meeting was not a gendered one. I remember being interested in our gendered differences as being a key part of the work we would do together, but in three words – Chisato meets Simon – you reminded me that my interests and assumptions are built around fragile understandings of the world and people.

And so, I started to collect our similarities, the things that place us *together*. But at the same time, I think I stopped believing in metaphors, or perhaps there are simply none left? And what if, in this choreography, there are no metaphors and no representation? Just you – Chisato Ohno – moving, dancing, a very simple act of generosity towards these people who have gathered here today.

But at the same time, you and the way you move, are not beholden to anything, or anyone. Certainly not to me.

So, dear Chisato, this letter is only a beginning and that's all. It sounds a bit serious, and I wish I could write a joke into it to make you smile, but it might cramp your style.

Dance well Chisato, and I'll see you soon.
Simon

Wednesday 26 December 2012: Conquer

Dear Chisato

On our last meeting we went for a simple meal together instead of going to the studio. It was a chance to take stock, to see how – or even *if* – we should continue to work together, and if so, how to make that happen.

You seemed interested – enthusiastic even – to keep working, and I think I tried to play it a bit cool, even though I remember leaping (on the inside) at the possibility of what we might do, and what we might make.

My notes from that meeting consist of one word: *conquer*, but I don't really remember how it was that you (or was it me?) came to say this word. This letter, then, is (as ever) a fabrication or construction, a chance to try and make sense of something that doesn't really make sense, by writing about it.

I imagine that the word was related to either *fear* or *doubt*: to *conquer* fear; to *conquer* doubt. But this seems ridiculous, doesn't it? Because we were just talking about two people meeting in a dance studio in order to make a dance together, and for one person to be responsible for performing it. But perhaps fear or doubt are manifest in the most benign situations? Forget about war, or violence, or the places we normally associate with these words; what if it is the most simple or everyday encounters with fear and doubt that demand the most consistent action or actions? The fear of solitude? To doubt one's own ability to complete something? To doubt love? To fear our limitations? To doubt the words of others?

And so, Chisato, this letter is a simple way of saying that this dance we have made together is now yours to complete. It is yours to perform with pleasure and with heart. I give it to you willingly and with abandon.

Dance well, and I will see you soon.
Simon

Saturday 12 January 2013: Habits and Desire

Dear Chisato

Happy New Year to you!

We worked together in the studio this morning for the first time in a month or so. We discussed habits, and also the desire as a performer to extend beyond not so much our physical habits but the limits we place on what we are prepared to be seen doing or being.

I'm more and more aware of when to step in or add ideas when you are dancing in the studio. I recognize the delicacy and simplicity of what it is that you are doing. You walk into the middle (or edge sometimes) of the space and then start searching for things that make you curious. Often you worry about whether they might be interesting from the outside (that is, for me as the one-person audience) but I try to discourage this kind of self-consciousness.

And now, here you are. Ready to dance for this different audience of more than one. What a pleasure, for you – and for them – to have these minutes to do and experience something that doesn't involve either screens or noise.

By gifting this letter to you, I'd like to fully give this dance to you. It is a collection and distillation of the work we have done together. I hope that it reflects your strength, your experience, and your tenacity.

Dance well Chisato.
Simon

Saturday 19 January 2013: Details

Dear Chisato

How are you? I'm writing on a snowy winter's day here in London and through my window the grey of the sky is muted by the white glare of the snow on the parks. And on these parks dogs are running with abandon, barking and revealing so much about how uptight adult humans tend to be.

But I suspect telling you this is just a way of avoiding what this letter is really about. Today we briefly talked about people who move and people who don't. On reflection, it's as if one of the privileges of being a dancer (or having had a life in dance) is how accessible the *idea* of movement is. Sometimes I want to yell at the world, 'LOOK AT WHAT YOU ARE MISSING OUT ON? DON'T YOU UNDERSTAND?' But I'm not really a yelling type of person, and I doubt you are either.

So, then, here you are, about to dance, and watched by a group of people who are all sitting down, relatively still, relatively inert. But they are not missing out, because over these last months it has been such a pleasure to watch you revel in the deepest details of how a human being can be with her body.

This letter is a way of marking my absence without wanting to get in the way. Tricky isn't it? This is your dancing, for these people, today.

I wouldn't have it any other way.

Simon

PS Dance like nobody's watching, or maybe dance like everybody's watching.

References

Ashwell, C. (2014, November 27). *Solitude with – Charlie Ashwell*. Retrieved from https://pauselisten.wordpress.com/2016/06/22/solitude-with-charlie-ashwell/

Barthes, R. (1977). The death of the author. *Image, music, text* (pp. 142–148). London: HarperCollins.

Bergoffen, D. (2004, August). Simone De Beauvoir. *Stanford encyclopedia of philosophy*. Retrieved from http://plato.stanford.edu/entries/beauvoir/

Bergson, H. (2007). *The creative mind* (M. L. Andison, Trans.). Mineola, NY: Dove.

Brown, T. (1976, January). *Solo olos*. New York [Performance].

Cage, J. (1961). *Silence*. Middletown, CT: Wesleyan University Press.

Cash, L. (2014, October 7). Time within time – Lucy Cash. https://pauselisten.wordpress.com/2016/06/22/time-within-time-lucy-cash/

Caspersen, D., & Steinwald, M. (2007, March). Methodologies: Bill Forsythe and the Ballett Frankfurt by Dana Caspersen. Retrieved from http://blogs.walkerart.org/performingarts/2007/03/09/methodologies-bill-forsythe-and-the-ballett-frankfurt-by-dana-caspersen/

Crisp, R., & Herbertson, H. (2015, March 13). *The boom project*. Melbourne, VIC [Performance].

de Beauvoir, S. (1944). *Towards a morals of ambiguity, according to Pyrrhus and Cinéas*. Paris: Gallimard.

de Beauvoir, S. (1987). Selections from towards a morals of ambiguity, according to Pyrrhus and Cinéas. *Social Text, 17*, 135–142.

Ellis, S. (2010). Anamnesis (remembered). *Journal of Media Practice, 11*(3), 267–280.

Ellis, S. (2014, September). Chisato Ohno and Jackie Shemesh. *Pause. Listen.* London: The Place [Performance].

Ellis, S. (2015). Jealousy, transmission and recovery. *Performance Research, 20*(6), 95–100.

Forsythe, W. (1984). *Artifact*. Frankfurt, Germany [Performance].

Forsythe, W. (1996). *Sleepers guts 3*. Frankfurt, Germany [Performance].

Gardner, S. (2007). The dancer, the choreographer and modern dance scholarship: A critical reading. *Dance Research, 25*(1), 35–53.

Grosz, E. (2005). *Time travels*. Durham, NC: Duke University Press.

Hall, G. (2016). *Pirate philosophy*. Cambridge, MA: MIT Press. https://doi.org/10.2307/j.ctt1bz3w33.

Herbertson, H., & Cobham, B. (2008, October 13). *Sunstruck*. Melbourne, VIC [Performance].

Ingold, T. (2000). *The perception of the environment*. London: Routledge.

Kolb, A. (2013). Current trends in contemporary choreography: A political critique. *Dance Research Journal, 45*(3), 31–52.

Larson, K. (2013). *Where the heart beats*. New York: Penguin.

Martin, R. (1990). *Performance as a political act*. New York: Bergin and Garvey.

Martin, R. (1998). *Critical moves*. Durham, NC: Duke University Press.

Núñez-Fernández, G. (2014, October 13). Different ears – Guadalupe Núñez-Fernández. Retrieved from https://pauselisten.wordpress.com/2016/06/22/different-ears-guadalupe-nunez-fernandez/

Parkinson, C. (2014). Tribal currencies. In C. Parkinson & J. Peeters (Eds.), *The dancer as agent collection*. Brussels, Belgium: Sarma. Retrieved from http://repo.sarma.be/Dancer%20as%20Agent/Parkinson.pdf

Parkinson, C., & Peeters, J. (Eds.) (2014). *The dancer as agent collection*. Brussels, Belgium: DOCH School of Dance and Circus. Retrieved from http://oralsite.be/pages/The_Dancer_As_Agent_Collection

Prigogine, I. (1997). *The end of certainty*. New York: The Free Press.

Roche, J. (2015). *Multiplicity, embodiment and the contemporary dancer*. Basingstoke, UK: Palgrave Macmillan.

Chapter 11
Beauty in Disability: An Aesthetics for Dance and for Life

Aili Bresnahan and Michael Deckard

Introduction: Beauty Reconsidered

Arthur C. Danto notes in his book, *The Abuse of Beauty: Aesthetics and the Concept of Art* (2003), that one of the great advances in the philosophy of art has been to understand that not all good art is beautiful. He cites Henri Matisse's painting *Blue Nude* (1907) as a case in point (p. 36). He also says, however, that:

> … beauty is the only one of the aesthetic qualities that is also a value, like truth and goodness. It is not simply among the values we live by, but one of the values that defines what a fully human life means. (p. 15)

In *On Beauty and Being Just*, Elaine Scarry (1999) also points to Matisse's paintings as examples that expand the capacity of our minds to change and accommodate new forms of beauty (pp. 46–47). Scarry also credits Matisse for showing us how beautiful persons or things lead the perceiver "to a more capacious regard for the world" (p. 48). Like Danto and Scarry, rather than claiming that beauty is an outmoded idea, we hold to the need for this important concept.

This chapter is an attempt to reconsider the idea of beauty in a way that broadens it to include the possibility that there can be beauty in disability when the perceiver learns to expand their regard for the world through dance-based and other social interactions with disabled persons. This broadening is not a watering-down of the idea of beauty, but rather an enriching of it in a way that is true to what is happening in both dance and in non-dance life. In reconsidering beauty, we will first look to the historical origins of the dominant contemporary understanding of beauty. From there we will show how historical accounts of beauty can be traced through

A. Bresnahan (✉)
Department of Philosophy, University of Dayton, Dayton, OH, USA
e-mail: abresnahan1@udayton.edu

M. Deckard
Department of Philosophy, Lenoir-Rhyne University, Hickory, NC, USA

K. Bond (ed.), *Dance and the Quality of Life*, Social Indicators Research Series 73,
https://doi.org/10.1007/978-3-319-95699-2_11

developments in dance history in connection with finding beauty in the dancing human body. Finally, we will show how experiencing beauty through contemporary dance expands both the idea of beauty and the quality of life by leading us to greater mutuality with others who exist with us in the world (see Albrecht & Devlieger, 1999). In short, disabled dance allows us greater access, via experience and interactive communication with others who are different from us, to both beauty and an expanded quality of life.

In the history of aesthetics, ugliness and bodily deformity were linked. Eighteenth-century philosophers and thinkers such as the Third Earl of Shaftesbury, Francis Hutcheson and David Hume suggested that bodily deformity could not be beautiful. In contrast to these thinkers, Edmund Burke (1730–1797) provides a model in which perfection or proportion were not necessary for beauty. In this chapter, we propose a perspective on beauty-in-experience rather than a classical or neoclassical conception of beauty in which perfection or proportion are necessary. Our view of beauty builds from a Burkean perceptual model rather than a Kantian judgment model.

When a human being encounters another human, an animal or plant, a work of art, or a natural scene, a certain feeling is conveyed between the object and the perceiver. What is at work behind such perception? What does the body have to do with such experiences? A present-day philosopher, Roger Scruton (2009) sets up this problem under the term "judgment" (after Kant), suggesting that what matters is a judgment of taste "for which the technical term 'aesthetic' is now in common use" (p. 17). Unlike Scruton, the Burkean perceptual model might describe beauty in biological or evolutionary terms *avant la lettre*, where a certain experience of bodily features like webs, wings, breasts, hips or muscular tone create a perception of beauty. As we will see, this perceptual model is not clearly tied to a judgment or rational claim about the object being perceived.

Classical Beauty

The classical ideal for beauty appears in both its Ancient Greek and European (Renaissance through nineteenth century) versions. In short, this idea held that the standard for beauty is one of harmony, symmetry, and proportion, and that this form of beauty imitates or is found in the perfection of the gods or of the universe. This latter line of reasoning (usually associated with German philosophy of the eighteenth century) regards perfection as the basis of beauty. Following Leibniz, Moses Mendelssohn defined beauty as an intellectual (and thus rational) perfection of an object (see Bourke, 2015, p. 133ff; Hochman, 2014, p. 39f.). Although written in a literary form, Mendelssohn's (1761/1997) *Letters on Sentiments* is an important discussion of this issue at the very origin of aesthetics as a discipline. The principal contrast in this text is between sensual perfection and rational perfection. Two of the characters of this dialogue stand for each of these ways of interpreting beauty: Euphranor supports a sensual (English) perception of beauty and Theocles the intellectual (German) perception.

Ancient Greek Beauty

Proportionality, a classical ideal, concerns ratios, numbers, and a beautiful form. Basing beauty on proportionality tends to exclude any element of feeling or property of the mind. From Plato to Shaftesbury, beauty primarily concerns the property of an object that is symmetrical and orderly – with proper mathematical ratios. For the Greeks, beauty is not an autonomous field of inquiry nor is it primarily applied to art. Instead, for Plato, beauty concerns *eros*, the desire for something lacking in oneself (Hyland, 2008; Kraut, 2008). The important point for Plato (and Neoplatonism) is how *auto to kalon*, "beauty itself," is a perfect and eternal form unchangeable and divorced from bodies. Eros is meant to lead us to this perfect form. We can begin to see how much this conception of beauty has changed since the Renaissance.

Ancient Greek Beauty and the Origin of Ballet Owen Smith (2005) points out that the classical standard for Western theatre dance has long been the Apollonian model of corporeal harmony, proportion and verticality. Indeed, Jennifer Homans' (2010) book on the history of ballet is titled *Apollo's Angels*. There Homans points out that Gaetan Vestris was known as "the god of the dance" for having a body that approximated the Apollonian ideal, with a "long, lean, elegantly apportioned body with physical stature and beauty" (pp. 26–27). Ballet is one of the main vehicles for the classical ideal of the body (Novack, 1993).

Ballet's aesthetic values derived from Ancient Greece show a Platonic as well as an Apollonian ideal for beauty. When Catherine De Medici married Henri II she brought ballet to France from Florence, after which it was developed by the French monarchies in order to combine their Christian beliefs, which included a body-transcendent love of God, with the ideal, Platonic world of the forms (Homans, 2010). Their Neoplatonic idea was to reveal God and His secret, ideal realm by shifting their attention away from passions and physical desire and towards the beauty of number, proportion, and design (p. 6).

Classical ballet has had a profound influence on the development of Western theatre dance overall, including its idea of beauty. Petra Kuppers (2000) observes that ballet is often cited by dance biographers as the form of dance that initially attracted their imagination and that this has an effect on their idea of the "dancerly body" as one that is "perfect" or "ideal" in a classical way (pp. 122–123).

Neo-classical Beauty

In Western culture and the ballet that became part of that culture, the idea of beauty progressed and developed from a classical to a neo-classical standard over time, one that changed the idea of beauty in classical proportionality to one that included fitness for function. Anticipating evolutionary theory of the nineteenth century, the

Third Earl of Shaftesbury (1671–1713) speaks of a spider and a fly in the following way: "The heedless flight, weak frame and tender body of this [fly] fits and determines him as much a prey as the rough make, watchfulness and cunning of the [spider] fits him for rapine and the ensnaring part" (Shaftesbury, 1711/1997, pp. 18–19). The important point for Shaftesbury is that there is a structural analogy between species, but also between limbs and organs. "And in the structure of each of these animals," he notes, "there is as apparent and perfect a relation to the other as, in our own bodies, there is a relation of limbs and organs or as, in the branches or leaves of a tree, we see a relation to each other and all, in common, to one root and trunk" (p. 168). In neo-classical beauty, the function of the organ or body as it relates to the whole becomes part of the thinking at the origin of aesthetics in a manner that, at the time, had not previously been emphasized.

Neo-classical Beauty in Aristocratic Europe and Ballet The purpose of classical ballet, as taught in the French Académie Royale de Musique et de Danse, established by Louis XIV in 1661, was to teach noblemen the bearing, carriage, posture, and grace that befitted the aristocratic class in Western Europe (Homans, 2010; Smith, 2005). This was part of a trend across Europe during Shaftesbury's time in which aesthetics as a discipline was born (Klein, 2004; Vermeir & Deckard, 2012). Classical ballet sought to teach this comportment not only as an aesthetic property to be experienced as pleasing or beautiful, but to include the moral quality of how one should conduct oneself in society. Thus, from its inception beauty in ballet included both the aesthetic property of beauty and the idea of beauty as a human ethical value. The standard for the posture and type of body that was best for ballet can be seen in Leonardo da Vinci's geometrical drawing of *The Vitruvian Man* (1490) man (Fig. 11.1) where the ideal body was taken to reflect universal laws of nature, proportion and harmony (Homans, 2010, p. 134).

Nineteenth-century Romanticism gave rise to the ballerina as female and sylph, with Marie Taglioni being admired both for encapsulating this ethereal ideal as well as for her "bourgeois propriety" (see Homans, photo inserts following p. 134). Indeed, the development of pointe shoes increased both the line of the ballerina's leg and elevated her towards the heavens. Homans notes that Taglioni's foot on pointe was even an object of romantic fantasy (p. 141). It is this balletic aesthetic of beautiful ethereality, what Petra Kuppers (2000) calls "the form's insistence on lightness and immateriality," that creates the "hypervisibility" of the disabled body, since what does not fit with this ideal is thrown into high relief (p. 124). Kuppers' theory of disability will be discussed further towards the end of this chapter.

Beauty in Balanchine Ballet

George Balanchine was a direct inheritor of ballet as an aristocratic art form. Born in St. Petersburg in 1904 he learned ballet at the Imperial Ballet Theatre under the reign of Tsar Nicholas II, where he both boarded and was taught his academic

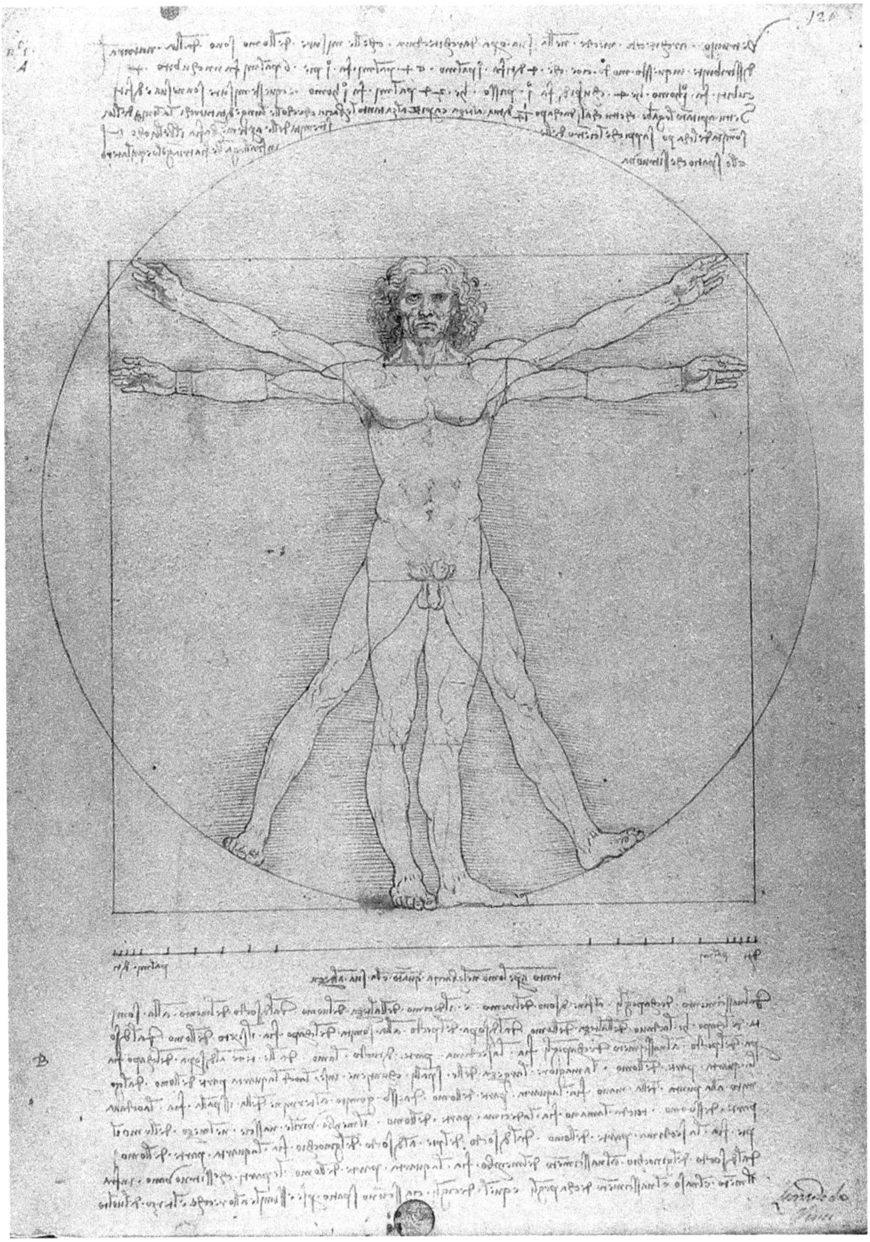

Fig. 11.1 Leonardo da Vinci *The Vitruvian Man* (1490)

subjects. He also trained as a musician at the St. Petersburg Conservatory. During the Communist revolution, the Imperial Ballet fell into disrepair and the students were often hungry and cold. Balanchine fled to Paris, where he spent a number of years dancing and choreographing ballets for various dance troupes. Lincoln Kirstein discovered Balanchine at Diaghilev's *Ballet Russes* and brought him to America in 1933. Together they founded the New York City Ballet (NYCB) (Volkov, 1985). The NYCB arguably reached its heyday in the 1960s, '70s, and '80s, before Balanchine's death, a period of time following the emergence of the avant-garde movement that made beauty unnecessary for philosophy's concept of art (Danto, 2003). Philosophers and critics who declared a beauty crisis in art could not have been those in the audience who were in the thrall of a Balanchine ballet.

The beauty of Balanchine ballet is classical in many aspects even though Balanchine called his style "neo-classical ballet" to distinguish it from older classical styles like Enrico Cecchetti's. His ballets contain order, unexpectedness, inevitability, economy (Euclid and Pythagoras according to Osborne, 1984, p. 295), and "coherent harmoniousness" with music under a unifying Idea (Plotinus, 1964, pp. 34–36). This classicism is particularly in evidence in the ballets he created with Igor Stravinsky (1936), a composer who acknowledged

> …a profound admiration for classical ballet, which in its very essence, by the beauty of its *ordonnance* [arrangement of elements] and the aristocratic austerity of its forms … represents the triumph of the studied conception over vagueness, of the rule over the arbitrary, of order over the haphazard. (pp. 99–100)

Stravinsky noted that for *Apollo* Balanchine designed "groups, movements, and lines of great dignity and plastic elegance as inspired by the beauty of classical forms" (p. 143). Indeed, in classical philosophers like Plotinus (1964) we find "the beauty [that] craftsmanship confers upon a house … and all its parts" (p. 36). Balanchine ballet might also be said to commune "with the intelligible realm" by its ability to be appreciated with the "faculty that is peculiarly sensitive to this beauty" and then judged in accordance with that faculty's "own inner Idea, which it uses as a canon of accuracy" (p. 36) (Fig. 11.2).

Towards Beauty-in-Experience

In this section we discuss the philosophical background to our reconsidered standard of beauty – one that treats what we will here call "beauty-in-experience" as a development of, rather than departure from, conceptions of beauty that are found in Western philosophical aesthetics. We show how Edmund Burke's eighteenth-century philosophy, for example, can provide a connecting link between traditional, perfection- and fitness-based standards of beauty and the contemporary idea of beauty-in-experience that is being developed by disability studies and disability-integrated dance companies.

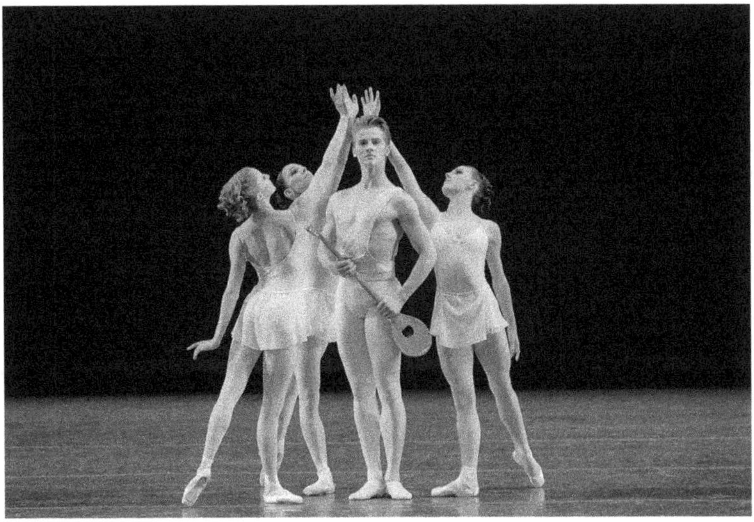

Fig. 11.2 Chase Finlay as Apollo with Sterling Hyltin as Terpsichore, Tiler Peck as Polyhymnia, and Ana Sophia Scheller as Calliope. (Choreography George Balanchine © The George Balanchine Trust Photograph: © Paul Kolnik)

A Burkean Theory

Edmund Burke (1730–1797) questioned many of his culture's deeply held beliefs about beauty – in particular its having to be perfect or proportionate. Interpreters have not taken his view of beauty seriously, though, because of his gendered categories, and some of this hesitation may be justified. However, this chapter aims to defend a Burke-inspired experiential account of the *origin* of our ideas of the beautiful. Fundamentally, at the level of efficient cause, beauty refers to a corporeal relaxation rather than a tension (as in the sublime).

While the English and the Scots upheld a theory of beauty based in proportionality and fitness, and the Germans one of intellectual perfection, the French constructed theories of beauty on more subjective matters, such as that of taste (*goût*) (Vermeir & Deckard, 2012). Burke is best read within a culture (as an Irishman in Great Britain) in which nerves and sensibilities as well as mores and manners become part of the philosophical vocabulary. Whereas the seventeenth century focused on the rationality of passion, the eighteenth century, and Burke in particular, speak in terms of bodily sensibility and experience. Following John Locke, who was a medical doctor, but also Richard Brocklesby's (1722–1797) experiments on animals, Sarafianos (2005) explains that,

> [Brocklesby's] research produced a new anatomical map … skin, nerves, and innervated parts were sensitive but motionless, while muscle fibers and membranes were insensible but moving …. Th[e] integrated perception of sensibility as a universal and omnipotent phenomenon of the body provides an immediate connection between Burke's *Enquiry* and later manifestations of vitalist thinking. (p. 63)

Burke's experiential theory of beauty is described here in anatomical, psychological and neuro-physiological terms, and as Sarafianos notes, this is a new way of describing the body. This medical background provides useful distinctions for our analysis. In looking specifically to dance, something Burke does not write about, we apply his theory of tensed nerves and relaxed solids – simply speaking, whether the body of the viewer is experienced as tense or relaxed – in a way that has not been done before.

In part I, section X, of *Philosophical Enquiry*, "Of Beauty," animals are treated as incapable of the sense for beauty as they are interested in sex only as a means of reproduction. "But man," Burke (1757/2015) writes, "who is a creature adapted to a greater variety and intricacy of relation, connects with the general passion, the idea of some *social* qualities, which direct and heighten the appetite which he has in common with all other animals" (p. 67). This social quality applies to both genders equally and is the very basis of beauty in human nature. "I call beauty a social quality; for where women and men, and not only they, but when other animals give us a sense of joy and pleasure in beholding them, (and there are many that do so) they inspire us with sentiments of tenderness and affection towards their persons" (p. 67).

The most significant criticism of Burke concerns his theory in which beauty is feminine and the sublime is masculine – this is viewed as too gendered (O'Neill, 2007). Here is the crucial and controversial passage:

> This quality [of beauty], where it is highest in the female sex, almost always carries with it an idea of weakness and imperfection. Women are very sensible of this, for which reason, they learn to lisp, to totter in their walk, to counterfeit weakness, and even sickness. In all this, they are guided by nature. Beauty in distress is much the most affecting beauty. (p. 88)

This passage needs to be taken in its socio-historical context. Burke's is not a normative claim regarding *how* women *should* act, but rather it is describing an empirical example to support the claim that, "the appearance of beauty effectually causes some degree of love in us, as the application of ice or fire produces the ideas of heat or cold" (p. 74). While Burke would have agreed with Shaftesbury's (1711/1997) claim that "it is not merely what we call *principle* but a *taste* which governs men," he contrasts Shaftesbury's neo-classical (and aristocratic) claim that "if in the way of polite pleasure the study and love of beauty be essential, the study and love of symmetry and order, on which beauty depends, must also be essential in the same respect" (p. 414). The perception of weakness is thus tied to beauty, which in the eighteenth century was connected to feminine mores.

It is thus in the context of mixed sentiments combined with the rise of the aesthetic in Francis Bacon, Thomas Hobbes, John Locke, and Shaftesbury, among others, that a culture of taste and manners contributed to a deepening in the contrast between beauty and ugliness, or fitness and deformity (Bourke, 1757/2015, Ch. III; Hochman, 2014). To situate Burke within this eighteenth-century context is to make a claim about beauty and disability that recovers beauty as a perceptual quality in place of a rational conceptual relation. What is it in this time of the rise of aesthetics that shifts the language from reason to feelings such that "abnormal" bodies may now be perceived anew? Later in the nineteenth century, romantic notions of beauty take over and, as Danto (2003) and Scarry (1999) have pointed out, by the time of the twentieth century, the ideals of the beautiful had all but died out. Philosophical definitions had eclipsed the Platonic origins of *eros* and love, and as Deckard (2011) has shown, Burke is interpreting Plato's love (and beauty) in terms of *philia* rather than *eros*. But in reconsidering beauty, the Burkean lens is a fruitful one through which to view contemporary dance, a form of dance developed from modern dance that offers dancers and audiences the opportunity to feel beauty by experiencing the ways that non-idealized bodies can move in ways that are afforded to them.

Burkean Application

The fundamental question underlying a rejection of the neo-classical in favor of a beauty-in-experience perspective is the following: What is it that makes a body attractive in perceiving it? While there are other possible angles, let us take two possibilities here: size and shape, and movement. Since the background of Burke's theory in particular is partly medical, with respect to nerves and the efficient cause already mentioned, we will attempt this application before turning to dance.

What might the difference in size and shape of human bodies say about our perceptions of beauty? Here is one passage from Burke (1757/2015): "The neck, they say, in beautiful bodies should measure half the calf of the leg; it should likewise be twice the circumference of the wrist" (p. 78). According to Burke, as much as proportion and perfection had to be true of attractive bodies, it can just as likely be true of ugly bodies. He continues,

> You may assign any proportions you please to every part of the human body; and I undertake, that a painter shall religiously observe them all, and notwithstanding produce if he pleases, a very ugly figure. The same painter shall considerably deviate from these proportions, and produce a very beautiful one. (p. 78)

He says the same of sculpture before turning to the male and female body:

> Consider how much difference there is between the measures that prevail in many similar parts of the body, in the two sexes of this single species only. If you assign any determinate proportions to the limbs of a man, and if you limit human beauty to these proportions, when you find a woman who differs in the make and measures of almost every part, you must conclude her not to be beautiful in spite of the suggestions of your imagination; or in obedience to your imagination you must renounce your rules; you must lay by the scale and compass, and look out for some other cause of beauty. For if beauty be attached to certain measures which operate from a principle in nature, why should similar parts with different measures of proportion be found to have beauty, and this too in the very same species? But to open our view a little, it is worth observing, that almost all animals have parts of very much the same nature, and destined nearly to the same purposes; an head, neck, body, feet, eyes, ears, nose and mouth; yet Providence…has worked out of these few and similar organs, and members, a diversity hardly short of infinite in their disposition, measures, and relation. (p. 79)

This long passage is quite remarkable, since Burke is critiquing a long tradition of proportion when it comes to size and shape, predicting an evolutionary standard – the animal kingdom (including humans) have different shapes and sizes and even some of the same "features" as humans.

Again, what makes a body disproportionate? Are there dancers' bodies that are attractive, but not proportionate according to a classical ideal? According to Burke, it is not a mathematical proportion or rational perfection that makes one attractive. Some may have perfect proportionality and not be attractive and some may have imperfect proportions and be very attractive. Thus, the size and shape of a body may have to do with beauty according to a "principle in nature," but it is not pure mathematical relations that evoke the feeling of beauty. Furthermore, this is not a static standard, but rather can be adapted by different perceivers, of both classical and contemporary dance, including dance that includes disabled dancers. We turn now to a discussion of how disability studies suggest that we can learn to perceive differently through alteration of experience.

The Contribution of Disability Studies

Disability studies go further than does Burke in suggesting that beauty is more than the perception of an ideally proportioned object or body, thereby adding a great deal to how we might claim beauty as something that can appear in disability, in both dance and in non-dance life. In the sections below we discuss the ways that disability studies, and the incorporation of some of its tenets (such as the social concept of disability to be discussed below) by the dance world, has contributed to this broader concept of beauty.

The Social Versus Medical Model of Disability

We use Petra Kuppers' view of the social model of disability to frame the discussion in the rest of this chapter. Kuppers (2003, 2011, 2014) explains that *disability* is a discursive construct that lies within the interaction between the person with atypical biology and the social environment, where a person is only labeled "disabled" when they cannot function adequately within dominant social structures and norms (see also Herman & Chatfield, 2010). If a public building is only accessible via a flight of stairs with no ramp, for example, a person who needs to use a wheelchair for access to the building will then encounter an obstacle that will signal their "disability." This locates disability in the social landscape rather than in the differently-abled person. In a world with sufficient ramps, for example, the person using a wheelchair is not disabled; there is just a diversity of persons who can function in society, those who use legs and those who use wheels.

The contrasting model is "the medical model of disability," where the medical world sets the standard for "normal" biology. "Normal" might be a person with two legs, two arms, vision and hearing ability who can achieve certain tasks, etc., the standard for vision being 20–20. This model would locate any departure from this norm in the biology of the person who does not meet it (Herman & Chatfield, 2010; Kuppers, 2000, 2014). Kuppers (2014) credits this medical model of disability with either creating or being part of the discriminatory social phenomenon known as "ableism," in which the disabled person is characterized as inferior or in need of change (pp. 23–24; Zitomer & Reid, 2011). Shelley Tremain (2015) links Foucault's idea of biopower or biopolitics to disability studies. Understanding the dichotomy of "abled" and "disabled" as a function of normative regimes and values, which we have claimed might follow historically from a Burkean concept of beauty, paves the way for disability-inclusive dance to be beautiful in a way that increases the quality of life for those who experience this dance through bringing us into greater connection with and understanding of the movement qualities of differently-abled human beings.

Disability-Inclusive Dance's Contribution

As shown above, classical and neo-classical ideals of beauty are still alive in ballet companies like the NYCB. The disability-inclusive dance on which this chapter will now focus has developed out of the contemporary dance tradition. Contemporary dance in the 1960s and '70s, like its precursor, modern dance, sought to counter the European, aristocratic ballet tradition by experimenting with new movement styles that explicitly connected with emerging social ideas and widened the idea of how a beautiful dance body should look (Novack, 1990). (Remember here that Burke allowed that social ideas affect the experience of beauty.) Dancers no longer had to be princes and princesses with elongated bodies made longer by thinness and pointe shoes. Dancers could now have bodies with strength and weight, and they could perform guttural and grounded movements in bare feet. Modern and contemporary dance companies opened the door to disability-inclusive companies by allowing dance to establish its own codes for movement, and for who could perform that movement, that were no longer tied to aristocratic norms (Anderson, 2008).

In recent years many forms of dance, including ballet, have tried to expand their audiences and respond to social pressures for inclusiveness by incorporating disabled dancers. The number of international dance companies and organizations that feature either all disabled dancers or are integrated or disability inclusive include (in alphabetical order and in addition to the ones we will describe more fully below): Ability Unlimited (India), Adugna Potentials (Ethiopia), AMICI (UK), Blue Eyed Soul (UK), Cleveland Ballet Dancing Wheels (US), Dance Integrated (Australia), Danza Sin Limites, (Argentina), Disabled People's Performing Art Troupe (China), Diverse Dance (Canada), Genesis of Entertainment (Japan), Grupo Alma (Argentina), Grupo Pulsar (Brazil), HandiCapace Tanz Kompanie (Germany), Infinite Flow (US), Infinity Dance Theatre (US), Le Ballets C. de la B (Belgium), Light Motion (US), Mobility Junction (US), MoMo Dance Theatre (Canada), Motion House (UK), Núcleo Dança Aberta (Brazil), Oiseau Mouche (France),

Paradox Dance (US), Remix Dance Project (South Africa), Stop Gap (UK), The Dance Laboratory (Norway), Tokounou Dance Company (US), Touch Compass Dance Trust (New Zealand), Vertigo Dance Company (Israel), and Wheelchair Dance Project (Turkey). Below, we briefly describe various approaches to dance and disability represented or pioneered by several dance companies, in particular Candoco (U.K.), AXIS Dance Company (U.S.), and DanceAbility (U.S.), all contemporary companies that use a social model of disability to inform their work.

AXIS Dance Company, Candoco, and DanceAbility

AXIS Dance Company (started in 1987 in Oakland, California) was one of the first contemporary dance companies to help pave the way for integrated and mixed-ability dance worldwide (AXIS Dance Company, 2016). Integrated dance exists where the contributions and movement styles of all dance participants, those with and without physical or mental impairments, are given equal weight (Benjamin, 2002). Like other integrated and mixed-ability companies and programs, AXIS includes contact improvisationas a method for sharing and engaging differently-abled persons' experience of movement and dance. Davies (2008) describes one dancer's experience of exploring contact-improvisation based techniques with AXIS and choreographers Bill T. Jones and Stephen Petronio. Contact improvisation was initiated by Steve Paxton in the early 1970s. In this heuristic method, improvising dancers are joined through ever-changing points of contact that enable them to move together and to share and shift weight and energy from one person to another (Pallant, 2006).

Founded in London in 1991, Candoco (named to place focus on what differently abled bodies *can* rather than *cannot* do) was the first professional touring company to integrate differently-abled dancers in Europe employing both contact improvisation and Graham-based techniques (Benjamin, 2002). Adam Benjamin began Candoco with Celeste Dandeker, a former professional dancer with London Contemporary Dance Theatre who was injured onstage, leaving her with little ability to move her legs. They wanted to explore a form of dance that incorporated Dandeker's new way of moving in a wheelchair (p. 4).

Beginning with what a non-standard body *can* do initiates dance training, movement, and choreography development from the vantage point of a body who is already different from an Apollo or a sylph. As noted above, this development was potentiated by early modern dancers' rejection of traditional ballet standards at the beginning of the twentieth century. Such an approach opens up the possibility that the graceful flow of a wheelchair moving seamlessly across stage or the staccato movement of a person with tremors due to Parkinson's might be perceived and termed "beautiful" along neo-Burkean lines (Fig. 11.3).

DanceAbility International is an organization devoted to training teachers how to teach mixed-ability dance classes. It was founded by Alito Alessi in Eugene, Oregon in the late 1980s. Among other principles, DanceAbility holds that everyone should

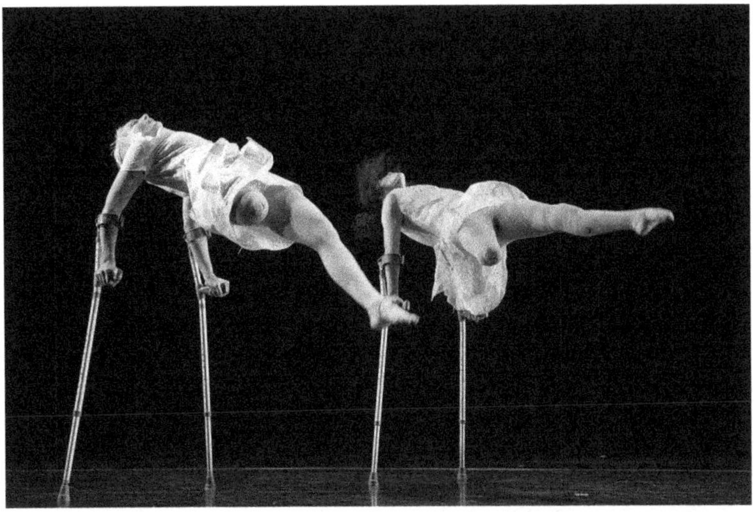

Fig. 11.3 Candoco Dance Company performs an Unlimited commission, *12* by Claire Cunningham at Southbank Centre's Unlimited Festival. (Photographer: Rachel Cherry, 2012)

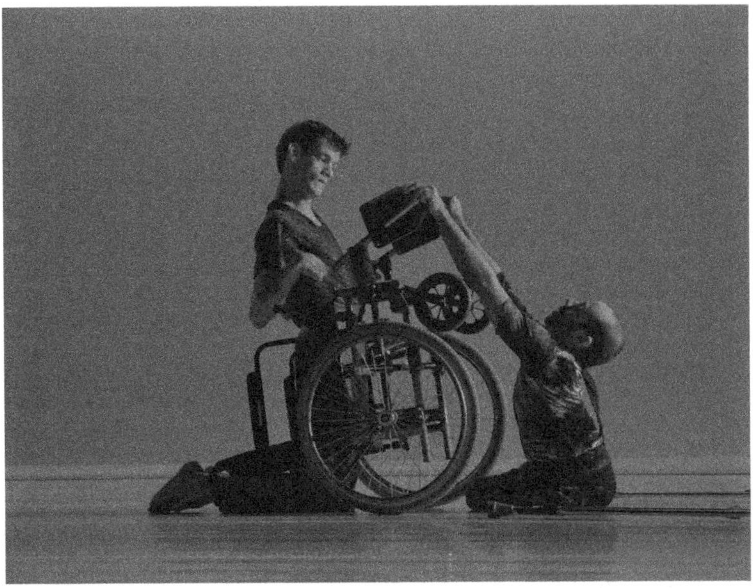

Fig. 11.4 DanceAbility International, photo by Gil Grossi. (From Sao Paolo, Brazil)

be able to dance (that dance is not for medically-termed "fit" or classical bodies only) and that dance has the social ability to breakdown prejudices (Herman & Chatfield, 2010). Here, dance education is acknowledged to affect not just the dance world but non-dance life as well (Fig. 11.4).

These innovators in dance and disability, among many others, instantiate a social model of disability through the medium and mode of dance. By doing so they are not just expressing the value of inclusiveness but showing through performance that beauty may be perceived in dance and in dancers performing with non-classical bodies, capabilities, and movement styles. As Benjamin (1993) stated:

> If contemporary arts and contemporary dance in particular is to reflect contemporary society, it must, just as it did when black dancers first appeared on stage in this country, open its doors and its eyes to perceive beauty and worth where it has hitherto been unable. (p. 46)

The question then becomes how the perception of the viewer might be changed so that they can see beauty where hitherto they could not.

Reconsidering Beauty as Beauty-in-Experience

We have so far discussed the various concepts of beauty, which can be listed as: classical beauty; neo-classical beauty; Burkean beauty; and beauty-in-experience. What do we mean, precisely, by beauty-in-experience? Clearly disabled dance and persons can both create and fail to create this experience (as can able-bodied dance and persons); not every experience with disability in dance or in life is necessarily beautiful. Beauty applies where there is a perceptual experience of beauty in the viewer. To expand one's perceptual scope may require education to "see" differently. Beauty, as Burke might agree, is something one identifies when perceiving or feeling it in experience. It may be related to a sort of movement economy of the dancer's particular body or the aids the dancer is moving with (such as the efficient movement of a dancer on wheels or using crutches or "walking" on their hands if they have no legs and feet). It also includes the idea that one can experience beauty through moving and dancing either as or with a differently-abled person (such as in a class, dance, or contact improvisation exercise).

In a study funded to examine dance students' experience of learning dance in "dance technique" classes that she conducted with her own students at Coventry University, Sarah Whatley (2007) sought to give voice to disabled dancers "who can so often feel silenced through their struggle to conform to normative representations of the dancing body" (pp. 6–7). This group of 15 female students from ages 18–26, including two students who are wheelchair users, reflected and reported upon their experiences in technique classes, both verbally and in writing, over a period of 9 months. Whatley also conducted research on levels of participation by disabled dance students in University dance classes across the UK, from which 13 of nearly 200 students identified as disabled (pp. 8–9). As a result, Whatley identified five "viewing strategies" (a term she uses following the work of Louise Kateraga and Petra Kuppers) used by dance students without disabilities to view dance performed by dance students with disabilities (p. 18). She found that these viewing strategies spanned a continuum of distant to empathic to transformative:

1. passive oppressive: where the viewer takes a voyeuristic stance;
2. passive conservative: where the viewer has internalized a classical aesthetic perspective;
3. post-passive: where the viewer looks to see how the disabled dancer transcends the disability;
4. active witness: where the viewer allows disability to open up new ways of seeing and interpreting the body in dance that includes a radical shift in aesthetic stance; and
5. immersion: where the non-disabled viewer experiences their own "becoming" through engaging with the disabled dancer's experience in a more fully immersive way. (pp. 18–20)

This framework shows how perceptions of disabled dance and disabled dancers' bodies might be changed through an interpretive mode of viewing; the viewing strategies described in (4) and (5) show how the idea of beauty might be expanded on the viewer/perceiver end to include such dancing under beauty-in-experience. In contrast, viewing strategy (1) suggests a way of viewing dance that treats the disabled person's body as "on display" as spectacle, and (2) views the disabled body with a classical aesthetic perspective. Both are experienced as alienating by the disabled dancer who is the object of this othering gaze (see pp. 18–19). Viewing strategy (3) seems to be what Ann Cooper Albright (1998/2013) refers to in her charge that disabled-inclusive dance companies sometimes remain within a traditional representational frame, "emphasizing the elements of virtuosity and technical expertise to reaffirm a classical body in spite of its limitations" (p. 301).

In fairness, Albright also notes that in the ballet *Gypsy*, Cleveland Ballet Dancing Wheels extends "the aesthetic heritage of nineteenth-century Romantic ballet into several intriguing new directions" (p. 315), which presumably included movements that are organic to wheelchair users. In addition, Albright points to contact improvisation as a promising way to achieve the immersive, experiential lens described in (5). Indeed, she suggests that contact improvisation differs from other methods of seeing and using disabled bodies because it succeeds in "pulling the audience in as witness to the ongoing negotiations of that [the disabled dancer's] physical experience" (p. 315).

Kuppers (2000) comments on how dance education might become better at training viewers to "see" differently. Suggestions include attending more carefully to spaces that disabled dancers have opened up through performance and complying with these performances' request that they become more aware of themselves as spectators (see pp. 126–129). Here she cites the Magpie and Retina Dance Company's 1997 performance for the London Blitz '97 festival that emphasized the company members' experiences with how they are treated as persons with learning disabilities (p. 126). She also cites performances by Bilderwerfer, a Viennese performance group that focuses on how audiences "read dance" in terms of what they believe is "natural" by disrupting these readings through the use of texts, music, glass screens, and other methods in public spaces (p. 127). This approach is one that fits with the work of Zitomer and Reid (2011), who found that children's perceptions of dance and disability change after immersion in an integrated dance program that includes children with and without physical differences.

Beauty-in-experience includes both how beauty appears to the viewer and how it feels to participants in the dance. Introducing her book on disability culture and community performance Kuppers (2011) discusses a workshop on physically integrated dance practice led by AXIS Dance Company where the instruction was to "find a strange and twisted shape" (p. 1). At first, she struggled to apply this direction. She explains,

> On the ground around me are plenty of people who live in twisted bodies, to whom the twist is not strange, but a deeply familiar way of experiencing their bodies' everyday frontality, location, or elevation while standing or sitting. (p. 1)

As the workshop went on, however, she realized that the disability-inclusive format of the workshop gave her explicit permission to:

> …translate the instructions into my own limbs, find twists that do feel strange, that stretch my bodily imaginary, that lead out of the comfort zone of my personal dancerly base-line. The category confusion passes. (p. 31)

Kuppers reconsidered "strange and twisted" in one of the ways that this chapter suggests that beauty can be reconsidered. The starting point was her own body's "dancerly base-line" and how movement *feels* rather than just how it looks. Thus, one might feel, as well as perceive, beauty.

This idea that beauty can be felt in both lived experience and in perception, not just in the viewing but in the process of "being," "becoming," or "dancing," is echoed in Sara Houston's (2015) article, "Feeling Lovely: An Examination of the Value of Beauty for People Dancing with Parkinson's." Carroll, a person with Parkinson's, remarks that an inclusive ballet class sponsored by the English National Ballet made her "feel lovely" and "beautiful again" (pp. 27–30). After considering this auto-ethnographic account along with the work of Arthur Frank, Michael Bury, Petra Kuppers, and others on the social and felt impact of disability, Houston suggests that the experience of beauty may be associated in part with the feeling of bodily control that dance can provide (pp. 33–34). Further, even though guided by balletic movements, this control is not an imposition from classical ballet, but the sort of control that is relative to the person's uniquely abled body with Parkinson's or any other body-movement affecting condition or biology. This is an experiential, or organic, sort of beauty. A non-disabled person dancing in a contact improvisation exercise with Carroll might also feel beauty through Carroll's body, carrying that experience and knowledge into other non-dance social realms where it can change new perceptions and experiences of beauty in disability (Fig. 11.5).

On Keeping Beauty

In conclusion, we would like to keep the term "beauty" because we believe – with Danto, Scarry, and Burke – that the experience of beauty is necessary to a full, rich, and "quality" life. It is no longer the case that only classical and neo-classical

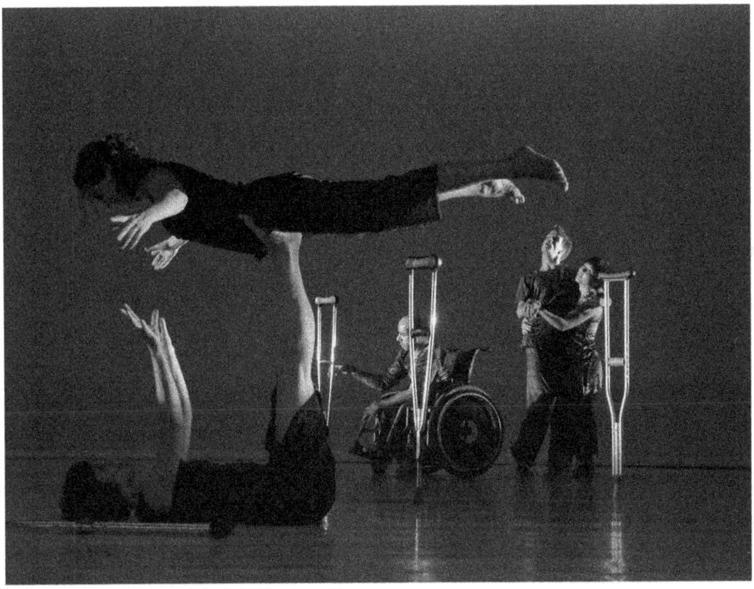

Fig. 11.5 DanceAbility International, photo by Gil Grossi. (Sao Paolo, Brazil)

dancers are eligible for the designation of *beautiful*. Disability-inclusive and non-disability inclusive dance companies have been offering performances and workshops that demonstrate how disabled bodies can both look and feel beautiful. Our goal in this chapter has been to trace the cultural development of a theory of beauty that can account for this change or enable us to see these companies as working with traditional concepts of the beautiful beyond the classical and neo-classical. We suggest that one point of departure from the classical norm resides in Edmund Burke's philosophy, which includes social awareness as part of the grounding for experiences of beauty. Disability studies has also expanded the meaning of "cultural perception" to include awareness of how the latter can be limited by factors that are more social than aesthetically necessary. We have also noted how dance practices such as contact improvisation and dance education have helped to change experiences and perceptions of dance and of dancers who are differently-abled. Finally, we have termed this kind of beauty, one that includes disability, as beauty-in-experience, so named to include the experience of beauty in both dance and non-dance life. Beauty-in-experience allows for a more "capacious regard," as Elaine Scarry (1999) puts it, in aesthetic and everyday encounters with others (p. 48).

References

Albrecht, G. L., & Devlieger, P. J. (1999). The disability paradox: High quality of life against all odds. *Social Science and Medicine, 48*, 977–988.

Albright, A. C. (2013). Strategic abilities: Negotiating the disabled body in dance. *Engaging bodies: The politics and poetics of corporeality* (pp. 297–317). Middletown, CT: Wesleyan University Press. (Original work published 1998)

Anderson, J. (2008). *Ballet and modern dance: A concise history* (2nd ed.). Hightstown, NJ: Princeton Book/Dance Horizons.

AXIS Dance Company. (2016). Retrieved from http://www.AXIS.org

Benjamin, A. (1993). In search of integrity. *Dance Theatre Journal, 10*, 42–46.

Benjamin, A. (2002). *Making an entrance: Theory and practice for disabled and non-disabled dancers*. New York/London: Routledge.

Bourke, R. (2015). *Empire and revolution: The political life of Edmund Burke*. Princeton, NJ: Princeton University Press.

Burke, E. (2015). *A philosophical enquiry into the origin of our ideas of the sublime and beautiful*. Oxford: Oxford University Press (Original work published 1757).

Danto, A. C. (2003). *The abuse of beauty: Aesthetics and the concept of art*. Chicago/La Salle, IL: Open Court.

Davies, T. (2008). Mobility: AXIS dancers push the boundaries of access. *Text and Performance Quarterly, 28*(1–2), 43–63.

Deckard, M. F. (2011). Wonder and beauty in Burke's *Philosophical Enquiry*. *Studies in Burke and His Time, 22*, 45–80.

Herman, A., & Chatfield, S. (2010). A detailed analysis of DanceAbility's contribution to mixed-abilities dance. *Journal of Dance Education, 10*(2), 41–55.

Hochman, L. (2014). *The ugliness of Moses Mendelssohn: Aesthetics, religion, and morality in the eighteenth century*. London: Routledge.

Homans, J. (2010). *Apollo's angels: A history of ballet*. New York: Random House.

Houston, S. (2015). Feeling lovely: An examination of the value of beauty for people dancing with Parkinson's. *Dance Research Journal, 47*(1), 27–43.

Hyland, D. (2008). *Plato and the question of beauty*. Bloomington: Indiana University Press.

Klein, L. (2004). *Shaftesbury and the culture of politeness: Moral discourse and cultural politics in early eighteenth-century England*. Cambridge: Cambridge University Press.

Kraut, R. (2008). Plato on love. In R. Kraut (Ed.), *The Oxford handbook of Plato* (pp. 286–310). Oxford: Oxford University Press.

Kuppers, P. (2000). Accessible education: Aesthetics, bodies, and disability. *Research in Dance Education, 1*(2), 119–131.

Kuppers, P. (2003). *Disability and contemporary performance: Bodies on the edge*. New York: Routledge.

Kuppers, P. (2011). *Disability culture and community performance*. New York: Palgrave Macmillan.

Kuppers, P. (2014). *Studying disability arts and culture: An introduction*. New York: Palgrave Macmillan.

Mendelssohn, M. (1997). *Philosophical writings*. Cambridge, MA: Cambridge University Press. (Original work published 1761)

Novack, C. J. (1990). *Sharing the dance: Contact improvisation and American culture*. Madison: University of Wisconsin Press.

Novack, C. J. (1993). Ballet, gender and cultural power. In H. Thomas (Ed.), *Dance, gender and culture* (pp. 34–48). London: Palgrave Macmillan.

O'Neill, D. I. (2007). *The burke-Wollstonecraft debate: Savagery, civilization, and democracy*. University Park: The Pennsylvania State University Press.

Osborne, H. (1984). Mathematical beauty and physical science. *The British Journal of Aesthetics, 24*(4), 291–300.

Pallant, C. (2006). *Contact improvisation: An introduction to a vitalizing dance form*. Jefferson, NC: MacFarland.
Plotinus. (1964). Beauty [from the Enneads]. *The essential Plotinus* (E. O'Brien, Trans., 2nd ed., pp. 33–44). Indianapolis, IN: Hackett Company, Inc.
Sarafianos, A. (2005). Pain, labor, and the sublime: Medical gymnastics and Burke's aesthetics. *Representations, 91*(1), 58–83.
Scarry, E. (1999). *On beauty and being just*. Princeton, NJ: Princeton University Press.
Scruton, R. (2009). *Beauty*. Oxford: Oxford University Press.
Shaftesbury, Third Earl of. (1997). *Characteristics of men, manners, opinions, times*. Cambridge, MA: Cambridge University Press. (Original work published 1711)
Smith, O. (2005). Shifting Apollo's frame: Challenging the body aesthetic in theater dance. In C. Sandahl & P. Auslander (Eds.), *Bodies in commotion: Disability and performance* (pp. 73–85). Ann Arbor: The University of Michigan Press.
Stravinsky, I. (1936). *Igor Stravinsky: An autobiography*. New York: W. W. Norton.
Tremain, S. (Ed.). (2015). *Foucault and the government of disability*. Ann Arbor: University of Michigan Press.
Vermeir, K., & Deckard, M. F. (Eds.). (2012). *The science of sensibility: Reading Burke's philosophical enquiry*. Dordrecht, The Netherlands: Springer.
Volkov, S. (1985). *Balanchine's Tchaikovsky: Interviews with George Balanchine* (A. W. Bouis, Trans.). New York: Simon and Schuster.
Whatley, S. (2007). Dance and disability: The dancer, the viewer and the presumption of difference. *Research in Dance Education, 8*(1), 5–25.
Zitomer, M. R., & Reid, G. (2011). To be or not to be – Able to dance: Integrated dance and children's perceptions of dance ability and disability. *Research in Dance Education, 12*(1), 137–156.

Part IV
Dancing Gender, Dancing Family

Chapter 12
"Just Me and Daddy"

Byron Richard

Gendered patterns of social, educational, and work life have been documented in the United States and remain unchanged over decades. These patterns show men distanced from aesthetic pursuits as well as from professions requiring skills in health, education, administration and literacy. Simultaneously, shifting patterns show women making slow but steady progress in education and work life, recently in the fields of science, technology, engineering and mathematics (Reeves & Sawhill, 2015). This chapter joins the gender discourse in dance education, asking: *What happens when a group of men and their male family members are invited into aesthetic and pedagogical experiences unanticipated by prevailing gender-based life patterns?*

Dancing and learning about dance are not typical pursuits for men in the United States (Oliver & Risner, 2017; Risner, 2008, 2009), a society where the number of women graduating from dance programs in higher education is approximately ten times that of men (United States Department of Education, 2013). This gendered pattern of participation is in addition to marginal access to dance education generally (NDEO, 2004). In public schools, for example, while student access to education in the arts is shrinking across arts disciplines, opportunities for students to engage in dance education are only a fraction of those for music and visual art learning (Parsad & Spiegelman, 2012).

Even more unusual are dance learning experiences in settings that include fathers and sons. With the goal of examining the aesthetic and pedagogical experiences of a community of highly social, verbally acute, literate and preliterate male children and their fathers, I designed a multi-week series of dance classes to investigate dance education with an intergenerational group of related males. I was interested

B. Richard (✉)
Independent Scholar, Minneapolis, MN, USA

K. Bond (ed.), *Dance and the Quality of Life*, Social Indicators Research Series 73,
https://doi.org/10.1007/978-3-319-95699-2_12

to know about this group of men and boys as a possible example of aesthetic community (Bond, 2008), a community engaged in expressing and mediating individual style and dispositions through a group process that afforded shared aesthetic meanings and development of a group style.

Research Methodology

Focusing on questions of the qualities and meanings of pedagogical interactions, I conducted a multi-modal, qualitative inquiry (Denzin, 1998). I sought pragmatic flexibility through reflective practice in an emergent curriculum design (Bond, 1994a, 1994b, 2001; Bond & Deans, 1997), and the study's small scale and practice orientation, resulting in local knowledge of particular situations and relations, aligns with action research (Bond & Richard, 2005; Carr & Kemmis, 1986; Schön, 1991). Autobiographical elements including teacher self-reflection, parenting and teaching in action and in reflection, and critical reflection on prior educational experiences salient to the study are aligned with narrative inquiry in educational research (Clandinin & Connelly, 1991, 1995). Finally, data collection and analysis were informed by phenomenological principles and strategies (Giorgi, 1992; van Manen, 1997).

Sources include audio and video documentation of participants' dance education experiences during each session, transcriptions of these materials noting movement and linguistic content, a field journal, and recorded interviews with parents and children. Further, a wealth of child and adult statements and pictorial representations of meanings through captioned, post-session drawings augmented triangulation of sources (Denzin & Lincoln, 2005). Bond's (1994b, 2008) articulation of personal and group style in terms of rhythm, gesture, and movement mannerisms also informed my analysis of participant engagement in dance. The study was approved as ethical human subjects research by Temple University's Institutional Review Board.

Transcriptions of session video-recordings were the basis for a line-by-line analysis of the entire sequence of dance education sessions. I treated the culminating interview transcripts similarly, helped by the organizing categories provided by my interview questions, and analyzing these transcripts for the kinds of language used by participants to describe their experiences, and for how their experiences changed over time. I also examined this material for reports and descriptions of particularly memorable dance experiences, and used it to dialog with and add perspective to other evidences and points of view toward these experiences.

After reading the entire video transcript to achieve a sense of the whole, I performed a phenomenological analysis, parsing each session description into units by listening for shifts of meaning in the text. To stay open to the possibility of new understandings, I attempted to bracket, or set aside my prior knowledge of the described phenomena, a discipline of phenomenological practice (Giorgi, 1992; van Manen, 1997). Each meaning unit included a brief description, an interpretation of the unit, questions about the unit, and reconstruction of my own lived experience of my body, space, time, and relationship during the episode (van Manen, 1997).

Analysis of video and interview transcripts resulted in over 1000 anecdotal units of descriptive meaning, which I organized into broad categories: participant interactions, movement interests and patterns, teacher concerns, emotions and feelings, and examples of language used by participants in sessions. I also performed a descriptive analysis of images and language in participants' drawings, which revealed each participant's perceptions of key events, activities, and objects in the series as well as the range of interactive dynamics among the participants and with me (Bond, 2001; Bond & Richard, 2005).

As a result of these systematic processes, the interpretations presented as findings strive for what Denzin (1998) calls descriptive realism, incorporating real-life dialogue, intimate voice, multiple perspectives, interior monologues, and scene-by scene narration that places the interpretation in a context full of multi-voiced interactions among its participants. One value of including multiple kinds of evidence is the potentially rich, nuanced reading of situations and relations they can afford. In other words, what I can transcribe about an interaction from the kinesthetic and audio portions of a videotape can be layered with content available from reflective, post-session captioned drawings. For example, son Carl's classroom interactions with dad Todd are augmented by his graphic depictions of the two in class and by his statements and actions during his culminating interview, which look back to dancing with his father and include kinesthetic recreations of prior incidents in the moment of interviewing.

"Just Me and Daddy"

Fourteen males in six family groups met together on seven Saturdays in a small community north of Philadelphia, Pennsylvania. Participants ranged in age from 5 years to 45 years. To teach this group I relied on my knowledge and experience of Laban Movement Analysis (Laban, 1988) as a source of theory and practice for developmental dance education, a body of theory often applied to creative movement for primary aged children. I also drew on my dance making and performance experience, which included dance improvisation, performance, and choreographic processes. My family and community life as a parent of two young children, one of whom, Wyatt, participated in the class, was the ever-present pedagogical setting I worked to understand as a source for teaching and learning.

In my career as a dance educator I have taught in universities, in open community dance classes in New York and Minneapolis, and in K-16 classrooms in Minnesota and Pennsylvania. I have also participated in parent education classes in the company of adults only where, in contrast to dance teaching and learning *among* family members, our young children were separated from us to receive early childhood experiences from trained educators and to allow adults to concentrate on parenting.

Our Saturday morning dance classes briefly liberated participant households of their male child and adult members, an unanticipated benefit identified by participating families. Fathers and sons danced in a large open space with vaulted ceilings in a neighborhood church, ringed with brightly colored indoor playground equipment used by a weekday preschool. I worked to match my internalized knowledge of dance teaching with my hunches about what would engage these men and boys and to revise this practice knowledge with what I was learning in reflection. As I interacted with participants during dance sessions, and in reflection after teaching, my private thoughts and reactions helped reveal my assumptions and biases as I co-created our emergent curriculum. Clearest of these initial sensations was my disdain for and concern about the play equipment lining the room and my expectations for child cooperation and compliance with my plans and direction (especially my son's).

With a sense of doubt about my prior assumptions and my curiosity about the emerging dance interests of this group, I found myself responding in the moment to changing conditions and participant responses with growing flexibility, moderating physically stressful activities for the middle-aged dads, altering groupings to support younger children, while researching child interests between classes in an attempt to increase their engagement with dancing. Children and adults worked frequently with commitment and vitality, mirroring Bond's (2008) finding that her nonverbal child participants with severe sensory impairments "worked hard," as observed in extended focus, commitment to content, and increasing engagement in social interaction with both peers and adults" (p. 416).

Development of the seven sessions fell into three distinct phases. The first phase, *Towering Adventures*, included sessions one to three in which fathers negotiated intense child interest in stacking and moving through play equipment while pursuing a curriculum of drumming and sharing dance in family and whole group contexts. The second phase, *Fathering while Teaching and Dancing*, encompassed sessions four and five in which a subset of the group explored father and son relationships through dance, story, and drawing. Active reflecting about the qualities of father and son relations and family life, using dance, extended into the next phase. With an emphasis on animals, environments, and journeys, the third phase, *Shaping the World*, included the final sessions six and seven, culminating in dances about landscapes and in family journey dances.

Pedagogical Sources Family relationships and the content of home life were ready sources for pedagogy and curriculum. Many parents know how powerfully children can transform adults' sense of themselves, their priorities in life, and their preoccupations with concerns of the world. Many teachers, too, experience the transforming effects young people have on their professional and personal lives. This powerful influence of children that can transform personal existence and radiate throughout an adult's life is what kindles…pedagogy (van Manen, 1991, pp. 11–12). This study seeks to reveal a network of pedagogical regard for the well-being and quality of life of family members and non-family dance class participants.

Aesthetic Community

New to the idea of pedagogy as tactful thoughtfulness about the wellbeing of others (van Manen, 1991), and to constructing curriculum in response to participant interests and evidence of learning (Bond & Richard, 2005), I adapted a flexible, ritual-like framework similar to Bond's (1994b, 2008) "right dance" (after Goodman's [1978] "rightness of fit" and Sparshott, 1988) to organize many of the temporal and spatial aspects of the classes. This structure aligned with my research commitment to recognize participants' meanings through reflection and to treat them as primary sources of dance ideas. Bond draws on physicists David Bohm and F. David Peat (1987), who distinguish between "an 'outside order of development' involving 'evolution in a sequence of successions' and a 'more inward order out of which the manifest form of things can emerge creatively'" (as cited in Bond, 2008, p. 409). The "right dance" (in current parlance, Bond views "right dance" as an aspect of "situated best practice") provides the iterative outside order of development through which individual aesthetic preferences merge creatively to form an aesthetic community (Bond, 1994b, p. 22).

In her germinal study with six young nonverbal children with deaf-blindness, Bond found that development of aesthetic community relied on a form of dance facilitation that affirms each participant's "aisthetic," or bodily sensory perception, as evidenced in their "personal style": "the characteristic bodily forms and modes through which human intents are conveyed" (p. 21; see also Maletic, 1982). Bond's implementation of "right dance" promoted participant engagement, self-transformation, and aesthetic community for children with severe learning disabilities.

The present study applied Bond's (1994b, 2008) prototype of "right dance" in a heuristic manner across a series of sessions for fathers and sons. Analysis of multiple sources of data illuminated participants' progression through the developmental sequence from individual aisthetic perception and response to aesthetic community (Fig. 12.1).

"Not…a Typical Interaction with Your Son[s]"

What follows sets the stage for a close description of the developmental journeys of two family groups, a subset of this group of participants. Both Todd and his sons Carl (five) and Ian (eight), and Paul and his sons Isaac (six) and Christian (eight), attended five of the seven sessions. I chose these families because each included three participating members, offering ample evidence of interaction by family members with each other and with other participants. Also, with a similar spread of ages and pattern of attendance, there was a solid foundation for comparing and contrasting the dance education experiences of each family. Todd's family also includes his wife Louise, daughters Sophia (six) and Bella (four), and 20-month-old

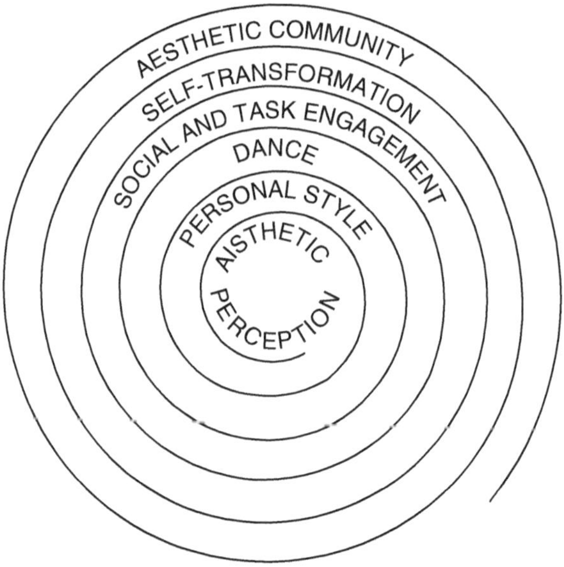

Fig. 12.1 A path to aesthetic community in dance. (Bond, 1994b, 2008)

Randall. Paul's family also includes his wife Jeanette. Both Louise and Jeanette offered comments about their husband's and sons' dance experiences.

The families' developmental journeys began with their initial responses and reasons to accept my unusual request for their participation in a "dads and sons" dance class. I first discuss members' initial meanings of the word *dance* and related vocabulary, along with any prior dance education experience. Progress of the two families through the seven classes is related through descriptions of episodes that reveal change and growth as perceived by the adult and child participants, including incidents of social mediation, mutual admiration, and persistence in dancing outside of class. I conclude with a discussion of reflective teaching practice, describe the interactions revealing the intersubjective tone of the classes, and present evidence of participants achieving a kind of aesthetic community through dance, also elaborating future lines of inquiry.

"Help Byron Out": A Reason to Start to Dance

Though initially Todd's family agreed to participate in the classes to, as he said, "help Byron out," family members engaged in substantial discussion about how to regard my invitation to a dance class for dads and sons. Todd described talking with his son Ian prior to the classes: "Beforehand, especially with Ian, we weren't allowed to call it dance. It was never dance, it was movement." He tested Ian's response to the word dance after several weeks of classes: "But then, after the first one or two [classes], I would do it sort of teasingly to see what he was going to do, and we'd call it dance and it didn't bother him." Todd asserted that by the end of the classes Ian's attitude had shifted. He suggested, "What we were doing wasn't necessarily what he thought of as dance, but it was dance, and it was moving, so he was okay with it."

Intrigued with her sons' responses to her early use of the word "ballet" to describe the sessions, Louise reported resistance: "My boys looked forward to going, as long as you did not call it ballet. It was a father and son class." She supported the idea of an out-of-the-house Saturday morning cost-free activity for her husband and sons enthusiastically. Jeanette was supportive also, joking "the price is right" in her interview. I learned through the neighborhood grapevine that a positive attitude toward the classes was shared among other mothers of participating families. Perhaps the unusualness of this experience fueled a sense of adventure and opportunity for enhanced relationship among these families that were already caring households.

Paul and Jeanette had briefly enrolled their sons in a private school focused on arts and experiential learning. They had also provided Christian and Isaac with workshop experiences in hip-hop dance. As such, dance and arts-based learning were not new experiences for Paul's family. He read the letter of invitation I sent to each family to prepare his two boys for the first class. Paul said, "They cracked up when I read…they just thought it was hilarious." Isaac clarified, "dads and sons was the name that was so funny."

In spite of early resistance, many participants used the word *dance* and its variants in their concluding interviews. Todd made statements including the words "dance," "dancing," and "dancer." Ian talked about "dancing" and described his dad as a "dancer." Though Carl never used the word dance, he responded freely to opportunities to dance as they arose in our conversation. Todd, Carl and Ian used the words "fun," "enjoy," "enjoyed" and "enjoyment" over 30 times in their concluding interviews to describe their dance experiences. Christian and Isaac used affective language sparingly, yet Isaac mentioned the word *fun* twice in relation to particular dance explorations. Louise also observed "enjoyment" of the sessions by her sons and husband. In contrast, Paul was the only one of his family members to use the word *dance*. As a linguist and Dutch language instructor, he referred to his own teaching experience to suggest improvements to my dance teaching strategies.

> With language classes, it's always good to have students do things in between because that makes them think of and use the language. For a dance class, it's the same thing I think. During the week, they will think about it.

Generously accepting my request for their participation, adult family members seemed to hold few expectations about the impact of family dancing on the quality of their family life. Aggravated by a medical issue, Paul admitted his unease prior to the classes, "I thought it was going to be too much dancing. I thought, 'I am not going to be able to do all that.' My second thought is always with Christian—will he cooperate…?" Todd commented on his initial sense of the unusualness of the class and his shift in his attitude.

> It was definitely different, not something you'd think of as a typical interaction with your son, but I think we're enriched for it. It was a much more positive experience than I thought it would be. When we weren't able to go, the two weekends that we went on vacation, I thought about it. You know, we would be dancing right now.

Adult Perceptions of Change and Growth

Todd's comments about his sons' dancing revealed his changing understandings of dance and his yearnings for his sons. At first, Todd guided Ian: "I remember encouraging Ian to just do whatever seemed to come naturally. He's a little bit older and a little more reticent maybe." Later, Todd spoke about seeing Ian dance and having an altered sense of his son:

> I remember Ian really enjoying the drumming…looking at him and thinking he almost seemed like he was losing himself in it. He didn't seem like the Ian I know. He was sort of becoming himself at an earthier level…primal in a way. I had never seen him in that light, or seen that sort of look come over him. I remember it in his face and eyes…an intensity and focus, and sort of lost in it as well, like he wasn't quite the little boy I know.

Referring to changes I made in later dance classes, I asked Paul how they affected his sons' experience. Paul responded, "Well you saw the landscape dance (in sessions six and seven), how he just opened up." I reflected back to Paul, "he just took off." "Yeah…I was so amazed to see Christian open up there," Paul agreed. I asked him what he noticed Christian doing. He responded: "Well, you showed the pictures. I think it was the Australian photographs where they think the animals shaped the landscape. He loved that. And then you had us."

My son, Wyatt, a social and kinesthetic learner, was highly stimulated by this group of people and often by the activities. Adventurous and unpredictable in his responses to movement explorations he built energy and cooperation among the boys for the sequence of tower dances that I eventually invited into the dance curriculum. In response to the tower dancing Wyatt played bells and drums with the other boys, then climbed to the top of the tower and waved his ribbon streamer. At the end of the class, Wyatt ran to the center of the room and leapt on top of a drum, roaring with energy to continue the exploration. As Paul helped the boys to reassemble the tower after class Wyatt shouted, "Let's bring everything to it." Wyatt's drawing that day showed two figures in a three-block tower, one figure on the lowest block and himself perched at the summit of the tower waving a streamer (Fig. 12.2).

Child Perceptions of Change and Growth

Ian's comments amplified his dad Todd's observations. Speaking of his experience of a series of sessions that involved building and then dancing on a play equipment tower, Ian commented, "I just wanted to be crazy and make up my own design. I didn't want to be copycatting. I was just a different [changed] guy…the guy who was jumping up and down on the tower."

Ian also described his drumming: "You just hit it and you feel like, oh, I just want to do this again…just want to do it again and again. It feels so confident." Ian's experience underscores the emergence of meaningful repetition, and the co-

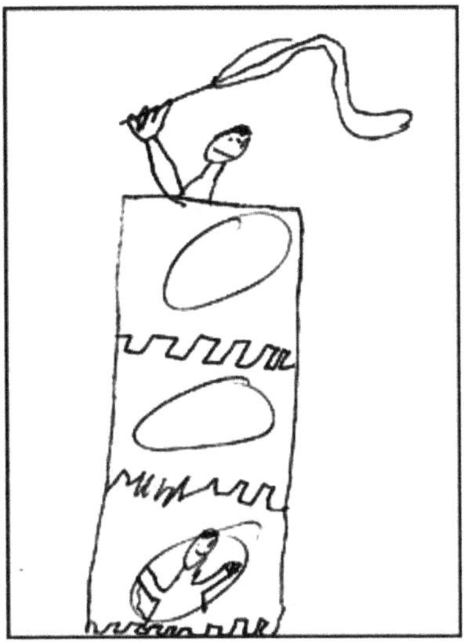

Fig. 12.2 Wyatt: Let's bring everything to it!

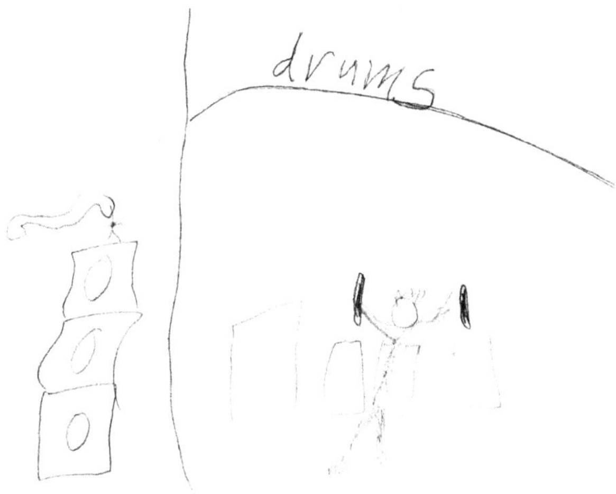

Fig. 12.3 Ian, son of Todd, brother of Carl: "Drums"

construction of dancing using large stacking blocks, a process that helped to bond this aesthetic community (Fig. 12.3).

Identifying the landscapes and masking tape pathways of dances about family journeys, as well as the tower dances, as the most memorable class episodes, Christian and Isaac acted out their enthusiasm with each other during the interview, chanting endlessly, "we want more, we want more…" I asked them what they would like to do for the next dads and sons class, and both responded immediately, "the tower," and then "landscape." Dance education researchers have documented rich evidence of young children's strong motivation to persist in dance learning and practice (Bond, 1994a, 2001, 2018; Bond & Richard, 2005; Bond & Stinson, 2000/2001, 2007/2016).

"He's a very good dancer…"

Father and son agreed that through dancing something shifted for Ian. These interactions suggest that dance can both inspire and reveal the way people in families change. During the interview, Ian brought his perceptions and learning directly to his father's awareness. Through Ian's comments we learned about his view of his father's dancing: "He's a very good dancer, that's for sure, honestly." "You're funny," Todd responded, deflecting the compliment. An often-serious child, Ian took his father's comment at face value: "I am? I never heard that before." During the exchange I asked Ian, "What did you see him (Todd) do?" Ian offered, moving his hips, "I liked when he did that…like that." His persistence in clarifying his appraisal of his father's dancing finally convinced Todd to accept his son's acknowledgement and admiration. "So you thought I was a good dancer, well thank you. I'll take that compliment."

Responding to my question, "How is your dad to dance with?" Isaac responded, "pretty good." Like Todd, Paul deflected the compliment and joked about needing more Beatles music. These two exchanges of admiration illustrate a sometimes-grudging participation in giving and accepting appreciation about dancing. A future goal for family dance education might be to make these exchanges more transparent, visible to the whole group and benefiting from the group's increasing articulation of dance and interpersonal qualities.

Carl and Todd's Dance of Everyday Life

Participant statements revealed how unusual these classes were, and I have shown how dance among these boys and men disrupts typical patterns of gender participation in dance education. Evidence from participant statements also pointed to reversals of leadership patterns in intra-family exchanges of dance. Carl decided to initiate dancing with his father in situations other than our dance sessions. Carl's father revealed:

> Carl keeps doing the sculpting. Every now and then if he sees me standing still, or if I'm sitting down, he'll clap his hands and say he wants me to move my foot or move my arm, and I'll play along. He gets cross with me now if I don't move my foot the way he wants me to move it. He'll say, "No, I want you to move it the other way."

Todd noticed the unique power it gave Carl to direct such moments: "He likes to be in charge and I think he likes the idea of having me do something. He's sort of calling the shots…" (Fig. 12.4). Todd suggested that in their large family, the dancing

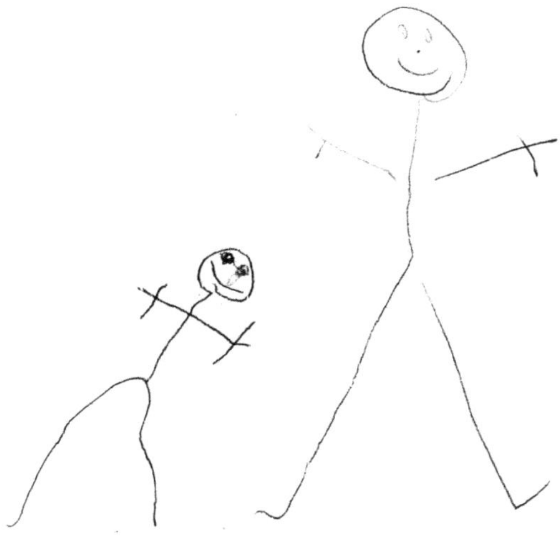

Fig. 12.4 Carl, son of Todd, brother of Ian
"I liked being the sculptor and my dad being the clay"

gave Carl a one-on-one experience with him. "It might just be a game for the two of us. You know, with as many kids as we've got it might just be something for him."During the interview, Carl and Todd demonstrated the shaping activity they had learned in class and Carl had been initiating at home. Todd began the exchange. "Carl, what does this mean?" Todd clapped and Carl moved. "And now he'll do it," Todd said. Carl clapped and his dad said, "now I have to move my head." Carl continued to demonstrate the sculpting activity, clapping to direct his dad's movements. "You liked doing that, didn't you? It was fun." When I asked him if his dad did a good job; Carl nodded, yes. Then I asked if he was always ready to do it? Again, he nodded. I asked, "Do you do it with anybody else?" Carl stated, "No. Just me and daddy." Resonating with Carl's dances of everyday life, several children in Bond's (2008) study initiated dance moments with adults between sessions (p. 416).

An Incident of Persistent Memory

Carl remembered other dancing he and Todd did together and suggested future dancing he would like to do with his dad. He recalled a North Pole dance they created together. Carl asked his dad, "remember when I was falling down?" His dad mentioned snowballs and Carl responded, "it's always snowing. Can we do the iceberg thing again?" Then, Carl began to illustrate by dancing. He said, "I did this move. I did that move." Carl made a shape with his feet up on his chair and his hands supporting himself on the floor with an opening beneath him. He accurately named the boys who danced through his shape, "Ben and Anker."

The detail of Carl's account of this dance learning experience was striking. With minimal assistance, he remembered both theme and sub-topics: snow and icebergs. He remembered where it happened in the studio, several dance actions, and relationships with other dancers, then launched from his description into actual dancing. This example is consistent with Bond (1994a, 2001), who has documented young children's detailed memories of dance learning, in one study 6 months after the dance program ended (Bond, 1994a).

If we focus for a moment on Carl's statements and dancing through the lens of standards-based arts education, this evidence of dance learning is substantial, pointing toward the potential of family dance education as a productive and accountable academic context. For example, his statements and dancing revealed that he knew dance could be done in reference to other ideas, such as features of the arctic environment. He also demonstrated the skill of dancing with others, and recreated how he and others danced together, describing his own actions and the actions of those with whom he danced. Most powerfully, by choosing dance as an activity to initiate with Todd, he demonstrated his aesthetic authority, an idea similar to how teachers understand student voice in arts standards-based arts education.

Discussion

Reflective Practice

This study demonstrates application of reflective practice to meet the needs and interests of an intergenerational group of dads and sons, a group identified as infrequent participants in dance education. The research adds to discourses that critique the usefulness of gender as a category for educators to reliably predict effective modes of instruction, curriculum materials or outcomes (Anttila, 2007; Bond, 1994a, 2017; Smith & Wilhelm, 2002). Analysis of multi-modal sources suggests that my reflective practice was a key sense-making resource helping me sort and update my responses to the accumulating flow of group interests and needs. Reflecting forward in time provided me with ways to modify and develop dance activities over several sessions, and to constructively respond to individual struggles.

From the perspectives of socio-economic status, race and gender, study participants appear remarkably similar; however, any initial notions I had about group homogeneity disappeared quickly, replaced by richly diverse needs and interests as I encountered the participants and their families. The emergent, idiosyncratic, and unanticipated nature of participants' responses underscored the dangers of treating any group from a monolithic perspective. A singular sense of boy interest or dad interest never emerged, though several centers of interest did arise in this particular aesthetic community.

I noticed my repertoire of available choices in the moment seemed to expand as a result of systematic efforts to notice and attend to participants reflectively. Most evident during a particularly problematic session, this elastic sense of possibility was built on reflecting in the present, backwards, and forwards. Planning, in the sense of instructional pre-planning to set up and facilitate particular learning situations using specific resources, and in the sense of holding an orienting question about a theme or participant, helped me teach with greater awareness and tact (van Manen, 1991).

Perhaps because of this "ethic of attention" (Freeman, 2015), my experience of teaching—moving through the ups and downs of each session—shifted toward curiosity and responsiveness. This sense of pedagogical mobility, characterized by a deepening of intersubjectivity in the group, was a very satisfying experience in my life as both teacher and parent of a child participant. In reflection, Wyatt helped me perceive more clearly, become more curious, less fearful and more empathetic in my dance pedagogy.

Intersubjectivity

The quality of intersubjectivity—the capacity for reciprocal experience with mutual impact (e.g. shared emotion, shared attention, shared intention) with others (Meltzoff & Brooks, 2007), was variously present among the child and adult sub-groups and families, manifested through tactile and kinesthetic, verbal and linguistic, and pictorial exchanges. Descriptive evidence highlighted how intra- and inter-generational pairings of participants, for example, mirroring, shadowing, sculpting and weight sharing, produced intersubjective exchanges that engaged participants across the continuum of development and often across generations. Detailed descriptions showed how these exchanges differed in quality from mimicry (Laverty, 2007), showing increasing empathy, understanding and connection. Ian's statements showed his sense of the urgency and authenticity of his dancing: "I just wanted to be crazy and make up my own design. I didn't want to be copycatting." His father, Todd, powerfully reflected back to Ian his own statements of admiration, a fulfilment of Todd's longing for his son to "let go."

Boys' linguistic capacities were almost continuously engaged through the sessions, while the adults were often less verbally expressive. The resulting social orientation of the boy group, and its developmental segmentation (younger, middle and older) introduced strong generational patterns of interaction, some of which led to satisfying individual and group expression, while others produced tension and resistance in the group. In light of this development, adult-child pairings seemed to moderate the provocative tone of some group interactions between children and adults. As an extension of paired dance exchanges, family members created portraits of each other using animal drawings as visual metaphors; this crossing of generational lines resulted in expressions of curiosity, insight, surprise, and admiration. Bond's (1994b, 2008) construction of aesthetic community with a group of nonverbal children with deaf-blindness and their teachers was also based on inter-generational partner dancing, with an emphasis on child leadership.

Aesthetic Community

Through these sessions, project documentation shows that family members experienced strong bodily perceptions, the emergence of personal style through dance, social engagement with each other in a variety of exploratory tasks that led to self-transformation, and the emergence of shared ritual forms and aesthetic meanings in this temporary dance community, providing qualitative validation of Bond's (1994b, 2008) theory of aesthetic community (see Fig. 12.1). Understanding the specific phenomena and conditions that evidence aesthetic community in this study of inter-generational dance education begins with a discussion about adults and children in pedagogical projects generally, and how the dynamics of age and authority played out in this study. Mouritsen (1998) describes a cultural predisposition toward children:

> Since modern childhood was shaped, an attitude to children that is in the broad sense educational has been a kind of "cultural law" in our relations with them. ... The children, inevitably, have directly and indirectly resisted and reacted to our role as agents of the pedagogical project. (p. 24)

Christian was perhaps the clearest voice of resistance in our group of boys, once complaining, "I have to do what teachers tell me all week. On the weekend, I want to do what I want."

In the face of cultural conflict, van Manen (1997) reminds us of our mandate as educators and parents "to help bring up and educate children in a pedagogically responsible manner" (p. 139). He refers to accounts of lived experience by Marcel (1978) and Langeveld (1987), pointing out the "importance of commitment and active involvement of the father in the child's life…fatherhood [is] a creative vow" (p. 75). Further articulating the pedagogical problem faced by adult participants in my study, Eeva Anttila (2007) states, "Educators as program initiators and leaders face a great challenge in respecting the participants' views on what is best for them and what their interests are" (p. 870).

How will we adults know what children need and how and when to provide it? Animated by our group's intergenerational tensions, we worked with our available knowledge of dance and dancing. Neither the participating fathers, nor I, had substantial childhood dance experiences; we relied on alternative sources of knowledge as we worked to discover what our group of eight boys needed. Adult knowledge sources included memories of being children, experiences of parenting, later life dance experiences and most directly, the evidence of child dance experience at hand during each session. I attempted to selectively read the evidence of participant interests and struggled to co-create and support an optimal dance experience for both children and adults.

Similar efforts were reported by other fathers. The pedagogical struggle, transformation and celebration evident in the narratives of the two families, speak to instances of sensitive tethering of their children in light of parental desires to do what was best for their sons and with respect for the authority and capacity of children to make choices, create dance, and make personal meaning. The themes, materials and processes of dance education, as applied in this adaptation of "right dance" (Bond, 2008), appeared to facilitate individual and shared dance meanings related to being and acting as a parent or a child in family and community groupings. Did it however, offer participants dance experiences through which individual aesthetic preferences merge creatively, and to what degree did we achieve Nelson Goodman's (1978) "rightness of fit" (as cited in Bond, 2008)?

Were We Dancing, and Did It Feel Right? Though Todd and Paul readily perceived our learning as dance learning, not all participants shared the opinion that we were dancing. One father commented, "it felt more like a movement class than a dance class." Another father, who had taken university dance classes, defined dance in terms of technique, clearly different from our fathers and sons dancing, which, like a number of other chapters in this volume, emphasized improvisation and creativity. Dads whose ideas of dance were different from those applied in class found it difficult to identify moments when they most felt they were dancing.

At the same time, adult participants agreed about the unusualness of dancing, and of our dads and boys' classes, in their lives. Perhaps the focus on individual and group creative authority and process helped distinguish this experience of dancing in ways that emphasized quality of life impacts with some depth. Though unusual, the parent and child setting for dance learning seemed to invite a sense of "naturalness." With one exception, adults expressed satisfaction with the "feel" of the class. Todd and other adults commented that we did things that "felt right."

Participant perceptions shifted over time. Paul's reflections about incidents early in the sequence contrasted with those of Todd and the other parents who found the session natural, and right feeling.

> It was moving in the wrong direction when it comes to Christian. Sometimes maybe you let them go too much. We had to chase each other, and it would end up being a chase. With two it is difficult already and I can't run that fast. I think they went off doing the wrong thing at some point. It was something we had to do very slowly, but they ran off.

Boys' comments were also varied. As noted above, Christian complained after the second class that I directed too much: "I spend my week listening to teachers tell me what to do…" Ian, interviewed at the end of the sessions, expressed satisfaction: "I think everyone had a good time. No one felt left out, or unappreciated…it was just perfect."

Christian's forthrightness and willingness to share his avid interest in hip hop dancing, animals, and life sciences helped me adjust my teaching to his needs. Until I developed more engaging content in response to Christian and Isaac, however, their powerful initiatives were sometimes provocative and centrifugal to the group experience of dancing, while sometimes central to it. For example, during the third session and continuing with remarkable persistence through the final session, Wyatt, Isaac and Christian developed a shoulder slouching, foot sliding, air guitar playing motif they sometimes referred to as "banjo playing." The trio found numerous places in group dancing to insert their motif, ranging from serious variations during our square dance to hilarious episodes during group mirroring exchanges that morphed flexibly into solo performances. In his interview comments Paul pointed to this exchange as a socially mediating development for Christian, as Wyatt had inspired this provocative and goofy signature movement. He also noted its endurance and commented that, "Wyatt trying to play the banjo, that is something even in between [sessions] they will talk about…so big an impression from so small an [action]."

Carl's adaptation of a dance interaction for his own purposes outside the dance class and the Isaac and Christian air guitar conversations, also outside of our sessions were, to my knowledge, unique in this group of boys. These incidents resonated with Bond's (1994b, 2008) findings that a group of nonverbal children with dual sensory impairments (and therefore significant learning challenges) were able to pursue their individual dance interests and communicate these interests authentically within a group composed of adult dance partners and peers.

The Spiraling Process of ***Right Dance*** Anttila (2007) reviewed recent research literature asking "to what extent is it possible to consider children as subjects, experts or active agents in researching dance education?" (p. 865). She references Bond (1994a, 2000, 2001), Bond & Richard (2005), Bond & Stinson (2000/2001), Hanna (1986), Lindqvist (2001), and others, illustrating examples of child-centered practices in dance education research that emphasize children's competence in artistic expression, personal transformation, and aesthetic growth. Lending specificity to Anttila's question, Mouritsen (1998) defines child culture as "artistic and other symbolic aesthetic products and forms of expression, and their context" (p. 4). Further, he distinguishes three distinct forms: culture produced *for* children by adults, culture created *with* children, and culture generated *by* children. The latter covers phenomena of culture that children produce in their own networks, and is closely related to play (pp. 5–6).

Applied to the social-aesthetic phenomenon of *aesthetic community,* Bond's (1994b, 2008) pedagogical framework of *right dance* appears to encompass all three of Mouritsen's categories: a dance prototype and process created *for*, *with*, and *by* children. A distinction between our respective projects came to light in terms of child leadership, an element of *right dance*. The child leadership design for the present study included distributed opportunities for leadership in adult sanctioned activities such as mirroring, shadowing, flocking, and sculpting, as well as "free dancing" in response to drumming or adult-initiated themes. Though culture *by* children did not inform my research design, child determined forms of expression were clearly manifest in the boys' interest in stacking and dancing on tower blocks, and in Wyatt's "banjo playing" motif. In addition, to these elements, Bond's design incorporated a structural component allowing the possibility of dance community to be created *by* children "in a field as free as possible from cultural coercion" (Bond, personal communication, April 30, 2017).

Since the dads and sons' "dance and life" research project, Bond has commented on her design of child, or more broadly, participant leadership in *right dance.* With regard to her program with nonverbal children with deaf-blindness, she reflects,

> I emphasized child leadership throughout, but there was a discrete segment of each session devoted to a reflective pedagogical attitude. We would "witness" and wait for children to initiate something, similar to "Authentic Movement" (see Pallaro, 1999). I think you are saying that you did not have the equivalent in your study, but I wonder… (Bond, personal communication, April 30, 2017)

At one point I asked what a step toward dance education culture *by* children might look like? She suggested, "Given the quality of verbal communication, could you have sat everyone down and said, okay now it's your turn, boys, to be completely in charge. What do you want to teach us dads today?" She adds, "Might this have brought Christian in sooner?" (Bond, personal communication, March 15, 2017).

This encounter about shifting/sharing pedagogical authority in dance education settings raises questions that I continue to ponder in my role as an action researcher concerned with student-centered pedagogy and its salience to family quality of life. For example, how might adults introduce this shift to promote child success? How might adult participants best support child leaders in realizing their interests? In large dance education groups, how can I ensure that individuals have equal opportunities to exercise leadership? From our supporting role, how can adults help make our learning visible to our child teachers?

References

Anttila, E. (2007). Children as agents in dance: Implications of the notion of child-culture for research and practice in dance education. In L. Bresler (Ed.), *International handbook of research in arts education* (pp. 865–879). Dordrecht, The Netherlands: Springer.

Bohm, D., & Peat, F. D. (1987). *Science, order and creativity*. New York: Bantam Books.

Bond, K. (2008). The human nature of dance: Towards a theory of aesthetic community. In S. Malloch & C. Trevarthen (Eds.), *Communicative musicality: Exploring the basis of human companionship* (pp. 401–422). Oxford, UK: Oxford University Press.

Bond, K. (2018). "Me … a tree": Young children as natural phenomenologists. In S. Fraleigh (Ed.), *Back to the dance itself: Phenomenologies of the body in performance* (pp. 205–232). Urbana: University of Illinois Press.

Bond, K. E. (1994a). How 'Wild Things' tamed gender distinctions. *Journal of Physical Education, Recreation and Dance, 65*(2), 28–33.

Bond, K. E. (1994b). Personal style as a mediator of engagement in dance: Watching Terpsichore rise. *Dance Research Journal, 26*(1), 15–26.

Bond, K. E. (2000). Revisioning purpose: Children, dance and the culture of caring. In J. E. LeDrew & H. Ritenburg (Eds.), *8th dance and the child international (daCi) conference: Extensions & extremities: Points of departure* (pp. 3–14). Regina, SK: University of Regina.

Bond, K. E. (2001). "I'm not an eagle, I'm a chicken!" Young children's perceptions of creative dance. *Early Childhood Connections, 7*(4), 41–51.

Bond, K. E. (2017). "Boys are morons!" "Girls are gross!" Let's dance! In W. Oliver & D. Risner (Eds.), *Dance and gender: An evidence based approach* (pp. 135–157). Gainesville: University Press of Florida.

Bond, K. E., & Deans, J. (1997). Eagles, reptiles and beyond: A co-creative journey in dance. *Childhood Education, 73*(6), 366–371.

Bond, K. E., & Richard, B. (2005). "Ladies and gentlemen: What do you see? What do you feel?" A story of connected curriculum in a third grade dance education setting. In L. Overby & B. Lepczyk (Eds.), *Dance: Current selected research* (Vol. 5, pp. 85–134). New York: AMS.

Bond, K. E., & Stinson, S. W. (2000/2001). "I feel like I'm going to take off!" Young people's experiences of the superordinary in dance. *Dance Research Journal, 32*(2), 52–87.

Bond, K. E., & Stinson, S. W. (2016). "It's work, work, work, work." Young people's experiences of effort and engagement in dance. In S. W. Stinson (Ed.), *Embodied curriculum theory and research in arts education: A dance scholar's search for meaning* (pp. 269–295). Dordrecht, The Netherlands: Springer. (Original work published 2007).

Carr, W., & Kemmis, S. (1986). *Becoming critical: Education, knowledge, and action research.* London: Falmer Press.

Clandinin, J., & Connelly, F. M. (1991). Narrative and story in practice and research. In D. Schön (Ed.), *The reflective turn: Case studies in and on educational practice* (pp. 258–281). New York: Teachers College Press.

Clandinin, J., & Connelly, F. M. (1995). *Teachers' professional knowledge landscapes*. New York: Teachers College Press.

Denzin, N. K. (1998). *The landscape of qualitative research: Theories and issues*. Thousand Oaks, CA: Sage.

Denzin, N. K., & Lincoln, Y. S. (Eds.). (2005). *The SAGE handbook of qualitative research* (3rd ed.). Thousand Oaks, CA: Sage.

Freeman, M. (2015). Beholding and being beheld: Simone Weil, Iris Murdoch, and the ethics of attention. *The Humanistic Psychologist, 43*, 160–172.

Giorgi, A. (1992). Description versus interpretation: Competing alternative strategies for qualitative research. *Journal of Phenomenological Psychology, 23*(2), 119–135.

Goodman, N. (1978). *Ways of worldmaking*. Indianapolis, IN: Hackett.

Hanna, J. L. (1986). Interethnic communication in children's own dance, play, and protest. In Y. Y. Kim (Ed.), *Interethnic communication, International and intercultural communication annual* (Vol. 10, pp. 176–198). Newbury Park, CA: Sage.

Laban, R. (1988). *The mastery of movement*. Plymouth, UK: Northcote House.

Langeveld, M. (1987). What is the meaning of being and having a father? *Phenomenology and Pedagogy, 5*, 5–21.

Laverty, K. (2007). Dance/movement therapy as part of a multi-family group program at the Children's Hospital of Denver. *American Journal of Dance Therapy, 29*(1), 9–35.

Lindqvist, G. (2001). The relationship between dance and play.*Research in Dance Education*, 2(1), 41–52.

Maletic, V. (1982). *On the aisthetic and aesthetic dimensions of the dance: A methodology for researching dance style (doctoral dissertation)*. Columbus, OH: The Ohio State University.

Marcel, G. (1978). *Homoviator*. Gloucester, MA: Smith.

Meltzoff, A. N., & Brooks, R. (2007). Intersubjectivity before language: Three windows on preverbal sharing. In S. Bråten (Ed.), *On being moved: From mirror neurons to empathy* (pp. 149–174). Philadelphia, PA: John Benjamins.

Mouritsen, F. (1998). *Child culture – Play culture*. Working paper 2, Child and youth culture, The Department of Contemporary Cultural Studies, Odense University, Odense, Denmark.

National Dance Education Organization (NDEO). (2004). *Statistics on dance education in the United States*. Retrieved from http://www.ndeo.org/content.aspx?page_id=22&club_id=893257&module_id=55774

Oliver, W., & Risner, D. (Eds.). (2017). *Dance and gender: An evidence based approach.* Gainesville: University Press of Florida.

Pallaro, P. (Ed.). (1999). *Authentic movement: Essays by Mary Starks Whitehouse, Janet Adler, and Joan Chodorow* (Vol. 1). Philadelphia, PA: Jessica Kingsley.

Parsad, B., & Spiegelman, M. (2012). Arts education in public elementary and secondary schools, 1999–2000 and 2009–10. (NCES 2012-014). National Center for Education Statistics, Institute of Education Sciences. Department of Education, Washington, DC.

Reeves, R., & Sawhill, I. V. (2015, November 15). Men's lib! *The New York Times,* p. SR1.

Risner, D. (2008). When boys dance: Cultural resistance in dance education. In S. Shapiro (Ed.), *Dance in a world of change: Examining globalization and cultural differences* (pp. 93–115). Champaign, IL: Human Kinetics.

Risner, D. (2009). What we know about boys who dance: The limitations of contemporary masculinity and dance education. In A. Shay & J. Fisher (Eds.), *When men dance: Choreographing masculinities across borders* (pp. 57–77). New York: Oxford University Press.

Schön, D. A. (1991). *The reflective turn: Case studies in and on educational practice*. New York: Teachers College Press.

Smith, M. W., & Wilhelm, J. D. (2002). *"Reading don't fix no Chevys": Literacy in the lives of young men*. Portsmouth, NH: Heinemann.

Sparshott, F. (1988). *Off the ground: First steps towards a philosophical consideration of dance*. Princeton, NJ: Princeton University Press.

United States Department of Education. (2013). *Table 318.30. Bachelor's, master's, and doctor's degrees conferred by postsecondary institutions, by sex of student and discipline division: 2011–12.* Retrieved from https://nces.ed.gov/programs/digest/d13/tables/dt13_318.30.asp

van Manen, M. (1991). *The tact of teaching: The meaning of pedagogical thoughtfulness*. Albany, NY: SUNY Press.

van Manen, M. (1997). *Researching lived experience: Human science for an action sensitive pedagogy* (2nd ed.). London, ONT: Althuss.

Chapter 13
Fathers, Sons and Encounters in Dance

Isto Turpeinen and Ralph Buck

Introduction

This chapter discusses relationships between fathers and sons in a dance project in Finland. With the guidance of Isto Turpeinen's studio teaching methodology he calls "raw-board-working," fathers are involved as active observers, teaching assistants, and as dancers. Briefly, raw-board-working values everyday "raw" movement and ideas, which are storyboarded by participants to create private and public performances. Since 2008, Isto has continued to develop this heuristic framework at the Theatre Academy Helsinki. From 2013 to 2016, he carried out a family dance project including stage performances. During this period, participants created three public performances—*Mother and Son* (2013), *Our Fathers* (2015), and *Hey, Father - Where are you?* (2016), each one dealing with boys' real life issues, aspirations, and needs, including their relationships with fathers. This chapter focuses specifically on father-son relationships during workshops, rehearsals and performances for this trilogy. The study replicates Isto's earlier work with only boys applying raw-board-working (Turpeinen, 2012, 2017).

In this collaborative endeavor, Ralph Buck takes the role of discussant. Ralph and Isto have shared an interest in male dance education since first meeting in Taiwan and Finland in 2012, and this project continues their conversation and collaboration. The chapter begins with brief discussion of the study's epistemological foundation, followed by an overview of research methodology and description of the practice-led method of raw-board-working as an artistic, pedagogical, and research modality (Arlander, 2013; Kirkkopelto, 2008). We then discuss and reflect

I. Turpeinen (✉)
University of the Arts Helsinki, Helsinki, Finland
e-mail: isto.turpeinen@uniarts.fi

R. Buck
University of Auckland, Auckland, New Zealand
e-mail: r.buck@auckland.ac.nz

K. Bond (ed.), *Dance and the Quality of Life*, Social Indicators Research Series 73,
https://doi.org/10.1007/978-3-319-95699-2_13

on some of the phenomena and meanings found in participants' danced stories and what they reveal about father and son relationships. The study found that as fathers and sons danced with each other in the open workshop process of raw-board-working, they re-constructed their relationships, both consciously and unconsciously.

Epistemological Foundations

An assumption informing pedagogy during the study was that growth (learning) comes through nurturing experience and reflection upon such experience with others. Essentially, an ethos of dialogue, democracy and equity underpin this constructivist epistemology (Freire, 1972; Greene, 1991; Vigotsky, 1962). Isto described these values to the boys as aiming for the ideal that "life should be good." That is, to lead a good life, you need to build identity and acknowledge your own physical and spiritual state. Moreover, the research embraces John Dewey's (1934) still influential notion of individuality as a created interaction between self and social environment. In other words, meanings of dance and self are constructed in dialogue with others, events and phenomena (Crotty, 1998; Eisner, 1998; Garrison, Neubert, & Reich, 2012; Merleau-Ponty, 1962; Neubert & Reich, 2012; Steffe & Gale, 2012).

Based on what Turpeinen (2015) calls in Finnish *kattoatmosfääri*, empathyand shared experience are important ingredients in nurturing growth in a teaching and co-working environment. The direct translation from Finnish to English includes the words *ceiling* and *atmosphere*. The relationship between these words might not be immediately obvious, but Isto sees a connection to Csikszentmihalyi's (1990, 1994) concept of *flow*. There are moments when the dialogical space allows for, or freely initiates happenings, such as dancing or storytelling. The atmosphere is positive, alive, and open to the "here and now." In discussing the notion of creating a positive classroom atmosphere, Ralph mentioned Mikhail Csikszentmihalyi's (1990) notion that an optimal flow of teaching and learning occurs when challenge and risk are well balanced (Bond & Stinson, 2007/2016). Eeva Anttila's (2003) construct of "embracing atmosphere" (p. 309) is also salient in its conception of dialogical relations (Buber, 1923/2013). Anttila (2003) describes an "array of dialogue" (p. 309); that is, more than one type of dialogue-in-action is operating at any one timein a dance lesson. She discusses possibilities for a person to first have a relation to body, sound, and image, and then to continue in relation with others, and finally to be part of a dialogical network.

Methodology: Providing Voice to Fathers and Sons

The aim of the study was to give voice to father/son relationships and to explore the role of dance as a means for facilitating that voice. A primary and compelling rationale for the phenomenological stance of this research is well stated by Juha Varto

(2012), arguably one of Finland's leading phenomenologists: "The knowledge in our flesh is where we all live and feel alive" (pp. 17–18). With Varto as a guiding voice, this research utilized a multi-modal research methodology.

As introduced above, an overarching constructivist epistemology emphasizes the dialectical relationships between researcher and participants, allowing for multiple forms of representing understandings and information (evidence) and for valuing diverse perspectives. Constructivism is a relativist ontology, meaning that multiple realities are created by individuals through consensus of social experiences, rather than a single reality waiting to be discovered (Guba & Lincoln, 1994). An assumption that there is no one way to be a father or a son underpins this study. Moreover, Isto and Ralph cannot ignore their own lived experiences as fathers and sons. Isto's son was initially involved in raw-board-working style workshops, and has gone on to become a professional dancer.

The research design was informed by Anttila's (2015a, 2015b) practice-based, embodied knowledge methodology that works in and through dance. Arlander (2013) reiterates that, "today we could claim that artistic research is an acknowledged field of research and knowledge production" (p. 153). As such, and with a long Finnish tradition of practice-led research (Arlander, 2013), we view practice-led research and participatory action research as appropriate methodologies for examining father and son relationships in dance.

Isto sought a methodological approach that would provide fathers and sons (especially fathers) opportunities to explore, reflect on and express their relationship. Artistic practice as a multi-modal research method was ideal, though we agree with Nelson (2013) that it "requires more labor and a broader range of skills to engage in a multi-mode research inquiry than a more traditional research process" (p. 9). Nelson points out that artistic practice as research demonstrates an equivalent rigor in concrete rather than abstract terms. The artist, in this case Isto, understands his artistic medium as a method for enacting and presenting research. He provides a research and artistic framework in which the dancers contribute their ideas and movement in an atmosphere where "anything" is valued in a safe environment. He values the "rawness" of ideas and movement, seeking to portray the dancers' authentic meanings. The artistic process may can also enable and articulate change—as a medium of invention and intervention (Borgdorff, 2010). Kirkkopelto (2012) notes that artistic research has institutional consequences. When an artist-researcher presents an "invention" or new work within an institution, the research has significance as it is regarded as production of knowledge (Arlander, 2013).

Complementary to practice-led, artistic approaches, participatory action research allows the researcher to "get in touch" with people in their own contexts (Eisner, 1998, p. 11). This study seeks to understand meanings of dance experiences of fathers and sons as they worked together in studio dance sessions, focusing on their "words and actions in narrative or descriptive ways…closely representing the situation as experienced by the participants" (Maykut & Morehouse, 1994, p. 2). Here, participatory action research processes captured "direct, intimate contact" (Eisner, 1998, p. 11) between fathers and sons.

A multi-modal approach scaffolds the collection of evidence through artistic processes, interviews, and observations (Bond & Stinson, 2000/2001; Bond & Richard, 2005). Further to the dance evidence that revealed lived experience and meanings, six fathers and five sons participated in semi-structured interviews (Holmes 1998; Tripp, 1983). Fathers were interviewed individually (Fontana & Frey, 2000), each one twice. All participants signed ethics forms, and interviews were recorded and transcribed. The first interview period was winter 2014–2015 when questions focused on families, father and son relationships, and masculinity. The second period was spring 2016 and highlighted such topics as my children, daily life, being a parent, being a son, arts and dance, acting and dancing together (father and son), performing together, and free space for discussion. The five boys in the study (ages 9–12) were interviewed in spring, 2016, individually or in pairs. All of the boys' interviews were recorded and parents provided ethics approval. A group interview including fathers was also recorded.

Further to the semi-structured interviews, raw-board-working included considerable verbal dialogue and opportunity to express ideas through movement (Holmes, 1998; Svendler-Nielsen, 2015). Isto wrote notes immediately after each studio session, all of which included space and time for individual verbal expression. Our interpretive circling between interviews and studio dialogues was a vital aspect of developing sensitivity of perception when searching for and distilling emergent research themes.

Another set of data was provided by videotapes of all dance classes, rehearsals and performances. As introduced above, the "fathers and sons trilogy project" was based on three practice-led artistic processes, approximately 10 weeks in autumn and 10 weeks in spring, during 2013, 2015 and 2016. The weekly 1–1½ h dance workshops typically included greetings, warm up games, and movement exploration and revision processes in preparation for performances. The timeline of the weekly workshop and performance trilogy was long, and videotaped materials included 16 tapes amassing to approximately 16 h of recording. This archive was invaluable in recalling information and analyzing meanings expressed by the fathers and sons. All data (semi-structured interview recordings, video recordings, and observations) were reviewed and through an inductive process, clustered into three descriptive categories (Maykut & Morehouse, 1994): the learning process, dance and performance, and fathers and sons.

Practice-Led Artistic Research: Raw-Board-Working as Medium

Artistic research directed by Isto and performed by boys and fathers presented key moments for generating, collecting and reflecting upon data. As represented in Fig. 13.1, the aim of this embodied research method of raw-board-working was to share experience through "action/dance," and to use this as the beginning point for

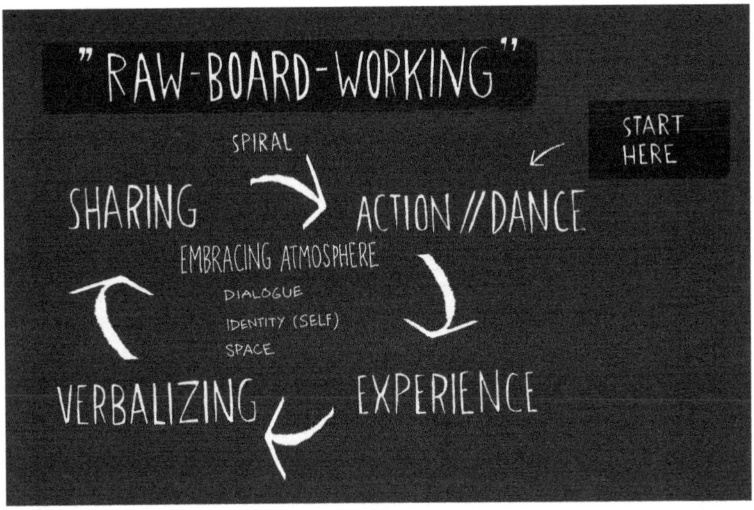

Fig. 13.1 Raw-board-working. (Turpeinen, 2015)

ongoing reflection, dialogue and action. Raw-board-working is a heuristic model that spirals around action (dance), dialogue and reflection. Its process embodies the present moment as meaningful experience that informs future action. An *experience*, here and now, will be perceived and *verbalized* or described (danced), and shared in a dialogical relation or network (Anttila, 2003). Re-presented experience continues the construction process through action in an ongoing spiralling process. This method creates a frame for investigation, respecting dance as a medium for sharing experience, and for developing awareness of relations between fathers and sons. Artistic processes and stages of this practice-led artistic research are framed as *episodes*, after Harré and Secord (1972), where the episode is a series of events that occur in a certain place and interval of time. An episode is defined here as an organized activity that has unity of focus, and was delineated in the "fathers and sons trilogy project" by processes and products created in workshops and performances.

Classes, workshops, and performances were regular meeting places where, in the frame of the episodes, we negotiated topics arising from shared experiences in and through dance. Raw-board-working provided space for experiencing, verbalizing, and sharing. Narratives and "embodied pictures" emerged from interactions in father and son partnerships, and these were developed into performances. Isto was intrinsic to these workshop and performance processes as researcher, participant, facilitator, and arts educator.

Artistic aspects of the research were framed in the theme *fathers and sons*. Key episodes in the study included the performances *Mother and Son* (2013), *Our Fathers* (2015) and *Hey, Father - Where are you?* (2016). Each performance premiered at the STOA Culture Centre's spring festival, ApinaFest! (MonkeyFest!), in East Helsinki, a forum for youth and experimental dance art held in cooperation with the Helsinki Theatre Academy Alumni Association and ARTSEQUAL research project.

Pedagogical Love

Key concepts of raw-board-working pedagogy are dialogue, experience, and creation of a teaching environment based on "pedagogical love." Providing a pedagogical environment that offers connections and an embracing atmosphere is respected beyond the classroom (Weil, 1949/2001). Notions of concern, care, and shared experience are resonant with those of a "good life," and fostering a nurturing atmosphere supports working towards a good life. Another way of thinking about this is to foster a kind of love. Within the present study, we are referring to *pedagogical love*, wherein Isto, as the facilitator, creates a teaching and learning environment in which fathers and sons are exploring their relationships consciously and unconsciously (Turpeinen, 2015, 2017).

Boys' relationships with their fathers has received scant attention in dance literature (Li, 2016; Richard, 2009; Chap. 12, this volume). Yet in terms of fathers offering social support, role models, encouragement, career advice and personal relationships advice (to name a few), this relationship is vital. Within their own dance backgrounds, both Isto and Ralph experienced the relative invisibility of fathers. This chapter discusses a small number of father and son relationships in relation to the emergent theme of *love* that surfaced in the "fathers and sons trilogy project." The focus on love within father and son relationships has sparked Isto's and Ralph's interest as they continue to collaborate on research within the Finnish Academy ARTSEQUAL research project.

Love is difficult to define and has stereotypical associations when related to fathers and sons. For example, the father-son relationship has been described as distant, and founded on reason and discipline (Pellegrini & Sarbin, 2012), while love is associated with intimacy, including a yearning for closeness (Real, 1997). Further, between men, especially in male groups, and between boys, there can be embarrassment or difficulty in talking about love, grounded in a background of coded masculinity, peer pressure, and (dis)respect (Burt, 2007; Connell, 2005; Lehikoinen, 2006; Li, 2016; Pollack, 1998; Risner, 2009; Turpeinen, 2015).

Love, like the good life, is difficult to account for in terms of pedagogy: "Here I am wondering whether 'my love' is my devotion to my work as a teacher, or in general my affection for human beings. How do you grab something that flows in constant movement?" (Turpeinen, 2015, p. 94). Lydia Amir's (2001) examination of Plato's theory of love provides some insights into Isto's comment above. Plato (385-370 BCE/1951) had several definitions of love, the first being, "love is desire for the perpetual possession of the good" (p. 86). Socrates, taking Plato's point and expanding upon it, stated, "the motive force in love is yearning for goodness, not just completion" (Amir, 2001, p. 7). Isto's comments regarding teaching towards a good life is about yearning for goodness in teaching and learning moments — seeking experience, things and beauty that will satisfy our needs, and in doing so provide happiness. Our position is that, ideally, dance education enables pedagogical love.

Amir (2001) notes the importance of understanding diverse meanings of and motivations for love, including *eros,* associated with erotica; *philia,* a brotherly, or in inclusive gender terms, sibling love; and, *agape* where love is altruism (385-

370 BCE/1951). In terms of pedagogy, the aim to foster a nurturing, loving, embracing teaching and learning environment is worth pursuing, and the word *love* need not be avoided simply because it — similar to the word *dance* (Bond, 2014) — has multiple meanings.

Isto has argued that reaching to hold or pursue an understanding of love is beneficial (Turpeinen, 2015). To Buber (1923/2013), love is inclusive and lies in experiencing the other. For phenomenologist Juha Varto (1991), love is a base for being human. Without love one will not live. Love permeates our lives and according to Varto is the "primal essence of all essences" (pp. 55–58; Vandenberghe, 2008). Logically, dance educators concerned with fostering mind, body, and spirit in embracing atmospheres are going to be concerned with pedagogical love.

Fathers and Sons Dancing Together

This section reflects on some key findings that emerged from the "fathers and sons trilogy project" including dance performances, interviews, and observations. Participant data clustered around three descriptive categories: the learning process, dance and performance, and fathers and sons.

The Learning Process

Fathers who were all new to creative process driven dance classes spoke about learning during their interviews and in the studio work. Firstly, they reflected on watching their sons dance, and secondly on learning by doing, i.e., dancing with their sons. All fathers were encouraged to enter the dance studio and watch their children dance. Isto used the idea of fathers being both participant and audience, and gave them free entry to the dance studio. Simply, fathers had the possibility to both witness their sons and dance with their sons. The workshops encouraged fathers to dance and make duets with their sons, which often included structured improvisation that included touching, leaning, contacting, lifting and carrying. Often as the workshops progressed more and more playful improvisation emerged.

Fathers on Observing Learning For Isto, fathers' responses to observing their sons in dance conveyed an element of *distance*. Prior to their embodied participation, watching their sons move, listening to their sons talk with peers and with the teacher, seeing their sons create, and feeling a son's body move seemed strange. When Ralph asked Isto if any fathers actually admitted to this feeling, Isto commented that, no, not at first. Initially, fathers tended to stay close to the studio walls and away from the dancing. It appeared they were distancing themselves. This changed, however, as the fathers felt more "at home" and welcome in the studio—as they began to see the meaning of dance within the raw-board-working process.

Evidence that revealed fathers increasing comfort and understanding was found in small comments made in "corridor chats": the ease with which they walked into the studio and how they watched what was happening with more interest. Learning by watching included observing dance actions, relations, and behaviors in the studio where the boys were revealing social relations and skills in the process of learning to dance. Fathers wanted to make sense of their sons' dancing in this particular studio: what was the working style and atmosphere, and most importantly, as one father noted (age 43, visual art teacher): "There is my son, embodied, succeeding, having spirit and emotions—that is all new to me" (personal communication, November 20, 2014).

Varto (2012) writes about human existence as co-existence. The closer people are to each other, the better they understand each other. When fathers carried their sons and played with them, they had memories of when their boys were babies or small children. For some, such reminiscing led to thoughts about how they "grew apart" and on how and when this distancing happened. As one father (35, application developer) observed, the small and seemingly "absurd endearments" are missing. When he contemplated the mechanisms of growing apart in daily family life, he experienced a wanting to be a different father than what his father was for him (personal communication, November 20, 2014). In his 2016 interview, he stated,

> I wanted to be more present with my son. But even though I am living in the same apartment and with my son for about 80% of the time, I noticed I was not able to play with him anymore. There was too much everything else…it's like I dropped to the role of being the adult male rather than being dad. I could not connect or break our respective "own circles." The contrast to when he was a little boy is…I miss it.
>
> In this dance project, I had to hold my son on my lap for a long time. The idea was to not do anything, just to stay still. He began to quietly lean into me. Maybe there was the closeness again, but not like a regression—a way that was good. I think he felt safe just to be. I think the safety is the biggest deal. The finest thing for me here was doing something together as equals. It is not the same in sport when I coach soccer or when I'm standing on the side of the sport field. In the Dance project, we are equal as dancers and art creators. (personal communication, April 14, 2016)

In contrast, some fathers reported that while their sons were showing self-confidence in the dance studio—learning and exploring, they themselves felt a lack of confidence or skill to participate. One father, a 52-year-old comic artist, said that unlike his sons he did not have "straight away know how" about dance (personal communication, April 21, 2016). Rauhala (2009) and Varto (2012) comment on skill and how it provides access to participation, also appreciating the inherent value of the activity (in dance). Without skill or engagement, fathers felt distanced from their sons' embodied and subjective knowing within the workshop process. However, this did change overtime, as the fathers and sons shared movements and ideas. Fathers learnt to own their movement and share it along with words that explained the movement. The boys from the outset worked with knowhow, enterprise and commitment. They achieved something intrinsic to the experience itself. In Varto's (2012) terms, parents may have felt far away from their own "fleshed knowing" (pp. 16–18).

Scholars observe that narrow and stereotypical notions of dance and gender are dominant factors informing dancing boys' marginalization (Anttila, 2013, 2015a; Bond, 2017; Li, 2016; Risner, 2009). We make assumptions about what is dance and who is a dancer, and when assumptions are not reflected on critically, boys can be quickly marginalized and stereotyped, which in turn can inform boys' willingness to participate in dance. Learning processes are in constant flux as different meanings enter and leave the dance studio. In the present study, fathers reflected on dance.

To understand dance, their own insecurity about dance and their sons' involvement, fathers desired a closer experience to share with their sons. As one father (56, engineer) reflected:

> It is nice to do together. Other hobbies have had "the door closed…come and get him in an hour." This dancing together allows for discussion and acquaintance between parents and children. And still, it is a part of everyday life. It is really a good thing. (personal communication, April 21, 2016)

In dance workshop rehearsals, participants were at situational crossroads: coming from somewhere, becoming something in the process, and leaving the crossroads, that is, being changed somehow (Rauhala, 2009). Several boys commented on the feeling of new intersections and new layers of experience, as well as hesitations. The above father's son (age 9) told about the change: "My father in the same rehearsals? It was first odd. I did not want to. But soon I wanted it. It was more fun to do things with my father than alone" (group communication April 21, 2016). His father reflected on the change also, emphasizing the experience of being closer and the possibilities to talk at a tacit level (Polanyi, 1958). He commented, "We could not talk about such things before … art, dance as visual" (group communication, April 21, 2016), and his son concurred, "And now, we are more together anyway." The father added that being separated from his son's mother caused difficulties with home life, but through dance they have committed to do more together.

Doing duets opened dialogical moments between fathers and sons. At the beginning, the boys had the advantage of knowledge and skills. They better understood the language and unspoken manners in the dance studio. As such, duets brought father and son into an interesting pedagogical relationship. First, there was hesitation about roles, but through dance and working together, traditional roles were put aside in action. Some fathers reflected on such moments as a kind of "profane meditation," as Rauhala (2009) puts it, where daily normality vanishes and mind empties. One part of this being is to be detached from daily life (pp. 284–290). In this "liminal" space, accepted roles and status positions may be transformed (Turner 1969, 2012).

One father (35, application developer) reflected, "So, fathering is telling the child to do-that-and-this. I now see we can be more equal in doing" (personal communication, April 14, 2016). He was surprised by his son's (age 9) behaviour while being carried on stage for some minutes during a performance: the boy was kissing his cheek secretly and sniffing his neck. He was profoundly moved by this and felt deep love and affection. He felt good in what he was giving his son. Writing about fathering relationships, psychotherapist Terrence Real (1997) describes a change in male culture. Instead of boys "walking wounded, denying difficulties," there is the possibility of a shift from, "'What will I get?' (boy's world) to 'What can I offer?' (mature male's world)" (p. 322). This father experienced déjà-vu when carrying his son. He remembered him as a baby swimming, being very close together. This insight prompted the questions of when do relationships change, and how and when does fathering or parenthood lose its embodied closeness to their child. The expression of intimacy between father and son was private, yet it informed how they relate, and in turn their willingness to teach and learn, in a reciprocal relationship. Both were asking in their action "what can I offer", and replying via a small kiss, "myself."

Dance and Performances

Turpeinen's (2015) raw-board-working (Fig. 13.1) can be understood as a spiral that starts from dance action. The action begins with walking, running, jumping, play and improvisation. The raw-board-working spiral collects more material that the participants' value and these provide starting points for ongoing development into dance sequences. The present moment is meaningful in a learner's life-world in relation to the past and the future. The shared present holds singular aspects—like reflecting roles of being a man, a father, or simply the relation to dance without previous skills. In some cases, these aspects point out and politicize relations in daily life—homes, schools and society. In the workshop atmosphere, space for discussion often prompted the group to talk about the Finnish elementary school's curriculum and arts education, or how much the boys are just sitting and playing mobile computer games. One continual topic was about working life — how careers have changed and how we do and don't balance time between work and family.

The boys, between nine and 12 years old, spoke about starting dance as a hobby. One boy (age nine) described, "My mother decided the hobbies I will start, and each day she informs me when we are travelling to the dance studio" (group communication, April 21, 2016). The boys all had more than one hobby, mentioning music and sport along with dance. In the interviews, parents and sons pointed out differences between sports and arts as a hobby, agreeing that competition was a defining difference. Competition was not an interest for all the boys. Some noted the "excitement" of high level activity and how it creates stress. Quite often a hobby was stopped because it was "too stressful." As one father (43, visual arts teacher) described: "it can be too demanding for a little child" (personal communication, April 12, 2016).

Each boy is a singular person with a voice and an opinion (Varto, 2012). The above-quoted visual arts teacher had two sons in the study (ages nine and 12). He thought dance would be a good hobby for his sons, a good means to approach daily life and a hobby offering wide opportunities. He also felt that dance might satisfy both of his sons' interests. One liked competition and strove to develop skills as a dancer and performer, while the other saw dance as a hobby without competition and struggle. This father observed, "We can think that we have succeeded in doing the right thing for our children, but they are all different" (personal communication, April 12, 2016). Another father (52, comic artist) had a similar experience with a non-competitive son (age 12) for whom football and visual arts did not work, but "dance as a hobby worked" (personal communication, April 21, 2016).

The first father mentioned in the previous paragraph (43, visual arts teacher) wanted to underline the point that the dance studio is relatively public. It involves group and individual work and is open to others, but at the same time "participation is singular (private), with the emergence of something public and new" (personal communication, April 12, 2016). He was intrigued by how the creative process worked in the dance workshops. As a visual arts teacher in a basic art education school, this father was using his new dance pedagogy experience in his own lessons. He was trying to understand the dance class teaching method, and wanted to pilot it in his own work as a pedagogue. For example, in his own visual art classes he used the rhythm of the process to help his art students value the process as product, and that the end points of a session can be the beginning points of the next session. This father had a different attitude about dance than the other fathers in the focus group, declaring quite firmly: "I do not dance." His siblings danced, but his areas are fine art and music. He enjoys collaborating, playing his banjo, and jamming with his 9-year-old son. The dance experience remained a puzzle for him but he conceded that he had new respect for his son as a dancer (and for the dance teacher). He also came to realise that he had limited meanings of what it is to dance and recognised that there are diverse meanings and ways to engage.

The second father (52, comic artist) stated that the work done with his son (age 12) empowered him (personal communication, April 12, 2016). Dancing opened "a positive opportunity" that had an impact in daily life by ameliorating stress. He observed, "My movements are rough…elegant movements do not exist in my body language." But dancing with his son started a process of empowering his body as it is, not as it should be. He used the phrase, "scrub and friction are good" to describe his self-described ungainly movement. He used the motto, "Toward that, my way" as a way to sum up his approach to dance. He was throwing himself into dance understanding that he could not do it all, or perfectly. As he said, "the forward rolls are not for me," but "butoh-walk" appealed to him as it was something like the "walking" in Samuel Beckett's plays.

There were two "fractures," or unplanned changes, to the workshop during 2015–2016. The fathers and sons workshop had to change rehearsal time, and hence one of the fathers could not continue. A mother (40) came to the group instead. The son (age 12) described the situation as, "fun. I had possibilities to dance with both parents" (personal communication, May 2, 2016). The group did not react or comment on this change in any way and the dynamics of the group did not vary. This workshop already had dynamics that differ from males in sports, for example (Tiger, 1970, 1999), especially ice hockey, and in violent street culture such as the Soldiers of Odin, an anti-immigration patrol group in Finland. The presence of dancing sons changed the potentially "masculine culture" of the male group. This observation suggests possibilities to further research the role of arts in shifting gendered behaviours (Bond, 1994, 2017).

The second fracture occurred at the beginning of spring 2016. A new father (54, audio-visual-coordinator) and son (age 10) joined the group. The father did not speak Finnish, so we started to use three languages in the studio—Finnish, Swedish and English. At first there was no reaction to this change, but eventually a tiny irritation was noticeable. Nevertheless, one father (43, visual arts teacher) declared this "a marvellous fracture," referring to opportunities that change brings. He observed that a new kind of otherness was in process (personal communication, April 12, 2016). The raw-board-working process presented a new horizon for the men to consider, where difference/change was presenting opportunity for "good" rather than "bad."

Fathers and Sons

The same father reflected on the difference between evening parent-teacher events at his son's school and participating in the dance workshops. He noted that in the dance workshop, the fathers "participate in actions as they are" (personal communication, April 12, 2016) or, one could say, holistically (Rauhala, 2009). In parent-teacher evening events, school based power relations are as "normally understood," with the father as parent and teacher as authority; the power relation between children and adults is asymmetrical. Another father (35, application developer) described the relationship between himself and his son (age nine) as "equal" in the dance workshop, but with variations or "leakages" at home (personal communication, November 20, 2014; April 14, 2016). Moreover, he observed that power relations between fathers and sons can change during the process. For example, especially "when we improvise," voices and opinions are offered by everyone. This father felt equal with his son when they were doing the same movement; he enjoyed it, noting, "it is just fun together." Later, he noticed that he sometimes reverted to norms of parenthood, like saying to his son, "do it well" or "practice." The common place for "leakage" was at home when they practiced their dance, as some others did. His mention of "fun" evidences a bonus for this father. Instead of just being his son's "transport" from one hobby to another, there was now common time with shared action. In sum, this father stated, "I want more of this kind of co-work, if time allows" (personal communication, April 14, 2016).

The comic artist (age 52) told stories about his role as a parent and about the fathering histories in his own childhood family (workshop, spring 2016; personal communication, April 21, 2016). Between the generations one can see how male temperaments are different and how aggressiveness appears. This father described himself as a "passive-aggressive" man—sometimes he feels himself being "hot-blooded" without any visible actions. In one instance, he became (passively) angry when his son (age 12) played videogames and did not stop when asked.

He reflected on his own father's behavior, which he remembered as quick-tempered: "He got angry suddenly, in 1 s, maybe not having an understandable reason." His grandfather had the same kind of temperament. He used a common expression to describe the classic Finnish male stereotype: "He chased the family outside with the axe into a snow blanket." World War II (1939–1944) did not help these men in Finland who went through a twofold contradictory personal and cultural experience: first the terrible personal experience of war and then the heroic attitude of the so-called "Winter War Miracle" (Rainio-Niemi, 2014). Between these two—the terrible and the heroic, a generation of Finnish fathers were wounded and silenced. There is truth in the quip, "don't talk about the war." This silence deserves another book and is beyond the scope of this chapter; suffice to say that notions of masculinity often require men not to feel, reflect, cry, and share. This is changing within Finland but slowly.

William Pollack (1998) wrote about the "boy code" in his book *Real Boys: Rescuing our Sons from the Myths of Boyhood.* Turpeinen (2015) suggests this kind of code is alive in Finland. One cultural phenomenon that illuminates the narrow construction of boy codes is found within art hobbies. As noted in the previous chapter, in dance education, males make up a small minority of enrolled students. More widely, the arts are not respected as a boy or male hobby. Scholars have described gender socialization in western cultural settings where boys and girls "halve themselves" (Real, 1997, p. 23; see also Keyworth, 2001). Boys are encouraged to develop their public, assertive selves while being pushed away both tacitly and consciously from the full exercise of emotional expressiveness and the skills for making and appreciating aesthetic connection (Bond, 2017; Connell, 2005; Lehikoinen, 2006; Turpeinen, 2015). This is seen in some of the stories from fathers in the dance workshop.

There are stories about fathers who have more respect for the walking wounded (men valorized for tolerating and surviving pain), separating from their children voluntarily, drinking too much alcohol, and denying difficulties. Interviews showed polarized male attitudes towards divorce. As noted earlier, issues of love, nurture, gender roles, and more come into play. Without doubt human relationships are complex, yet within this study fathers were willing to experience an activity that questioned behaviors and fostered relationships, and they acknowledged faults, histories of behavior, and aspirations for their sons. As such, we can imagine a possibility for better social relationships, and for dance to positively influence male social behavior.

Isto observed a degree of change throughout the project. Over the 3-year period slow change was evidenced by changes in participation. At the beginning the men were shy workshop participants and at the end they were proud to perform in public. Real (1997) discussed how fathers and sons tend to play out culture's values about masculinity. Men assessed as having warm, nurturing relationships with their children, however, were shown to be healthier, less depressed, and surprisingly, more successful in their careers than distant fathers. The present study is not as wide-ranging as Real's, but it opens the door for further research about the role of dance in social transformation in Finland and perhaps beyond (Fig. 13.2).

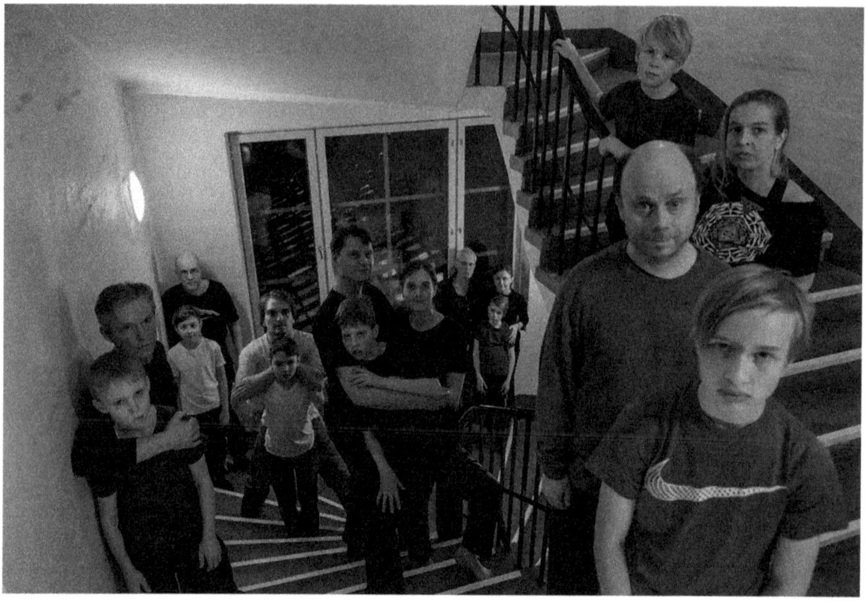

Fig. 13.2 The EXTRA workshop group in "The Living Photo Album" project (2017). (Photograph: Isto Turpeinen)

Conclusion

This research project engaged with a small number of father and son relationships and reflected on the emergent theme of love that surfaced through the raw-board-working dance workshop process. The study found that as fathers and sons danced with each other within a "safe" open workshop process, they re-constructed their relationships consciously and unconsciously. Diverse meanings of masculinity were found to both negatively and positively inform how relationships were expressed.

The study found that the dance experience revealed and celebrated stated and unstated love between fathers and sons. The raw-board-working process valued a teaching and learning environment based on pedagogical love. Through the workshop process boys and fathers noticed change in their relationships to dance, to each other and with ideas of masculinity; they grew to feel more connected and loving towards each other. The intimacy found in sharing embodied dialogue, studio space, and ideas — in a trusting and defined dance process that valued diverse movement offerings and experience—enriched fathers' and sons' relationships. Of great interest is that the word "love" is what fathers spoke about and in some cases yearned for.

In sum, this study found that the raw-board-working dance process provided fathers and sons some safe and open opportunities to question and express ideas and feelings. The significance of the finding might be in how they came to know each other better and how the love that underpins a father and son relationship can be re-kindled and affirmed.

What's Next? Fathers and Sons in ARTSEQUAL

Isto and Ralph's work with dancing boys and fathers continues within the ARTSEQUAL research initiative at the University of Arts Helsinki. ARTSEQUAL is funded by the Academy of Finland's Strategic Research Council through its Equality in Society Program (Project no. 293199). ARTSEQUAL addresses one of the central questions for future development of the Finnish welfare society: to rethink the role of the arts. Within ARTSEQUAL, Isto and Ralph are focusing on questions of gender and family in arts education. The ongoing research project asks: *What if the arts were understood more widely as a public service with equality as the starting point?*

As evidenced in this chapter, a pedagogical artistic research process called raw-board-working offered an open space that allowed for deconstruction of unquestioned realities about notions of love, men's experience, fathering, and so on. Further research will examine how to foster gender and culturally sensitive pedagogies in and through the arts, and investigate successful practices in basic arts education. An agenda driving ARTSEQUAL research is that opportunities to examine and model pedagogies that foster "a good life" are integral to arts education, specifically a life that nurtures equality, diversity, empathy, and happiness.

This study has strengthened our understanding that dance workshops and performances can provide ways for fathers and sons to reflect on how they relate to each other. Ironically (given the negative gender associations surrounding dance), dance can provide a safe space and activity that has scope to develop father-son communication and behaviours. This component of an ongoing study reinforces that dance has potential to transform a key human relationship within Finnish society. Fathers and sons can learn from each other via a holistic, democratic dance pedagogy such as raw-board-working. Our ongoing belief is that dance and the arts can foster healthier relationships and hence a healthier society.

References

Amir, L. (2001). Plato's theory of love: Rationality as passion. *Practical Philosophy: The Journal of Philosophical Practitioners, 4*(3), 6–14.

Anttila, E. (2003). *A dream journey to the unknown. Searching for dialogue in dance education.* Helsinki, Finland: Theatre Academy.

Anttila, E. (2013). *Koko koulu tanssii! Kehollisen oppimisen mahdollisuuksia kouluyhteisössä* [The entire school dances! The possibilities of embodied learning in a school context]. Helsinki, Finland: Acta Scenica 37.

Anttila, E. (2015a). "Entire School Dances!" Project generated new insights on embodied learning. *Nordic Journal of Dance: Practice, Education and Research, 6*(1), 67–69.

Anttila, E. (2015b). Dance as embodied dialogue: Insights from a school project in Finland. In C. Svendler Nielsen & S. Burridge (Eds.), *Dance education around the world: Perspectives on dance, young people and change* (pp. 79–87). New York: Routledge.

Arlander, A. (2013). Artistic research in a Nordic context. In R. Nelson (Ed.), *Practice as research in the arts.* Hampshire, UK: Palgrave Macmillan.

Bond, K. E. (1994). How 'wild things' tamed gender distinctions. *Journal of Physical Education Recreation and Dance, 65*(2), 28–33.
Bond, K. E. (2014). Dance and quality of life. In A. C. Michalos (Ed.), *Encyclopedia of quality of life and Well-being research* (pp. 1419–1424). Dordrecht, The Netherlands: Springer.
Bond, K. (2017). "Boys are morons" … "Girls are gross": Let's dance! In W. Oliver & D. Risner (Eds.), *Dance and gender: An evidence based approach* (pp. 135–157). Gainesville: University Press of Florida.
Bond, K., & Richard, R. (2005). Ladies and gentlemen! What do you see? What do you feel? A story of connected curriculum in a third grade dance education setting. In L. Overby & B. Lepczyk (Eds.), *Dance: Current selected research* (Vol. 5, pp. 85–133). New York: AMS.
Bond, K., & Stinson, S. (2000/2001). "I feel like I'm going to take off": Young people's experiences of the super ordinary in dance. *Dance Research Journal, 32*(2), 52–87.
Bond, K. E., & Stinson, S. W. (2016). "Its work, work, work, work:" Young people's experiences of effort and engagement in dance. In S. W. Stinson (Ed.), *Embodied curriculum theory and research in arts education: A dance scholar's search for meaning* (pp. 269–295). Dordrecht, The Netherlands: Springer. (Original work published 2007).
Borgdorff, H. (2010). The production of knowledge in artistic research. In M. Biggs & H. Karlsson (Eds.), *Routledge companion to research in the arts* (pp. 1–43). London: Routledge.
Buber, M. (2013). *I and thou*. London: Bloomsbury Academic. (Original work published 1923).
Burt, R. (2007). *The male dancer: Bodies, spectacle, sexualities*. London: Routledge.
Connell, R. W. (2005). *Masculinities* (2nd ed.). Cambridge, UK: Polity.
Crotty, M. (1998). *The foundations of social research: Meaning and perspective in the research process*. London: Sage.
Csikszentmihalyi, M. (1990). *Flow: The psychology of optimal experience*. New York: Harper & Row.
Csikszentmihalyi, M. (1994). *The evolving self*. New York: Harper Perennial.
Dewey, J. (2005). *Art as experience*. New York: Penguin. (Original work published 1934).
Eisner, E. (1998). *The enlightened eye: Qualitative inquiry and the enhancement of educational practice*. New York: Macmillan.
Fontana, A., & Frey, J. H. (2000). The interview: From structured questions to negotiated text. In N. K. Denzin & Y. S. Lincoln (Eds.), *Handbook of qualitative research* (2nd ed., pp. 645–673). London: Sage.
Freire, P. (1972). *Pedagogy of the oppressed* (M. Ramos, Trans.). Harmondsworth, UK: Penguin Education.
Garrison, J., Neubert, S., & Reich, K. (2012). *John Dewey's philosophy of education: An introduction and recontextualization for our times*. New York: Palgrave Macmillan.
Greene, M. (1991). Blue guitars and the search for curriculum. In G. Willis & W. Schubert (Eds.), *Reflections from the heart of educational inquiry* (pp. 107–122). New York: SUNY Press.
Guba, E., & Lincoln, Y. (1994). Competing paradigms in qualitative research. In N. K. Denzin & Y. S. Lincoln (Eds.), *Handbook of qualitative research* (pp. 105–117). Thousand Oaks, CA: Sage.
Harré, R., & Secord, P. (1972). *The explanation of social behaviour*. Oxford, UK: Basil Blackwell.
Holmes, R. M. (1998). *Fieldwork with children*. Thousand Oaks, CA: Sage.
Keyworth, S. (2001). Critical autobiography: "Straightening" out dance education. *Research in Dance Education, 2*(2), 117–137.
Kirkkopelto, E. (2008). New start: Artistic research in Finnish Theatre Academy. *Nordic Theatre Studies, 20*, 16–27.
Kirkkopelto, E. (2012, March 1). *Inventions and institutions: Artistic research as a medium of change*. Seminar presentation, Finnish Society for Aesthetics.
Lehikoinen, K. (2006). *Stepping queerly? Discourses in dance education for boys in the late 20th century Finland*. Oxford, UK: Peter Lang.
Li, Z. (2016). *Dancing boys*. Toronto, ONT: University of Toronto Press.

Maykut, P., & Morehouse, R. (1994). *Beginning qualitative research: A philosophic and practical guide*. London: The Falmer Press.
Merleau-Ponty, M. (1962). *Phenomenology of perception* (C. Smith, Trans.). London: Routledge.
Nelson, R. (2013). *Practice as research in the arts*. Hampshire, UK: Palgrave Macmillan.
Pellegrini, R. J., & Sarbin, T. R. (Eds.). (2012). *Between fathers and sons: Critical incident narratives in the development of men's lives*. New York: Routledge.
Plato. (1951). *The symposium* (W. Hamilton, Trans.). New York: Penguin. (Original work published 385-370 BCE).
Polanyi, M. (1958). *Personal knowledge: Towards a post-critical philosophy*. London: Routledge & Kegan Paul.
Pollack, W. (1998). *Real boys: Rescuing our sons from the myths of boyhood*. New York: Henry Holt.
Rainio-Niemi, J. (2014). *The ideological Cold War: The politics of neutrality in Austria and Finland*. New York: Routledge.
Rauhala, L. (2009). *Henkinen ihminen. Henkinen ihmisessä & Ihmisen ainutlaatuisuus*. Helsinki, Finland: University Press.
Real, T. (1997). *I don't want to talk about it. Overcoming the secret legacy of male depression*. New York: Scribner.
Richard, B. (2009). *"Daddy, root me in:" Tethering young sons in the context of male, intergenerational, child-centered dance education*. Doctoral dissertation. Retrieved from ProQuest Dissertations and Thesis database (ATT 3359701).
Risner, D. (2009). *Stigma and perseverance in the lives of boys who dance: An empirical study of male identities in western theatrical dance training*. Lewiston, NY: Edwin Mellen.
Steffe, L. P., & Gale, J. (Eds.). (2012). *Constructivism in education*. New York: Routledge.
Svendler Nielsen, C. (2015). An embodied and artistic-based research methodology to study processes of learning and change in dance education. *International Yearbook for Research in Arts Education, 3*, 147–150.
Tiger, L. (1970). *Men in groups*. New York: Vintage.
Tiger, L. (1999). *The decline of males*. New York: St. Martin's.
Tripp, D. (1983). Co-authorship and negotiation: The interview as act of creation. *Interchange, 14*(3), 32–45.
Turner, E. (2012). *Communitas: The anthropology of collective joy*. New York: Palgrave Macmillan.
Turner, V. (2008). *The ritual process: Structure and anti-structure*. New Brunswick, NJ: Aldine Transaction. (Original work published 1969).
Turpeinen, I. (2012). Dance and gender. Is there any change? In S. W. Stinson, C. Svendler Nielsen, & S-Y. Liu (Eds.), *Dance, young people and change: Proceedings of the daCi and WDA Global Dance Summit*. Taipei, Taiwan: Taipei National University of the Arts. Retrieved from http://www.ausdance.org.au/publications/
Turpeinen, I. (2015). *Raakalautaa ja rakkautta. Kolme sommitelmaa oman elämän tanssista*. Helsinki, Finland: Theatre Academy.
Turpeinen, I. (2017). Raw board working style, pedagogical love and gender. In C. Svendler Nielsen & Susan R. Koff (Eds.), *Exploring identities in dance. Proceedings from the 13th World Congress of Dance and the Child International*. Retrieved from http://ausdance.org.au/publications/details/exploring-identities-in-dance
Vandenberghe, F. (2008). Sociology of the heart: Max Scheler's epistemology of love. *Theory, Culture, Society, 25*, 17–51. Retrieved from https://www.researchgate.net/publication/240708618
Varto, J. (1991). *Laulu maasta. Luennot etiikasta*. Tampere, Finland: Tampereen yliopisto.
Varto, J. (2012). *A dance with the world. Towards an ontology of singularity*. Helsinki, Finland: Aalto University.
Vigotsky, L. S. (1962). *Thought and language*. Cambridge, MA: MIT Press.
Weil, S. (1949/2001). *The need for roots. Prelude to a declaration of duties towards mankind*. London: Routledge.

Chapter 14
Friction: Male Identity and Representation in Umfundalai

C. Kemal Nance

Umfundalai is a contemporary African dance technique created from the movement vocabulary of dance traditions throughout Africa and the African Diaspora. In Kiswahili, Umfundalai means "essence" or "essential." For Kariamu Welsh, Umfundalai's progenitor, the technique is an artistic medium for exploring an African essence – an aesthetic commonality that binds Diasporan dance traditions and Black people to an African cultural continuum. Since 1970, Welsh has been developing Umfundalai with predominantly female dancers.

Welsh describes Umfundalai as "an approach to movement that is wholistic and body centric" (K. Welsh, personal communication, December 21, 2012), language that ideologically shifts African dance from its originative traditions to the embodied persons who inhabit the movement. Umfundalai's first dance master, Glendola Yhema Mills (1995), describes Umfundalai as a "women's continuum continuing to be" (p. 6). Yet, 15 men have danced in and out of Umfundalai's evolving tradition over the last 46 years. What "continuum" does Umfundalai perpetuate with its dancing men?

This chapter presents a collective and interpretive autoethnography (Denzin, 2014) that "queers" Umfundalai, illuminating what Sara Ahmed (2006) calls the "oblique existence" of eight men, including the author, who have studied and performed this contemporary African dance technique. Aligning with sociologist Carolyn Ellis's (2004) definition of autoethnography, the chapter also reflects "research, writing, story, and method that connect the autobiographical and personal to the cultural, social, and political" (p. xix). The narrative is "collective" in that it starts with the author's lived experiences and goes on to include the perspectives of other Umfundalai dancing men (see Kidd & Finlayson, 2010). It is interpretive in that it "allows the researcher to take up each person's life in its immediate particularity and to ground the life in this historical moment" (Denzin, 2014, p. x).

C. K. Nance (✉)
University of Illinois, Urbana, IL, USA
e-mail: cknance@illinois.edu

K. Bond (ed.), *Dance and the Quality of Life*, Social Indicators Research Series 73,
https://doi.org/10.1007/978-3-319-95699-2_14

This qualitative inquiry is sourced by open-ended interviews with the eight men and informed by personal communication with Kariamu Welsh and Glendola Yhema Mills.

Methodologically, the study is informed by Max van Manen's (1997) hermeneutic phenomenology, specifically his guidelines for capturing lived experience description through interviewing, and Norman Denzin's (2014) interpretive perspective, in which the researcher moves back and forth between past and present to release possibilities for new knowledge. With collective hindsight and a critical, inductive lens, the research illuminates the complexities of dancing men's lived experiences of gender in Umfundalai. and how these support men's placement along an African continuum, a gendered agency (Hays, 1994) that looks beyond whiteness for its definition.

Mills offered the following comments about her experience of learning Umfundalai from Kariamu Welsh:

> So, when you talk about the culture, the intangible stuff, in the studio, … the dance I'm going to do is important. I'm a person entering the dance and that is going to affect you and I dancing together, dancing with other people, us—the teacher, the choreographer being inspired by what we do. That was new, that idea that I'm just as important in the creative process to the choreographer as they are to me. (Y. Mills, personal communication, May 19, 2013)

Mills has an important role in this study as a conduit of the Umfundalai tradition for many of the men who have studied the technique. She made the above comments in response to my question about the culture of Umfundalai upon her entry. They provide a context for the "intangible stuff" that pervaded Umfundalai studio practice, including a gendered discourse for Umfundalai's dancing men.

Some of our dancing men's "life stories" (Denzin, 2014) speak to a friction enflamed by our socialization as African American males, and our participation in a female dominated dance tradition. I endeavor to identify the "problems connecting meaning (culture) and action (social interaction)" (Gagnon, 2004, p. 140) that emerge from men's engagement with Umfundalai's transmission of dance culture.

The Friction of Representation

In Umfundalai, Stafford C. Berry, Jr. and I are leading men in both the characters we dance in repertory and the gender roles we perform in its evolving tradition (see Nance, 2014). Prior to January 1993 when we both joined Kariamu & Company after having studied Umfundalai at our respective undergraduate institutions (Berry at Temple University and I at Swarthmore College), there was no consistent male presence, and we both felt this absence. I recall having conversations before and after rehearsals about how we might alter certain movements for our tall male bodies – how we wanted to represent our gendered selves in the technique, folklore, and choreography of Umfundalai.

Without masculine role models, Berry and I sought resources to inform how we wanted to present ourselves on the concert stage. Sometimes, to express the physicality of our male bodies, we would incorporate movement vocabulary from our concurrent neo-traditional West African dance training with Hodari Banks, for example, phrases from *Doun Doun Ba* of Guinea. Whenever there was an opportunity to personalize Welsh's choreography or to improvise during the rehearsal for the audience participation portion of our concert, we would find ways to demonstrate our facility for these specific West African dance styles. We both wanted access to the high level of performance of our female peers – as men. To this end we interrogated what we thought were the conventions of Umfundalai. Welsh recalls our beginning days with the company:

> Particularly you and Staff were vocal about things I would do. You were very funny. I don't know how the female dancers felt, but I would laugh because a lot of the humor was based on truth. And a lot of what I was doing that had already been done you wanted to do. When I did it for women it wasn't because it was a female dance – that's just what I had to work with. When you all came in, you just wanted to do it, and I would see you do it. I said, "That's great. I like that!" It gave me more options… (K. Welsh, personal communication, December 21, 2012)

During Kariamu & Company (K & C) rehearsals, whoever was directing assigned the dancers' parts based on what she felt were their movement strengths. In our beginning days, Welsh would see Berry and me only in the dances that Umfundalai teachers Mills and Joylynn Ama Houtman thought best suited our skills. However, we would learn everyone's parts and dance them on the periphery of the studio during our 'rest time.' We liked to exclaim how we could do the 'other' parts. We imitated other dancers, exaggerating their movements to resemble hip-hop dances of the late 1980s. In tandem, we found any opportunity to laugh and dance. Welsh thought our antics were "disarming" and "funny."

Two statements in Welsh's reflections above illustrate the culture of Umfundalai at the time. The first, "I don't know how the female dancers felt but I would laugh," suggests there might have been a difference between how she viewed our behavior in Umfundalai and how the women experienced us. We spent most rehearsal times learning repertory from other dancers and trying to understand the culture of Umfundalai in performance. Our interactions with Welsh as artistic director would usually happen near the end of the creative process. I recall palpable tensions between Welsh's vision of her work, the senior dancers' interpretation of that vision, and Berry's and my sometimes-comedic interrogation of Umfundalai that the women only seemed to enjoy and participate in when we shared meals after rehearsals.

When we joined the company, the seasoned company members – all women – warned us that our laughter and perpetual joking during and after rehearsals were inappropriate. They advised us to get it out of our systems before Mama (Welsh) arrived, but we disobeyed and felt that Welsh's hearty laughter at our jokes, her smile, and subsequent conversations showed that she appreciated our humor. Nevertheless, there was a tacitly gendered company culture that Berry and I "troubled" (Butler, 1990). At the time, we viewed this culture as female and thought the dissonance was due to our being men. This social aspect of Umfundalai was evolving without Welsh's presence and independent of her direction.

Welsh's statement, "...that's just what I had to work with," is also telling. It appears that what Berry and I interpreted as an intentional women's company came to exist for pragmatic reasons. Recalling conversations with Berry when we joined K & C, we inferred that we were in a women's company from three factors: (1) the choreographer (Welsh) was a woman; (2) women were the company's content experts; and (3) much of the thematic material focused on what we considered women's discourse.

In 1993, K & C's repertoire consisted of newly choreographed and selected older works from Welsh's tenure with the Black Dance Workshop in the late 1970s including *Aluta Continua* (1976), the story of how women of southern Africa protected their homeland while men were at war; *Raaahmonaaah!* (1989), a biomythography of a 1985 bombing in Philadelphia and the sole adult survivor Ramona Africa; *Women Gather* (1991), a dance that explored the idiosyncratic communication of Caribbean women; and *The King Must Die* (1992), an ancient Kemetic tale about a king who was killed by his community because of his physical inability to rule and his head wife's reign after his demise. While Welsh had worked with male dancers prior to Berry's and my arrival, they often danced specific roles as guest artists rather than as full company members.

Essentially, Welsh created work with the dancers she had access to. Until this moment in our separate and concurrent careers – specifically, our first year with Welsh's company, Berry and I had yet to experience her creative process. We had been affected solely through her artistic production, from watching her work in University of the Arts students concerts, her annual February concert at Temple University, and other selected performances throughout the year. While enamored with her artistry, we were convinced that she choreographed works about women to advance an unspoken feminist agenda.

The familial aspect of Umfundalai, as Mills describes above, taken together with dances about women and a visibly female dance culture, created fertile ground for the male seeds that Berry and I sowed during our early years in the company (1993–1997). Here is Berry's recollection of our beginning in K & C:

> They had this little sister circle. I am sure it was nurturing for them and it came from Mama on down. I hated to be the person to break all that up [*said with a facetious grin*]. ... It was a challenge for them...we were treated like annoying little brothers. They didn't take us seriously. For them there was this nurturing happening...but we didn't need all that. And when we were invited to come in, they were like, "Well, who are they?" It didn't blow up... they eventually accepted us...we became like family. But we were bringing the male essence up in there...a different energy. We weren't just annoying little brothers. We brought something that did not exist before and that was huge! I don't think we realized it then. We are the male folks up in here now! (S. Berry, personal communication, May 11, 2012)

Sister Circle

"Sister circle" seems an apt metaphor for the social dynamic of female company members. Even the anecdotal histories of the company and Welsh's deportment as leader, which have been passed along through generations of dancers – what I think of as the company's folklore – were conveyed through vernacular and gestures of "girl talk." Senior company members would share anecdotes amidst playful slaps on each other's arms and "gurl!" and "chile" designations, replete with adolescent giggles and whispers. Throughout the rehearsal process, dancers would recall instances of "Mama's wrath" or reminisce about performing with dancers who shared "sisterly" bonds. I often heard expressions like, "That was my gurl! She was my sistah!" as they described dancing in previous seasons.

We were new and we were men. I perceived condescension in how the women answered my questions about the technique and the meanings of movements and rituals. Yet, they often laughed with Berry and me in our joking, like the way siblings might do when parents are absent. When Welsh attended rehearsals, however, our joking stopped being as funny: four of the ten women and the four men who comprised the company would place themselves strategically at the front for company class and volunteer to teach repertoire to us and other new dancers. In Umfundalai training, maintenance of community is an important value, and the seasoned dancers were responsible for teaching and acculturating newer dancers. Perhaps their "willingness" to teach us was a way to assert leadership, or to win favor with "Mama Kariamu," or maybe this was an example of the broader phenomenon of gender's "hidden curriculum" in American dance studio settings (Bond, 2017; Stinson, 2005). I recall how complicit Berry and I were in our annoying little brothers "performances" (see Denzin, 2014). We would even sometimes imitate the women's speech, performing their idiosyncrasies as a way to poke fun.

I asked Mills to describe any cultural shifts she perceived on Berry's and my arrival as males. She recollects talking with Welsh about me when I was taking their classes as a first-year graduate student in the master of dance education program at Temple University in 1992:

> Mama said, "We're going to have to tame him." You were a real energy! To me, the energy was good…playful. We would get serious, but you were always mocking somebody. Even if it was just the face… There was this lightness…laughter…even in class. Especially when she would critique you. You were thinking you were wearing something out and she would show you what she *really* wanted. You'd be like, "Whoa! Whoa, okay!" (Y. Mills, personal communication, May 19, 2013)

Speaking as an older brother, Mills' description of my behaviors does sound like the antics of a younger sibling. I recall clearly how my brother's laughing and mimicry would annoy me. Berry and I participated in the "girl talk" of the company but also satirized it as males. During rehearsals, we did drag impressions of the dancers and of Welsh at least once a week. After Carrie Noland (2009), I consider that these acts of resistance reflected the inherent autonomy of dancing bodies (see also Louppe,

2010). Noland (2009) argues that through extension of gestures, which she conceives as any movement practice, is how agency is enacted. She writes:

> I intend to privilege corporeal performance and the sensory experience it affords in the hope of yielding a theory of agency fully implicated in embodiment, which I take to be that ambiguous phenomenon in which culture both asserts and loses its grip on individual subjects. (p. 7)

As outlined above, many factors could have informed Umfundalai female dancers' reception of Berry and me. We were new and our proficiency in dancing Umfundalai had been achieved only recently. In retrospect, I wonder whether the new female dancers felt a similar alienation from the sister circle. In any case, in the years that followed, Berry and I became principal dancers in K & C and therefore integral to the continuing development of Umfundalai.

We Wear the *Shokatoes*

While 1993 marked our first year of dancing with K & C, the company did not perform a full season again until 1996 when Welsh changed the name to Kariamu & Company: Traditions. Between 1993 and 1996 Berry and I ran our own company while studying and performing neo–traditional West African dance with Ibeji Performing Arts Company under the direction of Hodari Banks and Jeannine Osayande. We would take classes with them twice a week and perform at selected engagements. Neo-traditional African dance aims to replicate movement practices of traditional African societies in contemporary venues, including the American concert stage (Shujaa & Shujaa, 2015). The prefix 'neo' acknowledges that the dances change once they are removed from their traditional social, cultural, and often religious contexts in Africa, and as noted by Welsh (2010), "are not bound to the aesthetic and cultural rules" of the original society (p. 18).

However, as a teacher Hodari Banks insisted that we learn the male canon of movements within the dances of the Old Malian Empire (thirteenth to seventeenth centuries ACE). These were the dances he had performed as a young artist in neo-traditional companies in both California and Washington, DC. We received an intentionally gendered education on how to dance like men, a stylization of body that aligned with masculine gender performances of the dances' African societies of origin. I found Hodari's pedagogy abrasive but valued his investment in grooming our "masculine presence" as performers. Berry reflects:

> He could be a meanie and belligerent and hyper-masculine, aggressively masculine. … I didn't take him personally. I took him seriously but not personally… I loved when he taught. Up until then we'd had female teachers and I was used to that. But he made me appreciate…doing the crocodile or putting flips and somersaults in the movement. Not that I could do any of that. He made me appreciate the more athletic, traditional African male movement. For that, I love and respect him. That's a part of African dance that I love to this day, the athletic and physical. (S. Berry, personal communication, May 11, 2012)

In retrospect, I also came to appreciate what Hodari gave me and grew to love him. Initially, however, I suffered through classes that might include Hodari having Berry and me go back and forth across the floor by ourselves until we were exhausted, and then dancing in front of us – showing us up – during our fourth or fifth crossing. Yet, he was giving us an education that informed our performance quality in both neo-traditional African dance and as male dancers in Umfundalai.

Umfundalai depends on the essence of each dancer who performs it. In other words, it relies on the phenomenology of the dancer – what "constitutes" them pre-reflectively as a singular individual – as well as a shared nature that binds them to other individuals (Husserl, 2012). Welsh explains, "The essence of the technique is individual and collective allowing artistic room for the one and the many" (K. Welsh, personal communication, February 12, 2014). On an earlier occasion, she described the male essence in African dance throughout the Diaspora as "physical and athletic" (K. Welsh, personal communication, December 21, 2012). Hodari's teaching focused on our athletic abilities. Our weekly interactions with him as dancers in his company, allied with our quest to find our own artistic voices, provided impetus to interrogate masculinities in Umfundalai. I asked Berry to clarify the ways we depended on each other for support in articulating maleness dancing Umfundalai.

> We sure did depend on each other—in three ways. One, we were always trying to figure out how to adjust Umfundalai to our bodies. It was not always a neat fit. Two, we were always trying to incorporate what we were learning from Jeanine and Hodari. He was always on our cases about dancing like men. We tried to bring some of that to Umfundalai. Three, we were always trying to personalize the vocabulary. Remember how we used to ululate [*laughing*]? Berry and Nance in the house! (S. Berry, personal communication, September 25, 2013)

Our neo-traditional African male dance education emphasized upper body strength, speed, and jumping high while the women did hip twisting. With the exception of the *Mbende* dances (Zimbabwe), distinctions between male and female movement were non-existent in Umfundalai at that time. Masculine ideologies prevalent in West African dance were fun to explore but felt artificial to me; they failed to narrate the African-American male-hood I had lived. It felt empowering to learn dances like *Mandiani* and their origins in that they associated me and my dancing with imagined African men; as an urban African American man, however, I could not relate to how a community – much less men – could celebrate dancing young women's entry into puberty in East Guinea.

While Umfundalai vocabulary drew on cultural sources from my African American upbringing, its "maleness" was hard to identify. Even though there were vestiges of traditional dances throughout the Diaspora, there was also vocabulary from *my* African experience, the one I lived in Chester, Pennsylvania. Among them, The Temptations' preparation for Umfundalai's "African Triplet," named after the African American singing group, brought memories of dancing with my mother while watching *Soul Train* on TV. This preparation is performed exactly like the rocking movement members of the Temptations would dance when they sang heir hit single *My Girl* (Robinson & White, 1964). The "Ring Shout" took me to "the

Smurf," an African American social dance of the early 1980s, and the "Baltimore Cracker Jack" made me recall a 1960s social dance my mother taught me.

As alluded to earlier, in Umfundalai classes and K & C rehearsals Berry and I would inquire about movement origins, particularly movements that required us to move our hips. We also challenged the absence of men in company repertory, specifically *Raaahmonaah!* (Welsh, 1989). In response, Welsh began to stylize movement in ways that created space for us to explore masculinity. Mills taught us most of the beginning repertory and listened to our questions about gender roles and choreographic intention. She developed the male arm variation of "Nigerian Stomp" for men during the 1994–95 academic year, which was approved by Welsh in July, 1995. She took an interest in helping male dancers achieve maleness in dancing, employing physiological and cultural references to convey how she felt the male should dance in this contemporary African dance form.

Machismo

Some of Mills' attempts were more successful than others. Berry recalls this critique of our dancing:

> I was never aware of my gender until it was pointed out. Yhema would say, "Staff and Kemal, y'all *machismo* it!" I remember thinking, "What the hell does she mean by that?" I kind of stuck my chest out and put on a placed physique. I remember her saying, "You know when you see the Ailey barrel chest...I'm talking about that." I remember thinking, "Chile, I ain't no Ailey dancer. You may be saying 'barrel' but 'bird' is what you gonna get" [*chuckling*]. … Not that I am not gonna try, but I am not an Ailey dancer. I am not going to pretend. Why use the Ailey male dancer as a model for Umfundalai? … We're not doing *Cry*. Yes, we're all dancing, but this is different, so why do I need to look like an Ailey male? (S. Berry, personal communication, May 11, 2012).

At the time, I shared Berry's confusion about Mills' *machismo* and Ailey's chest. Some years later in an interview with Mills, I asked if she remembered what she meant by *machismo* all those years ago.

> *Machismo*! Come on! Pull it up [*lifting her shoulders*]. We know what *machismo* is… upright with strong shoulders. I don't mean stiffening, but there's a confidence…a broadening of the chest. There's a strength. It's like the guy in the hood. "Yeah! There's a brother right there." By the carriage of his body…I don't mean rigid. I mean a strong upright posture–how Black men walk. That is the uprightness I wanted him to maintain in the dance. It goes back to strength and power. (Y. Mills, personal communication, May 19, 2013).

Mills cannot recall what she was trying to get across with the "Ailey barrel chest" metaphor, but practical reason suggests she may have been commenting on Berry's slender build – a distinct contrast to the muscular upper bodies that Mills associated with Ailey male dancers. While *machismo* evolved into a global meme, neither Berry nor I were aware of its social import in the context of contemporary African dance.

During a K & C rehearsal in Philadelphia during winter 1998, after Berry left the company to join Chuck Davis's African American Dance Ensemble in Durham,

North Carolina, I heard Mills use *machismo* again to describe what two of her younger male students at Freedom Theater were lacking in their performance of her choreography. (She had only just left them moments before arriving at our rehearsal.) Only through this autoethnographic inquiry, however, have I begun to understand that Mills was trying to get the men of K & C to articulate a masculinity that was distinct from the strength and power of Umfundalai's dancing women. For Mills, *machismo* was a way to encourage dancing men to find an agency in their danced gender that captured the masculine archetypes that pervade the African aesthetic.

I asked Mills if during her years of teaching experience, she had observed any common challenges men face in embodying Umfundalai. She answered,

> Maybe it's more my challenge than theirs, but I would say it's a challenge of maleness. If we take the posturing of the hands, here is where I am. You know how we do it with the hands swinging on the pelvic drop sequence? I pull the elbows back because I don't want them to look like me. I want them to do movement like men, males. So, *machismo*, that uprightness, is a male aesthetic. Using the hips, there is this as opposed to this [*demonstrates*]. If you come into class and I size you up and say, "Okay! That's his maleness," I want to see that in all of the work. I don't want to see you shift your aesthetic, how you move, so that it looks like me. (Y. Mills, personal communication, May 19, 2013)

This disclosure indicates that for at least two decades Mills has strived to ensure that her "intangible me" is not cloned by male dancers, but rather that males embody a masculinity uniquely informed by their personhood. Despite the confusion that *machismo* caused Berry and me, Mills was also offering a physiological approach to training – emphasizing our physical strengths and how these might be manipulated to achieve a level of performance on par with the more skilled female dancers in the company.

As her definition of *machismo* reflects, Mills was trying to help us embody a representational masculinity. However, this was a masculinity that she desired, not one we could achieve with our uniquely gendered, phenomenological selves. This "challenge of maleness," as she put it, affected my carriage as a conduit of Umfundalai, and in turn has affected the men who have learned from and danced with me. I view the first challenge of maleness as cross-gender mimicry.

Beginning dancers emulate their teachers. The young men who had problems "*machismo*-ing" Mills' choreography were 16 and 17 years old. Berry and I were 24 and 23 respectively when we joined K & C in 1993 after studying Umfundalai for 5 years. Personally, I imitated everything Welsh did as my instructor (and still do). I wanted to be good at dancing, and it appeared that the key was to dance like her as well as the other female dancers in class.

Dancing Like a Female

A critical point for me occurred in 1991 during a Cultural Arts Safari with Chuck Davis in Gambia, West Africa, when a male teacher commented that I danced like a woman. Something about what I had embodied through Kariamu Welsh, or something that dancing Umfundalai brought out of me resonated as female for this continental African man. Perhaps this quality is what Hodari Banks later fought to correct in teaching me neo-traditional West African dance; I needed to change something to become a dancing man who dances like a man. A male dancer who imitates his female dance teacher may risk disturbing the connection between the man he experiences when he dances and the man the audience sees while he is dancing.

As a young boy, dancing brought me much joy, as it does for many young people across cultures (Bond, 2000; Bond & Stinson, 2000/2001; Chaps. 5, 6, 13, 19 and 31, this volume). I felt alive, vital, and spiritual. When I danced, I could go to another place. While I was not familiar with the idea of spiritual transcendence as a child, my memory of the feeling of dancing is much like the trance I have experienced as an adult dancer. When I was dancing, nothing mattered besides the moving and the music. I felt powerful, which I associated with boyish virility – the energy of having control over my body and willing it to create rhythms.

Yet, I recall many instances in my childhood when my dancing was viewed as feminine. Wanting to learn Janet Jackson's choreography from music videos rather than play basketball was an aberration in my community. Moreover, my ability to imitate Janet Jackson with finesse was deemed weird, or peculiar at best, as evinced by the nervous smiles of my male friends and jeering looks from others. I loved to move, lived to dance, and was impartial about how. This expressive freedom of movement outside of the heteronormative sexual displays narrated by "slow-dragging," or the demonstratively urban "street culture" illusion characterized by b-boying and breakdancing, meant that for many of my male and female peers, I danced like a girl.

For me, therefore, the second challenge of maleness has been the pursuit of *maleness* itself in a mode of expression that my peer socialization classified as non-masculine. My mother encouraged me to do anything that made me happy but unfortunately, her parenting was not enough to neutralize the social rules of gender performance that I had received from a larger community. Devoid of male mentorship in Umfundalai, Berry and I depended on each other to find a danced maleness – one uniquely ours that could accommodate the strong man archetypes of traditional African dances while leaving room for us to create the men we wanted to be. Nonetheless, by the time I started dancing professionally as an adult, I had some residual concern that audience members would see something other than the 'man' I experienced when I danced.

In traditional African dance, movements are linked to social roles within a given society, many of which are differentiated along gender lines (Salamone, 2005; Welsh, 2010). This allows one to be a "man" by nature of their physical execution of culture. In the West African canon, for example, masculinity is achieved through one's ability to accurately dance the traditional male movement in a way that is congruent with the masculine gendered performances of continental Africa. In contrast, Umfundalai, dancers do whatever movement the teacher or choreographer can imagine. This means that a man has to draw on something more "organic" to achieve a masculine gender performance; their source material is a myriad of expressions within the African continuum that could be gendered and/or otherwise informed by their social/cultural origins.

While Welsh generated much of Umfundalai's vocabulary from traditional male dances, she avoids viewing movement through a gendered lens: movement is movement.

> That's something you do beautifully [the *Kananga* arm series with hip articulation]. I've seen many women who can't do it. So, it's like all of a sudden I have this palette of all kinds of things and I can have men embody my movements. I don't think of pelvic movements as being necessarily female. Even the female dancers don't do what I would call overtly feminine movements. So there wasn't a separation with you all. (K. Welsh, personal communication, December 21, 2012)

In the above passage, "separation" references the gendered distinction that occurs in traditional and neo-traditional African dance, a difference that Banks upheld vehemently. Moreover, separation refers to Berry's and my attitude toward dancing. From Welsh's perspective, we exhibited no apprehension in executing movement as she gave it to us. While we interrogated the dances, this did not impede our willingness to perform them, an enthusiasm we modeled for others.

Taken together, inter-gender mimicry along with the pursuit of maleness through gendered movement assignation challenged me as a young dancer and teacher of Umfundalai. Welsh gave her protégés license to be creative in the technique with her mantra, "Umfundalai belongs to you." Allied with concurrent experiences in neo-traditional African dance, this permission compelled me to champion a "male element" in Umfundalai. I incorporated and stylized traditional West African dances in my classes so that there would be a gender distinction, specifically, to allow for what I viewed as more "masculine" expression. Much like the way Mills offered movement stylizations to evoke maleness, I was intentional about conveying movement to my male students in a way that freed them from any worries that their expression might be viewed as non-masculine.

For the dancing men who followed me, this new gender separation created a space of both tension and empowerment. The next section features the "life stories" (Denzin, 2014) of six of the 13 dancing men who entered Umfundalai's evolving tradition between 1993 and 2014. These six represent African American dancing men who have studied Umfundalai for more than 3 years, performed in Kariamu & Company: Traditions (Umfundalai's demonstration company) and were available to participate in two-session individual interviews.

Brothers of the Bah Yah!

Derrick Perkins holds a prominent position in the lineage of Umfundalai men in that he, along with Stafford C. Berry, Jr. and myself – C. Kemal Nance, danced during the 1996 season of Kariamu & Company: Traditions, when men danced principal roles for the first time. In his interview, Perkins refers to this premier season as the "heyday" of Umfundalai, a time of exceptionally skilled dancers and familial relationships in the company. I suggest that he was also finding his gendered agency in what became an unfolding masculinity in Umfundalai. Perkins describes,

> Dancing Umfundalai, I am very aware of my maleness. The movements are distinct; they are defined by gender-associated occupations in Africa or whatever. I am aware of it through the way I walk, the upright posture, and the groundedness of the movements. "The Nigerian Stomp," yes. Absolutely, I'm so a dude, I'm so the man! (D. Perkins, personal communication, May 15, 2012)

Perkins' reference to upright posture is not only about the position of the torso in "The Nigerian Stomp," but relates to a broader meme of masculinity in African American culture. As vernacular expression, uprightness speaks to a masculine aesthetic. Phrases like "keep your head up" or "stay up" refer to a tenacity and, as Perkins described, a "boldness" that Black men are socialized to embody in response to tacit racism (Conners, 1995). They are also a reaction to an American masculinity of acquired wealth and financial autonomy that many African American men have struggled to achieve (Alexander, 2006; Majors & Billson, 1993; Matua, 2006; Neal, 2006).

Many of Umfundalai's emergent masculinities reside in the stylization of its core movement vocabulary, and in the development of choreographies that depict stories about men and also feature male dancers. In Umfundalai, Welsh taught us that the "The Nigerian Stomp" makes a statement. Mills, in her adaptation, would often suggest that each time our heels touched the earth we were sending a message to the ancestors. For Perkins, this statement of communion with the ancestral world reified boldness and virility.

Charles Tyson was a dancer in Kariamu & Company: Traditions when I was the company's associate artistic director in 2000. In his interview, I asked him if he could recall a moment when he felt he had to dance gender. He responded,

> There are gender specific variations of movement, so yes, I've had to dance gender. I like that there's a special way to do things that only I can do, that it's only correct if I'm doing it that way. "The Undressing" is an example. I like that I get to do a different version. (C. Tyson, personal communication, October 9, 2012)

Tyson found this stylization of male movements empowering. "The Undressing" is a back undulation in which the dancer moves their body like a wave of water. Typically, it is done with arms unfolding from shoulders to the sides of thighs, repeating in synch with each undulation. Tyson refers to "liking" Mills' stylization in which men extend arms away from the torso from the shoulder. For Tyson, having access to gender-specific movement in a situation where he is one of few or the only male provides him with a movement experience he can enjoy.

For Harvey Chism, a K & C dancer from the 1998 and 2000 seasons, however, gender-specific movement instruction raised questions in Umfundalai. He stated,

> I'm aware of my gender when different movements are given to men. When I'd see movement put on women, I'd be, "Oh, I can wear that out!" (but that's not your part). When it wasn't presented as my part or as intended for men, I would be, "Oh no! That's not how we move" (*chuckling*). There were adaptations of movements and instances when the movements would be completely different if you were a male versus a female. "Why do the girls get to do that?" (H. Chism, personal communication, June 15, 2012)

Chism is responding to a class structure experienced while a student at Swarthmore College, one that made him feel that dancing deemed as female was unavailable to him. I was so preoccupied with having male students take on my contrived notions of masculinity in order to accentuate maleness that I projected a gendered hierarchy of movement. When I gave movements with rigorous hip action to the women in my class, I would concurrently give the men something that looked athletic. Chism's parenthetical comment, "but that's not your part" implies that the movement he saw the women perform was not appropriate for him. "That's not how we move" underscores a social expectation I created that inhibited him from dancing a movement he wanted to explore.

Like Chism, K & C dancer and former Umfundalai student at Swarthmore College Jumatatu Poe, was aware of being limited to certain gendered movement qualities. In his interview, Poe referred to me as the "male body of Umfundalai," while admitting, "I didn't like being told that I had to do something because of something that I couldn't help, like being a guy" (J. Poe, personal communication, November 24, 2012). I was Poe's and Chism's first dance teacher. In my attempt to create a space in the tradition where they could have the option to "dance like men," much like Mills' *machismo,* I imposed a masculinity that these two questioned. Moreover, I replicated the friction I myself experienced choosing dance as a career when my socialization suggested that dance was a non-masculine endeavor.

For Khalil Munir, a dancing man from K & C's 2000 season, the class structure was a portal for male experience that transcends sexual orientation. He feels power and strength in his dancing and visceral carriage, which he describes as "masculine."

> I always feel masculine in class. Any time we would go across the floor, the first walk, walking series, to walk with strength and confidence, just that alone, I felt powerful, really masculine. I remember Shawn Lamiere saying to us, I don't care what your sexual preference is, a man dances like a man, and a woman dances like a woman, and that kind of stuck with me. So it just translated into Umfundalai. (K. Munir, personal communication, October 17, 2012).

Like Munir and Lamiere, I was preoccupied with dancing like a man. I taught classes so that men, regardless of sexual orientation, could relate to the danced masculine archetypes in Umfundalai. For Munir, the "Walk Strong" part of class was a place and time where he could exhibit power. In Umfundalai, the across-the-floor portion of the class is a moment of critical distinction. Men dance in the back, which means they are the last to move across the floor, a practice Welsh uses to assist organization of the class when the movement being taught is gender specific. Female dancers see the men moving together as they bring up the rear. For Tyson, this is a moment of pressure as the women's eyes focus on the men. According to him, "you simply must be good."

Twan Claiborne, an African American man with a distinctively African physique – dark complexion, thick thighs, full buttocks – highlights another aspect of Umfundalai's evolving male aesthetic. Unlike Berry and me in the late 1980s, Claiborne can go to a dance class and see himself in the instructor. In this movement tradition in which only 15 men have studied the technique for three or more years and performed in its professional company, this young man, who has been the only male in most of his dance and dance education experiences, can see a reflection of himself as a dancing African American man. My presence as a dancing Black man and master teacher in Umfundalai eased the friction of Claiborne's entry: "Because I saw a lot of myself, I didn't feel the pressure." The following remarks from Claiborne underscore the gendered Umfundalai emerging from Welsh's dance tradition:

> I'm all about legacies and how I'm connected and part of this larger tree. If I'm part of the tree of Nance, I've got to step everything up 100 times because he's like over there and then over here, and I'm like right here and still right here. But eventually, I got over there. (T. Claiborne, personal communication, December 16, 2012)

Khalil Munir offered a description of both Berry's and my roles in his dancing life:

> You were the men I looked up to growing up as a dancer in the genre…the figures I was able to emulate…like a blueprint. They've done this before and—you are someone we can ask for advice and connect with in an artistic sense and in everyday life situations. I haven't had that before, not in African dance. (K. Munir, personal communication, October 17, 2012)

Much like Berry and me before him, Munir was looking for male mentorship in dance. Neither Berry nor I had predicted that we would influence future male dancers.

Conclusion: JA LI TU NE

Berry's and my vocal and kinetic presence in Umfundalai created a space for us to dance. With "familial" humor and exported movement from our neo-traditional African dance training, we projected a critical perspective that facilitated a *maleness* in Umfundalai. In my own efforts to develop a way for men to move in Umfundalai, however, I incidentally modeled a way for some "not to move," reinforcing stereotypes of a larger American society. Both Mills and I shaped gendered "scripts" (Gagnon, 2004) that align with the masculinities of many societies. These are the "cultural myths of masculinity" that Chris Blazina (2003) references, even as dancing men seek to locate themselves in an evolving African movement tradition whose male gender roles are literally works in progress. Mills and I reified what we had seen and heard in our respective communities and posited these as "natural" among Umfundalai's dancing men.

In spite of such "machismo-ing" projects, however, the evolving masculinities in the Umfundalai dance tradition that the presented interview data reflect underscore the multiplicity of dancing men's lived experiences – the "contours of masculinity," as Anthony Shay (2016) advocates. They avail Umfundalai's men to dance a gendered agency in an African dance tradition. Even a superficial survey of literature on African American masculinity would reveal an ideological dependency on a mystical white patriarchy that white men themselves cannot fully embody (Matua, 2006). Yet, these African American dancing men are "contouring" their gender in a movement tradition that centralizes their racial and cultural orientation. It might be "ethno identity dance" at its best, "the genre of stage and presentational traditional, folk, and popular dance…, which constitutes a single phenomenon with many reasons for its performance" (Shay, 2016, p. viii).

As a metaphor, *friction* offers dancing men the potential for gender performativity in the Umfundalai dance tradition and for the pursuit of gendered agency in Umfundalai dance culture. It might be the quintessential modality through which a Hegelian "thesis-antithesis-synthesis" process of cultural agitation (Blazina, 2003, p. xiv) gives way to newer "contours" (Shay, 2016). Based on phenomenological interviewing supporting an autoethnographic inquiry, my sense is that Umfundalai's impact on the quality of life for dancing men could be, ultimately, spiritual, as it is for me.

Theorizing spirituality as the way by which Africans survived the oppression of slavery and subsequent racism in North America, Dona Richards (1990) explains:

> We look around us and, while in the Caribbean and in the black communities of South America, African retentions are often visible, black existence in North America is problematical. "How are we Africa?" we blacks ask. *We do not know where to look for likeness* [emphasis added]. Not knowing ourselves, we have not known how to recognize manifestations of our heritage. (p. 207)

I reflect: might the "likeness" Richards refers to be found in the agency Berry and I offer as male presences in Umfundalai? Perhaps the friction, as it were, serves to unearth the multifarious male essences situated in an Africanist paradigm, one not dependent on a white antecedent but emergent from the Black men who dance it. I title this conclusion "JA LI TU NE," the truncated Kiswahili syllables with which Umfundalai teachers begin movement phrases to suggest a commencement. I reflect further: is the quality of life that this intracultural dancing men's discourse avails a fundamentally spiritual one? Accordingly, perhaps the male ways of embodying Umfundalai will emerge more clearly in the dancing men who have yet to enter the studio.

Negotiation of masculinities, locally and globally, will possibly exist as long as people dance in the societies where they dwell. I propose, however, that "friction," as a perennial investigation of gendered embodiment, can avail a rich palette of African-centered maleness from which future dancing men might find "likeness."

References

Ahmed, S. (2006). *Queer phenomenology: Orientations, objects, others*. Durham, NC: Duke University Press.

Alexander, B. K. (2006). *Performing black masculinity: Race, culture and queer identity*. Lanham, MD: AltaMira.

Blazina, C. (2003). *The cultural myths of masculinity*. Santa Barbara, CA: Praeger.

Bond, K. E. (2000). Revisioning purpose: Children, dance, and the culture of caring. Keynote address. In J. E. Le Drew & H. Ritenberg (Eds.), *Proceedings of the 8th dance and the child international conference – Extensions & extremities: Points of departure* (pp. 3–14). Regina, SK: University of Regina.

Bond, K. (2017). "Boys are morons" … "Girls are gross" Let's dance! In W. Oliver & D. Risner (Eds.), *Dance and gender: An evidence based approach* (pp. 235–257). Gainesville: University Press of Florida.

Bond, K. E., & Stinson, S. W. (2000/2001). "I feel like I'm going to take off!" Young people's experiences of the superordinary in dance. *Dance Research Journal, 32*(2), 52–87.

Butler, J. (1990). *Gender trouble*. New York: Routledge.

Conners, M. (1995). *What is cool? Understanding black manhood in America*. New York: Crown.

Denzin, N. (2014). *Interpretive autoethnography*. Thousand Oaks, CA: Sage.

Ellis, C. (2004). *The ethnographic I: A methodological novel about autoethnography*. Walnut Creek, CA: Altamira.

Gagnon, J. H. (2004). *An interpretation of desire: Essays in the study of sexuality*. Chicago: The University of Chicago Press.

Hays, S. (1994). Structure and agency and the sticky problem of culture. *Sociological Theory, 12*(1), 52–72.

Husserl, E. (2012). *Ideas: A general introduction to pure phenomenology*. Hoboken, NJ: Taylor & Francis. Retrieved from http://Trico.eblib.com/patron/FullRecord.aspx?9=958202

Kidd, J., & Finlayson, Z. P. (2010). *Mental illness in the workplace: A collective autoethnography*. Retrieved from http://web.b.ebscohost.com

Louppe, L. (2010). *Poetics of contemporary dance* (S. Gardner, Trans.). Alton, UK: Dance Books. (Original work published 1997).

Majors, R., & Billson, J. (1993). *Cool pose: The dilemma of black manhood in America*. New York: Simon & Schuster.

Matua, A. (2006). *Progressive black masculinities*. New York: Routledge.

Mills, G. Y. (1995). *Dancing in my mother's mother's body: The transmutation and synthesis of African dance culture in Kariamu Welsh-Asante's Umfundalai dance technique* (Doctoral dissertation). Temple University, Philadelphia, PA.

Nance, C. K. (2014). *Brothers of the Bah Yah!: The pursuit of maleness in the Umfundalai tradition of African dance* (Doctoral dissertation). Temple University, Philadelphia, PA.

Neal, M. A. (2006). *New black man*. New York: Routledge.

Noland, C. (2009). *Agency and embodiment: Performing gestures/producing culture*. Cambridge, MA: Harvard University Press.

Richards, D. (1990). The implications of African-American spirituality. In M. K. Asante & K. W. Asante (Eds.), *African culture: The rhythms of unity* (pp. 207–231). Trenton, NJ: Africa World Press.

Robinson, S., & White, R. (1964, December 21). *My girl* [Recorded by The Temptations]. [Seven-inch single]. Detroit, MI: Gordy.

Salamone, F. (2005). Hausa concepts of masculinity and the "Yan Daudu". In L. M. Ouzgane (Ed.), *African masculinities: Men in Africa from the late nineteenth century to the present* (pp. 75–86). New York: Palgrave Macmillan.

Shay, A. (2016). *Ethno identity: Dance for sex, fun and profit – Staging popular dances around the world*. London: Palgrave Macmillan.

Shujaa, M. J., & Shujaa, K. J. (Eds.). (2015). *The SAGE encyclopedia of African cultural heritage in North America*. Los Angeles, CA: Sage.

Stinson, S. (2005). Why are we doing this? *Journal of Dance Education, 5*(3), 82–89. https://doi.org/10.1080/15290824.2005.10387290.

van Manen, M. (1997). *Researching lived experience: Human science for an action sensitive pedagogy*. Albany: State University of New York.

Welsh, K. (2010). Dance as a reflection of life. In *African dance* (2nd ed., pp. 13–37). New York: Chelsea House.

Part V
Health, Wellbeing, Ability

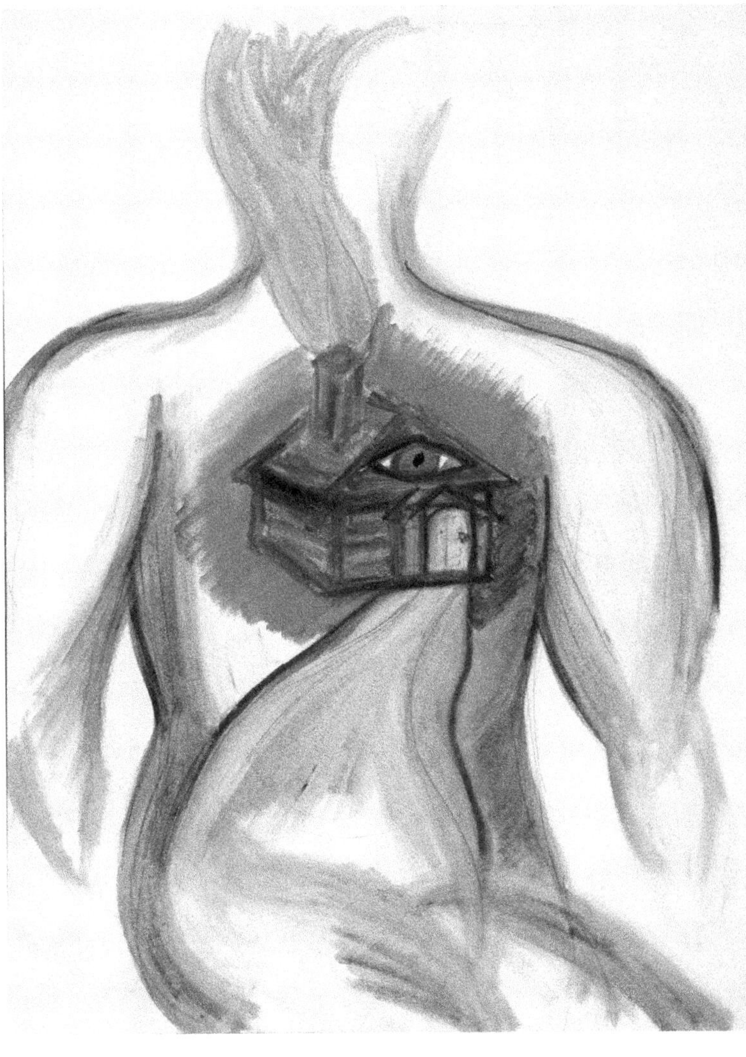

III Heart Home Eye River (M. Shanahan)

Chapter 15
The Impact of Community Engagement Through Dance on Teen and Young Adult Dancers

Miriam Giguere

Introduction

As both an artistic discipline and an educational field, dance puts a great deal of emphasis on connection and communication between human beings. Whether this is through choreography and performance, where the communication is between stage and audience, or between partners participating together in a dance, interpersonal communication plays an important role. Many young dancers in their teen and early adult years love to teach dance: they want to share their love of movement with others. Further, a belief that dance participation enhances quality of life drives many to engage in community dance projects.

Universities with dance programs, including the institution in which this study is grounded, encourage community based learning, sometimes referred to as community outreach or community engagement. Kronick, Lester, and Luter (2013) define anchor institutions as a "large spatially immobile, mostly non-profit organization that plays an integral role in the local economy" (p. 659), noting that universities often function as anchor institutions for a community. As a result, institutions of higher education are often engaged in some kind of community partnerships. This allows a university to broaden its platform for research and scholarship, which in turn increases the institutional value of community engagement (Kronick et al., 2013). University dance programs become part of this cycle of research and engagement.

As a faculty member in one such university dance program, I have often wondered about the specific effects that community engagement experiences are having on my students. Fairly regularly a student tells me that these experiences have been valuable to them in understanding how dance helps them connect to others, or define their career aspirations or other life enhancing effects. Universities promoting civic

M. Giguere (✉)
Drexel University, Philadelphia, PA, USA
e-mail: mgg22@drexel.edu

K. Bond (ed.), *Dance and the Quality of Life*, Social Indicators Research Series 73,
https://doi.org/10.1007/978-3-319-95699-2_15

engagement often make claims that these kinds of activities increase empathy, and I have heard dance teachers remark on the increase in self-esteem that community projects engender. Such statements peaked my curiosity into examining student experiences more closely. What is it about community engagement in dance that so deeply affects artistic understanding and career aspiration, and does this differ from other kinds of civic involvement? Can a rise in students' self-esteem or empathy be documented? These are the questions I ask in this study.

Background Literature

The literature addressing community dance participation intersects with the discourse of civic engagement, which addresses many forms of what is also termed service learning, community based learning, and community engagement. I use these terms interchangeably in this chapter. The concept of community, in this context, refers to a group aligned by geography, physical or socio-economic circumstance (Furco, 1996). According to civic engagement scholar Barbara Jacoby (2015), service learning is "a form of experiential education in which students engage in activities that address human and community needs, together with structured opportunities for reflection designed to achieve desired learning outcomes" (pp. 1–2). Service learning differs from volunteerism by the reciprocal nature of the activity; the former is designed to benefit the community or community members and the student in equal measures.

Theoretical foundations of service learning are credited to John Dewey, a common ancestor to dance education theory. Dewey's turn-of-twentieth-century philosophy advocated for education to be focused on the child's experience as opposed to curricular subject matter. One key concept in Dewey's (1933) model of education is the importance of reflection on experience: "Critical reflection is the active, persistent, and careful consideration of any belief or supposed form of knowledge in light of the grounds that support it …" (p. 9). This kind of deep reflective practice is structured into civic engagement activities and may be responsible for some of its documented outcomes (Jacoby, 2015; Pigza, 2010; Rama & Battistoni, 2001). Reported outcomes germane to this study include psycho-social and identity development constructs such as self-efficacy, emotional maturity, and development and clarity of values and life purpose (Jacoby, 2015).

Critical reflection in the context of civic engagement does not attempt to disguise social inequities between university and local populations, which was a significant factor in this study. The research setting was a large urban university located immediately adjacent to a federally recognized Promise Zone, a funding and assistance designation given to the poorest areas in America. Reflection throughout this study acknowledged the inappropriateness of homogenizing or stereotyping the identities of participants, whether local children involved in the dance activities or the university dance teachers. This points to another posited benefit of community engagement for high school and university students – the opportunity for development of ethical maturity. Flanagan and Levine (2010) see civic engagement as an important factor in the development of moral and political conscience as these issues are salient when adolescents are engaged civically. Developmentally, this is appropriate since teens and young adults are "taking stock of the values they live by and the kind of world they want to be a part of" (p. 160).

Broad claims have been made about the impact of community based learning projects on personal development. Eyler and Giles (1999) found a positive effect on personal and interpersonal growth for college students engaged in this practice. Similarly, Moely, McFarland, Miron, Mercer, and Illustre (2002) and Moely, Mercer, Ilustre, Miron, & McFarland (2002) found that students engaged in service learning tested higher on interest in civic and community issues, problem solving, political awareness, leadership skills, social justice attitudes and diversity attitudes. Students have reported that service learning was a vehicle for modifying career decisions (Flanagan & Levine, 2010; Payne, 2000) and achieving a greater level of self-knowledge (Eyler & Giles, 1999).

Researchers have associated self-knowledge with self-esteem. Laguardia and Ryff (2003) define self-esteem as "one's feelings of self-worth and the extent to which these feelings are externally imposed demands...versus internally valued components of self" (p. 49). Self-esteem is often defined as either high or low, which relates to a status of secure or fragile. It is generally considered stable, while also context dependent. An individual can experience high self-worth in one situation and low self-worth in another, which is referred to as intra-individual self-esteem. Self-esteem can also be measured between individuals as a way of assessing difference (Robins & Trzesniewski, 2005).

Service learning researchers also report an increase of student empathy through community engagement (Jacoby, 2015; Kendall, 1990; Stanton, 1990). In the case of service learning in dance, the principle of kinesthetic empathy might also apply, that is, a physical rotation into another's point of view or spatial frame of reference can induce a more empathetic response (Ehrenberg & Wood, 2011).

Community Dance

The activity studied in this research is not just community based learning, but community dance as well. Many testimonials and research findings indicate that community dance participants reap the benefits of skill development in mentorship, nurturing, and collaboration (Green, 2000; Houston, 2005; Lomas, 1998; Stinson, 1998/2016). While a clear definition of this specific field is elusive, most advocates agree that community dance includes, as dance scholar Jill Green (2000) describes,

> ...an emphasis on working with people from the community who may not see dance as a professional goal. The idea that everyone can dance is paramount, and many of these programs attempt to serve the needs of the community. For this reason, community dance has often been linked with disenfranchised populations such as the elderly, inner city, those

with special needs and physical disabilities, those with health needs and "at-risk" children. (p. 54)

Dancer and community practitioner Christine Lomas (1998) attributes the effectiveness of community dance to the idea that this kind of practice offers ways for dancers to make sense of themselves, creating a sense of achievement. In this way, community dance affords an authentic experience and *communitas*. This last term comes from anthropologist Victor Turner's (1973) theory of social bonding that occurs during liminal or transitional periods when role hierarchies may be reversed. Specifically, Lomas appears to be referencing *existential communitas*, a condition whereby a group of people consider themselves to be a connected, homogeneous unit pursuing collective goals (Turner, 1973).

Community dance is antithetical to the competitiveness often associated with commercial or studio dance and individual achievement. Most often the community dance class more closely mirrors the larger society, with greater diversity of participants and a wider spectrum of needs and expectations than one finds in a typical private studio dance class. For new teachers, understanding leadership in this setting may come with a set of more complex issues to navigate. This is a place where we can gain newfound confidence and humility in our leadership skills (Stinson, 1998/2016).

Research Design and Methodology

A mixed method action research design was employed to examine the changes in attitudes and opinions of my students over a 3–8 month period as they engaged in service learning in community dance settings. For purposes of this study community dance is defined as dance that is relevant and evolving from the common characteristics of a community. The connection can be based on geography, age grouping, socioeconomic status, sexual orientation, or other factors such as neighborhood advocacy interests or medical diagnosis (Barr & Giguere, in press).

I consider this study as affiliated with action research since I am undertaking it in order to reflect deeply on my own community of teaching and learning in the university dance setting. Action research is less a specific method or technique of conducting research than a methodology that values the epistemology of reflective practice. Closely akin to reflective dance education practices (Bond & Richard, 2005; Giguere, 2014), action research involves thinking carefully about what one is doing, so that, as McNiff (2013) explains, "it becomes *critical* self-reflective practice" (p. 23). [author emphasis] It is rooted in the philosophical traditions of John Dewey (1938) who believed that cycles of action and reflection, which included both students and teachers, were the key to educational reform. His charge for reflective educators was championed by many in the field of education over the decades, (Elliot, 1991; Schön, 1995), particularly those who found value in looking at the environment of the learning, such as Stephens, Barton, and Haslett (2009) who call for research that "recognizes and integrates the influence of the environment into the enquiry process" (p. 473). This study pays special attention to contextual factors, namely what role the community plays in dance activity for university students.

Reason and Bradbuty (2008) describe three approaches to action research: first person, second person, and third person. First person action research is when an individual participant reflects on his or her own personal practice. Second person action research happens when people inquire about others and how to address areas of mutual concern. Third person action research is an individual researching with a wider community. Noffke and Somekh (2009) refer to these same three categories, giving them the labels of personal, professional, and political. The present study fits most closely into the professional category, since students and researcher have related interests in seeing how community engagement affects the university participants.

In the sphere of service learning research, the mixed method, or quantitative-qualitative, approach has been referred to as an explanatory design. Simons and Cleary (2006) suggest that mixed methods studies can further the researcher's conceptual framework through integrative analysis of qualitative and quantitative data. Quantitative results are used to generate questions and provide context for the qualitative analysis. This description could also apply to the integrated analysis of data gathered in the present study through surveys and interviews.

The Participants

Seventeen female university and private studio dance students of multiple ethnicities between the ages of 16 and 21 took part in the study. Participants were engaged in one or more of three different community dance projects that occur in two different community settings near Drexel University. The first two projects, collectively named Wheelchair Dance, take place at HMS School for Children with Cerebral Palsy, and the third at an urban community center, the Dornsife Center for Neighborhood Partnerships.

Wheelchair Dance is a weekly project run since 2009 in collaboration with the HMS School, a residential school a few blocks from campus. Conducted by a dance-movement therapist, the program partners Drexel University dancers with wheelchair bound teens for a yearlong process to create dances that are later performed at the HMS School and again at Drexel University. Dancers keep the same partner all year long, and some Drexel dancers have been involved with the same HMS partner for as long as 4 years. A local dance company, DanceFusion, has a youth arm, Fusion II, which participates weekly in a similar project with HMS. Three of these high school age dancers were also part of the study. Ten of the 17 students in the study were involved in one of these wheelchair dance projects.

Dornsife Dance is the umbrella name for Drexel's partnership with the Dornsife Center to offer free after-school dance technique classes for youth and seniors in West Philadelphia. Drexel dance students and alumni teach weekly dance classes while being mentored by Drexel dance faculty who support their teaching practices and provide opportunities for reflection on these experiences. Ten of the 17 students in the study participated in Dornsife Dance, with three students participating in both projects. Commitment to these projects, all of which involved attendance once a week, ranged from 3 months to 8 months. This was a first-time engagement for ten students and the second or third year of engagement for seven participants. Table 15.1 shows dancers' ages and length of participation (HSW indicates high school wheelchair participant).

Research Questions

My central research question was to understand more fully the impact and experiences of high school and college students involved in community engagement through dance. Sub-questions guiding the research design came from my experiences as a facilitator and organizer of these community engagement activities. Specifically, I hoped to shed light on:

Table 15.1 Participant information

Subject	Age	Years dancing	Years in community dance engagement
Wheelchair			
W1	18	12	1
W2	18	16	1
W3	30	27	3
W4	21	10	1
W5[a]	20	17	3
W6[a]	21	18	1
W7[a]	21	17	4
HSW1	16	12	2
HSW2	17	12	1
HSW3	17	14	3
Dornsife			
D1	18	13	1
D2	18	15	1
D3	20	17	2
D4	20	17	3
D5[a]	21	17	4
D6[a]	20	17	3
D7	18	16	1
D8	18	10	1
D9	20	18	1
D10[a]	21	18	1

[a]Students who participated in both activities

- the impact of participation on self-esteem
- the impact of participation on empathy
- the impact of participation on defining dance itself
- the impact of participation on perceiving a difference between dance engagement and other kinds of civic or community volunteerism
- the impact of participation on career choice

Several approaches were used to investigate the research question and sub-questions in this mixed method study. Data sources include surveys and interviews with 17 dancers (ages 16–21) who had volunteered more than 40 h in a dance related project with a community population.

Mixed Methods

Surveys Surveys consisted of two quantitative measures, the *Rosenberg Self-Esteem Scale (RSES)* (Rosenberg, 1965) and the *Balanced Emotional Empathy Scale (BEES)* (Mehrabian, 1996). A self-report survey on confidence and sense of control in the world, the *RSES* is a widely-used, validated 10 question instrument with a Likert scale of four choices: strongly agree, agree, disagree, strongly disagree. It is scored from 1 to 30 with a score of 15 indicating low self-esteem. The *BEES* (Mehrabian, 1996) contains two parts: one with 22 questions and the second with 15 questions, using a Likert scale with five options. Higher numbers are associated with higher empathy and general positive outlook on the world. My home institution, among others, uses this test (pre- and post-) to assess the impact of civic engagement on participating students in terms of empathy toward community members (J. Johnson, personal communication, 2015). Participants completed both surveys pre- and post- their engagement in one or more of the three community projects. Survey instruments for both the *RSES* and the *BEES* were administered at the time of the pre- and post- interviews.

Interviews To broaden and strengthen the study beyond descriptive statistics, I conducted interviews with each student before and after the projects in which they participated. All study participants were interviewed the week before they began participation and again the week after the projects were completed. I recorded and transcribed the 34 interviews, which lasted approximately 20–30 min each.

Interview questions asked participants for their definition of dance, the importance of dance in their lives and what differences, if any, they saw between dance-focused community engagement and other types of volunteerism in which they had been engaged, and about their career aspirations, mirroring the sub-research questions of the study. The same questions were asked in both the pre-participation and post-participation interviews. Interviews were transcribed and then analyzed by the following procedures:

1. Each answer from pre- and post- community involvement interview questions was analyzed to find a key descriptor that encapsulated the answer for each subject for each question.
2. The key descriptors were then compared for each participant looking for differences and similarities in pre- and post- answers to the same questions. I refer to the result of these descriptor comparisons as "statements of difference."
3. Statements of difference were then sorted by the participant group (Wheelchair or Dornsife) and question, yielding six categories of meaning.
4. I summarized the findings of these six separate analyses in the qualitative findings section presented below.

Self-Esteem and Empathy Results

Wheelchair Dance participants' *Rosenberg Self-Esteem* scores ranged from 17 to 23 pre-experience with a mean score of 21.2 and a standard deviation of 2.82. The same participants scored from 15 to 30 in post-experience testing, with a mean of 21 and a standard deviation of 4.86. The change in scores creates a p-value of .9320, clear evidence of no significant change, statistically-speaking. For Dornsife participants, *RSES* scores ranged from 18 to 30 pre-experience, with a mean of 23.5 and a standard deviation of 4.5. Post experience these same participants' scores ranged from 19 to 30 with a mean of 23.8 and a standard deviation of 4.9. This change creates a p-value of .89, again, a statistically non-significant change.

While I might perceive "growth in confidence" for students who participate in extra-curricular dance projects, these survey results do not support a claim that self-esteem was increased as a general phenomenon, at least not by the measures used. Perhaps students who are more affected by the experience and/or are more verbal are the ones who talk openly about how they are feeling with their teachers, skewing perceptions. There is a great deal happening in the lives of 16–21 year olds, (Csikszentmihalyi & Larson, 1984) and many factors might have been influencing self-esteem that had nothing to do with this activity; as it stands, these quantitative measures do not support claims or assumptions about the connection of community-based learning in dance and self-esteem, as assessed by the *RSES*.

Dancers' composite scores on the *Balanced Emotional Empathy Scale* showed a similar pattern to those for the Rosenberg. Wheelchair Dance participants had scores ranging from 60 to 102, with a mean of 81 and a standard deviation of 11.2 in pre-experience testing. In post-experience testing, these same participants' scores ranged from 60 to 104 with a mean of 79.3 and a standard deviation of 13.9. The p-value of this change is .47, and not statistically significant. For Dornsife participants, pre-experience scores ranged from 74 to 96, with a mean score of 84.1 and a standard deviation of 7.3. Post testing, these same participants' scores ranged from 66 to 104, with a mean of 82.3 and a standard deviation of 11.9. Again, this yields a p-value of .89, a non-statistically significant change in scores. As with the Rosenberg scale, it is not possible to demonstrate quantitatively that students gain empathy or a positive outlook on life in general from these experiences.

One rationale for a mixed method research design is to be able to delve deeper into quantitative results and potentially understand more through detailed qualitative analysis of the phenomenon (Simons & Cleary, 2006). Although negative results for change in self-esteem and empathy were found through quantitative analysis, following an explanatory design (Simons & Cleary, 2006), I continued with a qualitative investigation to uncover a more complete story of the dancers' experiences. These findings are described next.

Qualitative Findings

As detailed earlier, I conducted qualitative interviews with each student before and after their community engagement project. I transcribed and analyzed all interviews for significant categories of meaning that relate to changes or lack of change in participants' (1) definitions of dance, (2) perception of the difference between dance and other community engagement, and (3) career aspirations. These categories appear in italics in the following discussion.

Definition of Dance

Eight of the ten Dornsife participants changed their articulated definition of dance in some way during this community dance project. Definitions changed in three ways, all of them expansions of original definitions, rather than a total change. Two individuals expanded their definitions to include the idea that *dance could be cathartic*. For example, D9 began with:

> Dance is being able to express how you feel and being able to move in ways that make your body feel good and make your soul feel good...

In the post-project interview, she elaborated:

> Dance is being able to express yourself and express how you are feeling, and a therapeutic way of working through things and being able to experience new things and put things out there that you want to tell other people but may not know how to tell them.

Three other participants expanded their definitions to include the idea of *connecting with others*, a concept related to the idea of dance as therapy, but still distinct. D4, for example, said pre-experience:

> Dance can be anything that kind of a) has movement and b) has evoked something for the person doing it, has some kind of importance to them, even if it's just walking in everyday life, because it has a purpose that makes it dance to them.

Her post-interview response showed more reflective depth:

> Dance is a means of communication, in general it communicates individual thoughts and feelings as well as connects everyone to each other in a very personal way because it does communicate individual thoughts and feelings. It makes you very vulnerable in a way that we can all relate to, so it makes a giant community. I've always loved that about dance become you are part of this community and you become very close, on a level that you are not with other family and friends.

Finally, three other participants from this group changed their definitions of dance to include the idea that *we all have individual answers* to this question and that it is not a universal understanding. For example, before Dornsife D5 defined dance as follows:

> For me it is always changing, but at this point in my life it is a necessity, the best way I can express myself and where I feel most comfortable. A way of living. And a way of exploring.

After Dornsife she felt unable to define dance:

> I can't define it. I think it is up to the individual to define, which is why I like it so much. For some people, it's a way to express their creativity, for some people it's a way to express their emotion, or thoughts or feelings, for some people it's an outlet for other things.

For the remaining two participants in the Dornsife group, there was virtually no change in definition, although wording was not identical.

All ten Dornsife participants included the idea of *self-expression* in their definitions of dance both pre- and post- participation. This could be related to why they elected to participate in the community dance program, although regrettably this is not one of the specific questions I asked the students. As a general observation, it appeared that students in this group learned about individual differences and that people can connect through dance.

For Wheelchair Dance participants, there seemed to be less change overall in their definitions of dance pre- and post- participation. Four of the ten dancers had unchanged answers, although two used significantly more vocabulary. The other six expanded their definitions to include *a focus on others*, especially including the function of dance to communicate and build relationships. For example, before engaging in Wheelchair Dance FW2 defined dance as follows: "It's a movement, it's an art in the form of movement used to either perform or strengthen the body." Afterwards she reflected,

> Dance is like any kind of movement or communication that is not necessarily through talking, movement or voices, or can be to music but it doesn't have to be. To me a dance is more than just about the movement it is about the community of relationships that you build with the people you dance with and how you improve yourself and get to be a better dancer.

All ten Wheelchair participants referred to dance as *communication and personal human expression* in their post-interview definitions.

Difference in Civic Engagement Involving Dance

The second area investigated through qualitative interviews related to how dancers perceived the difference, if any, between community engagement that involved dance as compared to other kinds of community engagement or volunteer community work. By asking the students to reflect on the distinction between volunteer or community work that is not dance focused, and the embodied project they were engaged in, this question seeks to understand how dance functions for these dancers as they engage with others in a helping role.

Four participants at the Dornsife Center said that dance-focused community work was more about *making a connection with others* than other experiences they had in volunteer work. Four others had thought it would be the same as other volunteer work they had done because it was a population they didn't know about, but changed to seeing it as *making an impact on individuals.* Witness the following pre- and post- interview responses of D7:

> I think that it will be a little different, because I'm an assistant and usually I am the head of the game. I don't care, because I want to do this. I think it will be the same. I'm really happy to do it, honestly. (Pre-project interview)

> Way different. Because you know…when you're in the studio you are focusing on yourself, but when you are teaching other kids you are focusing on them and their improvement. It makes it feel like what you are doing in the studio because you are able to share your hard work in your life and you get to give it to kids that they would never get to experience without Dornsife It doesn't matter what you are teaching, what you are sharing with them, it something that you are fortunate to have been given to you. (Post-project interview)

There seems to be something in these answers that suggests that prior to their dance-based community engagement, students sensed an otherness in the community members they would be interacting with. After participating in the Dornsife dance project, however, students saw their community members as individuals with whom they had a shared humanity.

Two other Dornsife participants pre-project anticipated that dance would be more interactive, but noted post-project that the difference was in the *amount of authority* they had in a leadership role, or in some way referenced power dynamics. For example, when D9 was asked about how volunteering in general and through dance are different she responded pre-project about volunteering in general:

> It's not as interactive and doing something and interacting with community members, it's like we are raising money for something or cleaning a park or its kind of like things that would help with other people but not necessarily interacting with them.

In the post-project interview, she stated:

> They are equally rewarding and equally fun, but they feel different because one is teaching and the other is support. Dornsife teaching was more me being in charge of something, but volunteer work is I am giving back to someone. I am enhancing someone's life, and I know that is the same with teaching, but I feel more like I am in charge when I am teaching something.

Wheelchair Dance participants seemed to have a similar experience to their Dornsife counterparts. Four of the ten went into the activity believing that the difference between dance based and other community service was *being more connected to others*, *being more hands on with others* and being *more personally gratifying*, and continued to feel that way after the project's completion. W7 articulated the difference in existential terms:

> I think there's a reason I don't do non-dance volunteer work, because the dance outreach work means so much more to me. HMS changed my life forever…when you volunteer in dance you just get a whole other level of communication with people because it's so personal and people don't really realize that.

Of the six participants who changed their ideas of the difference in this kind of community work, two came to see it as *deepening a connection with others*, one saw it as *sharing the power dynamic* with the community members, one saw it as *needing a great deal of patience* to do, and two saw it as being about *pride and hope for the community members*. As an example of the last group, FW3 said pre-project:

> Very different in the fact that these people at HMS are still people, they are disabled but they are still a person--they just can't do as much as we can. I interact with them the same way as the other people in volunteer work.

After the Wheelchair Dance project, she reflected:

> It's different because they don't have the same meaning as with HMS, you are dancing with someone who doesn't get to dance every day or doesn't know how to express as normal… well they are just different. I feel like I get back more at HMS because it makes me feel proud and I know it makes them proud and have hope.

Notably, in both projects the college students had a view of the community as "other" prior to participating and saw the importance of building connections with individuals after the project was completed.

Career Aspirations

In general, the career aspirations of both groups showed little change. Most of the changes were a *narrowing in identifying which populations* the students wanted to work with, or in what setting they saw themselves working. Since this was a self-selected group of community volunteers, it seems likely that these students were already interested in careers that in some way related to the care of or interactions with others. Three of the ten Dornsife dance volunteers stayed completely consistent in their stated aspirations before and after the project: nurse anesthetist, health science administrator, and teacher. The other seven provided more specificity of age group or population, while maintaining the same general career goal. For example, D3 said before the project, "I want to be a dance therapist," but after the project elaborated to explain:

> I still want to be a dance/movement, but I want to try working with adults now that I've had so much experience working with children, just to see how different the experience would be, but I still feel that working with children with special needs, more so, would be my top choice.

It is not surprising that experiences related closely to a chosen field of study would yield a more nuanced answer.

For Wheelchair Dance participants, three had no change of career aspirations as dance/movement therapists (two) and teacher – both careers closely tied to the activity. Similar to the Dornsife experience, five Wheelchair Dance volunteers retained their career goals, but narrowed the populations of interest. For example, W2 says simply: "Dance/movement therapy" in her pre-activity interview, but post activity reports:

> Still want to be a D/MT. I think this opened up a new door and let me see new paths in life that I didn't know before or didn't fully understand completely. It opened up new opportunities.

The remaining two Wheelchair dance participants were the only respondents out of both groups who expressed interest in changing careers. One was a high school student, one of the youngest dancers in the study, who was less certain of her career choices both before and after the activity. She expressed an interest in media and business in the pre-activity interview and an interest in communication and photography in the post-activity interview. The other participant who changed her career aspirations went from an interest in physical therapy to an interest in education, both careers intensive in personal interaction and taking on a helping role with others. She (W5) explains that her community volunteer work was "definitely what changed me," explaining,

> I think learning the program and then repeating it every week, and finding new entry points in it. I learned new things in it and new ideas about education. That is definitely what pointed me in the right direction.

It should be noted that the respondent was simultaneously experiencing struggles and dissatisfaction with the required science courses for the physical therapy curriculum, so her community experiences were a change of direction that she might have been searching for.

Discussion

Community dance practice is a complex and impactful experience for the adolescents and young adults involved, although not necessarily what we would anticipate or claim it to be at first blush – such as a reliable way to enhance empathy and self-esteem. This study does not refute such claims, but rather illuminates with meaningful detail how dancers experienced their engagement in community dance service. One way the study documents change is in how these young adults transformed their definitions of dance. For most participants, change can be described as an expanded definition of dance, which includes communication, human expression and a connection with others as individuals. Post-community engagement definitions tended to encompass more of the psycho-social and cathartic aspects of dance as a healing art and the ability of movement to create community amongst the participants. Many of the dancers had only seen dance in relation to self and performance prior to this study; now they have perceived dance in relation to others and to group experience rather than just performance.

A similar change in experience can be seen in the qualitative findings related to how dance based community service differs from other volunteer activities. Students came to see the community more as a collection of individuals than a monolithic "other," and dance as a way of connecting with others. The idea of dance as a way to create *communitas* (Turner, 1966); that is, collective goal setting and a feeling of non-hierarchical homogeneity within a group (Bond, 2008), became more tangible and personal for these dancers.

While shifts in viewpoint on dance and its ability to connect with others was documented, the "how" of this process was not fully illuminated by this study. The literature on service learning indicates that critical reflection plays an important part in effective civic engagement. If we begin with this premise, then the study design itself might have been part of the reason for the changes noted in the qualitative findings of the study. There was no consistent procedure for formal reflection across the two community dance settings. Students teaching at the Dornsife Center were closely mentored by a faculty member at the participating university, giving them ample opportunity to discuss and reflect on what was happening in their classrooms. However, the approach to reflection was student led and thus inconsistent across settings. For example, some students reflected on the context of community dance, while others were more pragmatically interested in classroom management issues.

Similarly, the facilitator of the Wheelchair Dance class checked in with the dancers monthly to see if they had any concerns or questions about the process, but deep or critical reflection was not a structured part of the activity. Students were invited to reflect deeply in pre-and post- interviews, however, and this may have contributed to the articulation and subsequent self-understanding of personal growth experienced by participating dancers. This is consistent with an action research model, which is in itself a critical reflection practice intended to lead to potential action (Bond & Richard, 2005; Giguere, 2014; McNiff, 2013; Stephens et al., 2009).

That critical reflection and civic engagement changed the dancers' conceptions of dance is an anticipated result. However, that the more quantitative survey data would indicate no influence on participants' self-esteem and empathy was not expected. One possible explanation is that the *Rosenberg Self-Esteem Scale* (Rosenberg, 1965) and the *Balanced Emotional Empathy Scale* (Mehrabian, 1996) were not sensitive enough to capture change in this study, since most respondents already had fairly healthy self-esteem levels and fairly high measures of empathy. Students' extant self-esteem and empathy might have contributed to their high-quality self-reflection in the projects. Further, these adolescents and young adults' sense of self and interest in others could have inspired their involvement in these initiatives, although regrettably I did not question students about their motivation. It would be informative to conduct the same tests on a larger sample of community dance participants who were assigned to the activities, rather than elected to participate, if such a population could be identified or created.

Another explanation for the negative quantitative results for increasing self-esteem and empathy is that I might have been looking for the wrong thing. Maybe it is not self-esteem or empathy *per se* that are enhanced, but rather these dancers' transition to adulthood. Seeing the world in a more comprehensive or realistic way, especially with respect to socio-economic realities or the perspective of a differently-abled population, might not have measurably increased self-esteem or empathy, but instead raised ethical self-awareness. It would not necessarily make a young adult feel better to know that he or she comes from a position of relative privilege, and this is arguably not a negative result. People have differing levels of self-worth depending on their environment and relationship with others (Kernis, 2003; LaGuardia & Ryff, 2003). Such fluctuation can be healthy; instability in self-esteem can inspire reflection and re-examination, in turn affecting growth, re-evaluation of self-concept, and ability to understand others (Leary, 1999).

While most assessments of self-esteem categorize people as either secure or fragile, based on assessment scores of high or low, LaGuardia and Ryff (2003) suggest that self-esteem is a layered concept, not a dichotomous one. Rather than evaluate self-esteem, these authors propose a focus on authenticity, a concept with two parts: awareness and action. They define awareness as "an openness to work on one's self – an openness to allow experiences to emerge, and then to take an interest in them and explore how they coalesce with or come into conflict with other core aspects of the self" (p. 49).

This authenticity perspective seems useful in the present study where young adults' self-reflection indicated willingness to see themselves and others in a different way in light of their community dance experiences. This is the action part of authenticity, defined by LaGuardia and Ryff (2003) as the "motivation processes by which one activity promotes or inhibits awareness processes" (p. 49). This is consistent with Lomas' (1998) observation that community dance practices create authenticity and *communitas*. As college dance educators, claims of increased self-esteem amongst our students might better be claims of increased authenticity, which relate also to the integrative intellectual, emotional, and social growth we hope to foster through artistic and educational practices. LaGuardia and Ryff (2003) suggest:

> Authenticity speaks to the relative integration of self-concepts and is intricately connected to intrapersonal growth and actualization as well as interpersonal connectedness. (pp. 49–50)

Regarding empathy, what seems to be engendered in these community dance projects is a tolerance for diversity and a reduction of stereotyping, a documented benefit of service learning (Simons & Cleary, 2006). According to Phillips (2003), empathy involves identification and imagination, grounded in perception; perhaps this is the mechanism at play in community dance. From infancy, we develop the ability to perceive and identify with other people and contexts (Chap. 31, this volume). The next step – imagination, is uniquely appropriate to the arts. Dance provides the opportunity to activate imagination, Phillips' (2003) other suggested ingredient in the development of empathy. Community dance can facilitate an appreciation for other and different human beings' creations, offering the conditions for one's natural empathy to develop (Greene, 2001). This can lay the groundwork for empathy skills to mature in young adults. The timetable of development might be longer than the duration of a community project, as assessed by quantitative methods, but through the interview data we can see the necessary perceptual structures for empathy to grow.

To supplement survey instruments, interview data offered a layered picture of the impact of community dance engagement on adolescents and young adults. Data were sourced by the specific questions asked and the abilities of participants to reflect articulately on their experiences. From this perspective, interviews can limit information, either by not asking the specific questions that will yield rich information or by the ability of the subject to articulate their experiences. A participant could be developing Phillips' (2003) requisites for adult empathy, but not yet have the reflective capacity to communicate this in interview. Each method has its strengths and drawbacks so that the mixed method approach used here has both the advantages and weaknesses of its component approaches. Just as dance as a performing art becomes marked by fusion and hybridization of genres, dance scholarship, too, can be a place for mixed method approaches. For dance, both artistically and scientifically, fusion has strengths and flaws.

One fusion that I am not questioning in the practice underlying this study is the combination of community dance and reflection. Perhaps reflection on embodied practice is, in fact, the lynchpin for change in these young adults. Landmark American pragmatist philosopher and educator John Dewey (1916) espoused that reflection leads to seeing the underlying issues or conditions of social unrest and poverty, for example, and is therefore a foundation of educational practice and development of self. The experience of dance in community with others, along with reflection on experience, might be a pivotal fusion that supports growth in young adults.

References

Barr, S., & Giguere. M. (in press). Community dance introduction. In K. Schupp & D. Risner (Eds.), *Case studies in dance education*. Jefferson, NC: MacFarland.

Bond, K. (2008). The human nature of dance: Towards a theory of aesthetic community. In S. Malloch & C. Trevarthen (Eds.), *Communicative musicality: Exploring the basis of human companionship* (pp. 401–422). Oxford, UK: Oxford University Press.

Bond, K., & Richard, B. (2005). "Ladies and gentlemen! What do you see? What do you feel?" A story of connected curriculum in a third grade dance education setting. In L. Overby & B. Lepczyk (Eds.), *Dance: Current selected research* (Vol. 5, pp. 85–134). New York: AMS Press.

Csikszentmihalyi, M., & Larson, R. (1984). *Being adolescent: Conflict and growth in the teenage years*. New York: Basic Books.

Dewey, J. (1916). *Democracy and education*. New York: Macmillan.

Dewey, J. (1933). *How we think: A restatement of the relation of reflective thinking to the educative process*. Lexington, MA: Heath.

Dewey, J. (1938). *Logic: The theory of inquiry*. New York: Henry Holt.

Ehrenberg, S., & Wood, K. (2011). Conference report: Kinesthetic empathy – Concepts and contexts. *Dance Research Journal, 43*(2), 113–117.

Elliot, J. (1991). *Action research for educational change*. Buckingham, UK: Open University Press.

Eyler, J. S., & Giles, D. E. (1999). *Where's the learning in service learning?* San Francisco: Jossey-Bass.

Flanagan, C., & Levine, P. (2010). Civic engagement and the transition to adulthood. *The Future of Children, 20*(1), 159–179.

Furco, A. (1996). Service learning: A balanced approach to experiential education. In *Expanding boundaries: Service and learning* (pp. 2–6). Washington, DC: Corporation for National and Community Service.

Giguere, M. (2014). Dance education and action research: A twin study. *Research in Dance Education, 16*(1), 16–32.

Green, J. (2000). Power, service, and reflexivity in a community dance project. *Research in Dance Education, 2*(2), 53–67.

Greene, M. (2001). *Variations on a blue guitar*. New York: Teachers College Press.

Houston, S. (2005). Participation in community dance: A road to empowerment and transformation? *New Theatre Quarterly, 21*(2), 166–177.

Jacoby, B. (2015). *Service learning essentials*. San Francisco: Jossey-Bass.

Kendall, J. C. (Ed.). (1990). Combining service and learning: An introduction. In *Combining service and learning: A resource book for community and public service* (Vol. 1, pp. 1–28). Raleigh, NC: National Society for Experiential Education.

Kernis, M. (2003). Toward a conceptualization of optimal self-esteem. *Psychological Inquiry, 14*(1), 1–26. Retrieved from http://www.jstor.org/stable/1449033

Kronick, R. F., Lester, J. N., & Luter, G. (2013). Conclusion to higher education's role in public school reform and community engagement. *Peabody Journal of Education, 88*(5), 657–664.

LaGuardia, J. G., & Ryff, C. (2003). Self esteem challenges. *Psyhological Inquiry, 14*(1), 48–51.

Leary, M. (1999). Making sense of self-esteem. *Current Directions in Psychological Science, 8*(1), 32–35. Retrieved from http://www.jstor.org/stable/20182550

Lomas, C. (1998). Art and the community: Breaking the aesthetic of disempowerment. In S. B. Shapiro (Ed.), *Dance, power, and difference: Critical and feminist perspectives on dance education* (pp. 149–170). Champaign, IL: Human Kinetics.

McNiff, J. (2013). *Action research principles and practice*. Florence, KY: Routledge.

Mehrabian, A. (1996). *Manual for the Balanced Emotional Empathy Scale (BEES)*. Available from Albert Mehrabian, 1130 Alta Mesa Road, Monterey, CA, USA 93940.

Moely, B. E., McFarland, M., Miron, D., Mercer, D., & Illustre, D. (2002). Changes in college students' attitudes and intentions for civic involvement as a function of service learning experiences. *Michigan Journal of Community Service Learning, 9*(1), 18–26.

Moely, B. E., Mercer, S. H., Ilustre, D., Miron, D., & McFarland, M. (2002). Psychometric properties and correlates of the civic attitudes and skills questionnaire (CASQ): A measure of student's attitudes related to service learning. *Michigan Journal of Community Service Learning, 8*(2), 15–26.

Noffke, S., & Somekh, B. (2009). *The SAGE handbook of educational action research*. London: SAGE.

Payne, C. A. (2000). Changes in involvement preferences as measured by the community service involvement preference inventory. *Michigan Journal of Community Service Learning, 7*, 41–53.

Phillips, L. C. (2003). Nurturing empathy. *Art Education, 56*(4), 45–50.

Pigza, J. (2010). Developing your ability to foster student learning and development through reflection. In B. Jacoby & P. Mutascio (Eds.), *Looking in, reaching out: A reflective guide for community service-learning professionals* (pp. 231–253). Boston: Campus Compact.

Rama, D. V., & Battistoni, R. (2001). *Service-learning: Using structured reflection to enhance learning from service*. Retrieved from www.compact.org/disciplines/reflection

Reason, P., & Bradbury, H. (Eds.). (2008). *The SAGE handbook of action research* (2nd ed.). London: SAGE.

Robins, R., & Trzesniewski, K. (2005). Self-esteem development across the lifespan. *Current Directions in Psychological Science, 14*(3), 158–162. Retrieved from http://www.jstor.org/stable/20183012

Rosenberg, M. (1965). *Society and the adolescent self-image*. Princeton, NJ: Princeton University Press.

Schön, D. (1995, November–December). Knowing-in-action: The new scholarship requires a new epistemology. *Change, 27*, 27–34.

Simons, L., & Cleary, B. (2006). The influence of service learning on students' personal and social development. *College Teaching, 54*(4), 307–319.

Stanton, T. K. (1990). Service learning: Groping toward a definition. In J. C. Kendall (Ed.), *Combining service and learning: A resource book for community and public service* (Vol. 1, pp. 65–67). Raleigh, NC: National Society for Experiential Education.

Stephens, J., Barton, J., & Haslett, T. (2009). Action research: Its history and relationship to scientific methodology. *Systems Practice Action Research, 22*, 463–474.

Stinson, S. W. (2016). *Seeking a feminist pedagogy for children's dance. Embodied curriculum theory and research in arts education: A dance scholar's search for meaning* (pp. 31–52). Dordrecht, The Netherlands: Springer (Original work published 1998).

Turner, V. (1966). *The ritual process: Structure and anti-structure*. New York: Aldine de Gruyter.

Turner, V. (1973). The center out there: Pilgrim's goal. *History of Religions, 12*(3), 191–230. Retrieved from http://www.jstor.org/stable/1062024

Chapter 16
Understanding Quality of Life Through the Experiences of Dancers with Parkinson's

Sara Houston and Ashley McGill

We are sitting in a circle with seven others. We've just been dancing – Popping, to be specific. We are listening to a small group of men and women in their 30s and 40s who live in South West London, UK. They are speaking about why they dance. They have been coming to the Popping class for about a year. Led by Italian dance artist and musician Simone Sistarelli, we practised tensing and releasing our muscles, moving to Herbie Hancock's *Ready or Not*. Popping is a sub-genre of Hip Hop, characterised by a staccato-like ripple in various parts of the body as muscles contract and release. Often associated with a number of different styles, such as locking, electric boogie and breakdancing, and with a Hip Hop sub-culture that spreads from graffiti, dance, music and rapping to clothes, dialects and behaviours, Popping is part of a global youth culture.

Yet, our fellow dancers that evening have what they describe as "an old person's disease." All have been diagnosed with the debilitating condition of Parkinson's, known in some countries as Parkinson's Disease. They have developed the condition at a substantially younger age than is typical. They talk of the "distress" that having the condition brings emotionally and physically. Parkinson's is a common neurodegenerative disease that affects the person's body movement, typically striking after the age of 50. Movement and cognition slow down, muscles become rigid, tremors may appear and postural instability is common. People with Parkinson's are at risk of falling and also of developing depression and dementia. Further symptoms, such as drooling, slurred speech, constipation and insomnia mean that this disease is not just a movement disorder. Social isolation is common, either because people feel embarrassed about their symptoms, or they feel unable to do activities that they had previously been able to do, or they are unable to socialise in the same way. Indeed, their social circle often contracts. There is as yet no cure for this degenerative disease that does not kill, but gradually progresses, slowly or quickly, for the

S. Houston (✉) · A. McGill
Roehampton University, London, UK
e-mail: sara.houston@roehampton.ac.uk; Ashley.McGill@roehampton.ac.uk

K. Bond (ed.), *Dance and the Quality of Life*, Social Indicators Research Series 73,
https://doi.org/10.1007/978-3-319-95699-2_16

rest of a person's life. Although there are medications to help with several symptoms, these diminish in effectiveness over time and can have their own set of debilitating side-effects.

Our conversation with the Popping class that evening continually returns to the idea that dancing gives them something back that they thought they had lost. One woman describes how her feet usually feel like they are encased in 'moon boots,' but dancing gives her back sensation and articulation. A fellow dancer perceives a lessening of tremor and an increase in feeling relaxed. Another argues that after a period of not exercising since diagnosis, going dancing is contributing to her overall fitness and giving her the confidence to try out other physical activities, such as yoga and Pilates. Dancing, the group explains, is a positive, pleasurable force in their lives. They have a better social life, connecting with dancing peers who understand what they are going through. They are not alone. Dance groups for people with Parkinson's exist in Europe, North and South America, Australasia, Asia and the Middle East (http://danceforparkinsons.org). Dance for Parkinson's is a growing dance phenomenon that is captivating people living with Parkinson's and dance teaching artists. Across the river in Central London another dance group for people with Parkinson's takes place in the studios of the large-scale company, English National Ballet (ENB). Here, participants move with the principles of ballet in mind and they dance to the music and themes of the works the company performs. We have studied this dance for Parkinson's group since 2010 in two consecutive studies (2010–2011; 2011–2014) to examine the physical, social, intellectual and emotional experiences that dancing offers. The ENB group may belong to a different demographic – older, mostly retired participants, many of whom are becoming frail, but there are connections between the ballet programme and the Popping group. Although Popping and ballet have different principles of moving, and the groups are dissimilar in age, in each group participants point to changes in how dancing makes them feel, how they approach everyday life, and how they approach their condition (Houston, 2015; Houston & McGill, 2013). With these experiences in mind, it is worth exploring how they may help us to understand the link between dancing and quality of life.

Regarding the concept and meanings of quality of life we draw on philosophers Martha Nussbaum and Amartya Sen (1993) who argue that discussion of quality of life generally speaking will explore what elements are important in life to be able to thrive in and across specific societies. Thriving is not about surviving, but about those factors that bring added value and meaning to one's life in order for it to be able to flourish. These may include political and social systems that allow a person freedom of movement and speech, or it could relate to how a society or individual opportunities can allow a person with limited functioning to be capable. Thriving might involve giving and receiving pleasure and emotional sustenance, or focus on physical and mental health. Within this general description of quality of life, we have taken the World Health Organisation's framework for assessing disability (WHO, 2001) as a way of examining issues that relate to quality of life, specifically, the relation between body functioning, daily life and participating in society (McGill, Houston, & Lee, 2014).

The case of dancing with Parkinson's is interesting as the dancers studied have an incurable, degenerative condition. The disease threatens the quality of their lives as it progresses by its physical, social and emotional consequences (Solimeo, 2009). Coming for many in the twilight of their lives, there may be other accompanying illnesses, bereavements and social change that also put pressure on people's resilience and material or emotional comfort and pleasure.

It might be tempting to conclude that since dancing seems to be pleasurable and seems to make people fitter, it should automatically give people better quality of life. Indeed, many projects report participant pleasure in and motivation to dance in health contexts (BUPA, 2011; Dance Factor Lincolnshire, 2015; Mason, Bone, & Cameron, 2013; Urmston, 2012; Watts, 2013). Gardner, Komesaroff, and Fensham (2008) present a qualitative account of the varied motivations that young people have to dance, many unconnected to exercise (see Chap. 26, this volume). As we discuss below, however, we cannot take better quality of life for granted, particularly when the dancers have Parkinson's. The first question that this chapter raises is whether we can talk about quality of life as being influenced by dance in a context where there are multiple variables. People's environments and lives are complex and Parkinson's is a disease that fluctuates month-to-month, daily and hourly. We will address this question by discussing the methods used to gain information about quality of life in dance for Parkinson's research in relation to our own analysis of dance's effectiveness in developing and maintaining quality of life. In this way, the chapter addresses how, as researchers, we need to open up the discussion about what might tell us more about dance's effects.

The second question to be addressed is equally challenging and important. Given that our dance participants have Parkinson's, what does it mean to have quality of life improved through dance when one has a chronic degenerative disease? To explore this question, the chapter will draw upon our research with the ENB Dance for Parkinson's group, highlighting participants' experiences. We will argue how these experiences may link to increased quality of life for individuals by situating their dance involvement within their everyday lives. By exploring what it means to have quality of life when one has a chronic degenerative disease, and how dancing can influence one's sense of being able to thrive, the chapter addresses significant issues about dancing as a participatory and communal experience and about the importance of dance activity for coping with chronic disease.

Research Methods in the University of Roehampton Study

The second of our mixed-methods studies, undertaken in 2011–2014, utilised qualitative and quantitative methods to assess the efficacy of dancing with Parkinson's. The University of Roehampton study has been discussed in other publications that probed dance for Parkinson's from multiple positions (Houston, 2011, 2015; Houston & McGill, 2011, 2013, 2015; Jones & Houston, 2011; McGill et al., 2014). Ethics clearance was granted by University of Roehampton's Ethics Committee and we used a quasi-experimental design (Harris et al. 2006) – a pre- and post-test, non-randomised study design, for the quantitative measures, including a control group of people with Parkinson's who did not dance.

Data collection included biomechanical measures of gait (step and stride variability, trunk coordination, and trunk range of motion), the *Unified Parkinson's Disease Rating Scale (UPDRS),* which assesses progression of motor and non-motor symptoms, and the *Dance for Parkinson's Questionnaire* (DPQ) mplied by Cynthia McRae and Bob Rubin based on McRae's 2004 study. The DPQ assesses changes to symptom and quality of life issues for people with Parkinson's after participation in dance. It is a 10-part scale compiled from a number of different validated scales, and includes a dance questionnaire based on work by Quiroga Murcia, Kreutz, Clift, and Bongard (2010). Formulated specifically to address people with Parkinson's who dance, the DPQ took the most relevant sections from several clinical scales to be filled in by participants themselves.

In our investigation of the impact of weekly ballet classes for people with Parkinson's, we analysed data from a small group of people who completed the DPQ alongside multiple other quantitative and qualitative measures over a 12-month period. While the investigation took place across 3 years, the quantitative measures lasted for a period of 12 months only due to the difficulty of collecting consistent data from tests across a longer period of time. A total of 15 dancing participants were analysed for this measure. A further eight people with Parkinson's who did not take part in dance classes across the duration of the study formed the control group.

In addition to the quantitative measures, we collected data from the dancing cohort using qualitative methods. Multiple one-to-one, semi-structured interviews and focus group discussions were carried out with 72 dancing participants across the 3 year investigation. These participants included dancers from the ENB groups in Oxford, Liverpool, Ipswich and Cardiff. One of the questions asked of individuals was what they thought was important to maintaining or developing their quality of life. We also asked people to keep diaries documenting their daily lives and thoughts. Finally, as we took on the role of participant-observers, multiple informal conversations occurred with participants. These provided additional insights into how the dancing was affecting this group of people. The qualitative cohort study was a key part of the mixed-methods study.

The choice to conduct research using a mixed-methods approach was important, particularly for assessing quality of life. As Houston (2011) points out, both Parkinson's and dancing are complex phenomena. Parkinson's presents itself differently in each person diagnosed. There are many symptoms that may or may not appear, and depending on the hour, day, week, month or year may present differently, or may be able to be coped with or not. In addition, the manifestation of symptoms may depend on how stressed a person is feeling, what they ate that day, where they are in their medication cycle, or what medication they are taking. Dancing may be accessed on different levels depending on what motivates people to take it up, what emphasis the teacher conveys to the class and conventions of style. It can be at one and the same time physical exercise, movement to music, an imaginative, creative activity, a source of pleasure, a source of pain, an activity with many traditions and heritages, a solo or group activity.

Because of the multifaceted natures of both key phenomena involved, the field of research is what John Laws (2004) would call, "messy." Many variables can affect results. In order to cope with this environment, we decided to use multiple methods so that we could check and re-check differences and similarities in results as they came in. We wanted to be able to build understanding of the field and specific concepts, such as quality of life, that we wanted to explore. In addition, in order to measure 'disability' we used the WHO International Classification of Functioning, Disability and Health (ICF) framework, which incorporates the three levels of body functionality, tasks of daily living and social participation. Different measurements and analyses were necessary to cover these three levels. Using mixed-methods allowed us to build, or at least start to build, a three-dimensional picture of the quality of life for people dancing with Parkinson's and of the factors that affect their quality of life.

Influences on Quality of Life: Where Does Dance Fit In?

Recent research has suggested that factors such as depression, disability, instability, and cognitive impairment have the greatest influence on quality of life for those with Parkinson's (Schrag, Jahanshahi, & Quinn, 2000). Considering the importance placed on these issues, the field of dance for Parkinson's research has focused heavily on how dance, in a variety of forms, can positively impact physical, and at times, mental wellbeing. While these factors often play a vital role in one's quality of life, research should also concern itself with how these physical and mental changes are impacting upon activities of daily living and participation in society (McGill et al., 2014). If research does not concern itself with how these physical and mental changes affect one's ability to function and participate in daily life, it appears that we are missing an important part of the story in demonstrating how meaningful these changes are to the participants involved.

Earlier studies have demonstrated that reduced activity participation overall is correlated with reduced health-related quality of life (Duncan & Earhart, 2011; Everard, Lach, Fisher, & Baum, 2000; Levasseur, Desrosiers, & St-Cyr Tribble, 2008; Yeung & Towers, 2014). However, while factors such as disability and instability are important to quality of life, these factors might hold even more significance if improvements to them are helping individuals to cope better with their condition and continue to be active participants in society.

Studies by Foster and Hershey (2011) and Foster, Golden, Duncan, and Earhart, (2013) have shown that reduced activity participation can occur even when motor dysfunction is not severe enough to cause physical disability. It appears there are other factors that play an important role in maintaining levels of participation and thus quality of life. The idea that one's quality of life is not solely based on physical and mental functioning is also apparent in recent research surrounding methods of assessing quality of life aspects. Den Oudsten, Lucas-Carrasco, Green, and Whoqol-Dis Group (2011) suggest that quality of life might be better assessed via focus group discussions or interviews that take into account the person's own perception of health and wellbeing. Chiong-Rivero et al. (2011) agree that measures of quality of life should include the perspectives of persons with the condition.

Studies in the dance for Parkinson's field, however, have used self-reporting questionnaires to quantitatively assess changes in quality of life aspects after dance. The *Parkinson's Disease Questionnaire* (PDQ-39), one of the standard validated questionnaires used to assess health-related quality of life for people with Parkinson's, has 39 questions pertaining to activities such as cooking, dressing, catching public transport, feeling anxious, feeling ignored, and being unable to concentrate (Jenkinson, Fitzpatrick, Peto, Greenhall, & Hyman, 1997). However, limitations and problems can arise as a result of using questionnaires to assess these variables. Foddy (1993) suggested that the set questions and responses presented to participants in a questionnaire can prompt respondents to provide answers they would not normally think of or choose on their own. In this case participants are being guided to provide an answer even if the given choices are not the most meaningful to them with regards to quality of life. Nevertheless, analysis of numerical data from quantitative measures can help researchers to discuss how the results reflect the experiences of a wider group of people. Schensul, Schensul, and Le Compte (1999) state that, "both quantitative and qualitative data provide the cross-checks (triangulation) that ensure the numerical data are a valid and effective representation of the phenomenon being measured" (p. 5).

Westheimer, McRae, Henchcliffe, Fesharaki, Glazman, Ene, and Bodis-Wollner, (2015) utilized both quantitative methods – the PDQ-39 and the *Beck Depression Inventory* (Beck, Steer, & Brown, 1996) – and qualitative methods (interviews) to assess changes in aspects of quality of life across 8 weeks of twice-weekly dance classes. Their participants consistently reported positive physical, emotional, and social benefits in exit interviews but the study found no significant changes from baseline to post-intervention in the PDQ-39 or the Beck Depression Inventory. This finding suggests that the interviews provided additional insights into what participants gained from the dancing experience that were not as easily accessible through questionnaires. Each individual participant will experience dancing in their own unique way and may value different elements of the class, and interviews allow for these nuances and differences to be explored (Westheimer et al., 2015). If the two questionnaires were the only instruments of analysis, one would have to suggest from the available evidence that dancing does not improve quality of life, as defined within the parameters of Westheimer et al.'s study.

Our research results echo those of Westheimer et al. (2015). While we found no significant changes across time or differences between groups on any analysed subscales within the DPQ, comments from interviews, group discussions, and informal conversations suggested that the participants perceived that dancing was doing them some good. However, some of the interview results were also ambiguous. Specifics of what exactly was happening were often difficult for participants to verbalise. Several described the general feeling of being energised, rather than more specific physical changes.

> It's not just I'm in the mood, but physically I feel different. I don't think about it all the time, but suddenly I realise how much better I feel. More movement, more energy, certainly more energised... I want to stay positive and not think about Parkinson's.

For this participant, there is a link between feeling better, as in "more energised," and feeling positive about their health. For others, the positive aspect related to the social interaction inherent in dancing with others. When asked whether anything has changed for the better as a result of the dancing, one participant states:

> Yes, I think there are two things, one is physical and the other is social. Physically, as I said before, it is hard to distinguish the effect of dance but I think it does help and quite often it is the non-physical things that are helping as much as anything… I have no doubt it has helped on the good side not the bad side.

While indicating that the physical changes are often hard to distinguish, this participant makes clear reference to other benefits that he is gaining from the dancing experience.

Often the non-physical benefits were discussed more readily in interviews, group discussions, and informal conversations across the 3 year study. Participants were keen to stress the importance of the ballet classes as a place where they felt valued and where they could make friends. They reported on how important that bonded community was to their participation in the ballet sessions. One participant stated: "And that means a lot. Go to some place where you are genuinely wanted and the fact that you are disabled it doesn't mean a darn thing." Another commented,

> So just to meet with the other people, to enjoy the class is good in itself. And people always seem cheerful when they arrive. And that seems to me to be quite a big part of it, all that. And everybody seems to notice when someone is doing better than usual and they comment upon it, so there is quite a lot of support here for people.

Supporting people to take part is a key part of the longevity of participation in dance for Parkinson's and it is clear that dancers found this support invaluable.

To give another perspective, we asked interviewees individually what was important for their quality of life. We distilled the 75 different answers into five categories:

- having the confidence to do things
- having the ability to keep doing interesting activities
- having movement stability and capability
- being around loved ones
- having a religious belief

These five categories point to physical and more-than-physical factors, but in particular, most are concerned with emotional or spiritual sustenance, capability and social participation.

Although insignificant statistically, results from two subscales within the DPQ warrant further discussion in relation to the above quality of life categories. Subscale six assessed participants' level of certainty that they could maintain a positive future life inclusive of making new friends and developing a sense of community with other Parkinson's people. Subscale eight assessed if participants felt that their Parkinson's was interfering with important life aspects such as personal relationships and their sense of independence. Both subscales align with the categories concerned with being around loved ones, continuing doing interesting activities, and having capability.

Subscales six and eight within the DPQ saw divergent results from the control group and dance group. These measurements indicated a decline in positivity and independence across the 12 months for the control group, while measurements for the dancing participants demonstrated a strong trend towards positive change. In these instances, the interviews, focus groups and diaries back up the notion that dancing promoted the particular categories echoed in the DPQ and in the individual quality of life categories. For example, there were a range of comments around the idea of being able to participate in "interesting activities." Responses indicate that the dance programme acted as an adult education initiative where participants deepened cultural understanding. Visits to the theatre to see the ENB perform reinforced this aspect.

In other words, the programme developed interest beyond getting fit. One man noted that he was "really enjoying learning about the technical side of ballet" and another remarked: "It certainly is very illuminating, isn't it? Seeing the ballet movers do the dance and do the movements it has given me insight into stuff that I never thought of, that I never realised." Added to the interest cultivated, the class was tailored to participants' needs, using a method of teaching that adapted and differentiated movement for individuals, which meant that many could keep attending despite growing infirmity.

A participant commented: "I watch all the waltzing and tango on *Strictly Come Dancing* [a television dance show in the UK] and I feel sad because I can't do that anymore, but coming here, I am still a dancer, I still feel able." Another pointed out, "as our disease progresses, we are gaining skills." The loss of physical mobility with the onset of Parkinson's is seen in contrast to the accumulation of "illuminating" dance knowledge and skills. The dance programme enabled people with Parkinson's to keep doing an interesting activity that allowed for a positive expansion of physical skills and understanding of an art form.

From interview responses, participants reported that they felt more confident to do other activities alongside dancing. One man mentioned another activity that he now does and that, "I wouldn't have gone had I not got the confidence coming here." Another participant explained how the dance classes encouraged her to try Pilates and visit the theatre more regularly. So, as well as being an interesting activity that takes into account increasing disability of participants, the dance programme acted as a catalyst for the dancers with Parkinson's to try out further activities in the wider social arena. This is particularly pertinent given that many people with Parkinson's gradually become socially isolated.

These findings are particularly interesting when looking at results from subscale three, which demonstrates that the dancing group perceived their Parkinson symptoms had become more severe over the duration of the study. Furthermore, other quantitative measures of symptom severity used within the study did not show any significant improvement. Our research suggests that the dancing has possibly helped participants to find ways to cope better with their condition, despite the perception that their condition has become more severe.

Responses in interviews, focus groups and diaries contribute to this conclusion.

Themes of changing lives, enrichment, positivity, and community were apparent in participants' statements. Several spoke of the dancing giving them hope. One woman wrote: "You need to know there is a future and you need to know there's people who've got talents and ability to help you and to give you hope. The dancing is enhancing and enriching."

Another spoke of dance being her "life line." She added that dance has kept her moving and given her the capability to join in the dancing at a cabaret show, which she said would not have happened before she started the ENB classes. Another spoke about life "feeling normal again." She stated: "there's a reason to get up, go out, join in with people and achieve and meet lots of other people in the same boat." Another man wrote about how he was enjoying the sense of "group motivation" and encouragement from the group; indeed, someone else commented that her attitude towards herself had changed because the welcoming, non-judgemental atmosphere had allowed her to think there are "possibilities" despite being "crooked and falling over."

In the above statements the value of the dance programme links to how participants are creating a way of thriving, not just surviving. The enriching, life-enhancing quality created through people's participation might be a clue as to how the dancers are finding their own ways through the sessions to cope better with their conditions. The valuing of this activity by participants is very strong and is underlined by the many who have attended the programme regularly for several years.

Back in the studio in South London members of the Popping group explain why they feel their dance class is their own special activity. One man comments that, being young and newly diagnosed, he finds Parkinson's support groups distressing. Facing the reality of what Parkinsonian degeneration looks like is upsetting for him and not his life as he knew it. Someone else chips in, exclaiming, "we're young and trendy." It seems these young dancers have seized the chance to Pop is because it gives them a connection back to feeling young. Another Popper comments: "I was feeling like an old person, now I feel like a spring chicken with the rhythm of the music. I want to move to it and I feel a bit young – young in inverted commas."

Popping gives this group of people with young onset Parkinson's the feeling that they are not old before their time. They have taken on a style of moving to define themselves as they would like to be defined. In this way, they are more than just coping, or surviving as a patient with Parkinson's, they are pro-actively shaping their identity as South Londoners in their 30s and 40s. In this example, participants have appropriated a style of dance, music, and culture in a quest to find their own identity as a group and as individuals with a neurodegenerative condition. Dancing has given them this opportunity to thrive as people who have Parkinson's.

Conclusion

From our study it appears that, for people living with Parkinson's, perception of quality of life is not solely dependent on physical and mental functioning and that quality of life can improve, despite progression of symptom severity. Furthermore, measures of quality of life that allow participants to discuss what is most meaningful to them might help researchers to gain useful information about the impact of dance on this group of people. This conclusion tells us is that we must be cautious when discussing the effects of dance participation on quality of life where dancing acts upon chronic disease to augment physical health. What is evident from our study is that it is fundamental to consider what individuals find important in dancing and to not assume that quality of life through dancing will be linked to better body and mental functioning.

Ostensibly, the study examines dance in relation to health, but our results suggest that quality of life through dance is less about health in a narrow sense and more about living life to the fullest. This is not to belittle claims that dancing is beneficial by suggesting that it is merely a fun filled activity – rather the contrary. Dancing as a participatory activity has been shown to be important, particularly for people with Parkinson's, as it allows them to create a life that does not revolve around illness, but around activities they find interesting, that enrich their lives. In this small way, dancing may allow people to thrive, rather than merely survive.

References

Beck, A. T., Steer, R. A., & Brown, G. K. (1996). *Manual for the Beck Depression Inventory-II*. San Antonio, TX: Psychological Corporation.

BUPA. (2011). *Keep dancing: The health and wellbeing benefits of dance for older people*. London: BUPA.

Chiong-Rivero, H., Ryan, G. W., Flippen, C., Bordelon, Y., Szumski, N. R., Zesiewicz, T. A., Vassar, S., Weidmer, B., García, R. E., Bradley, M., & Vickrey, B. G. (2011). Patients' and caregivers' experiences of the impact of Parkinson's disease on health status. *Patient Related Outcome Measures, 2*, 57–70.

Dance Factor Lincolnshire. (2015). *Dance Factor Lincolnshire project report*. Sleaford: Dance Factor Lincolnshire.

Den Oudsten, B. L., Lucas-Carrasco, R., Green, A. M., & Whoqol-Dis Group. (2011). Perceptions of persons with Parkinson's disease, family and professionals on quality of life: A focus group study. *Disability & Rehabilitation, 33*(25–26), 2490–2508.

Duncan, R. P., & Earhart, G. M. (2011). Measuring participation in individuals with Parkinson disease: Relationships with disease severity, quality of life, and mobility. *Disability & Rehabilitation, 33*(15–16), 1440–1446.

Everard, K. M., Lach, H. W., Fisher, E. B., & Baum, C. M. (2000). Relationship of activity and social support to the functional health of older adults. *Journal of Gerontology Series B – Psychological Sciences & Social Sciences, 55*(4), S208–S212.

Foddy, W. (1993). *Constructing questions for interviews and questionnaires. Theory and practice in social research*. Cambridge, UK: Cambridge University Press.

Foster, E. R., Golden, L., Duncan, R. P., & Earhart, G. M. (2013). A community-based Argentine tango dance program is associated with increased activity participation among individuals with Parkinson disease. *Archives of Physical Medicine & Rehabilitation, 94*(2), 240–249.

Foster, E. R., & Hershey, T. (2011). Everyday executive function is associated with activity participation in Parkinson disease without dementia. *OTJR: Occupation, Participation and Health, 31*(1), 16–22.

Gardner, S., Komesaroff, P., & Fensham, R. (2008). Dancing beyond exercise: Young people's experiences in dance classes. *Journal of Youth Studies, 11*(6), 701–709.

Harris, A. D., McGregor, J. C., Perencevich, E. N., Furuno, J. P., Zhu, J., Peterson, D. E., & Finkelstein, J. (2006). The use and interpretation of quasi-experimental studies in medical informatics. *Journal of the American Medical Informatics Association, 13*(1), 16–23.

Houston, S. (2011). The methodological challenges of researching dance for people living with Parkinson's. *Dance Research, 29*(2), 329–351.

Houston, S. (2015). Feeling lovely: An examination of the value of beauty for people living with Parkinson's. *Dance Research Journal, 47*(1), 27–43.

Houston, S., & McGill, A. (2011). *English National Ballet Dance for Parkinson's: An investigative study*. London: University of Roehampton Retrieved from https://www.roehamptondance.com/parkinsons/articles/.

Houston, S., & McGill, A. (2013). A mixed-methods study into ballet for people living with Parkinson's. *Arts & Health: An International Journal for Research, Policy and Practice, 5*(2), 103–119.

Houston, S., & McGill, A. (2015). *English National Ballet Dance for Parkinson's: An investigative study, part 2*. London: University of Roehampton Retrieved from https://www.roehamptondance.com/parkinsons/articles/.

Jenkinson, C., Fitzpatrick, R., Peto, V., Greenhall, R., & Hyman, N. (1997). The Parkinson's disease questionnaire (PDQ-39): Development and validation of a Parkinson's disease summary index score. *Age and Ageing, 26*(5), 353–357.

Jones, D., & Houston, S. (2011). *Researching dance for Parkinson's. Animated, autumn* (pp. 23–25).

Laws, J. (2004). *After method: Mess in social science research*. Abingdon: Routledge.

Levasseur, M., Desrosiers, J., & St-Cyr Tribble, D. (2008). Subjective quality-of-life predictors for older adults with physical disabilities. *American Journal of Physical & Medical Rehabilitation, 87*(10), 830–841.

Mason, L., Bone, N., & Cameron, K. (2013). Dance and older people evaluation report. Creative Scotland. Retrieved from http://www.creativescotland.com/__data/assets/pdf_file/0018/26172/Dance_and_Older_People_-_Evaluation_Report.pdf

McGill, A., Houston, S., & Lee, R. Y. (2014). Dance for Parkinson's: A new framework for research on its physical, mental, emotional, and social benefits. *Complementary Therapies in Medicine, 22*(3), 426–432.

McRae, C., Cherin, E., Yamazaki, T. G., Diem, G., Vo, A. H., Russell, D., Ellgring, J. H., Fahn, S., Greene, P., Dillon, S., Winfield, H., Bjugstad, K. B., & Freed, C. R. (2004). Effects of perceived treatment on quality of life and medical outcomes in a double-blind placebo surgery trial. *Archives of General Psychiatry, 61*(April), 412–627.

Nussbaum, M., & Sen, A. (Eds.). (1993). *The quality of life*. Oxford, UK: Clarendon.

Quiroga Murcia, C., Kreutz, G., Clift, S., & Bongard, S. (2010). Shall we dance? An exploration of the perceived benefits of dancing on well-being. *Arts and Health: An International Journal for Research, Policy and Practice, 2*(2), 149–163.

Schensul, S. L., Schensul, J. J., & LeCompte, M. D. (1999). *Essential ethnographic methods: Observations, interviews, and questionnaires*. Oxford, UK: AltaMira.

Schrag, A., Jahanshahi, M., & Quinn, N. (2000). What contributes to quality of life in patients with Parkinson's disease? *Journal of Neurological Neurosurgical Psychiatry, 69*(3), 308–312.

Solimeo, S. (2009). *With shaking hands: Aging with Parkinson's disease in America's heartland*. New Brunswick, NJ: Rutgers University Press.

Urmston, E. (2012). *Go dance research report*. Ipswich, UK: East Youth Dance.

Watts, V. (Ed.). (2013). *Dance for lifelong wellbeing: Project report 2013*. London: Royal Academy of Dance.

Westheimer, O., McRae, C., Henchcliffe, C., Fesharaki, A., Glazman, S., Ene, H., & Bodis-Wollner, I. (2015). Dance for PD: A preliminary investigation of effects on motor function and quality of life among persons with Parkinson's disease (PD). *Journal of Neural Transmission, 122*(9), 1263–1270.

World Health Organization. (2001). *The international classification of functioning, disability and health (ICF)*. Geneva, Switzerland. Retrieved from http://www.who.int/classifications/icf/en/

Yeung, P., & Towers, A. (2014). An exploratory study examining the relationships between the personal, environmental and activity participation variables and quality of life among young adults with disabilities. *Disability & Rehabilitation, 36*(1), 63–73.

Chapter 17
Dance and Well-Being: Honoring Caroline Plummer

Uzoamaka Nwankpa and Stephanie Bevill

Introduction: Uzo

> Imagine a world where mothers, babies, family and all community members are moving and dancing together supporting mind, body, and spirit. (Uzo Nwankpa)

I identify as Igbo, a tribe located in Nigeria, West Africa. Music and dance are together translated as *Egwu* in the Igbo language – there is no distinction between the two. The power of music and dance is a presumed ancient fact in Igbo culture – for healing mind, body and spirit. As a Nigerian immigrant to the United States and a community health registered nurse, I have long been curious about ancient healing practices and how they might be integrated into western concepts of healing and innovative health approaches. My work in the US has included facilitating classes where dances, music, rhythms, songs and movements from various regions of Africa are explored as they were likely intended, such as for healing. My own quality of life has been enhanced through music and dance, for example, building my social health in a foreign land.

As recipient of the 2015 Caroline Plummer Fellowship in Community Dance (University of Otago, New Zealand), I was able to carry out a project that integrated Igbo traditions of healing through music and dance, the Māori concept of Hauora (wellbeing), components of western integrative medicine, and the nursing process within a community dance project in Dunedin, Aotearoa/New Zealand.

U. Nwankpa (✉) · S. Bevill
Samuel Merritt University, Oakland, CA, USA

K. Bond (ed.), *Dance and the Quality of Life*, Social Indicators Research Series 73,
https://doi.org/10.1007/978-3-319-95699-2_17

The Caroline Plummer Fellowship in Community Dance

The Caroline Plummer Fellowship in Community Dance was established in 2003 to honor Caroline Plummer (1978–2003), a member of the Dunedin, New Zealand community whose life was shortened by cancer. The Fellowship, housed in the University of Otago School of Physical Activity, Sport and Exercise Sciences, acknowledges Caroline's outstanding scholarship at the university, her passion for dance, and her vision for community dance in New Zealand. The annual 6-month fellowship is open to community dance practitioners, teachers, and researchers from New Zealand and around the world who have a proposed program of activity or project that furthers Caroline's belief and aspirations for community dance in New Zealand.

Working as a community health registered nurse in the field of maternal and child health exposed me to many challenges that new mothers and their babies face emotionally, socially and physically. In the USA, I developed the Uzo Method (https://theuzo.com/) of healing through dance, music and movement to support new mothers. The desire to explore concepts of wellbeing in a global context, plus a strong sense of affiliation with Caroline Plummers's beliefs about the importance of holistic healing through dance, prompted me to apply for Caroline's Fellowship. I was honored to become its tenth recipient in 2015 – and spent 6 months in Dunedin, New Zealand (July–November).

Plummer fellows are expected to engage community members in their project. While I had been connecting with various communities in the US since 2008, leading dance workshops and performances intended to foster experiences of healing through music and dance, these events were challenging due to the limited amounts of time available to gain trust with a community – to establish relationships with organizations, healthcare providers and community members. In New Zealand, my relationship with the community was enabled by the fellowship, which is highly valued by community members, even over the short time period of 6 months.

The Maternal-Child Community Dance Project The Maternal-Child Community Dance Project was conceived within the framework of nursing. Community health nurses are in an optimal position to screen, refer, and provide support to families at risk for mood and anxiety disorders. Nurses are often the first line of defense for early detection of patient concerns. While stigma and shame are often attached to mental health disorders such as anxiety, nurses can help alleviate stigma by supporting activities that are not medicalized, such as participation in music and dance. Segre, O'Hara, Arndt, and Beck (2010) report that nurse-led interventions for postpartum depression are readily accepted by patients.

My Caroline Plummer Fellowship project was to examine the influence of music and dance on the experienced wellbeing of postpartum women with children newborn to 24 months, a population at risk for mood disorders. Postpartum anxiety and depression are two of the many possible complications of childbirth. These conditions are under-diagnosed and can lead to numerous problems after the child is born

(Jacob & Storch, 2013), to be discussed later. Such conditions are being approached through integrative health practices, including music and dance therapies (Pylvänäinen, Muotka, & Lappalainen, 2015; Yang, 2009). Sichel and Driscoll identify five aspects of care that are necessary for recovery: nourishment, relaxation and rest, understanding, exercise, and spirituality (as cited in Blackmore, 2008, pp. 165–166). The Maternal-Child Community Dance project addressed the exercise, spirituality, understanding, relaxation, and rest components of the model, which connect to the physical, mental-emotional, family-social, and spiritual dimensions of Māori Hauora.

The Maternal-Child Community Dance Project was an 8-week music and dance program held at the Dunedin Parent Centre, a volunteer run community organization and leading expert provider of pregnancy and childbirth education. One hour dance sessions were offered twice a week and were open to postpartum women and their children. One weekly session was designated for participants with depression and anxiety symptoms, while the second session was open more broadly to parents with toddlers. Only mothers attended the sessions. A total of 31 participants attended 147 dance sessions, with over 50% attending more than one session a week. Additionally, at the post-partum maternal depression (PPMD) weekly gathering, the *Edinburgh Prenatal Depression Scale* (EPDS) (Cox, Holden & Sagovsky, 1987), a screening tool, was administered pre- and post-session. EPDS was used as means of self-reflection and to help participants identify if they might benefit from additional support. The Caroline Plummer fellowship provided support for a pilot project that addressed the imbalance of Hauora as a condition that could make the postpartum period more challenging, and investigated the possible interventions available through community music and dance.

The Māori Renaissance

The *Treaty of Waitangi,* New Zealand's founding document, was signed in 1840. The treaty was an agreement, in Māori and English, between the British Crown and about 540 Māori *rangatira* (chiefs). After the treaty was signed, the settler population grew to outnumber Māori. British traditions and culture became dominant and Māori were expected to adopt Pākehā (White) culture (Hayward, 2012). New Zealand was unofficially mono-cultural until the 1980s with government policies favoring Pākehā culture. Since then, a Māori renaissance has created renewed emphasis on biculturalism, based on the treaty (Hayward, 2012). In the 1980s, the government began to recognize the languages, cultures and traditions of both Pākehā and Māori, and some government reports advocated biculturalism (see http://www.mch.govt.nz/).

Hauora

As a visitor to Aotearoa – New Zealand, I came to understand the many layers of being on Māori land and the *tangata whenua* (the indigenous people of the land). I observed the use of certain biculturalisms by individuals, organizations, and government agencies, for example, the use of both languages – English and Te Reo (Māori), the honoring of Māori protocol, and acknowledgment of history. On arrival, I consulted with residents of Dunedin as well as healthcare providers – including midwives of Pākehā (white New Zealander) and Māori descent, who stressed the importance of honoring the *tangata whenua*. This prompted me to incorporate Māori Hauora (wellbeing) as the guiding principle of my maternal-child dance and music work in New Zealand, demonstrating respect and engagement with the community.

A philosophy of health unique to Aotearoa New Zealand. Hauora was first outlined in the *Whare Tapa Whā* model developed by Māori health expert Mason Durie in the early 1980s. Durie (1985) described the traditional Māori view of health as a "four-sided concept, representing the four basic tenets of life" (p. 483), including *te taha wairua* (spiritual wellbeing), *te taha hinengaro* (mental/emotional wellbeing), *te taha tinana* (physical wellbeing), and *te taha whānau* (family/social wellbeing), which are viewed as interconnected. This holistic framing of wellbeing is highly relevant to contemporary Māori and continues to be applied in health and community environments throughout the country (New Zealand Ministry of Education, 2015; Wirihana & Smith, 2014).

Moreover, Māori Hauora aligns with the western integrative medicine paradigm of care, which puts the patient at the center of treatment and addresses the full span of physical, emotional, mental, social, spiritual and environmental influences that affect a person's health (Duke Integrative Medicine, 2016). When in harmony, the four dimensions of Hauora support and influence each other to achieve wellness. A misalignment or imbalance of these dimensions, such as a traumatic event, can challenge the emotional, physical, social and spiritual state of the family and lead to disharmony (Wirihana & Smith, 2014).

Background Problem

Postpartum anxiety and depression encompass a range of disorders that include generalized anxiety disorder, obsessive-compulsive disorder, post-traumatic stress disorder, social phobia and panic disorder. New mothers are likely to have symptoms associated with anxiety more so than depression in the postpartum period (Indivero, 2013). In their review of literature, Jacob and Storch (2013) found that anxiety is often under-diagnosed during pregnancy and after the child is born. In the United Kingdom, Heron, O'Connor, Evans, Golding, and Glover (2004) assessed anxiety and depression at different intervals pre- and postnatally, confirming that anxiety in the prenatal phase usually overlaps and increases the possibility of post-natal depression. Symptoms of this range of disorders include significant distress, sexual fear or avoidance, harmful and intrusive thoughts, feelings of numbness, and detachment and powerlessness, which can lead to the mother's loss of attachment with child and family, as well as isolation, early weaning from breastfeeding, and depression (Jacob & Storch, 2013). Maternal stress is also linked to preterm birth, low birth weight, miscarriages, and smaller infant head circumference (Frazer & Stathas, 2015).

Perinatal mood and anxiety disorders affect many families worldwide, with up to 20% of women experiencing significant symptoms of anxiety or depression (http://www.postpartum.net/). For mothers in the Pacific region (including New Zealand), Abbot and Williams (2006) found that 16% of mothers had probable depression, with rates varying between different communities. A study of postpartum women in Auckland found that 16% of the 225 respondents scored above the cut-off for depression risk on the EPDS (Thio, Oakley Brown, Coverdale, & Argyle, 2006). When undetected or untreated, postpartum depression and anxiety can negatively affect women's ability to function (Ko, Farr, Dietz, & Robbins, 2012; O'Hara, 2009). As noted above, music therapy and dance therapy have shown to be promising complementary interventions for depression and anxiety (Pylvänäinen et al., 2015; Yang, 2009).

Community Music and Dance

There is evidence that music and dance can enhance individual and community wellbeing. Music is a nonthreatening, noninvasive modality that can be administered easily in community settings. Further, music can provide a familiar acoustic environment and distract attention from feelings of fear, act as a cue for relaxation, and become a masking agent for unpleasant distracting sounds from the outside (Mok & Wong, 2003). Music has been shown to decrease anxiety levels during labor (Simavli, Gumus, Kaygusuz, Yildirim, & Usluogullari, 2014) and to induce relaxation in hospitalized psychiatric patients (Yang et al., 2012). Dance/movement therapy (DMT) has been reported to improve quality of life (Goodill, 2005; Koch, Kunz, Lykou, & Cruz, 2013; Quiroga & Kreutz, 2012), lessen depression and anxiety in people with severe illnesses, facilitate expression of feelings, and deepen discussion of end-of-life issues (Graham-Pole, 2001). In such therapeutic contexts, dance is a medium that "furthers the physical and emotional integration of the individual" (Leste & Rust, 1984). Hence, the combination of music and dance seems a promising combined solution for postpartum anxiety.

Ancient Māori methods of healing such as *waiata* (song, chant, psalm), *mōteatea* (to grieve, lament, traditional chant, sung poetry), *haka* (dance, perform), and *whakawhanaungatanga* (process of establishing relationships) continue to be performed on a daily basis within Māori communities to sustain well-being. These practices are based on generations of tradition. Traditional narratives have the potential to support Māori wellbeing, including the healing of historical traumas of colonialism (Wirihana & Smith, 2014). Similarly, cultures around the world continue to embody the protection of socialization through community gatherings, which in some cases include music, songs, dance and movement.

The RICHER Model: Uzo

The 8-week music and dance program in Dunedin was based on the RICHER Model, which applies aspects of ancient healing practices to the socialization of caregivers and their babies through music and movement. I developed this model as a systematic way to engage participants in an integrative process that emphasizes connection of mind, body and spirit, patient-centered care, and alternative healing modalities. The following principles of integrative medicine compiled by Maizes, Rakel, and Niemiec (2009) inform the RICHER Model:

- Patient and practitioner are partners in the healing process.
- All factors that influence health and disease are taken into consideration, including mind, body spirit, and community.
- Effective care is based on solid evidence, inquiry-driven, and open to new modalities, for example, movement, stress management, and spirituality.
- The individual must decide how to proceed with health care based on values, beliefs, and evidence; along with treatment, broader concepts of health promotion and illness prevention are integral.
- Practitioners of integrative medicine exemplify its principles and commit to self-exploration and self-development. (p. 279)

In the Maternal-Child Community Dance Project, a private and safe space was provided for participants to engage in the five-part RICHER process: **R**eflection (pre), **I**ntervention, **CH**oreography, **E**valuation, and **R**eflection (post). As facilitator-researcher, I drew on nursing practice as an evidence-based guide for implementation. Table 17.1 outlines my integration of RICHER with standard nursing practice. RNs use systematic, dynamic ways to collect and analyze data about clients, patients or community, which consists of assessment, diagnosis, outcomes/planning, implementation and evaluation (American Nurses Association, 2017).

Phase One (Reflection: assessment/diagnosis) of the New Zealand project involved pre-session self-reflection in which participants assessed themselves using the *Edinburgh.*

Postnatal Depression Scale (EPDS) and responded to a qualitative self-reflection question: What word or phrase describes how you feel in this moment?

Phase Two (Integration: diagnosis/planning) involved engagement with Hauora dimensions of wellbeing. Participants were guided through meditative practices to engage the physical body. In conjunction with breathing techniques, I encouraged the women to release into their bodies, noticing any physical sensations and

Table 17.1 The RICHER model as integrative nursing practice

RICHER model	Nursing process	Time	Description
1. Reflection	Assessment/diagnosis	10 min	**Self-screening tool (EPDS) and self-reflection:** *What word or phrase describes how you feel in this moment?*
2. Integration	Diagnosis/planning	10 min	**Meditative practice consciously engaging the four dimensions of wellbeing:** Physical, mental-emotional, social-family, spiritual
3. CHoreography	Diagnosis/planning/ implementation	10 min	**Technical exercises, warm up and choreography**
4. Evaluation	Implementation/ evaluation	10 min	**Facilitator observation, improvisation and mirroring**
5. Reflection	Implementation/ evaluation	10 min	**Reflective cool down and post-session reflection**

emotions. Through guided visualizations, participants were invited to focus on aspects of wellbeing, bringing conscious awareness to areas needing support. I asked them to channel those areas into their expressive movements throughout the session. For example, a mother who stated, "I feel grumpy" was encouraged to identify where in her body the feeling was most prevalent.

Phase Three (Choreography: diagnosis/planning/implementation) involved facilitator-led choreography. During this phase, participants performed warm up and stretching exercises, mirroring my cues and calls, which aligned with rhythms of the music. Warm up and stretching exercises began with the major muscle groups, finishing with the minor muscles. Examples include neck and shoulder rolls, back isolations, torso isolations, hip and pelvic rotations and thrusts, and knee elevations and rotations. Group choreography incorporated Igbo culture and Pan-African inspired movements, progressing from low impact, low intensity to high intensity. The group mirrored my movements such as rotating the right arm, then the left arm, then a clap, then a vocal "hey" as we all clap our hands together as a group. I continued to assess the group throughout each session to ensure safety and make adjustments as necessary.

Phase Four (Evaluation: implementation/evaluation): While evaluation was ongoing, it was emphasized after the choreography phase in order to record any subtle or significant shifts in participants' behavior and affect. I observed the group while they were immersed in the activities. This is a skilled observation known to healthcare professionals and nurses who, for example, can assess breathing patterns, affect and gait, all while having a conversation with the patient. The goal of this phase was to assess body movements, tension, emotional shifts, response to baby, and response to music rhythm, noticing changes since implementation.

Participants created body movements through guided improvisation. The mothers' movements were drawn from their everyday caregiving actions, such as feeding, diapering, getting into the car, lifting baby out of the pram (stroller), chasing after the toddler, and so on. Participants compiled their movements into a complete group dance that they performed all together. I supported the group to materialize and manifest positive and negative emotions through their bodies. They physicalized both empowering thought processes and debilitating thought processes, expelling the latter through their bodily movements. Participants mirrored each other's expressions as validation and acceptance. At the end of this phase, the group would remove any negative energies from the space by physically "grabbing" and "throwing away" what was no longer needed.

Phase Five (Reflection: implementation/evaluation) contained post-session self-reflection consisting of low impact movements and breathing exercises for cooling down. Participants then completed the following post-session reflection question: *What word or phrase describes how you feel in this moment?* I invited them to reflect on their experience, including perceptions of their baby, who might have been carried on the front or back of their body. I encouraged the mothers to think about their initial response so that they could assess themselves and be aware of any changes. Discussion sometimes occurred between participants, supporting social connections.

Music Music is an important element of the RICHER model and is also conceived in phases. The first phase sets the space using the music, the second provides music of about 110 beats per minute for the warm up and stretch, and the third evolves from 120 to 140 beats per minute for the choreographic section depending on the energy levels of the group. The fourth phase – cool down, reduces the beats per minute to about 110. As facilitator, my preparation involved having music ready and playing about 5 min before the session started. The objective was to bring the entire group in synch energetically and musically using binaural beats composed by Jeremy Mayall, the 2015 Mozart fellow at the University of Otago.

Binaural Beats is a therapeutic tool used to entrain the brain. This technology has been used and investigated since the early 1800s (Huang, 2008). According to Lester Fehmi, Director of Princeton Behavioral Medicine & Biofeedback Clinic, binaural beats induce brainwave synchronization so that left brain and right brain operate in harmony. This synchronization can evoke a state of deep awareness and intense mental clarity (Licklider, Webster, & Hedlund, 1950). Reported effects of binaural beats include decreased anxiety and increased quality of life (Wahbeh, Calabrese, Zwickey, & Zajdel, 2007), improved sleep (Abeln, Kleinert, Strüder, & Schneider, 2014), and increased production of hormones related to longevity and wellbeing (Harris, 2009).

The Group

The 31 participants in the Maternal-Child Community Dance Project included Māori, Pākehā, and other immigrants who were local to Dunedin. All participated voluntarily and provided written informed consent. I was responsible for recruitment, eligibility assessment, and monitoring adverse effects. The co-author of this paper, Stephanie Bevill, collaborated on research design and data analysis. The

Edinburgh Postnatal Depression Scale (EPDS) was administered once a week to screen for mothers experiencing symptoms of depression and anxiety. The EPDS represents a clinically useful tool for the detection of depression risk in perinatal women. It does not, however, assess qualitative benefits of music and dance. A sign-in sheet for recordkeeping and self-assessment screening tools were freely available.

The group established ground rules, which were reinforced at the beginning of every session. These rules included: no social media sharing of photos unless agreed upon; respect for each other; no making fun of others; looking out for the safety of the mobile children; and agreeing to have fun. Over the 8 weeks, participants grew familiar with each other and their babies. The babies were worn on front or back carriers, or placed in their car seats, on floor mats or in the play area with age appropriate toys provided by the center. Participants attended to their babies' needs during sessions – physical, emotional, and social. I provided pieces of colored fabric for mothers to write down their responses to the following self-assessment question: *What word or phrase describes how you feel in this moment?* As introduced above, some participants described their baby's responses as well, which in some cases, they noted, influenced their own feelings.

The meditative practices of Phase Two: Integration always began in a circle, allowing for eye contact among participants. Mothers wearing their babies would typically bounce gently to comfort them and stimulate relaxation. We would start with yoga-based deep breathing exercises and I would then facilitate a guided visualization based on the session theme; examples included groundedness, joy, passion, growth, creativity, mindfulness, love and connection. Movement patterns included circular motions individually or as a group, movement toward and away from the group, lateral side movements, upper extremity extensions, lower extremity rotations, hip thrusts, body percussion, claps, waves and vocalizations.

The babies were mostly engaged during the sessions. Non-ambulatory babies were placed in the center of the circle and danced around when awake or held by a participant. Older children became inspiration for movements explored during the sessions. The toddler bounce and "arm swivel" were common base movements inspired by the children. One particular child always wanted to be carried on her mother's back and refused to come down until the end of the session. Another child would display movements from the previous week, meeting a developmental milestone for gross motor skills. The younger babies sometimes fell asleep on their mother while she danced carrying her or him.

Results of the Study

Participant recorded their anonymous responses before and after each dance session. At the end of the 8-week series, all responses from before and after each session were pooled. The co-author/researchers, blinded to whether responses were reported before or after a dance session, independently coded each response as *negative* or *positive*. The four components of Hauora (wellbeing) were then set as coding categories for the pooled responses, plus a fifth category, *ambiguous*, for responses that did not fit into one of the other four. We defined each category – *physical, spiritual, social, emotional*, and *ambiguous* – to be as all-inclusive and mutually exclusive as possible (see Table 17.2) and independently coded each response manually. Inter-rater reliability was calculated using Cohen's Kappa ($\kappa = 0.77$) indicating substantial inter-rater reliability; the few coder disagreements were resolved through random selection.

Qualitative data suggest that a music and dance intervention using the RICHER Model addressed multiple components of wellbeing. In terms of Māori Hauora, participants experienced enhanced wellbeing on a number of levels. Post-dance session responses to "*What word or phrase describes how you feel in this moment?*" were significantly more likely to be positive than negative ($p < 0.05$). Pre-dance, 38.5% of categorizable responses were positive, whereas post-dance, 91.3% of responses were positive. Further, many positive pre-session responses related to the upcoming intervention, evidenced in words such as *excited* and *enthusiastic*. A large proportion (58.8%) of participants expressed negative thoughts and feelings before sessions, while only 5.7% of the post-session responses were coded as negative. The most common negative post-dance response was "tired."

Participant responses indicated that their perceptions of social and spiritual health changed for the better over the course of each session of music and dance. Categorization of responses revealed that prior to a dance session, participants were most likely to describe their physical and emotional health, while after a session, responses had a more even distribution across all found domains.

Seven percent of responses were unable to be categorized into components of Hauora, and were coded as *ambiguous*. Notably, in the context of physical activity, participants' word and phrase responses were not exclusively related to the physical. Before each session, the majority of responses were in the emotional category, while post-dance responses were most likely to relate to the social category with feelings of belonging. Figure 17.1 displays the aggregate difference between categorizations before and after each music and dance session.

As already noted, one session each week was designated as a group for participants with postpartum mood and anxiety disorder (PMAD) symptoms. Although the same participants attended the community session and the targeted PMAD

Table 17.2 Categories of Hauora – wellbeing

Physical: The physical body (e.g. tired sweaty sore)
Emotional: Thoughts and feelings (e.g. happy sad excited worried)
Social: Self-perception and interaction with others: "the capacity to belong " "the strength to be who we are" (e.g. fun loved shy ugly)
Spiritual: The capacity for faith unseen and unspoken energies (e.g. hopeful invigorated alive wrong)
Ambiguous: Terms that are unable to be categorized or are not mutually exclusive such as good or "Yep"

New Zealand Ministry of Health (2015)

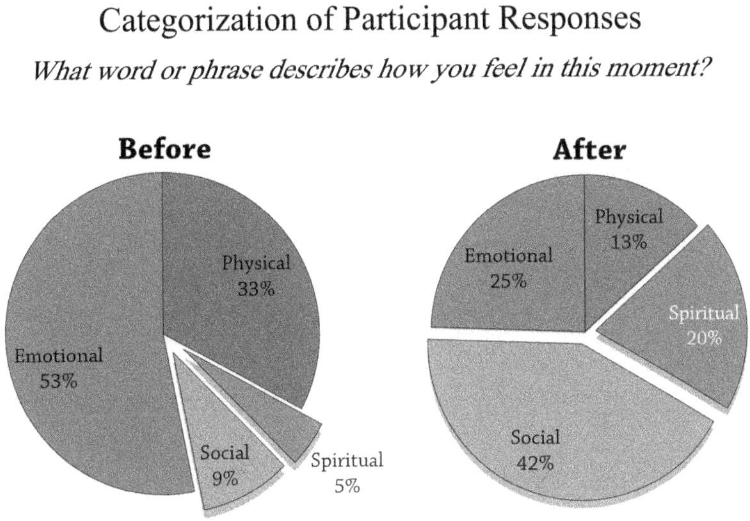

Fig. 17.1 Summary of participant responses

session, the PMAD group appeared more likely to disclose pre-intervention language that was intense and perhaps less "socially acceptable." For example, no participants in the general group used the words *angry, frustrated, stressed, challenged, or confused* pre-intervention, but those words were recorded in the PMAD group. This suggests that labeling the group as a safe place for people working through perinatal adjustments may have enabled them to share intense feelings. My commitment was to acknowledge, address, honor, and validate all affective expressions. After each dance session, PMAD participants wrote words like *energized, invigorated, happy, thankful, calm, and centered.*

Discussion

The Maternal-Child Community Dance Project examined dance and movement in a social setting and its impact on participants' wellbeing, understood holistically. In this small cohort, a dance intervention appeared to show promise in improving immediate feelings of wellbeing. Participant responses indicate that holistic dance program addressed more than physical fitness and that the RICHER Model can support the varied components of wellbeing, and most pertinent, appears to be a viable and useful component of interventions designed for perinatal women. This model differs from exercise methods where participants are required to learn certain dance steps and combinations, which for some can be overwhelming and self-defeating. Some participants described the room as "safe" and "comfortable." In the present study, my conception of safety includes freedom for participants to move their bodies privately and to share their felt realities of motherhood in writing and speaking.

This project yielded insights regarding the possibilities of realignment of a perceived imbalance of wellbeing (Hauora). Moreover, an emergent hypothesis is that The RICHER model's "freedom from failure" approach coupled with social interaction may result in improved self-concept. These results are a starting point to identifying the key components of a dance and movement-based creative expression program. Further investigation is needed to assess whether the intervention might be beneficial across various populations. Overall our study suggests that there could be real value in making community music and dance available to new mothers/parents and their babies. This intervention addresses multiple components of wellness and minimizes isolation of new mothers.

Limitations of the Study

In order to respect the privacy of participants and the open, organic flow of dance sessions, responses were not linked to participants, only to before or after each dance session, prohibiting statistical analysis of individual response trends. Further, as practitioner-researcher, Uzo was not blinded to participant responses, so there is the possibility of participant response bias as a coder. Finally, although care was taken in coding responses, there remains the possibility of cultural differences between intended meanings of responses and their interpretation by the researchers, as participants and interpreters had different countries of origin.

Conclusion

It is important for stakeholders and change agents to be aware of the implications of postpartum anxiety and depression, and the importance of prevention, early detection and intervention. The set of skills needed to implement the kind of program described in this chapter requires an organization committed to investing in the training of qualified health care providers as arts in medicine facilitators, utilizing existing mental health care providers, or hiring certified dance and movement therapists to work with health experts.

Participation in dance and movement-based creative expression has been documented to improve wellbeing within a variety of community groups (Koch et al., 2013). A prior study of the RICHER Model suggested a positive impact on mood and energy of postpartum mothers (Sheehan & Bevill, 2014). Sponsored by a Caroline Plummer Fellowship in Community Dance, the Maternal-Child Community Dance Project applied a broader focus to look at Māori Hauora's cornerstones of wellbeing. This group-based dance program for postpartum mothers and their babies demonstrated a likely experienced effect on the four components of Māori

Hauora: physical, mental-emotional, spiritual, and family-social. Although dance is a fundamentally physical modality, participant responses suggest that the RICHER Model dance intervention addresses holistic wellbeing – not just the physical. For a small cohort of new mothers, expressive movement and dance enhanced experienced feelings of wellbeing within each session. This project illuminates dancing as a component of holistic health, an ancient function of dance that continues today in cultures around the world.

References

Abbott, M. W., & Williams, M. M. (2006). Postnatal depressive symptoms among Pacific mothers in Auckland: Prevalence and risk factors. *Australian and New Zealand Journal of Psychiatry, 40*(3), 230–238.

Abeln, V., Kleinert, J., Strüder, H. K., & Schneider, S. (2014). Brainwave entrainment for better sleep and post-sleep state of young elite soccer players - a pilot study. *European Journal of Sport Science, 14*(5), 393–402. https://doi.org/10.1080/17461391.2013.819384.

American Nurses Association. (2017). *Nursing process*. Retrieved from http://www.nursingworld.org/EspeciallyForYou/What-is-Nursing/Tools-You-Need/Thenursingprocess.html

Blackmore, E. R. (2008). Postpartum mood and anxiety disorders: A clinician's guide. *Birth, 35*, 165–166.

Cox, J. L., Holden, J. M., & Sagovsky, R. (1987). Edinburgh postnatal depression scale (EPDS). *British Journal of Psychiatry, 150*, 782–786.

Duke Integrative Medicine. (2016). What is integrative medicine? *Duke Integrative Medicine*. Retrieved from https://www.dukeintegrativemedicine.org/about/what-is-integrative-medicine/#fn-410-3

Durie, M. (1985). A Mäori perspective of health. *Social Science & Medicine, 20*(5), 483–486.

Farr, S. L., Dietz, P. M., O'Hara, M. W., Burley, K., & Ko, J. Y. (2014). Postpartum anxiety and comorbid depression in a population-based sample of women. *Journal of Women's Health, 23*(2), 120–128.

Frazer, C., & Stathas, S. A. (2015). Mindfulness: Being present in the moment. *International Journal of Childbirth Education, 30*(2), 77–83.

Goodill, S. W. (2005). *An introduction to medical dance/movement therapy: Health care in motion*. London: Jessica Kingsley.

Graham-Pole, J. R. (2001). The marriage of art and science in health care. *Yale Journal of Biology and Medicine, 74*, 21–27.

Harris, B. (2009). *The science behind Holosync® and other neurotechnologies*. Beaverton, OR: Centerpointe Research Institute.

Hayward, J. (2012). Biculturalism. *Te ara – The encyclopedia of New Zealand*. Retrieved from http://www.TeAra.govt.nz/en/biculturalism

Heron, J., O'Connor, T. G., Evans, J., Golding, J., & Glover, J. V. (2004). The course of anxiety and depression through pregnancy and the postpartum in a community sample. *Journal of Affective Disorders, 80*(1), 65–73.

Huang, T., & Charyton, C. (2008). A comprehensive review of the psychological effects of brainwave entrainment. *Alternative Therapies, 14*(5), 38–49.

Indivero, V. (2013, March 20). Postpartum anxiety more common, less recognized than postpartum depression. *Penn State: News*. Retrieved from http://news.psu.edu/story/269398/2013/03/20/research/postpartum-anxiety-more-common-less-recognized-postpartum

Jacob, M. L., & Storch, E. A. (2013). Postpartum anxiety disorders. *Asian Pacific Journal of Reproduction, 2*(1), 63–68.

Ko, J. Y., Farr, S. L., Dietz, P. M., & Robbins, C. L. (2012). Depression and treatment among U.S. pregnant and nonpregnant women of reproductive age, 2005–2009. *Journal of Womens Health, 21*(8), 830–836.

Koch, M. E., Kain, Z. N., Ayoub, C., & Rosenbaum, S. H. (1998). The sedative and analgesic sparing effect of music. *Anesthesiology, 89*, 300–306.

Koch, S., Kunz, T., Lykou, S., & Cruz, R. (2013). Effects of dance movement therapy and dance on health-related psychological outcomes: A meta-analysis. *The Arts in Psychotherapy, 41*(1), 46–64.

Le Scouarnec, R., Poirier, R., Owens, J., Gauthier, J., Taylor, A., & Foresman, P. (2001). Use of binaural beat tapes for treatment of anxiety: A pilot study of tape preference and outcomes. *Alternative Therapy Health Medicine, 7*(1), 58–63.

Leste, A., & Rust, J. (1984). Effects of dance on anxiety. *Perceptual and Motor Skills, 58*, 767–772.

Licklider, J., Webster, J., & Hedlun, J. (1950). On the frequency limits of binaural beats. *The Journal of the Acoustical Society of America, 22*(4), 468. https://doi.org/10.1121/1.1906629.

Maizes, V., Rakel, D., & Niemiec, C. (2009). Integrative medicine and patient-centered care. *EXPLORE: The Journal of Science and Healing, 5*(5), 277–289.

Mok, E., & Wong, K. Y. (2003). Effects of music on patient anxiety. *Association of Perioperative Registered Nurses Journal, 77*(2), 396–410.

New Zealand Ministry of Education. (2015). Well-being, hauora. *TKI*. Retrieved from http://health.tki.org.nz/Teaching-in-HPE/Curriculum-statement/Underlying-concepts/Well-being-hauora

New Zealand Ministry of Health – Manatū Hauora. (2015). *Māori health models – Te Whare Tapa Whā*. Retrieved from http://www.health.govt.nz/our-work/populations/maori-health/maori-health-models/maori-health-models-te-whare-tapa-wha

O'Hara, M. W. (2009). Postpartum depression: What we know. *Journal of Clinical Psychology, 65*(12), 1258–1269.

Pylvänäinen, P. M., Muotka, J. S., & Lappalainen, R. (2015). A dance movement therapy group for depressed adult patients in a psychiatric outpatient clinic: Effects of the treatment. *Frontiers in Psychology, 6*, 980. https://doi.org/10.3389/fpsyg.2015.00980.

Quiroga Murcia, C., & Kreutz, G. (2012). Dance and health: Exploring interactions and implications. In R. A. R. Macdonald, G. Kreutz, & L. Mitchell (Eds.), *Music, health, and wellbeing* (pp. 125–133). Oxford: Oxford University Press.

Segre, L. S., O'Hara, M. W., Arndt, S., & Beck, C. T. (2010). Screening and counseling for postpartum depression by nurses. *The American Journal of Maternal/Child Nursing, 35*(5), 280–285.

Sheehan, C., & Bevill, S. (2014). *Mothers' oasis: Lessons from a grass roots community center for perinatal mental health*. PSI 27th annual conference. Chapel Hill: University of North Carolina Press.

Simavli, S., Gumus, I., Kaygusuz, I., Yildirim, M., Usluogullari, B., & Kafali, H. (2014). Effect of music on labor pain relief, anxiety level and postpartum analgesic requirement: A randomized controlled clinical trial. *Gynecologic and Obstetric Investigation, 78*(4), 244–250.

Thio, I. M., Oakley Browne, M. A., Coverdale, J. H., & Argyle, N. (2006). Postnatal depressive symptoms go largely untreated: A probability study in urban New Zealand. *Social Psychiatry and Psychiatric Epidemiology, 41*(10), 814–818.

Wahbeh, H., Calabrese, C., Zwickey, H., & Zajdel, D. (2007). Binaural beat technology in humans: A pilot study to assess neuropsychologic, physiologic, and electroencephalographic effects. *The Journal of Alternative and Complementary Medicine, 13*(2), 199–206.

Wirihana, R., & Smith, C. (2014). Historical trauma, healing and well-being in Māori communities. *MAI Journal, 3*(3), 197–210.

Yang, C., Chen, C., Chu, H., Chen, W. C., Lee, T. Y., Chen, S. G., & Chou, K. R. (2012). The effect of music therapy on hospitalized psychiatric patients' anxiety, finger temperature, and electroencephalography: A randomized clinical trial. *Biological Research for Nursing, 14*(2), 197–206.

Yang, M., Linjang, L., Haili, Z., Ivy, M. A., Shan, L., Zhou, W., & Ren, X. (2009). Music therapy to relieve anxiety in pregnant women on bedrest: A randomized controlled trial. *American Journal of Maternal and Child Nursing, 34*(5), 316–323.

Chapter 18
Somatic Movement Dance Education: A Feminist, Cognitive, Phenomenological Perspective on Creativity in Dance

Rebecca Weber

Introduction

Somatics is an umbrella term for the field of mind-body integration practices (Eddy, 1992; ISMETA, 2015). Because cognitive experiences (including attention, perception, problem-solving, and decision making) are "embodied," Somatics finds its scientific complement in the neuro-phenomenological theory of embodied cognition (Batson & Wilson, 2014; Varela, Thompson, & Rosch, 1991). Embodied cognition theories hold that the coupling of the sensate moving being with the environment gives rise to thinking, meaning, and personal agency (Gallagher, 2014; Robbins & Aydede, 2012; Shapiro, 2011). This understanding of sensing, moving, and meaning making is espoused in somatic practices and uniquely facilitated in Somatics' pedagogical environments.

In recent years, Somatics has become an integral part of dance education and training in the West, where it is known as Somatic Movement Dance Education, or SMDE (Eddy, 2006, 2016; Fortin, 1995; Mangione, 1993; Nettl-Fiol, 2016; Reed & Whatley, 2016; Tarlow-Morgan, Selver-Kassell, Lipman, & Brehm, 2016). It is widely held that dance gives rise to meaning, well-being, and quality of life (Batson & Wilson, 2014; Bond, 2014; Eddy, 2007; Fortin & Siedentop, 1995; Fraleigh, 2004; Halprin, 2000; Hanna, 2006; Henley, 2014; Sheets-Johnstone, 1999). However, the intentions and outcomes of traditional forms of dance training differ in significant ways from those of SMDE (Batson & Wilson, 2014; Shapiro, 1998).

Somatic movement is a unique mode of practice that extends some of the benefits of traditional dance training, particularly in terms of bodily sensation and perception (Enghauser, 2007; Nelson, 2008). Training in Somatics can also afford a sense of individual autonomy, allowing dancers to exercise more choices in dance making (Eddy, Williamson, & Weber, 2014; Fortin, Vieira, & Tremblay, 2009; Long, 2002;

R. Weber (✉)
Coventry University, Coventry, UK

K. Bond (ed.), *Dance and the Quality of Life*, Social Indicators Research Series 73,
https://doi.org/10.1007/978-3-319-95699-2_18

Williamson, 2009). In Somatics, philosophy and pedagogy are entwined (Eddy, 1992; Eddy et al., 2014; Green, 2002; Williamson, 2009); discussion of foundational philosophies in SMDE pedagogies (namely, feminist and phenomenological) enables me to address how Somatics practice can facilitate development of perception, attention, and individual authority.

This chapter poses the following questions:

- How do embodied cognitive processes support creativity in dance making?
- What cognitive psychological theories underpin the use of somatic practices in creativity?
- What distinguishes the pedagogical environment of SMDE from traditional dance education?
- How does the SMDE environment promote autonomous, creative dance-making capacities?

My approach to these questions examines SMDE within the discourses of dance studies and cognitive psychology. While acknowledging current theories of embodied cognition, where perception is viewed as an intersubjective process (Gallagher, 2014), this chapter highlights the individual, subjective aspects of perception, attention, and internal authority, or autonomy, which are the primary focus of Somatics pedagogies (Williamson, 2009). I propose that deepening one's abilities to engage with these cognitive processes in SMDE's unique pedagogical environment, described later in the chapter, can facilitate greater creativity in dance-making, or choreographic, practices.

The chapter begins with introduction to the field of Somatics, including its incorporation in dance education. I examine the benefits of somatic practices in dance education and discuss contemporary theories of cognition that illuminate meaning-making processes inherent in dance and Somatics. I acknowledge Somatics' epistemological base in existential phenomenology to connect somatic practices with theories of embodied cognition. I attribute SMDE's focus on individual development of refined sensory perception and sustained awareness to its foundation within this phenomenological framework – as Sondra Fraleigh (1996) notes, "a philosophy either implicit or actually stated in all somatic designs" (p. 18). Next, the chapter turns to SMDE's broad incorporation of feminist epistemologies and pedagogies (Burnidge, 2012; Eddy et al., 2014; Williamson, 2009), reflecting the field's assumption of the developmental importance of internal, subjective authority and autonomy. Finally, I introduce selected psychological theories of creativity that support my overarching argument that somatic practices, through their focus on deepening attention and strengthening internal authority, can facilitate greater creativity in movement generation and choreography.

Somatics: A Brief Overview

Derived from the Greek *somatikos,* for "of the body," the word *somatic* references the living body. The term was first used by Thomas Hanna (1970) to describe mind/body integration as experienced from the first-person perspective, and came to name the field of study related to the *soma* (body) as experienced through this perspective (Eddy, 2009). Somatic work is founded on the belief that *soma* is a fluid entity that responds plastically to both internal and external stimuli (Hanna, 1979). Perception of inner, felt-sensation is at the core of all somatic modalities practiced today under the umbrella term *Somatics* (Brodie & Lobel, 2006; Eddy, 2002, 2009). The terms *somatic* and *Somatics* are used discriminately by both practitioners and theorists, and there is some divergence in their application. In this chapter, I use *somatic* as an adjective according to its dictionary meaning: "relating to the body" (http://www.oxforddictionaries.com/definition/english/soma#soma__2). I use the capitalized form, *Somatics*, when referring to the field of mind-body integration practices identified above.

Somatics modalities cross a spectrum of codified to semi-structured to open-framework practices, including blended and hybrid approaches (Enghauser, 2007; Weber, 2009), and generally share basic principles of kinesiology and movement re-education, as well as goals toward greater well-being, awareness, expressivity, and efficiency in movement (Brodie & Lobel, 2004). All approaches share underlying ideologies that define them as Somatics, such as a global focus on principles over techniques of movement (re)education (Brodie & Lobel, 2012; Johnson, 1986), and an emphasis on individual agency rather than a 'set' of movement patterns. Indeed, there is such an overlap in founding principles that many people incorporate multiple modalities within their Somatic Movement Education (SME) and SMDE practices.

The professional field of SME began in the late 1960s (Eddy, 2009), centered largely in Australia, Europe, and the United States, and has grown in popularity and credibility with dance educators and those working in psychology and physiology. In recognition of the need for professionalism and integrity among practitioners and educators, a professional association, The International Somatic Movement Education and Therapy Association (ISMETA), was founded in 1988 by Jim Spira, PhD. Its mission is to grow the field of somatic movement education and therapy. In an effort to identify the shared scope of practice underlying the broad spectrum of Somatics disciplines, ISMETA (2015) names the following pan-modality educational objectives:

- focus on the body both as an objective physical process and as a subjective process of lived consciousness;
- refine perceptual, kinesthetic, proprioceptive, and enteroceptive sensitivity that supports homeostasis and self-regulation;
- recognize habitual patterns of perceptual, postural, and movement interaction with the environment;

- improve movement coordination that supports structural, functional, and expressive integration;
- experience an embodied sense of vitality and create both meaning for and enjoyment of life. (n.p.)

Somatic Movement Dance Education (SMDE)

After five decades of dialogue between somatic education and Western concert dance, SMDE – which combines dance education and SME – has become an integral part of formal dance training and performance, both technical and creative, particularly in higher education and professional-training settings, but also increasingly in pre-professional training schemes and the private sector. Though initially SMDE was perceived as more passive and therapeutic, advances in both SMDE and general dance education have led to more cohesion between the two (Batson & Wilson, 2014). As Somatics has grown and become more systematized through initiatives such as ISMETA, the field has gained presence in higher education, not only in somatic psychology and physical education programs, but especially in dance education programs internationally (Eddy, 2009; Long, 2002).

Morever, the research profile of Somatics has advanced since the field entered academia, including critiques (notably, Ginot, 2010) of the "unscientific" claims made for somatics practices. Ginot's seems a short-sighted claim, however. When she argues that Somatics "needs to affirm its value in accordance with society's belief in the objective truth of science" (pp. 13–14), she glosses over Somatics' grounding in phenomenological philosophies, which places it primarily within post-positivist paradigms. Furthermore, her qualms about the generalizability of individual accounts and case studies (which can be considered a subset of scientific reliability) ignore existing empirical studies that evidence the benefits of somatics within positivist frameworks dating back to the 1930s (Fairweather & Sidaway, 1993; Gamboian, Chatfield, & Woolacott, 2000; Krasnow, Chatfield, Barr, Jensen, & Dufek, 1997; Studd, 1983; Sweigard, 1939).

Most published research to date has focused on advocacy, that is, reasons to include SME in dance programs (Eddy, 2007; Kleinman, 1990), dance courses (Arnold, 2005; Batson, 1990, 2009; Batson & Schwartz, 2007; Brodie & Lobel, 2012; Debenham & Debenham, 2008; Fortin & Siedentop, 1995; Fortin et al., 2009), and in particular how to introduce concepts from somatics into dance technique classes (Brodie & Lobel, 2004; Eddy, 2006; Enghauser, 2007; Fortin & Siedentop, 1995; Long, 2002; Weber, 2009). Former dancers and current professors of kinesiology and dance Julie Brodie and Elin Lobel (2012) point to SMDE's pervasive implicit role within the dance classroom today:

> Many dance teachers and performers draw upon and reference somatic theory. … The somatic lexicon has become so intertwined with contemporary modern dance that for some, it has become the basis of the technique itself. (p. 5)

However, as stated, while there is overlap, the aims of traditional forms of dance training differ from those of SMDE (Batson & Wilson, 2014; Burnidge, 2012; Fortin, 1998; Shapiro, 1998). The following section offers a comparison.

Traditional Dance Training and SMDE Training

Though only recently gaining momentum in academia, numerous researchers have championed Somatics as a valuable addition to dance education (Batson, 1990; Batson & Schwartz, 2007; Brodie & Lobel, 2004; Burnidge, 2012; Eddy, 2009; Enghauser, 2007; Fortin, 1995, 1998). Somatic practices aim to facilitate a deep sense of embodiment and autonomy in dancers, in both connecting with self and exercising greater choices in dance making (Fortin et al., 2009; Williamson, 2009). SMDE's impact on dancers' agency, well-being, and aesthetic integrity is well-reported (Bond, 2014; Brodie & Lobel, 2004; Dyer, 2009; Eddy, 2009; Fraleigh, 2004; Sheets-Johnstone, 2013; Weber, 2009), and I acknowledge the relevance of these findings to quality of life discourse. Further contributing to quality of life, SMDE has been shown to enhance students' self-understanding and relationships with others (Rouhiainen, 2008).

More traditional dance training, for example, "the many forms of mid-twentieth-century western contemporary dance...largely destined for display" (Batson & Wilson, 2014, p. xv), might not offer adequate opportunities for consciously developing awareness and understanding of dancers' embodiment. As Glenna Batson (1990) noted almost three decades ago:

> In the act of learning something new, we [dancers] can strive so hard to learn the sequences, timing, phrasing, etc. that we forget to sense our bodies... We frequently even stop breathing; we lose our awareness, our sense of ourselves, as we (ironically) try to "make sense" of the movements. We give our full attention to movement, repeating steps at the expense of attending to the way we might accomplish them. Rather, we could be sensing our bodies exquisitely as we move, which would organize our motor system and in turn aid in our learning. (p. 29)

Rebecca Enghauser (2007) echoes this perspective, stating, "The structure of a traditional dance class does not currently offer sufficient opportunities for students to develop a sensitized relationship with their body" (p. 33). In contrast, SMDE emphasizes this through slowing down to "body temporality" (Williamson, 2009, p. 31), training dancers "to heighten both sensory and motor awareness to facilitate a student-client's own self-organization, self-healing, or self-knowing" (Eddy, 2009, p. 8).

Through bodily sensing, somatic modalities offer pathways for enhanced kinesthetic understanding and re-patterning of movement along neuromuscular pathways. However, as noted above, even though Somatics has infiltrated the current dance technique training climate, historical perspectives and culturally-ingrained training traditions persist in dance education (Lakes, 2005). Such methods can be critiqued for treating the dancer's body as a tool or object rather than the dancer as a sentient, whole being. The learning of codified, proscriptive movement patterns; the traditional hierarchy of teacher over pupil, where the teacher offers feedback on "correct" ways of moving; and the common setup of a room with mirrors, encouraging students to objectify their own bodies through an external gaze, are a few examples of how traditional dance training differs from somatic approaches. These key pedagogical differences' impact on dancers' perception and attention will be discussed later in this chapter.

Somatic methods incorporate strategies for addressing the lack of opportunities identified by Enghauser (2007) for students to develop a sensitized relationship with their bodies. For example, including rest periods in dance education (a practice shared by many somatic techniques) can aid in memory retention, motor recall, and performance (Batson, 2009). According to Martha Eddy, focusing on the feeling of movement rather than its outward appearance allows students to "perform so that the embodiment of a truly integrated statement is expressed" (as cited in Fortin & Siedentop, 1995, p. 6).

Moreover, Somatics training can help dancers move in healthier, more balanced, and more efficient ways, and thus suffer fewer injuries (Batson & Schwartz, 2007; Brodie & Lobel, 2004). Brodie and Lobel (2004) highlight that, "shifting the focus from product (skill acquisition) to process (what is actually happening in the body) can promote optimal functioning and help prevent injury" (p. 80). Further, the field of dance education is showing interest in SME for stress management (Adams, Caldwell, Atkins, & Quinn, 2012). In short, Somatics offers benefits to dancers in education programs; as Martha Myers famously said, "It is time to teach dance principles rather than dance steps" (as cited in Fortin & Siedentop, 1995, p. 6).

Having proposed that SMDE offers quality of life benefits beyond those provided by traditional dance training, a further question arises: *How* might the SMDE learning environment facilitate these benefits? Research from neurocognition sheds some light.

Neurocognition and Meaning Making in Dance

Both traditional dance training and SMDE acknowledge that dance is an inherently multimodal activity that engages kinesthesia and cognition in tandem. Beyond preparing dancers as athletes or communicative artists, or training bodies as artistic instruments, SMDE's primary focus is re-integrating mind and body, and as such is innately opposed to a Cartesian hierarchy of mental over physical. The field of *embodied cognition*, which holds that cognitive acts extend beyond the confines of the brain, helps to elaborate how SMDE might contribute to creativity in choreography.

Embodied Cognition

Like Somatics, the theory of embodied cognition calls into question Cartesian dualism, a hallmark of traditional cognitive psychology. To operate under this hierarchical assumption is to ignore the brain as an integrated dynamic system that responds to the moment-by-moment embodied dynamics of our lives. Cognitive scientist Raymond Gibbs (2005) highlights:

> Understanding embodied experience is not simply a matter of physiology or kinesiology (i.e., the body as object), but demands recognition of how people dynamically move in the physical world (i.e., the body experienced from a first-person, phenomenological perspective). The mind (its images, thoughts, representations) is created from ideas that are closely related to brain representations of the body and to the body's continued activities in the real world. (pp. 9–10)

A relatively recent stance in cognitive science, previously the brain was viewed mostly as a computational system, with processing happening in neural networks, and the body being an "output mechanism" with little effect on cognitive processing.

Batson and Wilson (2014) trace cognitive science through three historical periods: computationalist (1950s–1970s); connectionist – joining neural networks and dynamic systems theory (1980s–1990s); and situated cognition – embodied, embedded, or distributed (1970s–present). Even though the first two models are still widely recognized, since the 1970s cognitive scientists, as represented by Gibbs above, have increasingly theorized that cognition is situated, or contextual – of mind, but also of body and beyond. Since this realization, cognitive science has aligned with existential phenomenology (Gallagher, 2014). Neuro-phenomenologist Francisco Varela argues that mind is inseparable from subjective experience – its biological embodiment and its situated context in the world. Varela (1991) coined the term *embodied cognition* to include both the biological and contextual body in cognitive processes (p. 42).

A central premise of phenomenology is that meaning's ground is "lived experience" (Husserl, 1970/1990). Existentialism posits that self-responsibility creates meaning in life, and existential phenomenologists add that the ability to make meaning (or make sense) derives from bodily interaction with world (Fraleigh, 1987). French philosopher and developmental psychologist Maurice Merleau-Ponty (1962) asserted that movement doesn't "designate" thoughts but rather, *is* thinking (p. 182). These ideas will be elaborated later.

Dancer-philosopher Maxine Sheets-Johnstone (1981) has long critiqued cognitive science's predilection to view the brain as a computational information-processing system by arguing for the centrality of our animate form in human thought, stating,

> Perception is interlaced with movement to the point where it is impossible to separate out where perception begins and movement ends or where movement begins and perception ends; the one informs the other. (p. 402)

Sheets-Johnstone (1999) aligns with existential phenomenology, which,

> goes back into actual experience, to the things themselves—or more precisely, to us ourselves—thereby showing first how movement is the generative source of our primal sense of aliveness and of our primal capacity for sense-making. (p. 132)

The idea that movement is central to cognition is revolutionary in cognitive science, and in scientific thinking more generally.

As identified above, the term used to distinguish this integrative perspective from the dualistic empiricism of traditional cognitive science is usually *situated cognition,* which includes the subsets of *embodied cognition* or *distributed cognition*. The link between embodied cognition and dance, as an integrated form of meaning-making through movement, becomes evident immediately. While Sheets-Johnstone (2011) critiques the term "embodied cognition" as a tautology, I suggest that this semantic redundancy is needed to distinguish the current trend in cognitive science from previous dominant ideologies in which cognition was viewed as separate from, and superior to, body.

Further, Sheets-Johnstone's overarching philosophy that, "Mind is indeed a function of body" (p. 464) reflects prominent ideas in embodied cognition. For example, her claim that bodies affect perception through the "natural kinetic/proprioceptive capacities of animate creatures" (p. 455), and that animate beings "straightaway know kinesthetically and/or proprioceptively" (p. 464) the options available to them in an environment, has parallels (even though she critiques them) with Varela et al.'s (1991) enactive approach, where cognition depends on an organism's perceptual and bodily capacities, and meaning-making is based on how an organism moves through the world.

As Batson and Wilson (2014) encapsulate, "Movement deposes the brain from a privileged position of being the chief executive officer toward foregrounding movement as vital in co-creating thought and action" (p. 44). In somatic practices, creation of meaning is thought to occur at a place of integration and equalisation of movement and mind. Somatics and embodied cognition share a relative de-prioritisation of brain vis à vis body; meaning is created through rich interactions *between* brain and body in synergy. Bodily experience is not merely a product of or an input to cognition; rather, it is the foundation of meaning-making and consciousness in general. Then, what elements of cognition does SMDE affect, exactly? And what elements of a SMDE learning environment facilitate these effects?

Developing Attention and Perception in SMDE

As noted earlier, in SMDE, philosophy and pedagogy are intertwined (Eddy, 1992; Williamson, 2009, 2016). Cognitive processes such as planning, problem-solving, and decision making are "enacted" through the body, often through non- and/or preverbal stimuli (Adler, 2002; Stromstead, 2001); embodied cognition theories lend weight to the idea that the coupling of sensate moving body with environmental context gives rise to thinking and meaning (Robbins & Aydede, 2012; Shapiro,

2011). Honing sensory awareness or sensitivity to intricate bodily relationships is foundational in training SMDE practitioners as well as a quality they seek to elicit from clients and students (Johnson, 2000). Such awareness is evoked through a nuanced practice of attention, an embodied cognitive act. As Batson and Wilson (2014) state:

> The [SMDE] learning environment usually affords the space and time to awaken embodied consciousness, focus attention, observe and hone sensory awareness and reflect on thoughts, feelings and action. Learners attend to sensory information arising from: (1) their own movement and thoughts (improvised or prescriptive); (2) teacher-led verbally guided lessons in sensory awareness/attunement (through movement or stillness); (3) kinesthetic inter-subjectivity (the multi-layered experience of group learning contexts); and/or (4) the sensate qualities embedded within the environmental context. (p. 129)

Somatics educator and scholar Don Hanlon Johnson (2000) suggests that this fine-tuned sensory perception is the change-agent in SME, stating, "the education of [the participant] in more intricate levels of sensitivity provides the basis for healing" (p. 486). This makes rational sense, since without awareness of one's physical state, an autonomous choice to change (or retain) a state cannot be made; without fine-tuned sense perception, self-regulation would be imprecise if not impossible. Batson and Wilson (2014) claim that SME trains attention and assert, "Attending to sensory data is not simply a matter of noticing...the learning lies in noticing and registering *distinctions* and *differences* in the bodily status quo" (p. 130, emphasis original). As discussed, the body is active in cognition, so training in a well-focused awareness of one's physicality, and the ensuing ability to change it, allows for potential shifts in consciousness and opportunities for learning, growth, and development. Through Somatics, automatic habits and lack of awareness can be shifted into consciousness awareness (Hanna, 1970; Reeve, 2011).

In dance, somatic approaches emphasize sensory and perceptual processes underlying movement skills (Enghauser, 2007). As such, SMDE is a unique form of thinking that supports nuanced awareness of physicality in the movement moment, the fine-tuning of movement choices, and ultimately, skill in dancing and dance-making (Batson, 1990; Batson, Quin, & Wilson, 2012; Fortin, 1993, 1995). Habitual movement patterns developed over years of dance study or lifestyle can limit movement potential and mask individual limitations and strengths (Behnke, 1997), even leading to dysfunction or injury (Brodie & Lobel, 2004; Hanna, 1970). Alternatively, the deepening of embodied perception and skilled movement in SMDE may aid dancers in avoiding harmful patterning.

Attention and Perception: Philosophical Pedagogical Support

SMDE's pedagogical emphasis on personal experience in sensing, perceiving, and developing attention to bodily states stems from phenomenology and existentialism (Eddy, 2009; Fraleigh, 1987, 1996; Williamson, 2016). As Eddy (2009) notes, even prior to the formalization of first-generation Somatics modalities in the early twentieth century, experiential learning, sensory research, and general somatic inquiry were "buoyed by [the] growth of existentialism and phenomenology" in academic and scholarly culture (p. 6). In addition to prioritizing individual, subjective experience as a basis for meaning making, phenomenology holds that consciousness is consciousness *of* something, and therefore relies heavily on the present nature, or immediacy, of *intention* – what we ascribe importance to (Fraleigh, 1987); intention is what directs us towards meanings (Husserl, 1970/1990). Intentional sensory awareness is heightened in somatic practices, as they bring consciousness to the subjective lived experience of one's own (and others') body states and bodily relationships (Johnson, 2000). The existentialist notion of meaning making as a self-responsible process, occuring when one's physical body interacts with their environment – parallels Gibbs' (2005) theory of situated cognition, introduced earlier, which posits that cognitive processes extend beyond mind and body into the environment (see Robbins & Aydede, 2012; Shapiro, 2011).

SMDE's underpinnings in existential phenomenology shaped its pedagogical aims through its phenomenological roots. Emphasizing individual, subjective experiences rather than external authority, the processual nature of perception instead of a pre-ordained movement product, and periods of restful integration, SMDE supports meaning making. Through attending to a deeper engagement with our own movement, we make *sense* of our environment and experiences. Through use of these pedagogical tools, dancers might achieve a more fine-tuned perceptual experience of their bodies and movement than they experience in a traditional dance education setting. As discussed next, such refinement could have implications for creativity in movement generation.

Authority and Autonomy in SMDE

SMDE and Dance Technique: Some Distinctions

Obviously, dance education trains dancers to be aware of their physicality, as Enghauser (2007) highlights; however, Somatics offers a generally slower, more nuanced attention to embodiment and movement compared to conventional dance training's focus on the outer perspectives of teacher-as-authority, feedback from mirrors, and the shape and form of the *product* of their movement (Dyer, 2009; Green, 1999, 2001, 2002). Elements such as co-creation, shared authority (addressed in the next section), duration, sustained internal attention, and non-proscriptive movement are difficult to achieve fully in a setting where inner, felt experience is not the main goal. As Detta Howe (2016) identifies, in SMDE, "Each lesson allows space and time to rest, breathe and notice, and usually takes place in silence; none of the above you generally associate with the conventional dance class" (n.p.).

It is important to note that fine tuning of sensory perception, attention, and autonomy require in-depth practice before they can be applied with consistency and ease outside of the dance education context. I acknowledge, too, that dancers' awareness of the external perspective of their movement also requires development in a performing art that is typically perceived and received externally by audiences. However, for dancers to develop a more attuned awareness, a more sensitized perception, greater well-being, optimal functioning, and so on, twenty-first century dance educators are increasingly articulating the importance of supplementing objectification of dance students' bodies with education that prioritizes individual agency and the development of each dancer's internal authority or authorship. Agency and internal authority are closely associated with cognitive processes of choice, decision making, and subsequently problem solving and creativity. They are another way in which SMDE pedagogy, through its grounding in philosophical frameworks, can facilitate greater creativity in dancers.

Authority and Autonomy: Pedagogical Support

SMDE pedagogy is also backed by feminist principles (Burnidge, 2012; Eddy, 2002; Eddy et al., 2014). Feminist pedagogies seek to disturb and re-balance inequalities of power and question traditional epistemologies (Bond, 2017; hooks, 1994; Shapiro, 1998; Stinson, 1993); in feminist pedagogies and in SMDE, power resides in the individual as an authority in their own meaning-making processes – a subject who is active in that creation of meaning, rather than an object who didactically receives knowledge from an external expert (or who is subjected to the oppressive forces of society). In the 1990s, a germinal decade of feminist pedagogical thinking, Carolyn Shrewsbury (1997) stated, "Feminist pedagogy begins with a vision of what education might be like but frequently is not. This is a vision of the classroom as a liberatory environment in which we, teacher-student and student-teacher, act as subjects, not objects" (p. 166).

Emphasis on subjecthood can support a collaborative learning environment. This shift is apparent in dance classroom pedagogies that acknowledge students as teachers, perhaps influenced by the incorporation (implicit or explicit) of Somatics (Bacon, 2010; Bannerman, 2010; Burnidge, 2012; Dyer, 2009). Huddy and Stevens (2014) state that such changes "demand dance teachers to reconsider some of the traditional teaching methodology handed down by generations of dedicated teachers that may no longer be relevant in today's dance environment" (p. 2). Traditional teaching has been called the "sage on the stage" model of imparting knowledge (King, 1993) in a hierarchical or "subjecting" relationship of master to student (Foucault, 1977; Green, 2002). While there are different "waves" or schools of feminism, they share the same goals of questioning oppressive power hierarchies, especially related to gender, and seeking social change through communal efforts to recognize and resist hegemonies. Arguably, SMDE is feminist to its core.

Theorists have described features of feminist pedagogy. Shrewsbury's (1997) categories include empowerment, community, and leadership, all of which are applied to ameliorating inequalities of relationship and power. She states, "Our classrooms need not always reflect an equality of power, but they must reflect movements in that direction" (p. 168). She views classrooms as communities of learners where students develop agency and leadership. Diana Gustafson (1999) offers five premises of feminist pedagogy: (1) body as epistemological site, (2) body as political signifier, (3) explicit construction of knowledge – i.e. analyzing why and how we know and value what we do, (4) the reconstructing of self (or, in Somatics, "repatterning"), both personally and politically, and (5) discovering commonalities while supporting diversity.

These feminist pedagogical values are foundational to SMDE pedagogy (Burnidge, 2012; Eddy et al., 2014), which seeks to empower the individual to step outside of dominant cultural narratives of body subjugation and external authority and step into a sense of self-leadership and bodily autonomy (Eddy, 2002; Eddy et al., 2014; Fortin, 1995, 1998; Green, 1999, 2001, 2002, 2013). Further, a sense of internal authority – both mentally and physically – can become a kind of political positionality within a community of learners. In existential phenomenological terms, feminism's and Somatics' reverence for body as a source of knowledge indicates a shared valuing of both individual autonomy (or what Burnidge (2012) terms "empowerment") and intersubjective mutuality. Development of internal autonomy and authority is crucial in choice making and hence an important component of dance making and creativity. The feminist principle of explicit knowledge construction, combined with valuing subjective experience, means that somatic study invites transparency about one's geo-socio-cultural biases (Fraleigh, 2004). Johnson (1995) explains:

> My body—its sensibilities, movement styles, reaction patterns, and health—is not simply an individual reality governed by its own biophysical laws and idiosyncratic effects of my personal history. I am also a result of the ideologies within which I move. (p. 65)

Awareness of personal biases allows a dancer to choose to participate or resist them. As Howe (2016) states,

> When a student…is given the opportunity to feel their body in motion, to get to know themselves through trusting in the unknown, I propose that thinking changes, learning and ownership take place…informed by a history of life and movement but not confined by its rules. (n.p.)

Applying awareness of bias and choosing to resist convergent options (in thinking or movement) to seek the novel or divergent requires a developed sense of internal authority and the fortitude to stand up to the status quo. This perspective, again, is grounded in feminist pedagogical principles that acknowledge the subjective nature of meaning-making. In SMDE, strengthening the individual through their own internal authority to resist both habitual movement patterns and the aesthetics of their zeitgeist – a form of radical autonomy (Louppe, 2010), may foster enhanced creativity in choreographic choices as dancer-choreographers shed the "rules" and physical formations of existing techniques in favor of their own, individual creative movement.

Cognition: Creativity in Dance Choreography

So far, I have endeavored to demonstrate that SMDE is a unique form of embodied thinking with a variety of benefits to dancers. In particular, somatic movement education, through its pedagogical grounding in phenomenological, existential, and feminist philosophies, affords a deep sense of embodiment and autonomy (Fortin et al., 2009). SMDE's impact on dancers' health, well-being, and artistic or aesthetic integrity is well reported (Brodie & Lobel, 2004; Dyer, 2009; Eddy, 2009; Fraleigh, 2004; Sheets-Johnstone, 2013; Weber, 2009). Beyond these, however, I propose that gains in attention, perception, and internal authority have implications for creativity, a premise supported internationally by dance education advocacy organizations (Ausdance, 2012; NDEO, 2016). Through integration of these higher-order mental processes, dancers can gain greater access to autonomous choice making.

Within the field of creativity research, as it sits in cognitive psychology, creativity has been defined across domains as the creation of something both novel and useful (Amabile, 1996; Campbell, 1960; Koestler, 1964), for example, in problem solving, communication, and entertaining oneself and others (Franken, 1982/2006). Acknowledging that there is an extensive literature on creativity across multiple disciplines, here I will delimit discussion to one example, an enduringly popular theory on how one might produce something both novel and useful regardless of the domain of production: Campbell's (1960) theory of blind variation and selective retention (BVSR), a theory of combinatorial thinking later extended by other researchers, notably Simonton (2011). BVSR is widely valued within psychological discourses, as most creativity testing assesses divergent thinking, while most people in a shared culture tend to give the same first-response answer. In order to come up with something novel, convergent solutions have to be overridden through a process of *variation*.

In BVSR, one goes through a process of creating variations on the solution to a problem – or in dance, discovering ways to enact an intention in a fresh, engaging way – and then chooses the most useful. The usefulness criterion of creativity, in particular, requires more attention in relation to dance. As noted by Eddy (2009), "the growing body of research on creativity does not adequately address dance" (p. 22). Applying BVSR to dance, if a choreographer develops greater sensory awareness, and thus more options to choose from, it seems likely that this will increase the novelty and usefulness of their movement generation and their ability to selectively retain the most appropriate, or fitting, response. As Howe (2016) notes,

> When the movement is small and slow [as in SMDE], sensory distinctions can be made between movements and allow for mapping of the brain to be rewritten...slower movement leads to more subtle observation and map differentiation, so that more change is possible. (n.p.)

Furthermore, if Somatics practice develops a choreographer's sense of autonomy and self-authority, it might be easier for them to confidently choose divergently and override cultural pressures to adhere to societal norms; this could mean eschewing what is traditionally "right" or technically "correct" in favor of movement patterns that best fit the task at hand and the individuals performing them. Further, dance artists who override their habitual movement patterns in favor of those that are more beneficial to quality of life – choosing, say, less-injurious approaches, might foster a longer performing or choreographic career.

Conclusion

Dance education holds many benefits for the dancer-student, and somatic movement dance education (SMDE) can deepen and extend these benefits. Dance is a unique form of cognition in which movement makes meaning. SMDE supplements traditional dance technique to potentially strengthen higher-order cognitive processes of attention and perception, while reinforcing individual autonomy, internal authority, and agency – all of which are central to cognitive choice-making processes. Benefits of SMDE are holistic: physical, mental, affective, social, aesthetic, spiritual. These benefits can include, through a complex web of cognitive processes, the ability to choose more novel movement. If choreographic creativity sits at the intersection of novel and useful, then the quest for novelty is supported in SMDE through refinement of sensation and perception, while usefulness might be found in an individual's trust in their self-authority (whether solo or as part of a group). Both find their grounding in SMDE through pedagogies that draw on existential phenomenology and feminism, enacted and embodied in the unique Somatics learning environment.

Acknowledgements This research was funded by a Leverhulme Trust Research Project Grant for "In the Dancer's Mind: Creativity, Novelty, and the Imagination;" Coventry University's Centre for Dance Research, Chancellor's Fund, and Centre for Global Engagement; the Rebecca Skelton Fund; and the MARCS Institute at the University of Western Sydney.

References

Adams, M., Caldwell, K., Atkins, L., & Quin, R. (2012). Pilates and mindfulness: A qualitative study. *Journal of Dance Education, 12*(4), 123–130.

Adler, J. (2002). *Offering from the conscious body: The discipline of authentic movement.* Rochester, VT: Inner Traditions.

Amabile, T. (1996). *Creativity in context: Update to the social psychology of creativity.* Boulder, CO: Westview.

Arnold, P. (2005). Somaesthetics, education, and the art of dance. *Journal of Aesthetic Education, 39*(1), 48–56.

Ausdance. (2012). *Dance recognised as a valuable part of Australian lives.* Retrieved from http://ausdance.org.au/goals/details/dance-recognised-as-a-valuable-part-of-australian-lives

Bacon, J. (2010). The voice of her body: Somatic practices as a basis for creative research methodology. *Journal of Dance and Somatic Practices, 2*(1), 63–74.
Bannerman, H. (2010). A question of somatics: The search for a common framework for twenty-first century contemporary dance pedagogy – Graham and release-based techniques. *Journal of Dance and Somatic Practices, 2*(1), 5–19.
Batson, G. (1990). Dancing fully, safely, and expressively: The role of the body therapies in dance training. *Journal of Physical Education, Recreation, and Dance, 61*(9), 28–31.
Batson, G., & International Association for Dance Medicine and Science (2009). *Somatic studies and dance*. Retrieved from www.c.ymcdn.com/sites/www.iadms.org/resource/resmgr/imported/info/somatic_studies.pdf
Batson, G., Quin, E., & Wilson, M. (2012). Integrating somatics and science into dance training and practice. *Journal of Dance and Somatic Practices, 3*(1/2), 183–193.
Batson, G., & Schwartz, R. (2007). Revisiting the value of somatic education in dance training through an inquiry into practice schedules. *Journal of Dance Education, 7*(2), 47–57.
Batson, G., & Wilson, M. (2014). *Body and mind in motion: Dance and neuroscience in conversation*. Bristol, UK: Intellect.
Behnke, E. A. (1997). Ghost gestures: Phenomenological investigations of bodily micromovements and their intercorporeal implications. *Human Studies, 20*(2), 181–201.
Bond, K. E. (2014). Dance and quality of life. In A. C. Michalos (Ed.), *Encyclopedia of quality of life and well-being research* (pp. 1419–1424). Dordrecht, The Netherlands: Springer.
Bond, K. E. (2017). "Boys are morons"..."Girls are gross": Let's dance! In W. Oliver & D. Risner (Eds.), *Dance and gender: An evidence based approach* (pp. 135–157). Gainesville, FL: University Press of Florida.
Brodie, J., & Lobel, E. (2004). Integrating fundamental principles underlying somatic practices into the dance technique class. *Journal of Dance Education, 4*(3), 80–87.
Brodie, J., & Lobel, E. (2006). Somatics in dance, dance in somatics. *Journal of Dance Education, 6*(3), 69–71.
Brodie, J., & Lobel, E. (2012). *Dance and somatics: Mind-body principles of teaching and performance*. Jefferson, NC: McFarland.
Burnidge, A. (2012). Somatics in the dance studio: Embodying feminist/democratic pedagogy. *Journal of Dance Education, 12*(2), 37–47.
Campbell, D. T. (1960). Blind variation and selective retentions in creative thought as in other knowledge processes. *Psychological Review, 67*(6), 380–400.
Debenham, P., & Debenham, K. (2008). Experiencing the sacred in dance education: Wonder, compassion, wisdom, and wholeness in the classroom. *Journal of Dance Education, 8*(2), 44–55.
Dyer, B. (2009). Merging traditional technique vocabularies with democratic teaching perspectives in dance education: A consideration of aesthetic values and their sociopolitical contexts. *The Journal of Aesthetic Education, 43*(4), 108–123.
Eddy, M. (1992). An overview of the science and somatics of dance. *Kinesiology and Medicine for Dance, 14*(1), 20–28.
Eddy, M. (2002). Somatic practices and dance: Global influences. *Dance Research Journal, 34*(2), 46–62.
Eddy, M. (2006). The practical application of body-mind centering (BMC) in dance pedagogy. *Journal of Dance Education, 6*(3), 86–91.
Eddy, M. (2007). A balanced brain equals a balanced person: Somatic education. *SPINS Newszine, 3*(1), 7–8.
Eddy, M. (2009). A brief history of somatic practices and dance: Historical development of the field of somatic education and its relationship to dance. *Journal of Dance and Somatic Practices, 1*(1), 5–27.
Eddy, M. (Ed.). (2016). *Mindful movement: The evolution of the somatic arts and conscious action*. Bristol, UK: Intellect.

Eddy, M., Williamson, A., & Weber, R. (2014). Reflections on the spiritual dimensions of somatic movement dance education. In A. Williamson, G. Batson, S. Whatley, & R. Weber (Eds.), *Dance, somatics and spiritualities: Contemporary sacred narratives* (pp. 159–194). Bristol, UK: Intellect.

Enghauser, R. (2007). Developing listening bodies in the dance technique class. *Journal of Physical Education, Recreation, and Dance, 78*(6), 33–54.

Fairweather, M. M., & Sidaway, B. (1993). Ideokinetic imagery as a postural development technique. *Research Quarterly for Exercise and Sport, 64*, 385–392.

Fortin, S. (1993). When dance science and somatics enter the dance technique class. *Kinesiology and Medicine for Dance, 15*(2), 88–107.

Fortin, S. (1995). Towards a new generation: Somatic dance education in academia. *IMPULSE: The International Journal for Dance Science, Medicine, and Education, 3*, 253–262.

Fortin, S. (1998). Somatics: A tool for empowering modern dance teachers. In S. B. Shapiro (Ed.), *Dance, power, and difference: Critical feminist perspectives on dance education* (pp. 49–74). Urbana, IL: Human Kinetics.

Fortin, S., & Siedentop, D. (1995). The interplay of knowledge and practice in dance teaching: What we can learn from a non-traditional dance teacher. *Dance Research Journal, 27*(2), 3–15.

Fortin, S., Vieira, A., & Tremblay, M. (2009). The experience of discourses in dance and somatics. *Journal of Dance and Somatic Practices, 1*(1), 47–64.

Foucault, M. (1977). *Discipline and punish: The birth of the prison* (A. Sheridan, Trans.). Harmondsworth, UK: Peregrine.

Fraleigh, S. H. (1987). *Dance and the lived body: A descriptive aesthetics*. Pittsburgh, PA: University of Pittsburgh Press.

Fraleigh, S. H. (1996). The spiral dance: Toward a phenomenology of somatics. *Somatics, 8*, 14–19. Retrieved from http://digitalcommons.brockport.edu/dns_facpub/8

Fraleigh, S. H. (2004). *Dancing identity: Metaphysics in motion*. Pittsburgh, PA: University of Pittsburgh Press.

Franken, R. E. (2006). *Human motivation* (6th ed.). Belmont, CA: Thomson/Wadsworth. (Original work published 1982).

Gallagher, S. (2014). Phenomenology and embodied cognition. In L. Shapiro (Ed.), *Routledge handbook of embodied cognition* (pp. 9–18). London: Routledge.

Gamboian, N., Chatfield, S. J., & Woollacott, M. H. (2000). Further effects of somatic training on pelvic tilt and lumbar lordosis alignment during quiet stance and dynamic dance movement. *Journal of Dance Medicine and Science, 4*(3), 90–98.

Gibbs, R. (2005). *Embodiment and cognitive science*. Cambridge, UK: Cambridge University Press.

Ginot, I. (2010). From Shusterman's somaesthetics to a radical epistemology of somatics (A. Barlow & M. Franko, Trans.). *Dance Research Journal, 42*(1), 12–29.

Green, J. (1999). Somatic authority and the myth of the ideal body in dance education. *Dance Research Journal, 31*(2), 80–100.

Green, J. (2001). Socially constructed bodies in American dance classrooms. *Research in Dance Education, 2*(2), 155–173.

Green, J. (2002). *Foucault and the training of docile bodies in dance education*. New Orleans, LA: AERA Conference.

Green, J. (2013). American body pedagogies: Somatics and the cultural construction of bodies in the institution of higher education. *Paper presented at the Congress on Research in Dance*. https://doi.org/10.1017/S2049125500000157.

Gustafson, D. L. (1999). Embodied learning: The body as an epistemological site. In M. Mayberry & E. C. Rose (Eds.), *Meeting the challenge: Innovative feminist pedagogies in action* (pp. 249–274). New York: Routledge.

Halprin, A. (2000). *Dance as a healing art: Returning to health through movement and imagery*. Mendocino, CA: LifeRhythm Energy Field.

Hanna, J. L. (2006). *Dancing for health: Conquering and preventing stress*. Lanham, MD: AltaMira.

Hanna, T. (1970). *Bodies in revolt: A primer in somatic thinking*. New York: Holt, Reinhart, & Winston.

Hanna, T. (1979). *The body of life: Creating new pathways for sensory awareness in movement*. Rochester, VT: Healing Arts.

Henley, M. (2014). Dance and embodied intelligence. *Journal of Emerging Dance Scholarship, 1*(2), 1–20.

hooks, b. (1994). *Teaching to transgress: Education as the practice of freedom*. New York: Routledge.

Howe, D. (2016, April). *Undoing the danced body – Feldenkrais and awareness in motion. Dance in the 21st century: Questioning methods of practice, pedagogy and research*. Paper presented at DanceHE Early Careers symposium, Bedfordshire, UK.

Huddy, A., & Stevens, K. (2014). Dance teaching and learning in context: Activating the head, heart and hands. *Brolga, 39*, 20–26.

Husserl, E. (1970). *Logical investigations* (J. Findlay, Trans.). Abingdon, UK: Routledge. (Original work published 1900).

ISMETA. (2015). *International somatic movement education and therapy association*. Retrieved from www.ismeta.org

Johnson, D. H. (1986). Principles versus techniques: Towards the unity of the somatics field. *Somatics, VI*, 4–8.

Johnson, D. H. (1995). In S. B. Shapiro (Ed.), *Bone, breath, and gesture: Practices of embodiment*. Berkeley, CA: North Atlantic Books.

Johnson, D. H. (2000). Intricate tactile sensitivity: A key variable in western integrative bodywork. *Progress in Brain Research, 122*, 479–490.

King, A. (1993). From sage on the stage to guide on the side. *College Teaching, 41*(1), 30–35.

Kleinman, S. (1990). Moving into awareness. *Somatics, 7*(4), 4–8.

Koestler, A. (1964). *The act of creation*. London: Hutchinson.

Krasnow, D. H., Chatfield, S. J., Barr, S., Jensen, J. L., & Dufek, J. S. (1997). Imagery and conditioning practices for dancers. *Dance Research Journal, 29*(1), 43–64.

Lakes, R. (2005). The messages behind the methods: The authoritarian pedagogical legacy in western concert dance technique training and rehearsals. *Arts Education Policy Review, 106*(5), 3–18.

Long, W. (2002). *Sensing difference: Student and teacher perceptions on the integration of the Feldenkrais method of somatic education and contemporary dance technique*. Master's thesis, University of Otago, Dunedin, New Zealand.

Louppe, L. (2010). *Poetics of contemporary dance* (S. Gardner, Trans.). Alton, UK: Dance Books.

Mangione, M. (1993). *The origins and evolution of somatics: Interviews with five significant contributors to the field*. Doctoral dissertation. Retrieved from https://etd.ohiolink.edu/

NDEO. (2016). *Dance education in the United States*. Retrieved from http://www.ndeo.org/content.aspx?page_id=22&club_id=893257&module_id=19474

Nelson, L. (2008, February 1). Lisa Nelson in conversation with Lisa Nelson. *Critical Correspondence*. Retrieved from https://movementresearch.org/publications/critical-correspondence/lisa-nelson-in-conversation-with-lisa-nelson. (Original work published 2006).

Nettl-Fiol, R. (2016). How dance has helped situate academic fields of somatic inquiry: Case study, University of Illinois-Urbana. In M. Eddy (Ed.), *Mindful movement: The evolution of the somatic arts and conscious action* (pp. 165–180). Bristol, UK: Intellect.

Reed, S., & Whatley, S. (2016). The universities and somatic inquiry: The growth of somatic movement dance education in Britain. In M. Eddy (Ed.), *Mindful movement: The evolution of the somatic arts and conscious action* (pp. 149–164). Bristol, UK: Intellect.

Reeve, S. (2011). *Nine ways of seeing the body*. Axminster, UK: Triarchy.

Robbins, P., & Aydede, M. (2012). A short primer on situated cognition. In P. Robbins & M. Aydede (Eds.), *Cambridge handbook of situated cognition* (pp. 3–12). Cambridge, UK: Cambridge University Press.

Rouhiainen, L. (2008). Somatic dance as a means of cultivating ethically embodied subjects. *Research in Dance Education, 9*(3), 241–256.

Shapiro, L. (2011). *Embodied cognition*. Abingdon, UK: Routledge.

Shapiro, S. B. (1998). *Dance, power, and difference: Critical and feminist perspectives on dance education*. Champaign, IL: Human Kinetics.

Sheets-Johnstone, M. (1981). Thinking in movement. *The Journal of Aesthetics and Art Criticism, 39*(4), 339–407.

Sheets-Johnstone, M. (1999). *The primacy of movement*. Amsterdam: Benjamins.

Sheets-Johnstone, M. (2011). Embodied minds or mindful bodies? A question of fundamental, inherently interrelated aspects of animation. *Subjectivity, 4*(4), 451–466.

Sheets-Johnstone, M. (2013). Bodily resonance. In H. DePreester (Ed.), *Moving imagination: Explorations of gesture and inner movement* (pp. 19–37). Amsterdam: Benjamins.

Shrewsbury, C. (1997). What is feminist pedagogy? *Women's Studies Quarterly, 25*(1/2), 166–173.

Simonton, D. K. (2011). Creativity and discovery as blind variation: Campbell's (1960) BVSR model after the half-century mark. *Review of General Psychology, 15*(2), 158–174.

Stinson, S. W. (1993). Journey toward a feminist pedagogy for dance. *Women in Performance, 6*(1), 131–146.

Stromstead, T. (2001). Dancing literature: Authentic movement and re-inhabiting the female body. *Somatics: Journal of the Bodily Arts & Sciences, 8*(2), 20–39.

Studd, K. A. (1983). *Ideokinesis, mental rehearsal, and relaxation applied to dance technique*. Master's thesis, University of Oregon, Eugene, OR.

Sweigard, L. E. (1939). *Bilateral asymmetry in the alignment of the skeletal framework of the human body*. Doctoral dissertation, New York University, USA.

Tarlow-Morgan, K., Selver-Kassell, E., Lipman, L., & Brehm, M. A. (2016). Somatic movement and dance education in pre-K-12 education. In M. Eddy (Ed.), *Mindful movement: The evolution of the somatic arts and conscious action* (pp. 149–164). Bristol, UK: Intellect.

Varela, F., Thompson, E., & Rosch, E. (1991). *The embodied mind: Cognitive science and human experience*. Cambridge, MA: MIT Press.

Weber, R. (2009). Integrating semi-structured somatic practices and contemporary dance technique training. *Journal of Dance and Somatic Practices, 1*(2), 237–254.

Williamson, A. (2009). Formative support and connection: Somatic movement dance education in community and client practice. *Journal of Dance and Somatic Practices, 1*(1), 29–45.

Williamson, A. (2016). Reflections on phenomenology, spirituality, dance and movement-based somatics. *Journal of Dance and Somatic Practices, 8*(2), 275–301.

Part VI
Quality of Educational Life

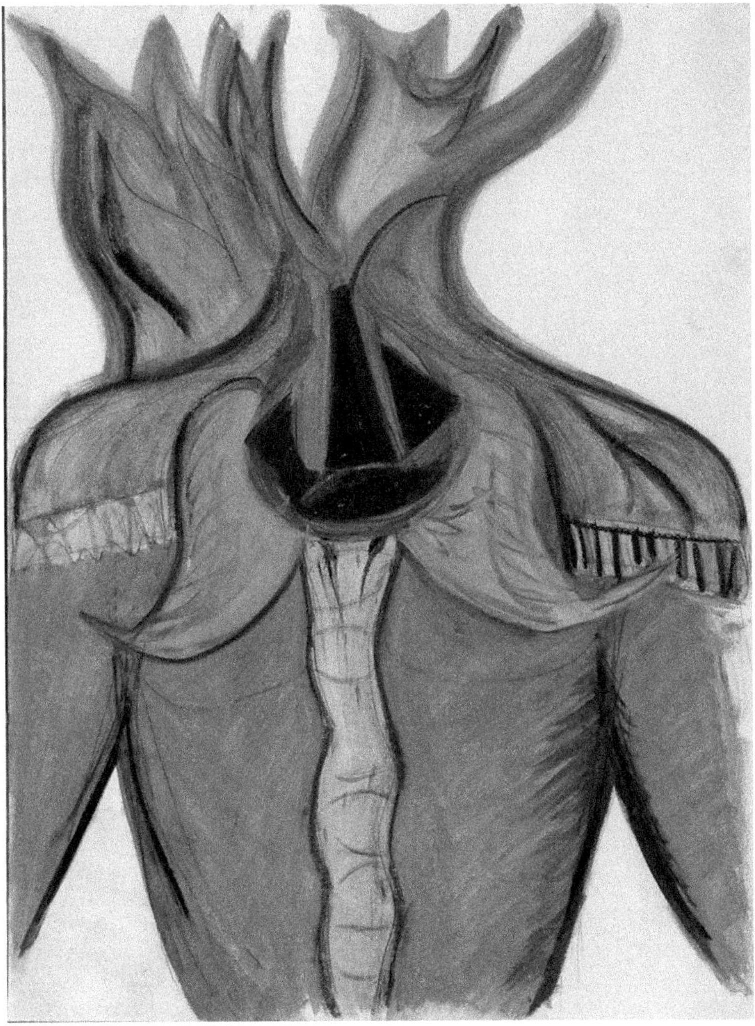

IV Flames, Snake with Wings (M. Shanahan)

Chapter 19
Dance and the Quality of Life at Schools: A Nordic Affiliation

Eeva Anttila and Charlotte Svendler Nielsen

Introduction

This chapter considers how dance can foster quality of life at schools. Writing together for the first time, we discuss dance as embodied learning, a topic we have both explored in previous research, and introduce Martha Nussbaum and Amartya Sen's (1993) philosophical framework for assessing quality of life into dance education research. We propose that this theoretical model – the *Capability Approach (CA)* – adds holistic substance to the often-claimed educational value of dance, and enhances understanding of conditions related to dance and quality of life (Nussbaum, 2011).

Our paths crossed first in the context of Dance and the Child International (daCi), an international organization aimed at providing access to dance for children and young people, and for dance educators and researchers from across the globe to exchange ideas and knowledge. During triannual daCi conferences, we have attended and presented in many of the same sessions, exchanging reflections on the significance of cultural contexts, cultural differences, the meaning of language within dance education practice and research, and on our Nordic connection. At the 2009 conference in Jamaica we made a decision to exchange data and together apply for research funding. After several attempts, we now have a formal possibility to collaborate, thanks to a research project titled "Art as Public Service: Strategic Steps towards Equality" (ArtsEqual, project number 293199), funded by the Strategic Research Council of Finland. ArtsEqual focuses on inclusion, participation, equality, and student well-being at schools – all quality of life indicators – through the lens of arts education.

E. Anttila (✉) · C. Svendler Nielsen
University of Copenhagen, Denmark, Finland
e-mail: eeva.anttila@uniarts.fi

K. Bond (ed.), *Dance and the Quality of Life*, Social Indicators Research Series 73,
https://doi.org/10.1007/978-3-319-95699-2_19

The Arts and Quality of School Life

To date, most studies on quality of school life are quantitative, using questionnaires and large samples. Some studies focus on effects of the arts, especially music. For example, Eerola and Eerola (2013) investigated 10 Finnish schools to assess whether music education can create social benefits in the school environment. Results indicated that extended music education enhances quality of school life, particularly in areas related to general satisfaction, sense of achievement, opportunity for students, and social life at school. The authors suggest that satisfaction in school is built on relationships between students in a particular study group, the class, and their teacher (p. 89). As a remedy for poor participation and lack of social cohesion within schools, curriculum researchers have suggested that schools make more room for voluntary subjects such as arts and sports (Pulkkinen & Launonen, 2005, p. 88).

For this chapter, we depart from educational evaluation models and move towards an interpretive, qualitative approach that leans on human rights and human development philosophy. Specifically, we apply the so-called "capability approach" (CA) model developed, most notably, by Martha Nussbaum and Amartya Sen (1993) for our analysis of qualitative data gathered from dance education settings in Finland and Denmark. The chapter concludes with commentary on how the capabilities generated by dance in relation to embodied learning may extend beyond subject areas and the world of school. These capabilities are related to being together and living together, to accepting oneself and others, to creativity and collaboration. The primary aim of this chapter is to discuss how these skills may enhance children's quality of life at schools.

The Dance Education Research Sites

Two dance education research projects in Nordic public schools are the source for this qualitative study: a 5-year dance education project in Finland (2009–2013) and a 1-year pilot study integrating dance and mathematics in Denmark (2013–2014). The collective findings, along with our critical reflection, suggest that dance, indeed, may enhance quality of life at schools.

Vantaa, Finland

The "Entire School Dances!" project took place at Kartanonkoski School, in Vantaa, Finland in 2009–2013, as part of "Aladdin's Lamp," a national arts education network funded by the Finnish Ministry of Education and the City of Vantaa. The project was carried out in collaboration with the Performing Arts Research Centre of the Theatre Academy Helsinki. A fulltime dance teacher was hired for 4 years to teach dance with all pupils at the school, and dance was integrated in the curriculum. The starting point for most dance classes was pupils' own movement. Tasks were based on creative dance and pupils' dance compositions, often created in small groups. In some classes, too, certain dance styles were introduced: for example, in dance classes connected to geography, dances around the world were explored. Most dance lessons took place in a visual art studio classroom, that was quite easily cleared for movement. In addition to dance instruction for pupils, the project included professional development days for the teachers, several dance performances, artists' visits and other events that included dance.

Teaching and research methodologies were intertwined in their concentration on embodied learning. The purpose was to articulate embodied learning and to see how dance might work in fostering a special form of embodied learning in the public school setting. The research design leaned primarily on collaborative action research (Reason & Bradbury, 2008). Participatory, or collaborative action research is conducted *with* rather than *on* people, and is based on participation of the entire community. This approach generated continuous feedback for developing the project and supported its pedagogical aims. A wide variety of data were collected from students, teachers, parents, and staff through interviews, written feedback, journals, observation, and videotaping. The data provided a broad and rich base for interpretative analysis (Anttila, 2013, 2015).

For this chapter, Eeva re-entered the hermeneutic circle with a fresh question, a new theoretical frame, a delimited source of data, and a cross-national Nordic collaborator, Charlotte, in order to examine dance education's possible contribution to a vital concern in education today, that of student wellbeing and quality of life at schools. Finnish data for this chapter include two sets of semi-structured interviews separated by two years. In both sets, children were interviewed in pairs – two boys and two girls from each grade level, for a total of 32 interviews. Excerpts from teachers' written feedback collected during professional development workshops are also included.

Elsinore, Denmark

The Danish research site for our "Nordic affiliation" was DanceMath, a pilot teaching project that took place in two sixth grade classes (12–13 year olds) of 23 and 24 students (approximately half boys, half girls) at two schools in the municipality of Elsinore, Denmark during the 2013–2014 school year. Half-day classes (when possible) were held weekly over a 4-month period. Inspiration for the project came from the Swedish Institute for Dance in Schools' development of "DanceMath" (Fridström, Björklund, & Andersson, 2011). Funded by the Danish Ministry of Education as part of a collaborative research project, "Learning through Movement," carried out by three Danish universities, DanceMath partnered the Danish National Center for Contemporary Dance, Dansehallerne (a national competence and performance center for dance), and the municipality of Elsinore. A teacher from each participating school collaborated to develop DanceMath with two dance educators employed by Dansehallerne to deliver the program at the two schools. The overall purpose of DanceMath was to experiment with new ways of learning in which body, movement, and creativity are central.

DanceMath lessons were inspired by a creative dance methodology (Smith-Autard, 1994) and used a five-part format: (1) Warm-up, (2) Improvisation, (3) Composition, (4) Performance, and (5) Appreciation/reflection. All parts of a lesson were focused on the mathematical theme of the day (for example, 'algebra'). One exercise in the composition part was to create certain mathematical phrases that the others had to guess (for example (a + a) + (b + b + b) = 2a + 3b) based on different ways of moving, which had been identified in the warm-up as a certain letter (a = jumping, b = rolling and c = stretching). Pupils had to find ways of doing the movements considering various elements of dance, for example, the timing or the level in space.

As in the Finland project, methodologies activated in the Danish DanceMath pilot concentrated on the role of embodiment in both learning and in researching; participating math teachers and dance educators were considered co-researchers (Reason & Bradbury, 2008). Data were collected through semi-structured interviews with students and teachers, usually held directly after DanceMath lessons. Student interviews sometimes included multi-modal exercises conducted by Charlotte (Svendler Nielsen, 2009, 2012). All 47 pupils chose to participate in interviews, which happened mostly in mixed gender pairs and threes.

Dance as an Embodied and Performative Practice

Our starting point in investigating the role of dance in fostering quality of life at schools is human embodiment, specifically *embodied learning*. We consider embodiment a focal concept in understanding the phenomenon of learning, and are interested in the notion of embodiment as the foundation for all learning. In our research on dance education in public schools, we use the term *embodiment* to refer to human existence as it becomes manifest through and in human bodies – as bodily sensations, lived experiences, and physical actions. This means that we are focusing on the human meanings that consciously embodied activities and experiences generate, especially in the context of dance.

We are aware of the breadth in how theorists from various fields use and define embodiment, including dance phenomenologist Maxine Sheets-Johnstone's (2010) critique that the concept of *embodied knowledge* is a tautology, since all knowledge – all learning, is embodied. While we appreciate the logic of this perspective, our intention as researchers is not to contribute to current epistemological debates, but to articulate *embodied learning* as a systemic and holistic process that takes place within the entire human being and between human beings, within the social and physical reality.

In order for learning to be experienced as embodied, and intentionally framed to be so, we assert that embodied activity must become a fundamental element in learning. Embodied activity refers to both actual movement and inner bodily sensations, experiences and physiological changes. In embodied learning, non-symbolic sensations generated by physical action and multisensory engagement become interconnected with symbolic knowing, leading towards complex meaning-making processes within the social and cultural world (Anttila, 2013; Katz, 2013; Svendler Nielsen, 2015). Through this process movement and concepts become connected in space and time so that reflection takes place simultaneously with action, and thus, "thought is placed in action and action is placed in the world" (Anderson & Harrison, 2010, p. 11).

We also acknowledge the complex nature of learning and education, and lean on contemporary approaches to educational research known widely as socio-material approaches. These approaches understand human knowledge and learning as embedded in material action and inter-action and trace how knowledge, knowers, and known merge together with/in activity (Fenwick, Edwards, & Sawchuk, 2011, p. 6). An example of this entanglement is how, in art and play, inanimate objects can become alive through artistic means and imagination.

Artistic activities and experiences related to appreciating art have the capacity to touch us deeply. We consider dance a modality that fosters learning and transformation in a special way. Dance connects non-symbolic, multimodal sensations with symbolic, cultural meanings in an embodied, performative way where multiple meanings can be shared, negotiated, and interpreted. The performance aspect of dance opens wide possibilities for learning that are grounded in embodiment and communicated through performative actions, thus connecting personal experiences with social life and cultural meanings.

The Capability Approach (CA): A Theoretical Lens for Dance Education Research

Nussbaum and Sen (1993) have worked towards a new theoretical paradigm for the development and policy world. It begins with a question: What are people actually able to do and be? What real opportunities are available to them? According to Nussbaum (2011), the capability approach (CA) is a counter-theory to models that steer development policy toward choices that go against widely shared human values. For example, crude measures of quality of life have given high marks to countries that allow alarming inequalities and encourage countries to work only for economic growth (pp. xi–xii).

In contrast, CA is allied with the international human rights movement, specifically, the idea that all people have core entitlements by virtue of their humanity. The ten central capabilities overlap with rights recognized in the United Nations' 1948 *Universal Declaration of Human Rights* (p. 62). Unlike human rights approaches, however, CA is a fully integrated theory of social justice that articulates the relationship between human rights and human dignity, between human entitlements and those of other species, and between human rights and duties (p. 63). Interested in the opportunities available to each person and personal freedom of choice, CA is pluralist about value (pp. 18–19). Thus, capabilities are opportunities to choose and act – through integration of personal abilities and the economic, political and social environment (p. 20). The ten central capabilities that Nussbaum claims are required for an existence worthy of human dignity include: (1) life, (2) bodily health, (3) bodily integrity, (4) senses, imagination and thought, (5) emotions, (6) practical reason, (7) affiliation, (8) other species, (9) play, and (10) control over one's environment (pp. 33–34).

We encountered CA in 2015 while exploring theoretical frameworks for equality in education as part of the ArtsEqual research initiative. On first exposure, it seemed clear to us that the central capabilities are integral to dance education, and that CA would provide a fruitful ground to investigate dance and quality of life at school. As a holistic modality that can be sustained throughout life, dance is arguably a form of bodily health in itself, supporting bodily integrity, engaging the senses, imagination, thought, emotions, and play, is intrinsically affiliative and playful, and facilitates environmental agency. While some might question the *other species* central capability as integral to dance education, our youngest dancers are particularly gifted in this capability and we can learn from them (Bond, 2001, 2018). Next, we reflect on each central capability in relation to our collective data from dance education projects in Finland and Denmark.

Life and Bodily Health

In the CA model, *life* refers to being able to "live to the end of a human life of normal length and not die prematurely" (p. 33). The *life* capability might seem a distant concern in a study focused on children who live in a peaceful democratic welfare society. Although the threat of premature death by outer forces (like war) is not apparent in the Nordic context, it is possible to conceptualize *life* as a central capability through association with *bodily health* (Bond, 2014; Hanna, 2006). Hence, we discuss the first two central capabilities – *life* and *bodily health* – together.

In interviews, Finnish students from across grade levels alluded to connections between dance and health.

> Dance is…refreshing. (2nd grade boy)
> Dance is agile and you get to sweat. (4th grade girl)
> I feel good because…movement is healthy. (6th grade girl)
> In dance you get to…move. You don't have to sit at your desk. (9th grade girl)

Some teachers started to incorporate dance exercises in their academic classes.

> The rhythmic structure supports balance, helps us to concentrate. We can get our brains to work in the best possible way. The children always join. They experience it as refreshing and maybe giving security. We count down, for example, in English and then in the end comes the lovely Zeroo! and they love the jumping and even arms come along when we say Zeroo! (2nd grade classroom teacher)

Moreover, a few teachers commented on dance as an alternative to PE:

> Some who are not engaged during PE take part enthusiastically in dance. (anonymous)
> Clumsy or reserved pupils in PE have enjoyed the dance classes. (anonymous)

In Denmark, sixth graders in the DanceMath pilot project made health connections also:

> We felt fresher when we were dancing. (girl)
> I got more energy. (girl)
> One of the best things was we got to move instead of sitting looking in a book. (boy)
> You can get very tired reading in a book. It gives more energy to move at the same time as calculating. (girl)
> You have to be ready for a lot, which is hard if you are not in a good shape. (boy)

A Danish dance educator noted,

> You don't fall asleep when you are jumping! When we work with our bodies we do not lose concentration, not from "I have to jump 5 times," so you jump and you are still active…

A Danish math teacher who is a yoga practitioner related her experience of "landing inside herself" to what she sees happening when students dance: "They have to inhabit their bodies, *be* their bodies, it is not something they *have*, it is something they *are*." This teacher broadens the notion of health as "being in good shape" to highlight an ontological perspective – we *are* our bodies. Another noted that DanceMath benefits her own quality of life at school: "Brain gym every day brings good feeling to my own body and to pupils (joy, smiles)."

With its emphasis on bodily sensing and communicating, dance has the potential to promote good health. Even when the purpose is artistic work, pupils' health may develop as a side effect. Also, when moving in new ways children are also sensing themselves and their surroundings in new ways, even if such experiences are never verbalized. Moreover, pupils who do not enjoy sports might have positive experiences of physicality in dance. Some may discover they are good at moving to music or inventing movements. By making sure that all pupils have a choice of diverse movement activities, we might inspire more children to be aware of their bodies and find more spontaneous interest in moving. Over time, it is possible that dance education could nurture more pupils to a life of movement, with the result of greater health, longevity, and quality of life.

Bodily Integrity

Nussbaum's (2011) notion of *bodily integrity* relates to being able to move freely in space without threat of harm (p. 33). While it is relatively safe in Nordic countries for children to move around independently, even in large cities, this capability has decreased in Finland over the past 20 years (Kyttä, Hirvonen, Rudner, Pirjola, & Laatikainen, 2015). Further, adolescence, peer pressure, and media can have negative effects on youngsters' body image and therefore their *bodily integrity* (Bond,

2017; Ricciardelli & Yager, 2016), in Scandinavia as in other (Western) countries. In its potential to build a positive body image along with sensory and spatial awareness, we suggest that dance education promotes the central capability of *bodily integrity*.

In Finland's "The Entire School Dances!" project, the dance teacher noted gender differences in students' courage to move freely in space: "Upper grade girls use a very limited movement range... If the boys are loud and take a lot of space, they do not dare" (see Young, 1980). Dance is, of course, a spatial art, and the dance teacher also reported positive development over time in how pupils were learning to use space:

> Half settled around the gym so that everyone had space around them. The other half withdrew along the walls, and despite my instructions, did not find courage to join. To the latter [pupils new to the school who had not had dance], the situation was anxious, strange…they sought security from each other and the walls.

She also reported that after initial hesitation, dance is "somehow pleasant to most." The pupils, in so many voices, welcomed the opportunity to move freely:

> It is just what I need, movement and action. (3rd grade boy)
> You get to move much more. (7th grade boy)
> You don't have to be quiet and sit and slouch at your desk all the time. (7th grade boy)
> You don't have to listen to boring stuff. (9th grade girl)
> You get to do things yourself and move. (9th grade girl)

In DanceMath, a 6th grade Danish boy reflected that, "it was fun with the music that made us move with such quiet and calm movements." Students experienced themselves moving in different ways than they are used to – sensing themselves differently. One math teacher observed:

> There are many side effects that this group in puberty can benefit from…here they seem to have high self-esteem. They don't seem critical towards themselves. They enjoy it and that seems to count more than any insecurity over what they might look like moving. It is the endorphins, so it's also physiological…their enjoyment moving. Their facial expressions are open. They concentrate…and it helps them to be less insecure, to remember…to enjoy learning.

Making dances involves imagination, multimodal learning, encounters with the physical and material world, and embodied interaction with others – which we suggest amounts to a kind of *bodily integrity* or agency. In educational dance, pupils practice autonomy and make choices in space. In these ways, *bodily integrity* relates to the next central capability – *senses, imagination, and thought,* as embodied learning.

Senses, Imagination and Thought

The central capability of *senses, imagination, and thought* refers to "being able to use the senses…use imagination and thought in connection with experiencing and producing works and events of one's own choice" (Nussbaum, 2011, p. 33). This includes freedom of artistic voice and the ability to "have pleasurable experiences…" (p. 33). In this study, pupils in both dance education settings described this capability, especially in relation to inventing and performing. Our first examples are from Finland.

> I hope our group can make up our very own performance. (2nd grade girl)
> You get to invent your own things and you don't have to do the same as others all the time. (4th grade girl)
> It would be fun to be able to suggest the different dances, street dance and others, and then, to choose and perform them. (5th grade boy)

Similarly, in the Danish DanceMath pilot project, participating 6th graders expressed that what they "liked best" was being asked to create a dance, practice, perform and watch each other:

> If we could just get the chance to be a little more creative than hop and slide and twist…if we could decide ourselves. (girl)
> I liked best when we created our own dances and performed them and the others watched and wrote down what we did. (girl)
> I liked when we performed with our group …when you practice a piece, for example this with the letters [a-b-c], and show it. (boy)

A Finnish classroom teacher observed inventiveness and performing as abilities that 'wait' for the opportunity to manifest:

> The class likes to go to R's dance class. They rehearse dance in hallways and in PE classes – especially girls want to perform the dances they have invented. (3rd grade classroom teacher)

Another teacher observed that pupils' ability to invent and perform improved in dance education: "Inventiveness…has developed. Children found courage in bringing forth their own ideas" (anonymous). The dance teacher highlighted the significance of performing, in seeing and being seen, musing, "Maybe self-confidence becomes stronger when you are visible all the time and create movement."

In terms of embodied learning as the integration of *sensing, imagining* and *thinking,* the following upper grade Finnish pupil's reflection is relevant: "In dance, you learn to remember things because you move at the same time" (6th grade boy). Other Finnish pupils noted similarly:

> When you do different movements, you remember things better…you have experienced yourself. (7th grade girl)
> I learn better…when I do something, and with some fun ideas and tasks the dance teacher is teaching. (8th grade girl)

A male student in Denmark appreciated how DanceMath was different from what normally happens in math: "It was very good that we got to move ourselves instead of just opening a book and sit and write."

A Danish math teacher highlighted the difference between "normal" math and DanceMath when she spoke appreciatively about the creative and aesthetic dimensions of moving, inventing, and performing:

> It is not just movement, it is also aesthetic…when they did the geometrical shapes and the movements across the floor. Something else happened—they felt that they created some-

thing…this was beautiful. I also sensed this among the students. They became quiet and aware—totally involved. (female)

This teacher's comments point to children's emotional capability to become fully engaged in dance – quiet and aware in their felt sensing, part of an affective community (see Bond, 2008), which the teacher described as "beautiful."

Emotions

As a central capability, *emotions* enable "attachments to things and persons outside ourselves…to love, to grieve, to experience longing, gratitude, and justified anger…not having one's emotional development blighted by fear or anxiety" (Nussbaum, 2011, pp. 33–34). One emotion – joy – stands out in the Finnish data for both pupils and teachers.

Movement and fun, joy, it always makes you glad. (1st grade girl)
You get…you get joy. (4th grade girl)
Children get joy from it and still they learn something. (4th grade boy)
I feel good…moving is fun. (6th grade girl)
Dance…different…good spirits. (9th grade girl)

Finnish teacher reports corroborate students' descriptions of joy, some noting their own emotional connection to dance.

After dance classes, happy faces, movements and turns in school. (6th grade classroom teacher)
The joy of dancing is visible. (anonymous)
I have followed with joy the dance classes that take place…, through the windows, when walking. (anonymous)

Danish math teachers observed joy and happiness in DanceMath sessions:

The students have fun doing the exercises…this motivates them to engage and to work with the math content. The physical aspect helps them to be less insecure…I think it simply gives them a sense of joy.
They have…thrown themselves on the floor, done all kinds of things…they are happy.

Sixth graders in the Danish project talked about the "good energy" in DanceMath classes. Many examples relate to music.

You get more good energy when you listen to music. (boy)
I like when it is music we know…I go faster and better if it is music I like. (boy)

Finally, the word "fun" seems to be a kind of global meme used by children to describe quality of learning at schools. The following Danish boy uses the word in relation to artistic agency: "It is fun when we can decide the dance ourselves."

Dance education researchers, notably Karen Bond and Sue Stinson (Bond, 2000, 2008; Bond & Stinson, 2000/2001, 2007/2016; Stinson, 1997) have examined students' associations between dance and emotions. Studying adolescent engagement, Stinson (1997) found that "the word most often used by the students to describe their dance classes … was *fun*" (p. 53). Through meta-analysis of verbal and visual material from approximately 600 young people ages 3–18, Bond and Stinson (2000/2001) found consistent use of the words *fun* and *happy* in relation to dance. In our projects, emotion seems closely connected with *play*, the 9th central capability, and we diverge from Nussbaum's order to discuss play next.

Play

Being able to invent and move freely stand out as qualities that pupils strive for. Nussbaum (2011) argues for protecting *play* as equally central as the other capabilities. She asserts, "what play and the free expansion of the imaginative capacities contribute to human life is not merely instrumental but partly constitutive of a worthwhile human life" (p. 36). As a central capability, *play* relates to "being able to laugh, to play, to enjoy recreational activities" (p. 34). Clearly, the importance of play cannot be underestimated when considering quality of life of children and youth at schools. One could say that play makes learning fun (for all ages). Not being able to play can generate negative emotions, like fear and anger (Panksepp, 1998).

We might ask, why would school as an institution not value play? A male pupil in Finland (4th grade) ponders a seeming paradox that dance "is like playing and school at the same time…it is school but it still feels fun." Echoing statements from pupils in both projects, a Finnish 1st grade girl said that dance is needed in schools "so that children can at times play and not have to sit and listen all the time."

Denying the value of play or fun in school can generate boredom and disengagement. Stinson (1997) suggests that play can be an attitude towards any activity, and that as an attitude play involves choice, freedom, intrinsic rewards, and heightened focus. Bond and Stinson (2007/2016) assert that distinctions between work and play, or achievement and fun are not straightforward. It seems evident that children enjoy being challenged in dance and other activities, and we suggest that playfulness can be present at school and in any learning situation, as well as in working life (see also Anttila, 2003).

Bond (2017) notes that, "theorists have long situated dance in play," (p. 153) citing *Homo Ludens,* Johan Huizinga's (1955/1949) treatise on the subject:

> The connections between playing and dancing are so close that they hardly need illustrating. It is not that dancing has something of play in it or about it, rather that it is an integral part of play: the relationship is one of direct participation, almost of essential identity. Dancing is a…particularly perfect form of playing. (as cited in Bond, 2017, pp. 153–154)

Sheets-Johnstone (2009) identifies rough and tumble play as an evolutionary marker of dance (p. 322).

Considering the important connection between play and social development, we next make another detour from Nussbaum's order to address *affiliation*, the 7th central capability. Schools are highly social environments and for both younger and older pupils, peer group dynamics and qualities of social interaction are strong indicators of quality of life at schools.

Affiliation

Nussbaum (2011) defines affiliation as follows:

> Being able to live with and toward others, to recognize and show concern for other human beings, to engage in various forms of social interaction; to be able to imagine the situation of another . . . being able to be treated as a dignified being whose worth is equal to that of others. (p. 34)

Students' desire to collaborate with classmates was strongly evident in both projects – moving, creating, performing, and making decisions together. Thus, affiliation as a capability was related to the "work" of dance (Bond & Richard, 2005; Bond & Stinson, 2007/2016), as well as to being together with friends. From the Finnish school study:

> I like when we do our own performances with friends, that is nice. (4th grade girl)
> You get to be with your friends and make decisions. (7th grade boy)
> You even get to talk to your mates. (7th grade girl)
> In dance everyone gets to do things together…group spirit. Then it is easy to perform. (9th grade girl)

Some Finnish students reported learning group skills through dance. A female 7th grader reflected, "Nowadays I can work better in a group," and a similar testimony came from an 8th grade male: "I think I have learned to do group work better since I have been 2 years in dance classes."

In the Danish DanceMath project, students reflected that through common experiences they could see others in new ways, which contributed to different and better relationships.

> Those that you were not used to being with…you saw different angles of them. Some I have become more friendly with. (girl)
> It is fun to watch others, how they dance…you get to know each other better. (girl)

Some mentioned that the creative processes and physical contact in DanceMath made it especially different from other kinds of social learning.

> Instead of having to do it alone…the way of working together in groups is different because we were dancing. (girl)
> We usually have to help each other with calculating and so on but suddenly you had to move some legs because they had to be in a specific angle. (girl)

Teachers in both projects described positive changes in social skills and group dynamics. Social development was observed across grade levels in Finland:

> I think the dance classes have increased group cohesion, a good atmosphere in the classroom, as we work together. (1st grade classroom teacher)
> The project has for sure had positive effect on the atmosphere of the school. (2nd grade classroom teacher)

> The boys do not have difficulties collaborating with the girls anymore. The group spirit gets better all the time and I have given more time to collaborative games. (3rd grade classroom teacher)
>
> The dance project has developed group cohesion. (5th grade classroom teacher)
>
> It brings communality to the school and dance close to each pupil. (dance subject teacher)

In Denmark, participating 6th grade math teachers agreed that DanceMath supported a special kind of group affiliation.

> This is a different kind of group work…they could not work on these exercises on their own. This is real group collaboration.
>
> When they solve tasks together they learn more about themselves, their bodies and the others. They dare to perform. Souls and minds are put into play through their bodies and their personalities stand forth.
>
> They have…moved each other's legs around without emotional barriers…they are close to each other, and they are happy.

One math teacher observed that dance's physicality expands possibilities for interaction and can influence social status in the class.

> Some touched each other, cuddling each other's hair. I have never seen that before. It was like the hierarchy changed…those with low status suddenly got new opportunities. This was very special, it was what I paid most attention to.

In Finland, the dance subject teacher reflected on the difficulties of affiliating for some children, and the possible role of dance in becoming a member of a group:

> A new pupil arrived in the middle of fall and it was a challenge for him. He withdrew: "I cannot, I cannot." But little by little he came forward…and he participated greatly in the end.

There is a plenitude of literature and research on how dance enhances social skills and creates communities (Bond, 2008; Bond & Etwaroo, 2005; Buck, 2015; Katz, 2013; Chaps. 10, 21, 22, 28, this volume). At the same time, we are aware that dance can also generate peer pressure, competitiveness and anxiety (Bond, 2017; Hanna, 2006). We return to this issue in the closing of this paper.

Practical Reason

For discussion of *practical reason*, we return to embodied learning and the bodily origin of reasoning. Nussbaum (2011) defines this capability as being able to form a conception of the good and to engage in critical reflection in planning one's life (p. 34). In dance education, *practical reason* seems closely related to *senses, imagination* and *thought*, as exemplified in the following quotes from Finnish pupils:

> I prefer doing dance and math together, because then you learn two things at the same time. (2nd grade girl)
>
> In dance you get to practice and learn new things, so it is not that same class work all the time. (4th grade girl)
>
> I have thought that dance comes to schools because it allows learning a different way. (5th grade girl)

> You can learn English, which is easy to connect to dance… and math, the number of steps, counts… (6th grade boy)
>
> You learn more when you are allowed to do things…with your body. You could learn much more. … If you really start to develop this, it would really work. (9th grade girl)

Similarly, Danish pupils highlighted that something abstract becomes more concrete and "easier to understand" (as well as "fun"); they remember math better when they have learned it with their own bodies:

> It is much more fun to dance it than to just sit and write…I understood it better than before. (girl)
>
> I like when the dance teacher uses people to show math…it is easier to understand. (girl)
>
> I find some math things difficult, but I understood it more easily when we had DanceMath. (girl)

A few Danish boys noted areas of math that they preferred to learn in a conventional classroom:

> To calculate with letters [algebra], for example a + a = 2a, that was easier, but equations became more difficult in DanceMath…harder to understand.
>
> I would have understood it better if I had worked with a book.

Tuning into their *emotional* and *affiliative* capabilities, a Danish math teacher recounted: "I recorded situations with my phone where I can see boys who expressed they didn't like it so much actually 'had a party.'" Math teachers commented directly on the value of embodied learning:

> Dancing math helped them understand, for example, if you stand with your legs like a rhombus, you will remember the shape in your legs.
>
> No doubt some remember through their bodies, recall a physical sensation that helps them remember.

A Danish dance teacher reflected,

> I felt from time to time that they understood and took it with them…when I built onto something and made it more difficult the next time, they were able to solve the tasks.

Other Species

Embodiment connects us with non-human agents. Nussbaum's (2011) 8th central capability, *other species,* refers to "being able to live with concern for and in relation to animals, plants, and the world of nature" (p. 34). As suggested early in the chapter, it is important to understand how non-human elements and materiality influence learning and school life (Fenwick et al., 2011). Although data from the two dance education projects highlighted here do not offer evidence of this capability's value, dance education research and curriculum literature is abundant with resources and depictions of children's identification with animals, as well as with "natural" and built environments (Anttila, 2003; Bond, 2001, 2018; Sansom, 2013; Chap. 5, this volume). Many pupils in pre-school and the lower grades perform this capability well. Unhesitant towards transformative play, they may readily embody, explore and perform the other-than-human world.

Control Over One's Environment

Nussbaum's (2011) 10th capability, *control over one's environment,* returns us to *bodily health* and *integrity*, that is, the ability to maintain health and move freely in the world. *Control over one's environment* is "being able to participate effectively in political choices that govern one's life…having the protections of free speech and association" (p. 34). Based on principles of democracy and pluralism, this capability nurtures and respects individual agency and social diversity.

As noted already, both Danish and Finnish pupils appreciated that in dance they were able to "decide on movements" and "do things yourself." We see a pattern in how pupils talked about their open possibilities in dance. In this section, we highlight in bold italics students' words that emphasize their agency and choice, beginning with the Finland project.

> You ***get to*** invent your own things and you ***don't have to*** do the same as others. (4th grade girl)
> You ***get to*** be with your friends and make decisions. (7th grade boy)
> You ***get to*** do things yourself—usually in learning you just have to write and you cannot try it out yourself… (7th grade girl)
> You ***can*** decide the movements, you are not compelled…you ***do not have to*** do something and you have influence (8th grade girl)

Like the many Finnish children, the Danish 6th graders also valued their individual agency:

> I like when we create our own dances, when we ***can*** decide ourselves. (boy)
> I like when we do our own things with our ***totally own*** movements. (boy)
> We ***could*** make up our own dances ***instead of having to*** do it the way the teacher decided… much more fun. (girl)
> It is always more fun when you ***can*** choose ***instead of having to*** do something someone else said…to have freedom to choose. (girl)
> I just prefer when I ***can*** decide myself. (girl)

Independence in choice of music was also valued. A female student in DanceMath reflected, "It was great when the teacher asked which music we wanted for our performances."

Educational research has illuminated dance's empowerment of children, youth, teachers, and communities (Bond, 2008; Katz, 2013; Martin, 2015; Rowe, 2016). Edited anthologies and conference proceedings offer global perspectives (Bresler, 2007; Shapiro, 2008; Stinson, Liu, & Svendler Nielsen, 2012; Svendler Nielsen & Burridge, 2015; Svendler Nielsen & Koff, 2017). In the present study, students' cross-national descriptions illustrate desire and capabilities for quality of life at schools. A Finnish pupil connects affiliation with emotions, practical reason, and more, illustrating the complex relationship between central capabilities: "Dance is needed so that there is some fun in school…collaboration and such. Fun studying and a bit different and we would have good spirits" (9th grade girl).

Conclusion

It has become evident to us that the power of dance at schools extends beyond visible outcomes in motor skills or in "measurable" academic success. DanceMath supports learning of mathematical concepts, but the dance in it gives opportunities for learning in a broader perspective relating to body consciousness, creativity, the courage to perform, and better social relations, i.e., in quality of life. Likewise, the Finnish "Entire School Dances!" project altered children's way of being in school, as well as the overall school atmosphere. Dance became a part of everyday life at the school, where interaction was enacted as embodied events and performative acts.

We are aware that not every school provides experiences that enhance the quality of school life. We suggest that quality of learning is enriched by multisensory experiences that engage the learner fully and are accompanied with reflective processes that strengthen student agency. We consider such learning as embodied learning, and that holistic engagement is an indispensable element of embodied learning. Hence, we connect high-quality learning processes with enhancing quality of life at schools.

In order to understand the potential power of dance in fostering quality of life at schools, it seems important to consider how individual, embodied and felt experiences intertwine with communal, shared life. Based on our analysis, pupils appreciate the possibility to make choices, invent movements, work creatively together, perform their own dances, and witness others' dances. The mutual recognition involved in performing, understood as seeing and being seen, seems a vital step on the path from bodily awareness to community. *Senses, imagination,* and *thought* intertwine with *emotions*, *play*, and *affiliation*, enhancing possibilities for pupils to act in the world and to become part of a community.

In DanceMath, community developed within specific classrooms, and in the Finnish project classroom communities extended and affected the entire school through common events and performances. When dance is introduced as a democratic, inclusive practice, it may bring about change that is not imposed, but created from within. Thus, practicing and performing dance is a social, shared event, and dance education is an inclusive, collaborative practice. This is how the capabilities generated by dance and embodied learning extend beyond subject areas and schools. These capabilities are related to being together and living together, to accepting oneself and others, and to creativity and collaboration.

References

Anderson, B., & Harrison, P. (2010). The promise of non-representational theories. In B. Anderson & P. Harrison (Eds.), *Taking-place: Non-representational theories and geography* (pp. 1–33). Surrey, UK: Ashgate.

Anttila, E. (2003). *A dream journey to the unknown: Searching for dialogue in dance education. Acta Scenica 14.* Helsinki, Finland: Theatre Academy. Retrieved from https://helda.helsinki.fi/handle/10138/33789

Anttila, E. (2013). *Koko koulu tanssii! Kehollisen oppimisen mahdollisuuksia kouluyhteisössä.* [The entire school dances! The possibilities of embodied learning in a school community]. *Acta Scenica 37.* Helsinki, Finland: Theatre Academy. Retrieved from https://helda.helsinki.fi/handle/10138/42322

Anttila, E. (2015). Dance as embodied dialogue: Insights from a school project in Finland. In C. Svendler Nielsen & S. Burridge (Eds.), *Dance education around the world: Perspectives on dance, young people and change* (pp. 79–87). New York: Routledge.

Bond, K. (2001). "I'm not an eagle, I'm a chicken!" young children's perceptions of creative dance. *Early Childhood Connections, 7*(1), 41–51.

Bond, K. (2008). The human nature of dance: Towards a theory of aesthetic community. In S. Malloch & C. Trevarthen (Eds.), *Communicative musicality: Exploring the basis of human companionship* (pp. 401–422). Oxford, UK: Oxford University Press.

Bond, K. (2018). "Me, a tree": Young children as natural phenomenologists. In S. Fraleigh (Ed.), *Back to the dance itself: Phenomenologies of the body in performance* (pp. 205–232). Urbana: University of Illinois Press.

Bond, K. E. (2000). Revisioning purpose: Children, dance and the culture of caring. Keynote address. In J. E. LeDrew & H. Ritenberg (Eds.), *Proceedings – Extensions & extremities: Points of departure* (pp. 3–14). Regina, SK: Canada: Dance and the Child International.

Bond, K. E. (2014). Dance and quality of life. In A. C. Michalos (Ed.), *Encyclopedia of quality of life and well-being research* (pp. 1419–1424). Dordrecht, The Netherlands: Springer.

Bond, K. E. (2017). "Boys are morons" … "Girls are gross": Let's dance! In W. Oliver & D. Risner (Eds.), *Dance and gender: An evidence based approach* (pp. 37–57). Gainesville, FL: University Press of Florida.

Bond, K. E., & Etwaroo, I. (2005). "If I really see you..." students' experiences of identity and difference in a higher education setting. In M. C. Powell & V. M. Speiser (Eds.), *The arts, education and social change: Little signs of hope* (pp. 87–100). New York, NY: Peter Lang.

Bond, K. E., & Richard, B. (2005). "Ladies and gentlemen! What do you see? What do you feel?" A story of connected curriculum in a third grade dance education setting. In L. Overby & B. Lepczyk (Eds.), *Dance: Current selected research (Volume 5)* (pp. 85–134). New York: AMS.

Bond, K. E., & Stinson, S. W. (2000/2001). "I feel like I'm going to take off!" young people's experiences of the superordinary in dance. *Dance Research Journal, 32*(2), 52–87.

Bond, K. E., & Stinson, S. W. (2016). "It's work, work, work, work:" Young people's experiences of effort and engagement in dance. In S. W. Stinson (Ed.), *Embodied curriculum theory and research in arts education: A dance scholar's search for meaning* (pp. 269–295). Dordrecht, The Netherlands: Springer. (Original work published 2007).

Bresler, L. (Ed.). (2007). *International handbook of research in arts education.* Dordrecht, The Netherlands: Springer.

Buck, R. (2015). Stepping back to step forward: Reflections on future directions on dance education. In C. Svendler Nielsen & S. Burridge (Eds.), *Dance education around the world: Perspectives on dance, young people and change* (pp. 161–167). New York: Routledge.

Eerola, P., & Eerola, T. (2013). Extended music education enhances the quality of school life. *Music Education Research.* Retrieved from http://www.tandfonline.com/doi/full/10.1080/14613808.2013.829428#preview

Fenwick, T., Edwards, R., & Sawchuk, P. (2011). *Emerging approaches to educational research: Tracing the sociomaterial*. New York: Routledge.

Fridström, H., Björklund, B., & Andersson, N. (2011). *Dansmatte för högstadiet. Att dansa matematik* [DanceMath for secondary level. To dance mathematics]. Västerrås, SE: The Department for Dance in Schools.

Hanna, J. L. (2006). *Dancing for health*. Lanham, MD: Rowman & Littlefield.

Katz, M. (Ed.). (2013). *Moving ideas: Multimodality and embodied learning in communities and schools*. New York: Peter Lang.

Kyttä, M., Hirvonen, J., Rudner, J., Pirjola, I. & Laatikainen, T. (2015) The last free range children? Children's independent mobility in Finland in the 1990s and 2010s. *Journal of Transport Geography, 47*, 1–12. Retrieved from http://www.sciencedirect.com/science/article/pii/S0966692315001271

Martin, R. K. (2015). The politics of dance education in post-revolutionary Cairo. In C. Svendler Nielsen & S. Burridge (Eds.), *Dance education around the world: Perspectives on dance, young people and change* (pp. 64–67). Abingdon, UK: Routledge.

Nussbaum, M. (2011). *Creating capabilities: The human development approach*. Cambridge, UK: Belknap.

Nussbaum, M., & Sen, A. (1993). *The quality of life*. Oxford, UK: Oxford University Press.

Panksepp, J. (1998). *Affective neuroscience: The foundations of human and animal emotions*. Oxford, UK: Oxford University Press.

Pulkkinen, L., & Launonen, L. (2005). *Eheytetty koulupäivä – lapsilähtöinen näkökulma koulupäivän uudistamiseen*. [Integrated school day: A child-centered approach to the reform of a school day.] Helsinki, Finland: Edita.

Reason, P., & Bradbury, H. (Eds.). (2008). *The SAGE handbook of action research: Participative inquiry and practice* (2nd ed.). London: SAGE.

Ricciardelli, L. A., & Yager, Z. (2016). *Adolescence and body image: From development to preventing dissatisfaction*. New York: Routledge.

Rowe, N. (2016). Threshold concept theory and nonformal education: Community-based arts learning in Palestine. *Educational Research for Social Change (ERSC), 5*(1), 94–106.

Sansom, A. N. (2013). Daring to dance: Making a case for the place of dance in children's and teachers' lives within early childhood settings. In F. McArdle & G. Boldt (Eds.), *Young children, pedagogy and the arts: Ways of seeing* (pp. 34–49). New York: Routledge.

Shapiro, S. (Ed.). (2008). *Dance in a world of change: Reflections on globalization and cultural differences*. Champaign, IL: Human Kinetics.

Sheets-Johnstone, M. (2009). "Man has always danced:" Forays into an art largely forgotten by philosophers. In *The corporeal turn: An interdisciplinary reader* (pp. 306–327). Exeter, UK: Imprint Academic.

Sheets-Johnstone, M. (2010). Body and movement: Basic dynamic principles. In S. Gallagher & D. Schmicking (Eds.), *Handbook of phenomenology and cognitive science* (pp. 217–234). Dordrecht, The Netherlands: Springer Science & Business Media B.V.

Smith-Autard, J. (1994). *The art of dance in education*. London, England: A & C Black.

Stinson, S. W. (1997). A question of fun: Adolescent engagement in dance education. *Dance Research Journal, 29*(2), 49–69.

Stinson, S. W., Liu, S., & Svendler Nielsen, C. (Eds.). (2012). *Dance, young people and change – Proceedings of the World Dance Alliance/Dance and the Child International Conference*. Retrieved from http://www.worlddancealliance.net/Publications.html

Svendler Nielsen, C. (2009). Children's embodied voices: Approaching children's experiences through multi-modal interviewing. *Phenomenology & Practice, 3*(1), 80–93. Retrieved from https://ejournals.library.ualberta.ca/index.php/pandpr/article/viewFile/19822/15340

Svendler Nielsen, C. (2012). Looking for children's experiences in movement. The role of the body in "videographic participation." *Forum: Qualitative Social Research, 13*(3). Retrieved from http://www.qualitative-research.net/index.php/fqs/article/view/1571/3449. ISSN: 1438–5627.

Svendler Nielsen, C. (2015). Exploring learning in dance as artistic-educational practice. In C. Svendler Nielsen & S. Burridge (Eds.), *Dance education around the world: Perspectives on dance, young people and change* (pp. 117–126). New York: Routledge.

Svendler Nielsen, C., & Burridge, S. (Eds.). (2015). *Dance education around the world: Perspectives on dance, young people and change*. New York: Routledge.

Svendler Nielsen, C., & Koff, S. (Eds.). (2017). *Exploring identities in dance – Proceedings from the 13th World Congress of Dance and the Child International.* Retrieved from http://ausdance.org.au/publications/details/exploring-identities-in-dance

Young, I. M. (1980). Throwing like a girl: A phenomenology of feminine bodily comportment, motility and spatiality. *Human Studies, 3*, 137–156.

Chapter 20
Discovering Freedom in Dance Education

Monica Jordan Cameron Frichtel

Introduction

My understanding of freedom in dance has developed in part through experiences as a dancer and dance educator and in part by dance philosophers and researchers such as Karen Bond (2008, 2013, 2017, in press), Sondra Fraleigh (1987, 1993, 2004), Danielle Goldman (2010), Maxine Sheets-Johnstone (1999, 2009), and Sue Stinson (2016). Dance freedom has been theorized as agency, autonomy, and authentic aesthetic expression and variously associated with *flow* (Csikzentmihalyi, 1990/2008), *peak experience* (Maslow, 1962), and *heightened engagement* (Bond, 1994, 2008; Bond & Stinson, 2000/2001). Such states have been illuminated through dance students' descriptive accounts (Alter, 1997; Anttila, 2004; Bond, 1994, 2008, 2013, 2017; Bond & Etwaroo, 2005; Bond & Stinson, 2000/2001, 2007/2016; Dyer, 2010a, 2010b, 2014; Frichtel, 2012; Kane, 2013; Martins, 2013a, 2013b; O'Flynn, Pryer, & Gray, 2013; Stinson, 2016). Experiential descriptions of dancing are laced with references to freedom.

From a young age, subjective descriptions of "dancing freedom" or "freedom dancing" are marked directly with words like *free, freeing,* and *freedom*, and indirectly through poetics, metaphor, and practical reason. An elementary school student combines both: "Dance was freedom…all big…like it was my house" (Bond & Stinson, 2000/2001, p. 60). Together such meanings: experiences of and reflections on freedom in dance, form the category of perception that I refer to as *freedom* in this chapter. I consider pursuit of freedom a core purpose of dance education for both students and teachers: freedom in movement and interpretation of movement, freedom in the ability to make choices, to respond and create, and freedom in relationships that evolve between individuals and the environment. Students' narratives of dancing sometimes include the particular language that I employ, creating direct

M. J. C. Frichtel (✉)
Temple University, Philadelphia, PA, USA
e-mail: mfricht@temple.edu

K. Bond (ed.), *Dance and the Quality of Life*, Social Indicators Research Series 73,
https://doi.org/10.1007/978-3-319-95699-2_20

associations between *free* (and its linguistic variations) and phenomena I include under the umbrella category of *freedom*. All such examples inform discussion.

This chapter presents a broad context for understanding subjective experiences of freedom in dance generally and dance education specifically. I engage with previous research investigating students' (pre-school through higher education) and adults' perceptions of freedom in dance. Further, students' descriptions and meanings of freedom are elaborated with dance philosophers' reflections on the idea of freedom. I also consider the role of phenomenological and critical pedagogy in facilitating students' autonomy, agency, aesthetic expression, and awareness of possibilities in dance education.

While much of the literature I discuss addresses research with student dancers in formal education, an exception is Rosemary Martin's (2013a, 2013b) work examining dance experiences of adult women in the southern Mediterranean region. Acknowledging there are many ways to participate in dance – different roles (e.g., choreographer, performer), purposes (e.g., religious, social, artistic), genres, and techniques that span cultures, for example – it is important to recognize that any given conditions could give rise to wide-ranging experiences of both freedom and limitation. The dance highlighted in this paper is concerned primarily with creative movement, improvisation, and western techniques and pedagogies. Exceptions include when students are introduced to non-western dance practices within a western educational framework.

Dance, Freedom, and Quality of Life

Dance philosophers have theorized freedom as lived experience arising from existential capacities and intentions. Several decades of phenomenological discourse on the lived experience of freedom in dancing include: Sondra Fraleigh's (1987, 2004) examination of the "lived body's" aesthetic pursuit of "intrinsic dance"; Maxine Sheets-Johnstone's (1999) framing of dance as a thinking, feeling, conscious act of emancipation; Karen Bond and Sue Stinson's (2000/2001) analysis of children's meanings of dance as freedom of flight, feelings, space, flow, spirit, and more; and Danielle Goldman's (2010) formulation of dance improvisation as a "practice of freedom" fraught with aesthetic and political constraints (after Foucault).

For Fraleigh (1993), bodily perceptions, sensations, and actions are fundamental to any experience of freedom. She writes, "the metaphysical ideal of freedom… defines dancing moments" (p. 110). Her understanding of freedom accounts for inherent conflict – biological, social, political, and other limitations and insecurities of life that define and influence one's understanding and experience of freedom. Perceiving one's body in comparison to other bodies, for example, affects the experience of self. Building upon previous ideas, Fraleigh (2004) writes of bodily experience:

> Alienation, the sense of separation from others, seems located precisely in this experience. Embodiment is thus the ground for all experienced values, for intimacy and alienation, freedom and limitation. (p. 17)

Dance is therefore, a *practice* of freedom – an intentional act of escaping the utilitarian actions of daily life to experience motional agency and possibility. Dance, both choreographed and improvised, can *ensure* bodily lived freedom in the temporary abandonment of everyday actions. In abandoning movement with utilitarian outcomes, one can focus on the embodied performance or creativity of dance. Such embodiment involves making choices to exercise creative freedom, which begins at a young age (Bond, 2000; Bond & Stinson, 2000/2001), some suggest from birth (Bond, 2018; Dissanayake, 2000, Coda, this volume).

Sheets-Johnstone (1999, 2009) builds a case for existential freedom that requires personal investment and felt risk. Drawing on Edmund Husserl, Sheets-Johnstone (1999) understands consciousness as rooted in doing – in moving. I move, therefore, I come to understand possibility. She explains, "Our very emergence as cognizing subjects is grounded in our original kinetic spontaneity" (p. 138) through which we come to know the world and ourselves as meaning making bodies and participants in life (Sheets-Johnstone, 2009). Any "awareness of corporeal powers" comes from *experiencing* movement – from the activity or "thing itself" (Husserl, 1919/1982) and not from *thinking* about such experience (Sheets-Johnstone, 1999, p. 134). Sheets-Johnstone argues that movement is the very basis of human life and *aliveness*. Movement itself generates kinesthetic awareness and thus the recognition of freedom in movement – the ability to vary, alter, and ultimately influence and control what is done. The personal investment or agency that Fraleigh (1987) claims is inherent to experiencing freedom entails risk and wonder (p. 37).

Goldman (2010) looks at the physical practice of freedom across diverse cultures through the genre of improvisational dance, drawing comparisons with political and social "tight spaces," where freedom is limited by socio-political forces of race, gender, sexuality, class, time, and artistic convention (p. 6). This notion is recognizable in Fraleigh's (1987) sense of the socio-political and other limitations that can shape perceptions of freedom. For Fraleigh and Goldman freedom is not the endpoint or goal, but something pursued and practiced, felt and experienced, while fundamentally unattainable in life. Experiences of freedom in dance are imagined, desired, sought after, felt, and valued by participants, and are consequently relevant to discourses on quality of life and well-being.

Goldman (2010) aligns with Michel Foucault's emphasis on the necessity of "practices of freedom" in the midst of an existence where there is minimal space for freedom (p. 144). She views improvisational dance as one such practice while challenging the sometimes taken-for-granted view that improvisational dance epitomizes freedom in its open invitation to create spontaneous movement. Recognizing the ever-shifting restraints of bodies and ideas, improvisational dance builds awareness of kinesthetic possibilities so that dancers might make choices reflexively when facing "tight spaces," exercising aesthetic autonomy. Goldman's contributions extend Fraleigh's and Sheets-Johnstone's ideas on dance as a practice of freedom accounting for agency and risk.

Dance education researchers have elaborated meanings of experienced freedom, including such phenomena as heightened engagement and affect, bodily empowerment, and transformation. Notably, Bond and Stinson (2000/2001) illuminate students' experienced freedom in dance across childhood and adolescence (ages 3–18), as in the following developmental sequence:

> I feel like I'm going to take off! (pre-school) (p. 60)
> Flow is if you do something you go with it and it just busts out. (elementary school) (p. 59)
> My goal, every time, is to get in that zone where everything around me just seems to dance and I can… just kind of let things go. (middle school) (p. 67)
> I don't have any limitations even though I do physically. In my mind, I have no limitations. (high school) (p. 60)

Some students' descriptions suggest altered perceptions of space and time. A high school student wrote, "I'm the only person in that little world. I have my own little world I can go to" (p. 67). Another high school student experienced deep engagement in dance to the level of "magic:" "When I move my body to a beat, or let it flow and ripple, I become engrossed in a magic spell" (p. 68).

All these varied depictions seem related to embodied freedom, illustrating breaks from the restraints of day-to-day challenges. The authors reflect that student dancers in their study place a high value on "bodily, emotional, intellectual, social, and spiritual" freedom and that they desire, seek, create, and find meaning in heightened experiences of engagement (p. 76). Becky Dyer (2010a) reports that, "images of 'taking flight,' 'birth,' 'transformation,' 'journeying together,' … were recurring themes in student discussions, writings and choreography" (p. 12) in her inner city high school dance class.

Dance engagement scholars calling attention to unique experiences of lived body in dance have drawn on Mihalyi Csikzentmihalyi's (1990/2008) theory of *flow,* where full investment in an act inspires a kind of all encompassing, or autotelic, engagement (Bond, 2013; Bond & Stinson, 2000/2001; Clark, 2016; Cowper & Michelle, 2013; Hefferon & Ollis, 2006; Stinson, 1997; Chaps. 13 and 30, this volume), and Abraham Maslow's (1962) theory of peak experience, or self-actualization (Bond & Stinson, 2000/2001, Cowper & Michelle, 2013; Li, 2016; Chap. 30, this volume). Together, notions of freedom, flow, and peak experience point to engagement that is intrinsically motivating and personally meaningful as unique experience that feels voluntary and significant.

Dance Education and Pedagogies of Freedom

Experiences of action, power, and agency as well as oppression, conflict, and limits influence our sense of physicality, shaping perceptions of what can and cannot be done – how one might act, move, or be an agent of opportunity. In dance education, students negotiate personal strengths and limitations, working together to create movement in time and space, while at the same time navigating the extant power dynamics in teacher-student relationships and educational institutions.

The "freedom and justice pedagogies" – phenomenological, critical, feminist, pluralist, have directly and indirectly influenced dance education theory and practice (Bond, 2017; Bond & Etwaroo, 2005; Dyer, 2010a, 2010b; Frichtel, 2012; Green, 2000; Ottey, 1996; Richard, 2009; Shapiro, 1998; Stinson, 2016). Oriented to social justice as well as to nurturing the unique in each student, phenomenological pedagogy supports existential freedom through a commitment to understanding the call of what it means to be a teacher (van Manen, 1982): "Phenomenology bids to cover reflectively the grounds which, in a deep sense, provide for the possibility of our pedagogic concerns…" (p. 298). A phenomenological attitude, then, can enable dance educators to facilitate students' experiences of agency, autonomy, authentic aesthetic expression, and awareness of possibility. Phenomenological pedagogy is grounded in a philosophy of action dealing with the practical and stressing the personal engagement of educator and student (van Manen, 1990).

The idea that active participation in the world is fundamental to the nature of existence is salient. Faced with multitudes of possibilities to move in the world we each face the privilege "to act upon our freedom, to move beyond, to transform our lives" (Greene, 1983, p. 399). The relationship between agency and freedom can be uniquely experienced in student-centered dance education, where each moment in time and space might be full of choices, often with no other purpose than multisensory poetics, or aisthetic transformation (Bond, 2008; Chap. 12, this volume). Manipulations of time, space, body, and energy affect the aesthetic experience of the dancer and those viewing the dance. Negotiations of bodies moving and finding stillness together, negotiations of intent, abilities and themes, and shifting and changing possibilities shape and nuance any given dance.

A critical pedagogical aim in dance education is to guide students towards critique of authoritarian practices and realization of autonomy and possibility (Duffy, 2014). For Brazilian educational philosopher Paulo Freire (1970/2018) and affiliated critical theorists in dance education (Greene, 1983; Shapiro, 1998; Stinson, 2016; Chaps. 5 and 23, this volume), liberation becomes possible only through practice of reflection directed towards transformation. After Freire, Darder and Baltodano (2009) suggest that critical pedagogy exists at the crux of overcoming fear of freedom in order to pursue the desire for freedom; this duality has to be resolved in order to pursue social transformation. Along with related transformative pedagogies, critical pedagogy values individual agency in construction of knowledge, while deconstructing the power structure that shapes perceptions and experiences of freedom.

Freedom's Dance/Dancing Freedom

Bond (2014) notes that, "A range of populations, including survivors of trauma and sexual abuse, prisoners, the aged, and children in educational settings, have reported that dancing creates an increased sense of freedom" (p. 1423). In this section, I attempt to fathom meanings of freedom from student dancers' reflections on what it means to dance. The human potential to experience freedom in dance lies outside of teaching styles, techniques, and cultural styles, despite western dance's relationship with the disciplinary aspects of training, technique, and pedagogy. Modern dance, in particular, often explores democratic themes of social justice and equality, pursuits of freedom and liberation, even while practices of training are sometimes entrenched in traditions of power, authority, control, and inequality (Bond, 2013, 2017; Bond & Stinson, 2007/2016; Fraleigh, 1993; Frichtel, 2012; Lakes, 2005; Martin, 2013a, 2013b; Shapiro, 1998; Stinson, 1997, 2016). Robin Lakes (2005) asserts, "The lay public may be amazed at the horrors inflicted in the name of dance, an art form that many associate with freedom, expressivity, passion, and abandon" (p. 3). Aligned with Freire's thinking (Darder & Baltodano, 2009), experiences of freedom can be desired and sought after as well as resisted and feared in dance (Goldman, 2010; Gottschild, 2003).

In this chapter, I examine the theme primarily through the multiple perspectives of university general education dance students enrolled in a dance pluralism course, a context of evolving research for over a decade (Bond, 2017; Bond & Etwaroo, 2005; Bond, Frichtel, & Gerdes, 2009; Bond & Gerdes, 2009; Frichtel, 2012). In response to a reading assignment, Bond and Etwaroo's (2005) research article about the course, a student wrote,

> I am not certain when I became afraid of my voice, but I am ready to lose that fear. I am also unsure of when I started being so passive about my feelings, but I want to move beyond that. I want to assert my distinctive spirit. (Frichtel, 2012, p. 111)

In this course for students who are not dance majors, many participants express excitement and desire, despite fear, to express themselves and share with others through movement and dance, regardless of varied previous dance education. Another student wrote,

> I expected to just do some reading and dance in class, but after reading this article and actually taking the class I realize that it is so much more. In this class I am not only on an educational journey, but also a spiritual, physical, and mental journey. (p. 104)

Freedom was first recognized in dance pluralism students' descriptions of dancing by Bond and Etwaroo (2005) and surfaced as an overarching theme in my in-depth study of students across five sections of the course (Frichtel, 2012); I quote particularly liberally from the latter data. Bond's (2017) study of dance pluralism students' writings about gender across 16 sections of the course (2008–2012) also includes references to freedom. Students have depicted dancing as the freedom *to be* and *to experience* ease, grace, release, presence, body, acceptance, friendship, difference, change, and caring for self and others, among other qualities of life. A student shared a sentiment recounted numerous times over the years: "This is the only class where I can be free and express myself. I don't feel judged" (p. 104; see Bond & Etwaroo, 2005, for similar student disclosures). Another described how bodily relaxation enabled a sense of freedom: "I relaxed and got lost in the Haitian style. I was free and not stressed or worried. I just danced" (pp. 137–138). These students represent many others across the studies noted above who experienced freedom's dance in pluralistic atmospheres of nonjudgment and relaxation from "stress and worry."

Experiential descriptions support the perspective that improvisational dance, the primary modality of the course, offers unique opportunities to embody freedom. One student wrote the following about an improvisation experience: "I felt things and expressed them in ways I never have" (p. 124). Others aligned their improvisational dance with freedom more directly: "I moved freely and individually. I was creative and not on display…" (p. 125); "I felt self-aware and free during the improvisation" (p. 126). The following reflection conveys a composite of awareness, expression, and communication with other and environment:

> This improvisation entailed feeling and responding to the music, as well as responding to others through wordless communication. … It was a spiritual experience; I connected strongly with myself, my partner, and the music. (p. 125)

Awareness or lack of awareness of one's *performing body* can also influence whether they feel free while dancing. The freedom of not being on display, for example, might suggest a body-self acting as an agent in their own practice, challenging, as Fortin, Long, and Lord (2002) posit somatic practices do, the contingent, "inscribed" body that dance scholar Susan Foster (1986, 1996) has long theorized.

For some, freedom is experienced in dance practices that are consciously defined and directed. Connecting with her Romany heritage, a dance pluralism student wrote, "I felt free dancing to rhythmic beats of the drums and brought out my Romany side. I explored the sounds of the music and various movements of my choice" (Frichtel, 2012, p. 138). While this student recognized a particular agenda of her own choosing, others described moments of freedom within movement structures established or put in place by others. The following exemplifies an experience of freedom that arose during spontaneous and collaborative choreography:

> When we altered my gesture, it took on a different meaning. We all crossed our arms and one-by-one we shook them faster and faster. By the end the last member of our group was shaking so fast her arms seemed almost like they would unhook. In this movement, I perceived freedom and breaking from the norm. (p. 121)

Analyzing university dance majors' perceptions of dance, Judith Alter (1997) recognized multiple meanings in relationships between freedom and expression and relatedness: "Dancing gave them freedom and joy; it gave them a chance to express themselves and a feeling of being unified" (p. 72).

It seems clear from the above and many other lived experience accounts that experiences and meanings of freedom in dance are multi-dimensional: bodily, emotional, intellectual, social, and spiritual. As introduced earlier, Bond and Stinson (2000/2001) found freedom tales and images spanning the educational spectrum from pre-school through secondary. Stinson (1993, 1997) identified freedom as a subjective experience of adolescent dance students in public school settings, citing descriptions of freedom in both middle school and high school dance. A high school student describes a complex state that she perceives as "freedom":

> I can let go of all my worries, all my inhibitions. It is very exhilarating to just move where the music takes me. I get a sense of freedom, I'm not constrained in any way, and that's beautiful. (Bond & Stinson, 2000/2001, p. 60)

Alexis Marimom, an 18-year-old male dance student at El Colegio del Cuerpo in Cartagena, Colombia tells a journalist (Moloney, 2008),

> For me, dancing means freedom. It allows me to escape and forget the violence and hunger around me. I know it sounds a bit fantastical but when I'm dancing I can drift into another world. Just with a simple deep breath or a long, slow stretch of an arm or leg, bad thoughts can disappear. (n.p.)

Alexis's teacher and director of El Colegio del Cuerpo, Alvaro Restrepo, comments:

> I believe that the body is … a means of expression that can improve the quality of life. Through dance we can teach kids to inhabit their own bodies as a territory of peace and dignity, and we can give them a means by which to face poverty. We can transmit to them another notion of wealth, a notion of dignity and a sense of the rights they have. (n.p.)

Tom, a participant in Zihao Li's (2016) research with boys in a Canadian high school dance setting, stated, "I like our class because it is not judgmental in any way. You are free to do whatever you want as long as you try and have a good attitude towards what you are doing" (p. 128), reminding us that freedom often has responsibilities.

Agency and Empowerment

Freedom to dance and in dance can afford agency and empowerment, that is, choosing and acting upon opportunities to make decisions and direct change. Any actual movement, like any actual thought, requires agency and motivation as shaped by experiences, current state, reflexive action, and bodily-kinesthetic and tactile experiences and knowledge (Sheets-Johnstone, 1999, p. 422). Opportunities to make choices and security in not being criticized for choices characterize students' experiences of freedom (Anttila, 2004; Bond & Etwaroo, 2005; Bond & Stinson, 2000/2001; Dyer, 2010b, 2014; Frichtel, 2012; Stinson, 1997; Stinson, Blumenfeld-Jones, & Van Dyke, 1990/2016).

In their study of young adolescent women's perceptions of dancing in private studios, Stinson et al. (1990/2016) found that students might have less actual freedom than what they perceive, at least in terms of *choosing* to dance. For these young women, dance was mostly something their parents chose for them, which continues today (Bond, 2017). Yet, Stinson et al. (1990/2016) note, "…our respondents clearly valued the idea of free choice in regard to whether or not one dances; several said that being forced to dance would ruin the experience…" (p. 209). It seems that for these advanced older adolescent private studio dancers, all female, the initial opportunity to study dance may have been by parental choice, but continuing was as an individual matter. In any case, children who never have the opportunity to study dance will arguably have less agency with movement and, ultimately, less opportunity to experience dance's freedom.

Transformation, a phenomenon with strong freedom associations, has been identified as a theme of dance student engagement (Bond, 1994; Bond & Stinson,

2000/2001; Frichtel, 2012; Stinson, 1997; Stinson et al., 1990/2016). Young dancers describe "being in the zone" and experiencing "altered awareness of space and time" (Stinson, 1997, p. 60), being "nowhere," a "moment of pure joy…unconscious of human limits" and "more of a soul" (Bond & Stinson, 2000/2001, pp. 67–71). The frequency of depictions raises the question of whether such experiences manifest through a kind of phenomenological bracketing that enables the dancer to practice existential freedom. The following description from a dance pluralism class depicts a student's experience of transformation as freedom-to-express: "In class I was transformed. I was free and I could express my ideas. I didn't have to be a professional to participate" (Frichtel, 2012, p. 91). Philosopher Francis Sparshott (1988) discusses the possibility of transformation through experiences of intense aesthetic engagement.

According to Anttila (2004), student dancers' experiences of empowerment are in themselves practices of freedom. Further, dancers make empowering choices while maintaining responsibility towards others. A dance pluralism student illustrates this relation between power and responsibility: "Outside we improvised movement, taking turns leading and following. I had an immense amount of power for a short amount of time when it was my turn to lead, and then I passed it on" (p. 134). Another student wrote, "I was free to dance for whatever cause I chose and not be judged. I felt an obligation to dance for my people and have their name be heard. It was freeing just to say the word…" (p. 149). This student was able to affirm her responsibility for others through a sense of agency dancing.

For some students, however, functioning as an independent force making constant movement choices is challenging: "It was difficult to continually invent new moves" (p. 126). Further, agency is not necessarily something that all students aspire to or believe they can achieve in dance:

> The gesture study makes me feel uncomfortable. A regular gesture is fine, but distorting it feels wrong. I don't like coming up with my own moves on the spot and I felt out of my element. If it's someone else's move I'll go along with it, but I prefer structure to free form. (p. 123)

Questioning whether agency is prerequisite for experiencing freedom, Becky Dyer (2014) extends the work of educational theorists committed to democratic, progressive, and transformative pedagogies, such as Maxine Greene, Paulo Freire, and bell hooks. She suggests that in developing the critical capacities of thinking through dance, students might develop greater "awareness of their individual freedom and the moral responsibilities that accompany that freedom" (p. 47). Dyer proposes that such a pedagogical framework requires creating opportunities for students to practice freedom and responsibility – to explore agency in making choices – and that such experiences can lead to transformation. In other words, critical, phenomenological and other progressive pedagogies that seek to promote student agency might lead to transformation among individuals and communities. Some participants value such experiences and take their learning beyond the classroom, but Dyer (2010b) notes that not all students readily accept the active engagement required of such pedagogies.

In the Freirean sense, critical pedagogy is framed by dialectics of power and freedom (Darder & Baltodano, 2009; Kincheloe, 2008). Critical pedagogy recognizes and critiques political power structures imbedded within education. It is concerned with domination and the various forms of social oppression related to race, class, gender, sexual identity, culture, religion, age, and ability. The ever-shifting premises of critical theory refute that "people are passive, easily manipulated victims" and support that individuals are agents in social communities (Kincheloe, 2008, p. 56). Critical pedagogy addresses the value of power when directed towards hope, change, transformation, and liberation. Power can be used to empower, engage, and effect change. Power "works to shape both the oppressive and productive nature of the human tradition" (p. 54).

Despite their expressed desires to experience freedom, some students acknowledge personal "discomfort" as a restriction (Frichtel, 2012, p. 217). A dance pluralism student wrote, "I was not comfortable enough with myself to perform full out in front of the class" (p. 143). Another described:

> I internalized the idea of an audience even though no one in class was watching me dance. I could not shake the feeling that I was on a stage. The invisible audience that I imagined was judging me and I wasn't fully present. I even laughed sometimes and pretended that I did not care that I was so horrendous at dancing. (p. 135)

In contrast, others described how feeling secure with their peers enabled them to participate in both speaking and dance invention: "I was free to say whatever I felt and not be criticized. I could actually talk, have a conversation, and learn from it" (p. 171); "Making my solo, I felt focused and excited…I didn't feel I would be judged by my classmates" (p. 145).

Similarly, Martin (2013a) recognized a spectrum of experience, noting that one of her students described a novel sense of freedom in her early improvisational dance experiences, while another felt a sense of alienation around being an agent of their own dance practice, in improvisation and other classes. Martin suggests that the differing contexts of these students' dance education – liberal arts vs. studio training – might have shaped their experiences. Her study also describes how mastering technical forms of dance can give students a sense of control over their own dance practices and artistry (pp. 206, 210), affording a kind of freedom. In this sense, engagement is associated with movement that *becomes* engrained through technical study and proficiency (O'Flynn et al., 2013, p. 135).

A common premise of nineteenth and twentieth century theories of creativity is that domains of artistic pursuits must first be understood and then unpopular ideas must be pursued that push the current frames of thinking and appreciating. In other words, learn the rules and expectations of a field, so that they can then be broken (Sternberg, Lubart, Kaufman, & Pretz, 2010). In dance, understanding the technique of particular dance styles enables the dance artist to move beyond expectations of a genre to make works that are novel and creative. It can be argued that the discipline of learning specific techniques fosters creative freedom by placing limits on practices of dance. The premise is that such limits can then be pushed, shaped, and negotiated through creative and artistic agency.

O'Flynn et al.'s (2013) discussion of "right" and "natural" movement proposes that what feels right is influenced by social relations as well as bodily and discursive meanings; further, the experience of dance can be "located in the idea of dance equating freedom" in contemporary western traditions (p. 135). The authors also suggest that descriptions of movement *becoming* natural suggest that the dance experience is qualitatively unique from other movement experiences. On the other hand, Bond's (1994, 2008) empirical research with nonverbal deaf-blind children supports a bio-aesthetic perspective that "personal style" in dance arises from non-discursive agency (Bond, 2018), an existential freedom that mediates engagement in the social and the cultural. In any case, movement that feels "right" or "natural" is arguably an experience of embodied freedom in dance (Fraleigh, 2004). Some dance pluralism students used the word *natural* for movement that *feels right.*

> Doing the dance, I felt powerful and natural, although I wasn't that good at it. With no male or female moves, we all moved together. There was no audience to please. My internal audience was gone. It was just the class and the dance. I was not worried about appearance or messing up like I usually am. (Frichtel, 2012, p. 136)

In a "just the class" context, students might both free up personal and social boundaries, and experience relief from everyday stresses of life.

> I completely forgot about the steps. I experienced others by noticing the movements they performed. I became comfortable and open with others, freely dedicating myself to them as they were to me. I felt like I had escaped the realities of work, school, family, stress, and issues that bog my life down. (p. 132)

Descriptions linked to feeling "powerful," "in control," "strong," or "comfortable" recognize dancers' experiences that fall outside of social norms of femininity and beauty. At the same time, Bond (2017) found that some female students relate the hard work of dance to "the freedom to feel feminine: "Ballet gave me the freedom to feel feminine because although I looked graceful and delicate, I was really straining and working very hard to keep up appearances" (p. 141).

Male students in Bond's (2017) study reported that they were not particularly drawn to stereotypically "masculine" activities such as sports and few of the males with previous dance experience recalled parental support. This differs from how many of the females discuss their experiences of being enrolled in dance by parents, usually mothers, at the age of two or three. *Continuing* to dance is perceived as a choice. Some males worry about gay stereotypes, but they enroll anyway. There is a unique freedom in *choosing* to dance without parental and peer support and encouragement.

Contradiction and Paradox

In dance, freedom means different things to different people and peoples. Collectively, ideas such as immersion, escape, presence, choice, obligation, alienation, liberation, need, control, power, flow, autonomy, privacy, connection, suspense, support, responsibility, and transformation co-exist under the umbrella of freedom. Fraleigh (1993) describes dancing as "pure presence" – a "radiant power of feeling completely present to myself and connected to the world" (p. 104). In contrast, "…we may forget ourselves, get lost; the motion consumes the mover" (p. 107). Freedom seems as elusive to define as dance itself (see Bond, 2014).

> Power is sometimes used to describe experiences of freedom dancing: Doing the dance, I felt powerful and natural…we all moved together. There was no audience to please. My internal audience was gone. It was just the class and the dance. I was not worried about appearance or messing up like I usually am. I felt more alone dancing than I ever had before despite many other people dancing with me. (Frichtel, 2012, p. 136)

Power and control are related ideas, and correlate to freedom. In this example, it seems that the student's experience of power is related to communal experience of dancing with others.

Considering the "paired opposites" of *freedom* and *control* that can co-exist in individual descriptions of experienced freedom, Brenda Dixon Gottschild (2003) suggests: "In some sense, we can say that dance of all kinds is about the literal and/or metaphorical play and balance between freedom and control" (p. 37). She applies a cultural lens, describing a difference between "Europeanist" and "Africanist" perspectives – within bodies and across cultures, where Europeanist ballet epitomizes the value of control, and Africanist dance forms emphasize the value of freedom. She also discusses Africanist dance's focus on energy, which is "often interpreted as a sign of liberation," stating, "So, the paradox: The people who endured four centuries of slavery in the Americas are the dancing emblems of liberation; a flexible dancing body implies freedom of the spirit" (p. 245). Bond and Stinson (2000/2001) cite a number of African-descended students' connections between freedom, spirit, and control, for example: "It felt like there was a god or a spirit inside of me. It was making me move. From where I know, I was flying" (elementary school) (p. 68).

Martin (2013b) describes the contrasting perceptions of students in improvisation and creative movement classes. Some find such experiences liberating, while others struggle to understand the purpose and seem to become trapped, not knowing what to do or how to exert their agency. Dance pluralism students in my own classes have also reflected on the challenges of creating and performing choreographed and improvisational dance, alluding to the tensions between freedom and restriction in creative practices such as dance. The following describes resistance to the class's improvisational method of guided discovery, stating, "Part of me wants to remain extremely uncomfortable when people get too close. I want my own way of self-discovery, not anyone else's. Last class, all I wanted to do was resist" (Frichtel, 2012, p. 157).

Similarly, Goldman (2010) discusses apparent contradictions in improvisational dance. Her navigation of socio-political "tight spaces" as a practice of freedom – pushing boundaries and discovering possibilities in places that do not immediately evoke freedom. Fortin et al. (2002) suggest that "creative self-fashioning" or the perception of "space to become," specifically, to challenge the authority encoded in technique, can be advanced through democratic practices that seek to empower students (p. 171). For this student, the dance experience takes her beyond the rigidity of performing the steps as well as the routines of daily life:

> I completely forgot about the steps. I experienced others by noticing the movements they performed. I became comfortable and open with others freely dedicating myself to them as they were to me. I felt like I had escaped the realities of work, school, family, stress, and issues that bog my life down. (Frichtel, 2012, p. 132)

Finding freedom where it does not seem to exist is perhaps intrinsic to creative work and pertinent to quality of life. Viktor Frankl (1946/2006), holocaust survivor, interned in Auschwitz, purports that the way one imagines purpose affects one's quality of life. His psychotherapeutic method of logotherapy requires the practitioner to imagine purpose and to then immerse in the creative process of imagining a positive outcome. Defined limits can challenge artists to work within confines or break free of restraints.

While seemingly contradictory, experiences of escape and "full presence" in dance can coincide in dance descriptions. The following example suggests both *escape* and *presence* when a student immerses herself in an improvisational exercise:

> Suddenly, I felt my imagination come alive and my movements were entirely reflective of the imaginary situation. It was an adventure through which I had to maneuver my way through with a series of obstacles. I moved from one situation to another so quickly that I had no time to consider the strangeness of my actions. It was just all very real and I felt suspense as to what would come next. (Frichtel, 2012, p. 123)

As introduced earlier, such depictions align with Csikszentmihalyi's (1990/2008) theory of *flow* and Maslow's (1962) construct of *peak experience,* both of which are grounded in phenomena of intrinsic motivation, engagement, autonomy, and personal power. Heightened engagement in creative practices can be perceived as both full presence or immersion and as escape from unrelated distractions. In what Csikszentmihalyi (1990/2008) describes as *optimal experience*, *flow* is associated with alertness, unselfconsciousness, and full involvement in the present. Release and constraint, surrender and resistance, contraction and flow, expressing authentic self while feeling responsibility for others – are all ways freedom can be experienced, perceived, and reflected upon in dance – spanning the bodily, emotional, intellectual, social, and spiritual potentials of life.

Closing Reflection and Vision

In this chapter, I have sought to expand discourse on perceptions of freedom as pertinent to quality of life, highlighting dancers', in particular student dancers' descriptive accounts of dance as freedom, or freedom as a dance. I propose that the "freedom pedagogies," teaching practices that are oriented towards personal change and social justice, are uniquely positioned to frame pursuits of freedom in dance education. As we have seen, freedom is associated experientially with bodily awareness, self-expression, confidence, heightened engagement, and agency, all salient to quality of life and well-being (Beghetto, 2006; Bond & Stinson, 2000/2001, 2007/2016; Csikszentmihalyi, 1990/2008; Ryan & Deci, 2001; Seligman, 2011). Furthermore, freedoms experienced, practiced, and valued in dance can support conceptions of freedom that arise through analysis, social learning, and reflection, spanning and integrating bodily, emotional, intellectual, social, and spiritual aspects of life (Bond, 2017; Dyer, 2009, 2010b; Risner, 2008; Shapiro, 1998; Stinson, 2005).

Dancing, relating, teaching, questioning: all these actions can be directed towards pursuits of freedom and change, and pedagogies that value exploration and facilitate discovery might serve such pursuits particularly well. Choice, skill, desirability of outcome, and intrinsic motivation are cited as key components of the experience of freedom (Csikszentmihalyi & Graef, 2014). Dancing can afford the agency to make choices, develop skill, compose, and create. Experiences of engagement in dance, as highlighted in this chapter, suggest intrinsic motivation and more broadly freedom (Bond, 1994, 2017; Bond & Etwaroo, 2005; Bond & Stinson, 2000/2001; Dyer, 2009, 2010a, 2010b; Frichtel, 2012; Martin, 2013a, 2013b). Phenomena of heightened engagement, transformation, community, and "creative self-fashioning," as Fortin et al. (2002) suggest (p. 171), correlate to perceptions of freedom and are salient to quality of life.

Dance artists and educators have been thinking and writing about dance as a practice of freedom since the early twentieth century (Berger, Serlin, & Siderits, 2007; Bond, 2013; H'Doubler, 1940/1998), reflecting a thread of continuity in how the arts are perceived as creative practices (Darder & Baltodano, 2009). Some contemporary scholars view freedom as an ethical imperative of dance and dance education (Bond, 2017; Bond & Stinson, 2000/2001; Goldman, 2010; LaMothe, 2015; Martin, 2013a, 2013b). Student-experienced freedom might be a goal of best practice in a dance education that values of agency, autonomy, authenticity, and possibility.

Recent dance education discourse has centered on critical, transformative, and somatic pedagogical practices as means to more egalitarian dance education (Barr & Risner, 2014; Bond, 2017; Dragon, 2014; Dyer, 2009, 2010a, 2010b; Fortin et al., 2002; Frichtel, 2012; Green, 2000; Risner, 2008; Stinson, 2016). Growing evidence suggests that dance can be a practice of freedom to realize change through aesthetic embodiment, discovery, analysis, reflection, and meaning-making. A dance education that calls students to dance and think in autonomous, critical, and reflective ways might indeed foster learning that recognizes pursuits and discoveries of freedom as essential to quality of life.

References

Alter, J. (1997). Why dance students pursue dance: Studies of dance students from 1953 to 1993. *Dance Research Journal, 29*(2), 70–89.

Anttila, E. (2004). Dance learning as practice of freedom. In E. Anttila, S. Hämäläinen, L. Rouhiainen, & T. Löytönen (Eds.). *The same difference? ethical and political perspectives on dance*, (pp. 19–62). Theatre Academy, Finland: Acta Scenica 17.

Barr, S., & Risner, D. (2014). Weaving social foundations through dance pedagogy: A pedagogy of uncovering. *Journal of Dance Education, 14*(4), 136–145.

Beghetto, R. (2006). Creative self-efficacy: Correlates in middle and secondary students. *Creativity Research Journal, 18*, 447–457.

Berger, M., Serlin, I., & Siderits, M. (2007). Dancing women's freedom: The story of Isadora Duncan. In E. Gavin, A. Clamar, & M. Siderits (Eds.), *Women of vision: Their psychology, circumstances, and success* (pp. 11–28). New York: Springer.

Bond, K. (2000). *Revisioning purpose: Children, dance and the culture of caring*. Keynote address presented at the dance and the Child international (daCi) conference, Regina, Saskatchewan, Canada.

Bond, K. (2006). *Course proposal. Embodying pluralism: Dynamics of race and diversity in American society*. Philadelphia: Temple University.

Bond, K. (2013). Recurrence and renewal: Enduring themes in children's dance. In T. K. Hagood & L. C. Kahlich (Eds.), *Revisiting impulse: A contemporary look at writings on dance, 1950–1970* (pp. 161–192). Youngstown, NY: Cambria.

Bond, K. (2017). "Boys are morons"… "girls are gross": Let's dance! In W. Oliver & D. Risner (Eds.), *Dance and gender: An evidence based approach* (pp. 37–57). Gainesville: University Press of Florida.

Bond, K. (2018). "Me, a tree": Young children as natural phenomenologists. In S. Fraleigh (Ed.), *Back to the dance itself: Phenomenologies of the body in performance* (pp. 105–133). Urbana: University of Illinois Press.

Bond, K., & Etwaroo, I. (2005). "If I really see you…": Experiences of identity and difference in a higher-education setting. In M. C. Powell & V. Marcow-Speiser (Eds.), *The arts, education, and social change: Little signs of hope* (pp. 87–99). New York: Peter Lang.

Bond, K., Frichtel, M., & Gerdes, E. (2009). *Embodying Pluralism: Dynamics of race and diversity in American society*. Paper presented at World Dance Alliance Conference, Madison, WI.

Bond, K. E. (1994). Personal style as a mediator of engagement in dance: Watching Terpsichore rise. *Dance Research Journal, 26*(1), 15–26.

Bond, K. E. (2008). The human nature of dance: Towards a theory of aesthetic community. In S. Malloch & C. Trevarthen (Eds.), *Communicative musicality: Exploring the basis of human companionship* (pp. 401–422). Oxford: Oxford University Press.

Bond, K. E. (2014). Dance and the quality of life. In A. C. Michalos (Ed.), *Encyclopedia of quality of life and well-being research* (pp. 1419–1424). Dordrecht, The Netherlands: Springer.

Bond, K. E., & Stinson S. W. (2000/2001). "I feel like I'm going to take off!": Young people's experiences of the superordinary in dance. *Dance Research Journal, 32*(2), 52–87.

Bond, K. E., & Stinson, S. W. (2016). "It's work, work, work, work:" Young people's experiences of effort and engagement in dance. In S. W. Stinson, *Embodied curriculum theory and research in arts education: A dance scholar's search for meaning* (pp. 269–295). Dordrecht, The Netherlands: Springer. (Original work published 2007).

Bond, K., Frichtel, M., & Gerdes, E. (2009). *Embodying pluralism: Dynamics of race & diversity in American society*. Madison, WI: World Dance Alliance Conference.

Clark, C. (2016). "We learned to perform by performing:" Ballet dancers in a beer hall. *Journal of Dance Education, 16*, 139–143.

Cowper, M., & Michelle, C. (2013). Dancing with inspiration in New Zealand and Australian dance communities. In C. McDonald & B. Sellers-Young (Eds.), *Belly dance around the world: New communities, performance and identity* (pp. 93–105). London: McFarland.

Csikszentmihalyi, M. (2008). *Flow: The psychology of optimal experience.* New York: Harper Perennial. (Original work published 1990).

Csikszentmihalyi, M., & Graef, R. (2014). *Flow and the foundations of positive psychology.* Dordrecht, The Netherlands: Springer.

Darder, A., & Baltodano, M. (2009). *The critical pedagogy reader.* New York: Routledge.

Dissanayake, E. (2000). *Art and intimacy: How the arts began.* Seattle, WA: University of Washington Press.

Dragon, D. (2014). Creating cultures of teaching and learning: Conveying dance and somatic education pedagogy. *Journal of Dance Education, 15*(1), 25–32.

Duffy, A. (2014). What would Liz and Larry say? Performing critical approaches to choreographic mentorship in American higher education. *Research in Dance Education, 16*(2), 114–127.

Dyer, B. (2009). Merging traditional technique vocabularies with democratic teaching perspectives in dance education: A consideration of aesthetic values and their sociopolitical contexts. *Journal of Aesthetic Education, 43*(4), 108–123.

Dyer, B. (2010a). Ruminations of a road traveled towards empowerment: Musing narratives of teaching, learning and self-realization. *Research in Dance Education, 11*(1), 5–18.

Dyer, B. (2010b). The perils, privileges and pleasures of seeking right from wrong: Reflecting upon student perspectives of social processes, value systems, agency and the becoming of identity in the dance technique classroom. *Research in Dance Education, 11*(2), 109–129.

Dyer, B. (2014). Exploring social and moral learning frameworks through collaborative inquiry. *Journal of Dance Education, 14*(2), 45–51.

Fortin, S., Long, W., & Lord, M. (2002). Three voices: Researching how somatics informs contemporary dance technique classes. *Research in Dance Education, 3*(2), 155–179.

Foster, S. L. (1986). *Reading dancing: Bodies and subjects in contemporary American dance.* Berkeley: University of California Press.

Foster, S. L. (1996). *Corporealities: Dancing knowledge, culture and power.* London: Routledge.

Fraleigh, S. (1993). Good intentions and dancing moments: Agency, freedom, and self-knowledge in dance. In U. Neisser (Ed.), *The perceived self: Ecological and interpersonal sources of self-knowledge* (pp. 102–111). Cambridge, UK: Cambridge University Press.

Fraleigh, S. (2004). *Dancing identity: Metaphysics in motion.* Pittsburgh, PA: University of Pittsburgh Press.

Fraleigh, S. H. (1987). *Dance and the lived body: A descriptive aesthetics.* Pittsburgh, PA: University of Pittsburgh Press.

Frankl, V. E. (2006). *Man's search for meaning.* Boston: Beacon. (Original work published 1946).

Freire, P. (1970). *Pedagogy of the oppressed.* New York: Herder and Herder.

Frichtel, M. J. C. (2012). *Freedom, transformation, and community: Student meanings of engagement in a dance-based general education course.* (Doctoral dissertation). Retrieved from ProQuest Dissertations and Thesis database. (ATT 3509061).

Goldman, D. (2010). *I want to be ready: Improvised dance as a practice of freedom.* Ann Arbor, MI: University of Michigan Press.

Gottschild, B. D. (2003). *The black dancing body: A geography from coon to cool.* New York: Palgrave Macmillan.

Green, J. (2000). Emancipatory pedagogy: Women's bodies and the creative process in dance. *Frontiers: A Journal of Women's Studies, 21*(3), 124–140.

Greene, M. (1983). Curriculum and consciousness. In H. A. Giroux & D. E. Purpel (Eds.), *The hidden curriculum and moral education* (pp. 168–184). Berkeley, CA: McCutchan.

H'Doubler, M. N. (1998). *Dance: A creative art activity.* Madison, WI: University of Wisconsin Press. (Original work published 1940).

Hefferon, K., & Ollis, S. (2006). "Just clicks": An interpretive phenomenological analysis of professional dancers' experience of flow. *Research in Dance Education, 7*(2), 141–159. https://doi.org/10.1080/14647890601029527.

hooks, b. (1994). *Teaching to transgress: Education as the practice of freedom.* New York: Routledge.

Husserl, E. (1982). *Ideas: General introduction to a pure phenomenology* (F. Kersten, Trans.). The Hague, The Netherlands: Nijhoff. (Original work published 1919).
Kane, K. (2013). Best practices in the performing arts: Transformation and flourishing in a progressive summer dance theater program for adolescents. *Journal of Dance Education, 13*(3), 71–77.
Kincheloe, J. (2008). *Critical pedagogy primer*. New York: Peter Lang.
Lakes, R. (2005). The messages behind the methods: The authoritarian pedagogical legacy in western concert dance technique training and rehearsals. *Arts Education Policy Review, 106*(5), 3–18.
LaMothe, K. L. (2015). *Why we dance: A philosophy of bodily becoming*. New York: Columbia University Press.
Li, Z. (2016). *Dancing boys: High school males in dance*. Toronto, ON: University of Toronto Press.
Martin, R. (2013a). Alienation and transformation: An international education in contemporary dance. *Research in Dance Education, 14*(3), 201–215.
Martin, R. (2013b). Pushing boundaries: Reflections on teaching and learning contemporary dance in Amman. *Journal of Dance Education, 13*(2), 37–45.
Maslow, A. H. (1962). *Toward a psychology of being*. New York: D. Van Nostrand.
Merleau-Ponty, M. (1962). *Phenomenology of perception* (C. Smith, Trans.). New York: Humanities Press.
Moloney, A. (2008). For me, dancing means freedom. *The Guardian*. (US Edition). 29 April 2008.
O'Flynn, G., Pryer, Z., & Gray, T. (2013). Embodied subjectivities: Nine young women talking dance. *Journal of Dance Education, 13*(4), 130–138.
Ottey, S. (1996). Critical pedagogical theory and the dance educator. *Arts Education Policy Review, 98*(2), 31–39.
Richard, B. (2009). *"Daddy, root me in:" Tethering young sons in the context of male, intergenerational, child-centered, dance education*. Doctoral dissertation, Temple University, Philadelphia.
Risner, D. (2008). The politics of gender in dance pedagogy. *Journal of Dance Education, 8*(3), 94–97.
Ryan, R., & Deci, E. (2001). On happiness and human potentials: A review of research on hedonic and eudaimonic well-being. *Annual Review of Psychology, 52*, 141–166.
Seligman, M. (2011). *Flourish*. New York: Free Press.
Shapiro, S. B. (Ed.). (1998). *Dance, power, and difference: Critical and feminist perspectives on dance education*. Champaign, IL: Human Kinetics.
Sheets-Johnstone, M. (1999). *Primacy of movement*. Amsterdam: John Benjamins.
Sheets-Johnstone, M. (2009). *The corporeal turn: An interdisciplinary reader*. Exeter, UK: Imprint Academic.
Sparshott, F. (1988). *Off the ground: First steps towards a philosophical consideration of the dance*. Princeton, NJ: Princeton University Press.
Sternberg, R., Lubart, T., Kaufman, J., & Pretz, J. (2010). Creativity. In K. Holyoak & R. Morrison (Eds.), *The Cambridge handbook of thinking and reasoning* (pp. 351–369). New York: Cambridge University Press.
Stinson, S. W. (1993). A place called dance in schools. *Impulse, 1*(2), 90–114.
Stinson, S. W. (1997). A question of fun: Adolescent engagement in dance education. *Dance Research Journal, 29*(2), 49–69.
Stinson, S. W. (2005). The hidden curriculum of gender in dance education. *Journal of Dance Education, 5*(2), 51–57.
Stinson, S. W. (2016). *Embodied curriculum theory and research in arts education: A dance scholar's search for meaning*. Dordrecht, The Netherlands: Springer.
Stinson S. W., Blumenfeld-Jones, D., & Van Dyke, J. (2016). Voices of young women dance students: An interpretive study of meaning in dance. In S. W. Stinson, *Embodied curriculum*

theory and research in arts education: A dance scholar's search for meaning (pp. 199–218). Dordrecht, The Netherlands: Springer. (Original work published 1990).
van Manen, M. (1982). Phenomenological pedagogy. *Curriculum Studies, 12*(3), 283–299.
van Manen, M. (1990). Beyond assumptions: Shifting the limits of action research. *Theory Into Practice, 29*(3), 152–157.
van Manen, M. (1997). *Researching lived experience: Human science for an action sensitive pedagogy*. London, ONT: Althuss.

Chapter 21
University Dance Students in Taiwan Step Out of Their "Bubble" of Elite Dance Training

Yi-jung Wu

Introduction

Forty-one college dance students took part in a Dance Teaching Practicum through a university in northern Taiwan. This chapter focuses on the challenges and accomplishments of these professionally-trained dancers over the yearlong course, during which they brought quality learning experiences to children who normally lack access to creative dance in school. Teaching creative dance for children enabled college dance students to reconsider the value of dance as a holistic modality and to reflect on teaching as a transformative experience in their own dancing lives.

Since at least the early 1990s critics have suggested that dance programs in higher education are not providing sufficient instruction in teaching (Kahlich, 1990; Risner, 2010a, 2010b). In 2010, the *Journal of Dance Education* published a special issue on post-secondary dance education (Risner, 2010b), offering a range of views on the state of dance teacher preparation in the early 2000s. Increasing numbers of teacher-researchers are advocating that dance educators must be capable of employing diverse methods within holistic curricular frameworks (Andrzejewski, 2009; Bond, 2010, 2013, 2017; Musil, 2010; Stinson, 2010; Svendler Nielsen & Burridge, 2015). Multiple chapters in this volume convey such values (see Chaps. 5, 12, 13, 18, 19, 20, 21, 23). It appears that quality of educational life in dance is becoming an important topic of discourse in the twenty-first century.

Risner (2010a) asserts, however, that since the end of the twentieth century, dance departments in the United States have deviated from the goal of nurturing dancers, teachers, and independent thinkers to that of training professional performers. Further, the growth of BFA Dance programs has resulted in a reassignment of funds and resources, leading to the downsizing or closure of non-profession-oriented programs and K-12 teacher certification programs. A Higher Education Arts Data

Y.-j. Wu (✉)
University of Taipei, Taipei, Taiwan

K. Bond (ed.), *Dance and the Quality of Life*, Social Indicators Research Series 73,
https://doi.org/10.1007/978-3-319-95699-2_21

Services (HEADS, 2011) survey confirmed that the number of both BFA and MFA dance degrees, which focus on practical knowledge of performance, choreography, and technical training, was increasing steadily.

Despite this phenomenon of artistic professionalization, research demonstrates that a majority of dance graduates make their livings primarily by teaching (Bennett, 2009; Montgomery & Robinson, 2003; Warburton, 2004), a situation that extends beyond the USA. Surveys of dance and theatre teaching artists in Australia, New Zealand, Southeast Asia, the United Kingdom, and the United States reveal that most feel inadequately prepared for teaching diverse learners and have to learn through trial and error (Anderson & Risner, 2014; Anderson, Risner, & Butterworth, 2013, 2014; Bond, 2010; Risner, 2012). Such studies suggest a world-wide trend toward the commodification of dance education, which might be instilling in students a sense of uncertainty about the viability of dance education as a career.

The Dance Teaching Practicum

Since 2006, I have led a course titled Dance Teaching Practicum for dance majors at a university in northern Taiwan, guiding students to design creative dance activities and lesson plans to implement in elementary schools. I have found that most dance majors consider teaching creative dance with children highly challenging, even when they themselves possess outstanding dance technical abilities. This observation inspired me to conduct pedagogical research with this demographic of dance education as a means to developing reflective and experiential approaches for the Practicum curriculum. This chapter recounts how a cohort of college dance majors in Taiwan reconstructed their ideas about teaching dance through an in-depth process of learning creative dance pedagogy, and how this process affected their quality of dancing and teaching life, and for some, life in general.

Local Context: Professional Dance Education Versus Creative Dance Pedagogy in Taiwan

In 1981, a professional dance education program was established in selected elementary, junior high, and senior high schools in Taiwan as part of an "arts talented track" (Tang, 2004). After implementation of the Arts Education Act in 1997, the program became the Art Capacity Class-Dance Group, or simply Dance Class, for students with interest in dance as an art form (Chang, 2011). An entrance screening procedure is used to assess physical condition, dance technique, and improvisation. Dance Class students receive professional training mainly in ballet, modern dance, and Chinese dance. Some are also provided with an improvisation and creation (composition) course. Graduates of Dance Class usually move on to study dance in higher education.

Although Dance Class has been praised for achieving a high caliber of education for young dance artists (Chang, 2011; Tang, 2004), I have observed that it over-emphasizes technical training and can contribute to a student's lack of interest in creative dance. Moreover, those who train in private dance studios instead of Dance Class have even weaker backgrounds in dance improvisation and dance creation.

In his work on modern prison systems, Michel Foucault (1975/1995) pointed out that human bodies and behaviors are trained by institutions, social systems, and norms to function compliantly according to certain values or standards. Dance educator and scholar Jill Green (2002–03) argues that student dancers are no exception, often being shaped into docile, compliant bodies by the ritual of dance technique class. Similar to the five graduate students in Green's study, some of my students also expressed that dance technique classes with clear aesthetic standards provide a sense of achievement and security. On the other hand, the improvisation and creation course in high school left them feeling frustrated and uncertain, with its minimal guidance and unclear objectives (Wu & Huang, 2011a).

While practitioners have ranging definitions of creative dance, most agree the term refers to a student-centered teaching approach where students create rhythmic movement phrases or short pieces that serve as physical expressions of their inner and outer worlds (Exiner & Lloyd, 1973; Gilbert, 2015; Joyce, 1994). Foreshadowing the theme of this anthology, *Dance and Quality of Life*, arts education advocate Charles Fowler (1977) articulated the importance of self-expression in dance education, stating,

> Dance education is a medium for enhancing the quality of life for children, youth, and adults. Every human being has the right to move in ways that are primal, expressive, imaginative, and transformational. (p. 45)

Many dance educators champion creative dance's value in education at every developmental stage, pointing to gains across physical, cognitive, social, and affective domains of learning (Cone & Cone, 2005; Lloyd, 2014). In Taiwan, researchers have studied the benefits of integrating creative dance with other school subjects for young students (Wu, 2012).

Since the mid-twentieth century, dance education specialists have published monographs to assist teachers in the development of lesson plans, units, and full curricula for creative dance and to effectively guide students in educational settings (Andrews, 1954; Boorman, 1969, 1971; Chang, 2007; Cone & Cone, 2005; Exiner & Lloyd, 1973; Gilbert, 2015; Joyce, 1994; Lloyd, 2014; Murray, 1975; Overby, Post, & Newman, 2005; Russell, 1975; Stinson, 1988). This genre of literature reliably covers the following topics: educational rationale, definition of creative dance, relevant developmental theories, curriculum/content design, and teaching strategies and resources. Cone and Cone (2005) note that learning activities of creative dance include improvisation, movement exploration, and creation. Students change, manipulate, select, connect, and organize movement in relation to elements of body, space, time, energy, and relation.

Despite advances in dance education methods and validation over the last half-century, creative dance concepts and practices do not seem to be easily adopted by my college students, who have been mostly immersed in teacher-centered, technique-oriented learning environments. According to Argyris and Schön (1974), "theories of action" are learned in practice rather than from textbooks. The theories formed through action govern a person's practical behaviors, especially when externally introduced "espoused theories" conflict with personal values. Indeed, I have observed that students come to my class unaware of their assumptions about dance teaching and learning acquired through previous educational experiences (Wu & Huang, 2011b), or their "apprenticeships of observation" (Fortin & Siedentop, 1995; Lortie, 1975).

Prior to taking my class, most students had not imagined that teaching a creative dance class, which might look playful and non-technical, requires thoughtful preparation. Mary Joyce (1994) notes the complex, generative aspects of teaching creative dance, saying,

> The individual is the first source; in teaching, you seek to reach the part of the individual that is a composer rather than a player, an originator rather than an interpreter, a creator rather than a performer. (p. 1)

It seems clear that teaching the complex pedagogy of creative dance requires more than simply textbook theories and strategies.

Aligning with educational psychologist Lee Schulman's (1986) perspective of *pedagogical content knowledge*, which is the adaption of content and pedagogical knowledge based on practical context, and Sylvie Fortin's (1993) and Carey Andrzejewski's (2009) applications of Shulman's theory to dance education, in 2010 I began to incorporate experiential learning activities in the Practicum framed in three epistemological goals:

- to enhance students' awareness of their existing assumptions about teaching based on their professional dance training
- to help students eliminate self-doubt about their dance teaching abilities
- to expand students' focus on technical training to include an interest in holistic dance education. (Wu & Huang, 2011a, 2011b)

Methodology: A Critical Hermeneutic Case Study

In order to formally examine the process of students' learning in the Dance Practicum, I devised a case study based on critical hermeneutic epistemology. Hermeneutic practices date to antiquity in the interpretation of biblical and other ancient texts. Maruizio Ferraris (1988/1996) defines hermeneutics as an art of interpretation that seeks the transformative nature of understanding rather than a fixed meaning or factual reality. The blend of hermeneutics and critical theory stresses the interpreter's constant reflection on and critique of taken-for-granted bias during the process of inquiry (Habermas, 1990). By entering the "hermeneutic circle" (Heidegger, 1927/1996), I hoped to understand how, after a year of education in creative dance pedagogy, my students appeared to transition from the docile, obedient, mimetic, and teacher-centered "products" of their professional dance training, and how some of them came to envision their future with a broader understanding of dance as art, education, and life.

The Case Study

As a research method, the case study investigates how a bounded system, e.g., a person, group, class, project, or multiple cases, functions in a specific context (Merriam, 1988; Stake, 1995; Yin, 2013). This case study examines a class of 41 college dance students (38 women and 3 men) who took the 1-year Practicum during the 2014 academic year. I selected this class as a research site for its updated course design. We met 4 h per week for 36 weeks. Prior to college, most students had received professional dance training in Dance Class during elementary, middle, and/or high school for 3–10 years, but had little or no experience teaching dance. All participants provided informed consent and the study was approved by the university's Institutional Review Board (IRB). Pseudonyms are employed to protect students' identities.

Fore-understandings of Researcher and Participants Drawing on Martin Heidegger's notion of the "hermeneutic circle," Hans Gadamer (1960/2004) suggests that understanding is formed from "fore-understanding" (p. 293), which is shaped by temperament, family background, education, and the individual's sociocultural context. Based on this critical hermeneutic perspective, I will first examine how the fore-understandings of my students and myself, in terms of dance learning and teaching, had been shaped before coming to the Practicum.

Fore-understanding of the Researcher As a child of the 1970s in Taiwan, the era just before Dance Class was established, I attended private classes taught by, in my view, an unacknowledged pioneer of dance education in Taiwan, Ms. Sue-ying Su, who offered a comprehensive program of improvisation, creation, technique, and appreciation. Ms. Su taught classes in her friend's loft until she could afford to invest in her own dance studio, which she named Feiyue, or Soaring. Compulsory education demanded long hours of sitting and studying, and I recall that the creative dance at Ms. Su's studio provided a refreshing outlet for my pent-up energies.

I did not officially enter a dance degree program until I pursued graduate studies in the United States, where I became even more convinced that creative dance can enhance a child's quality of life and should be part of childhood education. I held a vision that every child has the right to experience creative dance as I had. After earning a PhD in Dance (Wu, 2005), I returned to Taiwan to teach in higher education, where I gradually realized, to my surprise, that all I had learned about holistic dance education in the U. S. was quite different from what my professionally-trained students experienced and understood.

Fore-understanding of the Participants Most of my students began their professional dance educations in elementary, middle, or high school, with a minority having only private studio backgrounds. As introduced earlier, their dance education included technical training in ballet, modern dance, and traditional Chinese dance. Most of them had also studied improvisation and creation. Over the years, about two-thirds of my students revealed that their improvisation and creation classes provided little or no guidance or structure. For example, teachers commonly instructed students to create short dance pieces within about 20 min and present them to the class. Moreover, teachers seldom articulated assessment criteria, but nonetheless graded students' work. Students recalled feeling insecure, if not frightened, during improvisation and creation class. Thus, prior to attending Practicum, most students saw creative dance pedagogy as little more than throwing a topic to students, playing music, and asking them to dance.

Integration of Researcher and Participant Fore-understandings My redesign of the Dance Teaching Practicum in 2010 endeavored to accommodate students' preference for practical learning, and students in turn have been willing to learn creative dance in spite of their general preference for dance technique and performance-related courses. I refashioned the Practicum using learning strategies aimed at developing students' awareness of creative dance pedagogy as performance. I wanted to help students realize that the dance studio could be an alternative performance space – a place to practice the performing art of teaching (Sarason, 1999), as well as a site of holistic education. As dance teachers, they might come to envisage themselves as choreographers and the teaching setting as a rehearsal where they guide student dancers to practice "educational choreographies."

Table 21.1 provides a content outline and schedule for the 2014 Dance Teaching Practicum (Y.-J. Wu, Syllabus, September 24, 2014). Later in the year, 13 students form collaborative teaching groups and travel to designated elementary schools, where they teach two creative dance sessions developed with each other during the Practicum throughout the year.

Data Analysis

Data for the study consisted of student assignments: lesson plans, reflective journals, peer review records, and self-documented teaching films created during the 2014 academic year. A research assistant, Yuting Huang, and I also made written notes during the data analysis process, which included my reflections on teaching the course and of particular students and episodes. We adopted Strauss and Corbin's (1990) three-stage coding process for qualitative data – open coding, selective coding, and axial coding – to help identify and shape meaning clusters out of the data and support the process of critical interpretation. Data analysis took place after the students graduated from college.

After Yuting coded the qualitative data, we engaged in in-depth discussions to justify her interpretations – a process that prompted me to reflect on my own a priori

Table 21.1 Dance teaching practicum, 2014

First Semester

Week	Learning activities	Week	Learning activities
1	**Unit 1: Who am I?** Discussion: 1. What makes a good lesson? 2. Finding a teacher inside me 3. My educational beliefs	10	Micro teaching: The preparation (continued) Assignment: Week 1 lesson plan
2		11	Micro teaching: The development – building students' abilities (15 min per group)
3	**Unit 2: Who to teach** Field trip to elementary school Teaching demo: creative dance Lecture, video & discussion: Theories of child development	12	
4		13	Group interviews: Discussion and critique of the lesson plan
5	**Unit 3: What to teach** Teaching demo: Using movement elements in dance teaching Class design: Arrangement of activities Class design: Flying Dragon's eight steps to a lesson plan Role play: What if I were a choreographer? Discussion: Why do we need a lesson plan?	14	**Unit 5: Integration** Micro teaching: Teaching a full class Preparation + development + conclusion (40 mins per group) Final presentation – Self-assessment and reflection Assignment: Learning documentation
6		15	
7		16	
8	**Unit 4: How to teach** Micro teaching (peer teaching groups, video feedback): The preparation (8 mins per person)	17	
9		18	

Second Semester

Week	Learning activities	Week	Learning activities
1	**Unit 6: Oral movement description** Presentation: Transcription of peer teaching practice videos from unit 5 Presentation: Analysis and practice of oral movement description skills	10	Micro teaching: second class (continued)
2		11	
3	**Unit 7: Curriculum design** Lecture Brainstorm week 2 lesson plan Assignment: Week 2 lesson plan	12	
4		13	**Unit 10: School practicum sessions** Collaborative teaching groups visit their assigned school site Getting ready for teaching Teaching!
5	**Unit 8: Classroom management** Scenario: Solving classroom management problems Micro teaching: "What if things could be played back…?" re-teaching a revised section	14	
6		15	
7		16	**Unit 11: Sharing and conclusion** Sharing, reflection, and discussion
8		17	
9	**Unit 9: Refining and rehearsing** Micro teaching: second class (40 mins per group)	18	Dance teaching workshop: guest teacher Final presentation – Self-assessment and reflection Assignment: Learning documentation

assumptions. In the final stage of axial coding, I renamed the coding categories to better capture students' growing awareness of their fore-understandings, which I propose changed their artistic and pedagogical sensibilities and therefore their quality of life in dance. Table 21.2 summarizes the study findings as they emerged across the stages of analysis.

In the following section, I present a critical hermeneutic interpretation of how students' quality of artistic and pedagogical life changed during the Practicum. I scaffold the discussion according to the three identified phases of the learning process: fore-understandings, challenges encountered, and change.

Research Findings

From Emphasis on the Physical to Exploration of Verbal Potentials

Before taking the Practicum, students had been trained to emphasize their physical and performing skills to the neglect of other abilities, such as verbalization and writing. In the beginning of the Practicum, nearly half of the participants described negative feelings related to writing and speaking, of which feeling nervous, feeling challenged, and "difficulty" were the top three. This seems unsurprising given that

Table 21.2 Stages of data analysis

Coding Stages	Open coding (by Yuting)	Selective coding 1 (by Yuting)	Selective coding 2 (by Yi-jung)	Axial coding (by Yi-jung)
Categories of meaning	17 categories of meanings related to students' reflections on dance teaching and creative dance	1. Difficult oral expression	1. Body concept	1. From emphasis on the physical to exploration of verbal potentials
		2. Past dance learning experience vs. creative dance teaching experience	2. Technique training	2. From predictable to unpredictable
		3. The difficulty of collaborative teaching	3. Self-identity in relation to others	3. From subjectivity to inter-subjectivity
		4. Understandings from the tedious teacher training process	4. Visions of dance	4. From dance to educational and social issues
		5. Reconsidering the meaning of education		
		6. Becoming aware of issues outside of dance		
		7. Growth out of frustration and pressure	[embedded in all four categories above]	[embedded in all four categories above]

the Practicum is aimed at developing multiple capacities for creative dance teaching, a task for which most students are not primed. In addition, students take 14–16 h of dance technique, performance, and composition classes per week, as well as evening or weekend rehearsals, leaving little time to develop other capacities.

Eight of the 41 students (more than one sixth) expressed directly their dislike of teaching. Xiaohong admitted, "I never like kids and am not interested in teaching at all." More interested in teaching professional-track students than beginners, Anna pointed out, "I just want to dance in the future, maybe taking a part-time job for teaching." Students' dislike of teaching was reflected in a lack of interest in the Practicum, as Dehui admitted, "I never wanted to be a teacher, and was not motivated to do the Dance Teaching Practicum." While students indicated that their struggles in the Practicum were related to deficiencies in oral, writing, and interpersonal skills, they expressed most concern about their speaking abilities, as they do not normally speak while dance training. Lan noted the class's weakness after observing the first round of teaching practice:

> I noticed most classmates have more or less problems with oral expression. Like me, I tend to speak too fast. Some people cannot express themselves clearly, some lack logical organization, and some like to use difficult words or jargon. Many of us need practice.

Suwen was a clear example of poor oral expression. Even with her peer co-teachers' patient support, she had difficulty speaking, despite having written, memorized, and rehearsed the lesson plan. In her journal she wrote,

> At the beginning, I really didn't know what I was talking about. My head went blank when I spoke. After a couple rounds of teaching practice, it was like subtitles of what I was going to say were coming out of my head.

Mili noted the challenge of writing a lesson plan: "After coming up with a theme, an outline of activities or games, and step-by-step instructions, we realized that our instructions had nothing to do with the theme." Mili's experience might be typical of college dance majors. Andrzejewski (2009) observes that college dance students seem to carry a tacit fore-understanding, an epistemological bias, that privileges body over mind in professional dance education.

While early in the Practicum, as illustrated above, some students' experienced quality of educational life appeared to be challenged, they gradually developed their multiple abilities in the Practicum. For example, in the beginning of the course, Fei faltered in oral presentation, speaking with a weak, tentative voice. In the second semester, however, she developed her own teaching style, which was calm, clear, and focused. From Fei's journal: "In the second semester, I got a sense of achievement and began liking to teach. It is unbelievable!!…I have a bit of self-confidence."

Fei's peers described their changes less expressively, but many improved their speaking skills by developing strategies or receiving support from classmates. As Laya shared, "I typed my script, showed it to my peers, and discussed what to adjust so that I could teach in a clear and smooth manner." In fact, nearly everyone described growing confidence, noting developments in speaking, writing, comprehending, problem-solving, or interacting with children. Many acknowledged the benefits of this "tedious" course, as Raishian put it:

> I learned so much from this course. In the beginning, we discussed the topic and wrote and rewrote endlessly until we got our final version of the lesson plan. Then, we practiced our teaching with our peers, received all the reviewers' comments, and re-taught after revisions. Finally, we…taught the real kids! The process was tedious. But those experiences definitely helped me grow…We made our first step!

From Predictable to Unpredictable

Prior to the Practicum, learning dance was predictable – codified and with few variations in student-teacher interaction and class format. Ailin pointed out, "Dance teaching has been stuck in the mode of teacher demonstrates and lectures about movements and then [students] practice." In the beginning, many students held the conception that teaching is easy. Both Oubi and Lily reflected that previously they only, "went through what to teach in the head" and then "gave a lesson."

Most students, therefore, expected creative dance teaching to require minimal preparation and to be similar to the improvisation and creation course in high school where teachers provided a topic, played music, and told students to "respond freely." Fortin and Siedentop (1995) reference Lortie (1975) to assert that in dance, "the apprenticeship of observation supports the conservatism of teaching, as teachers replicate what they learned as students" (p. 9). Oubi's and Lily's initial confidence in their teaching abilities likely arose from the predictable routine of dance technique classes.

Encountering creative dance content and pedagogy, students were surprised by its unpredictable, or emergent content, and generally "child-centered" teaching approach (Bond & Deans, 1997; Gilbert, 2015; Joyce, 1994). Almost half of the students wrote about "stress" while facing a class situation "beyond control." Keren exclaimed, "We were kind of shocked because the kids…were dashing right up to us." Tingting reflected, "As soon as they entered the room, I could sense they were not so disciplined…." May shared, "I felt every second of the 40-minute class was like a year. I was so worried that problems might occur."

Moreover, students with lack of verbal confidence were concerned they might make inappropriate responses to children's unpredictable behaviors. Meichu exclaimed, "I often forgot what I was supposed to say, when an unexpected condition interrupted my teaching flow." Lirong realized, "We need to have richer vocabulary to gain a sense of control." Ninhua became aware of her taken-for-granted pre-conceptions about dance teaching and learning, "In an activity, we took things for granted and forgot those kids hadn't been trained (professionally) and thus might not respond when we asked them to change their formation."

I continuously reminded students to drop jargon, habits, and expectations for dance class protocols when interacting with school children: "You don't need to count 'five, six, seven, eight' when cuing children to start reciting a poem." Hanyu called this process "resetting a teaching mindset." Xinyi reminded herself, "They create their own movements according to our guidance. I hope I can get used to it."

All the learning activities I designed for the Practicum were aimed at nudging students out of their "bubble" of elite professional training by challenging their assumptions about dance education. Most participants began to recognize their limitations. As Dayu stated, "I realize that there isn't only one way to teach." Cilan reflected, "If we are dictatorial (as our teachers were), children may want to quit or feel nervous and restricted." Insights such as "change accordingly," "have to improve our problem-solving ability," "respond promptly," and "handle all kinds of situations" appear often in students' writings, evidencing a release from the norms of professional dance training and greater understanding of dance education as a broad realm of access and practice.

While many felt nervous or uneasy in an unfamiliar pedagogical environment, Ailin experienced a sense of relief. As a dancer with attention deficit disorder (ADD), Ailin acknowledged that professionally-oriented training, with its specific standards of physicality and codified aesthetics, was not for her:

> In my dance learning journey, I often made my teacher angry over my lack of attention…I couldn't do as well as others. Now we are learning this new teaching method… You give them guidance, helping them express their creativity with their own bodies. That makes them full of confidence.

"Amazed" by the children's involvement and innovative expression, one co-teaching group discarded biases about "ordinary" children's interest or ability to dance. As Vannie said, "The children were more enthusiastic and active than we had imagined." Kewei observed, "The children were as engaged as we were, and their creativity was expressed in a very open and pure manner." Several student teachers noted a connection between clear oral guidance and children's ability to move in innovative ways. Yanru said, "Very often the [children] just copied our movements. When we provided varied oral guidance or personal instructions, their movements became more diverse."

Observing children's engagement and creative expressions seemed to broaden my students' conceptions of what was possible in a dance classroom, bursting the bubble of conservatory dance technique that had encased them for so long. Stepping out, they were surprised by children's enthusiastic and unrestricted, albeit "artistically unpolished" expressions of movement that transcend the boundaries of stylized dance technique.

From Subjectivity to Intersubjectivity

Students of Dance Class usually work on personal body conditioning and technique in the dance studio, with minimal social interaction. Accordingly, many of my college students disliked teaching because of its interactive nature. Yuchi wrote, "I fell in love with dance, with myself, in my first dance class when I could simply imitate the movement of the teacher and classmates." Anna reflected, "I am not good at interpersonal skills. In the future, I just want to dance." Rouen recalled, "I don't like kids or teaching. To me, teaching a 40-minute class was like hell."

More specifically, my students are accustomed to a teacher-centered learning environment where one-way transmission of messages from teacher to student is the primary channel and mode of communication. Thus, for some the personal interaction required in the student-centered learning environment of creative dance was difficult to adopt. Chili wrote, "In our first teaching internship class, three of us were very nervous. The class was very noisy. We called out, 'Attention' throughout the class." Similarly, when faced with a loud class in an elementary school, Aimay and Dayu felt "bombarded" and "like crying," respectively.

Of all research participants, Junjie was possibly the most detached from children, emotionally and physically. Watching a video recording of his practicum teaching a group of kindergartners, Yu-ting recorded the following:

> He's tall and handsome. He looks like an elegant prince, standing erectly, either against the wall or next to one of his female peer teachers who is leading the class, exactly like the live supporter in classical ballet repertoire. He dares not get close to the kids. The teaching task mainly falls upon his two peers.

Junjie's classmates were not as detached from children as he was; however, many were unsure what school children might like or dislike – whether they would enjoy the activities they designed.

In the Practicum, students had to learn how to support children in creative dance. In doing so, more than one-third became sensitive to children's needs and came to understand the intersubjective nature of the creative dance classroom, and perhaps, by extension, the possibility for all dance classrooms. Although the learning process was not easy, most students had positive experiences interacting with children and appreciated children's interactions with each other.

Some did not realize their potential for intersubjective sensitivity until the Practicum. Limin reflected,

> I used to view school children as little devils and kept a good distance from them…I knew I had no patience… To my surprise, I found I was doing well. I could catch the children's attention all the time.

Like Limin, about a quarter of the students expressed relief that children were not as "terrifying" as they had imagined, or were surprised by children's "genuine," "adorable," "forgiving," or "courageous" nature, and by their enthusiasm for movement. For example, Mila felt "grateful" and "amazed," elaborating, "Children really like our class. Their enthusiastic responses and full attention made me really enjoy teaching." Yuchi pointed out, "I realized that the teacher's careful observation of children's responses and environment can help children get involved in the class." Juer was uplifted by a young girl who exclaimed, "This class is really a super fun class of the whole world." Her peer teacher Xinyi agreed:

> I learned more from children than from my teacher. Looking at their sincere smiles and contact with me in activities, I felt tremendous joy deep in my heart. It was like the audience's applause, which is invaluable and irreplaceable.

Dola was probably the most skilled in interpersonal relations. Her best "crisis control" occurred when a couple of boys' complaints about the unfair result of a game interrupted the class flow. She persuaded the boys with an easy smile, "Come on. It's just a game. The most important thing is we all had a good time, isn't it?" By sounding as if she was talking to her buddies, she helped the boys throw off their feelings of injustice. Dola's intersubjectivity might derive from her involvement in public affairs as president of the student government in the dance department. As well, she acknowledged the value of Practicum for helping her to understand children's developmental stages and behaviors and to promote proactive solutions:

> I used to teach in a private dance studio and could teach by just repeating what my teachers had done. From the course, I developed my teaching belief and learned the general behaviors and attitudes of children at different ages.

In addition to interacting with children, students had to engage in intensive relationships with their class peers during collaborative teaching tasks for an entire academic year. With three to four students per group, they worked through lesson planning, peer teaching, teaching in a school, and final presentations. Each process required in-depth discussion and negotiation of ideas and content. Moreover, when one person was leading a learning activity, the others had to stay alert and ready to assist. Vannie commented:

> In the beginning, we tried not to talk when assisting because we were afraid we might interrupt the leading teacher. Gradually we developed a tacit understanding and could jump in anytime to help make up a missing part and maintain the class flow.

All but two of the 13 co-teaching groups recounted intensive relationships of mutual support. An outstanding example was when Kewei, Ninhua, and Anna supported Suwen when she went blank while teaching. Kewei wrote, "We didn't give up on her. We kept encouraging her to continue practicing as we believed she could make it." Heping commented on the course's emphasis on productive interpersonal communication: "We learned how to make good use of each other's strengths to make the lesson plan better. Rather than just gossiping with friends, we learned how to hold a discussion during a meeting."

Achieving group equanimity could be difficult, however, when one member was particularly experienced in teaching. Fanny was an extraordinary storyteller with teaching experience and naturally took a leadership role, but in the name of group harmony, often apologized humbly for being arrogant. In another group, Rouen and Jully worked with Limin, who had honed his public speaking skills in high school contests. Rouen "felt like Limin's assistant," while Jully appreciated having two peers to correct her "awkward oral expressions." Bona tried to make the best of being in an uncooperative group, reflecting, "We might have uncooperative colleagues after graduating from college. Through practicum, I learned how to cope with this potential, and how to see a situation from the positive side."

From Dance to Education and Beyond

Practicum's directive is to prepare students for dance teaching jobs. Some had a head-start by having helped at their teacher's dance studio during and after the course. Yanru shared, "I was given a half hour to teach at the end of each class. Kids in that studio were very young and not professionally trained… I found creative dance helped a lot." Others, after teaching in an elementary school, began paying attention to what was possible with children, deepening their vision of dance teaching and dance education. For instance, Yifang, who attributed her "low self-esteem" to her dance teachers' "constant criticism of my poor technique," realized "the depth in the word *teacher*" in the course, suggesting, "Dance education should be what all dancers need to consider." Dola reflected, "To me, what's important is not to teach kids the subject. What's really meaningful is to bring them more concepts and right attitudes via creative dance."

Almost half the students said that teaching creative dance was difficult, requiring careful planning, clear procedures, knowledge, and sophisticated skills. As Binchi declared, "I finally realized that teaching children requires a series of systematic steps, a full lesson plan, and props to make a lesson complete." Naiyuan agreed, "I know better what 'learning by teaching' means." These responses indicated a change from disinterest in teaching to realizing the value of creative dance pedagogy.

Three co-teaching groups encountered educational or social issues in their schools, including bullying and children with special needs, which piqued their concern for the value of education and social justice for children. After dealing with a bullying event, Yuchi reflected,

> I know it is not just the bullies' problem. It also has to do with their family condition… But I felt sad for the victim, who had to experience that at such a young age… From this practicum, I learned the importance of family education and school education.

Although few encountered such issues during their practicum, the opportunity to teach creative dance in elementary school helped students to interact with the world outside their bubble of elite professional dance. Moreover, they gradually began to perceive the limitations of dance technique and their previously held assumptions about teaching, like Oubi who said, "In this course, I absorb what I would never have done or thought about." Cilan noted, "The course about creative dance pedagogy gives me teaching skills beyond professional dance training." Hanyu reflected, "Teaching creative dance is fun. Children got to create their own movements to show individual ideas. It's unlike professional dance technique that sets specific standards to achieve."

Ten students hoped to find careers unrelated to teaching. Nevertheless, they saw their study of creative dance pedagogy as a positive experience that could carry through to the future. For example, Chili planned to be a flight attendant after graduation and said, "Practicum was a training opportunity that no one can take away." Students wrote of greater confidence and enhanced abilities in oral expression, writing, interpersonal skills, planning, problem solving, creativity, and compassion, using language like "satisfaction," "sense of achievement," "making progress," and "becoming stronger" to reflect on their Practicum experiences. Importantly, whether teaching or not, most students realized that they did not want to be constrained by their taken-for-granted biases.

Closing Reflection

Reflecting on my initial motivation for changing the Practicum curriculum, I recalled that it was based on my perception of students' need for higher quality teaching resources and a stronger sense of personal and professional identity as "teacher." Especially helpful was Bond and Richard's (2005) advocacy for a *connected curriculum* that encourages dance teachers to recognize and follow their intuitive, felt responses to students' personal styles of movement rather than always adhering to external theories or fixed objectives. I hope this chapter will inspire other higher education dance faculty to research their own teaching and design short-term strategies for boosting students' skills and teaching confidence without abandoning long-term goals (Risner, 2010a). Accordingly, Bond (2013, 2018) recommends that, moving forward, children's perceptions and theories need to be recognized as foundational knowledge in philosophy, aesthetics, and for the future of dance.

Even after 4 years of revising Dance Teaching Practicum, when I entered the critical hermeneutic circle to examine the 2014 course, I questioned whether (again quoting my student Raishian), my "tedious" version of creative dance teacher education would simply become another type of training that creates "docile bodies" (Foucault, 1975/1995; Green, 2002–03). I concluded, however, that evidence from this study points to "no," echoing David Mead's (2011) case study of Taiwan's Cloud Gate Dance Theatre's educational program. Cloud Gate dance education aims to develop children's creativity and promote dance as a mode of education and life improvement. Every Cloud Gate teacher, most of whom had trained as professional dancers, found Cloud Gate's curriculum valuable, helping them to avoid the traditional teacher-centered approach of their own dance educations.

Mead (2011) concluded that the Cloud Gate curriculum provides "a form of scaffolding, supporting new teachers in particular in what may be [an] unfamiliar environment, and certainly an unfamiliar role" (p. 13). Similarly, the present study suggests that through a rigorous, sustained, and collaborative curriculum in creative dance pedagogy, students can shift away from their habitual focus on technical proficiency and assumptions about teaching. Nevertheless, both Cloud Gate's and Dance Teaching Practicum's aims of nurturing college dance teaching students' confidence and ability to design and implement diverse learning activities for creative dance continue to be atypical for mainstream dance education in Taiwan.

To achieve its goals, Dance Teaching Practicum offers a systematic structure of practice, feedback, and revision for each teaching strategy. This affords students the possibility to become familiar with holistic methodology in a consistent, confidence-oriented environment. More capable and confident, some students were ready to step out from the constraints of professional dance, while others had already begun. For all of these reasons, I consider that my students became engaged in quality of life transformations while practicing creative dance pedagogy at a university in northern Taiwan.

Acknowledgment I express my gratitude to research assistant, Yu-ting Huang. The research findings emerged and were clarified through our in-depth dialogue that occurred during the data analysis period.

References

Anderson, M., & Risner, D. (2014). Teaching artist responsibilities. In M. E. Anderson & D. Risner (Eds.), *Hybrid lives of teaching artists in dance and theatre arts: A critical reader* (pp. 183–199). Amherst, NY: Cambria Press.

Anderson, M., Risner, D., & Butterworth, M. (2013). The praxis of teaching artists in theatre and dance: International perspectives on preparation, practice and professional identity. *International Journal of Education & the Arts, 14*(5). Retrieved from http://www.ijea.org/v14n5/

Anderson, M., Risner, D., & Butterworth, M. (2014). Teaching artist communities. In M. Anderson & D. Risner (Eds.), *Hybrid lives of teaching artists in dance theater arts* (pp. 3–18). Amherst, NY: Cambria.

Andrews, G. (1954). *Creative rhythmic movement for children*. Englewood Cliffs, NJ: Prentice-Hall.

Andrzejewski, C. E. (2009). Toward a holistic model of dance teacher education. *Journal of Dance Education, 9*(1), 17–26.

Argyris, C., & Schön, D. A. (1974). *Theory in practice: Increasing professional effectiveness*. San Francisco, CA: Jossey Bass.

Arts Education Act. (1997). 10400151431 Hua Zong Yi Yi Zi § 8.

Bennett, D. (2009). Careers in dance: Beyond performance to the real world of work. *Journal of Dance Education, 9*(1), 27–34.

Bond, K. E. (2010). The benefits of dance, interpersonal skills and expression. In K. Vacarro (Ed.), *Dance in my life*. Reston, VA National Dance Alliance.

Bond, K. E. (2013). Recurrence and renewal: Enduring themes in children's dance. In T. Hagood & L. Kahlich (Eds.), *Revisiting impulse: A contemporary look at writings on dance, 1950–1970* (pp. 161–192). Amherst, NY: Cambria.

Bond, K. (2017). "Boys are morons"…"Girls are gross:" Let's dance! In W. Oliver & D. Risner (Eds.), *Dance and gender: An evidence-based approach* (pp. 135–157). Gainesville, FL: University Press of Florida.

Bond, K. (2018). "Me, a tree": Young children as natural phenomenologists. In S. Fraleigh (Ed.), *Back to the dance itself: Phenomenologies of the body in performance* (pp. 105–133). Urbana: University of Illinois Press.

Bond, K. E., & Deans, J. (1997). Eagles, reptiles and beyond: A co-creative journey in dance. *Childhood Education, 73*(6), 366–371.

Bond, K., & Richard, B. (2005). "Ladies and gentlemen! What do you see? What do you feel?" a story of connected curriculum in a third grade dance education setting. In L. Overby & B. Lepczyk (Eds.), *Dance: Current selected research* (Vol. 5, pp. 85–134). New York, NY: AMS Press.

Boorman, J. (1969). *Creative dance in the first three grades*. Don Mills, ON: Longman Canada.

Boorman, J. (1971). *Creative dance in grades four to six*. Don Mills, ON: Longman Canada.

Chang, C.-S. (2007). *A treasury of creative dance*. Taipei City, Taiwan: Taipei National University of the Arts.
Chang, C.-S. (2011). A century of dance development in Taiwan. *Journal of Aesthetic Education, 180*, 36–43.
Cone, T., & Cone, S. (2005). *Teaching children dance* (2nd ed.). Champaign, IL: Human Kinetics.
Exiner, J., & Lloyd, P. (1973). *Teaching creative movement*. Sydney, NSW: Angus & Robertson.
Ferraris, M. (1996). *History of hermeneutics* (L. Somigli, Trans.). Atlantic Highlands, NY: Humanities Press. (Original work published 1988).
Fortin, S. (1993). The knowledge base for competent dance teaching. *Journal of Physical Education, Recreation, and Dance, 64*(9), 34–38.
Fortin, S., & Siedentop, D. (1995). The interplay of knowledge and practice in dance teaching: What we can learn from a non-traditional dance teacher. *Dance Research Journal, 27*(2), 3–15.
Foucault, M. (1995). *Discipline and punish: The birth of the prison* (2nd ed.) (A. Sheridan, Trans.). New York, NY: Vintage books. (Original book published 1975).
Fowler, C. (1977). *Dance as education*. Washington, DC: National Dance Association/American Alliance of Health, Physical Education and Recreation.
Gadamer, H. (2004). *Truth and method* (2nd rev. ed.) (J. Weinsheimer & D. Marshall, Trans.). New York, NY: Continuum. (Original work published 1960).
Gilbert, A. (2015). *Creative dance for all ages*. (2nd ed.) Reston, VA: The American Alliance for Health, Physical Education, Recreation, and Dance (AAHPERD).
Green, J. (2002–03). Foucault and the training of docile bodies in dance education. *Arts and Learning Research Journal, 19*(1), 99–125.
Habermas, J. (1990). A review of truth and method. In G. Ormiston & A. Schrift (Eds.), *The hermeneutic tradition: From Ast to Ricouer* (pp. 213–244). Albany, NY: State University of New York Press.
Heidegger, M. (1996). *Being and time* (J. Stambaugh, Trans.). Albany, NY: State University of New York Press. (Original work published 1927).
Higher Education Arts Data Services [HEADS]. (2011). *Dance data summaries 2010–2011*. Reston, VA: Vault Consulting.
Joyce, M. (1994). *First steps in teaching creative dance to children* (3rd ed.). Palo Alto, CA: Mayfield.
Kahlich, L. (1990). *An analysis of the Master of Fine Arts degree as preparation for dance faculty roles in United States' institutions of higher education*. Doctoral dissertation. Philadelphia, PA: Temple University.
Lloyd, M. (2014). *Adventures in creative movement activities: A guide for teaching* (2nd ed.). Peosta, IA: Eddie Bowers.
Lortie, D. (1975). *Schoolteacher: A sociological study*. Chicago, IL: University of Chicago Press.
Mead, D. (2011). Creativity in dance teaching: It's not only about 'what', but also 'who,' 'where', 'when' and 'why'. *Taiwan Dance Research Journal, 6*, 1–30.
Merriam, S. (1988). *Case study research in education: A qualitative approach*. San Francisco, CA: Jossey-Bass.
Montgomery, S., & Robinson, M. (2003). What becomes of undergraduate dance majors? *Journal of Cultural Economics, 27*, 57–71.
Murray, R. (1975). *Dance in elementary education* (3rd ed.). New York, NY: Harper & Row.
Musil, P. (2010). Perspectives on an expansive postsecondary dance. *Journal of Dance Education, 10*(4), 111–121.
Overby, L., Post, B., & Newman, D. (2005). *Interdisciplinary learning through dance: 101 MOVEntures*. Champaign, IL: Human Kinetics.
Risner, D. (2010a). Dance education matters: Rebuilding postsecondary dance education for twenty-first century relevance and resonance. *Arts Education Policy Review, 111*(4), 125–135.
Risner, D. (2010b). The rise and fall of postsecondary dance education: Charting an expansive recovery. *Journal of Dance Education, 10*(4), 93–94. https://doi.org/10.1080/15290824.2010.529768.

Risner, D. (2012). Hybrid lives of teaching and artistry: A study of teaching artists in dance in the USA. *Research in Dance Education, 13*(2), 175–193. https://doi.org/10.1080/14647893.2012.677426.

Russell, J. (1975). *Creative movement and dance for children*. London, UK: MacDonald & Evans.

Sarason, S. (1999). *Teaching as a performing art*. New York, NY: Teachers College Press.

Schulman, L. (1986). Those who understand: Knowledge growth in teaching. *Educational Researcher, 15*, 4–14.

Stake, R. (1995). *The art of case study research*. Thousand Oaks, CA: Sage.

Stinson, S. (1988). *Dance for young children: Finding the magic in movement*. Reston, VA: The American Alliance for Health, Physical Education, Recreation, and Dance (AAHPERD).

Stinson, S. (2010). Questioning our past and building a future: Teacher education in dance for the 21st century. *Journal of Dance Education, 10*(4), 136–144.

Strauss, A., & Corbin, J. (1990). *Basics of qualitative research: Grounded theory procedure and techniques*. Newbury Park, CA: Sage.

Svendler Nielsen, C., & Burridge, S. (Eds.). (2015). *Dance education around the world: Perspectives on dance, young people and change*. London: Routledge.

Tang, S.-H. (2004). *The current condition and perspective of dance talented education*. Kaoshiung City, Taiwan: Fu-wen.

Warburton, E. (2004). Who cares? Teaching and learning care in dance. *Journal of Dance Education, 4*(3), 88–96.

Wu, Y.-J. (2005). *Dancing with little spirits: A journey towards enhancement of pedagogical relationship and intersubjectivity in a third grade dance education setting in Taiwan*. Doctoral dissertation. Philadelphia, PA: Temple University.

Wu, Y.-J. (2012). Bringing creative dance elements into school: A review of literature. In S. Stinson, C. Svendler Nielsen, & S.-Y. Liu (Eds.), *Dance, young people and change: Proceedings of the daCi and WDA global dance summit*. Retrieved from http://www.ausdance.org

Wu, Y.-J. (2017). *Theories and practices of creative dance teacher education*. Taipei, Taiwan: Yili.

Wu, Y.-J., & Huang, Y.-T. (2011a). The transformations of college dance students in dance teaching practicum. In L. Caldwell (Ed.), *In time together: Viewing and reviewing contemporary dance practice, proceedings of the 2010 world dance alliance global summit*. Retrieved from http://www.twu.edu/dance/world-dance-allianceproceedings.asp

Wu, Y.-J., & Huang, Y.-T. (2011b). A process of knowledge transference from educational theory to teaching context: Taking the teaching practicum of creative dance as an example. *Taiwan Dance Research Journal, 6*, 31–71.

Yin, R. K. (2013). *Case study research: Design and method* (5th ed.). Thousand Oaks, CA: Sage.

Chapter 22
"A Little Kind of Community": South African Students Dance for Self, Other and Society

Marelize Marx

In South Africa, we dance! We dance to establish identity, build community, and to foster collective healing. South Africans also dance in protest, such as the 2015 national "fees must fall" student protest where participants danced the *ukutoyiza*, commonly known as the *toyi-toyi,* a dance symbolising solidarity (Edwards, 2010; Glasser, 2000). South Africans dance for freedom, dignity, equality, human rights, public services, and fair wages (Bakare & Mans, 2003; Edwards, 2010; Glasser, 2000; Kothari, 2006; Onyeji, 2004; Wanyama & Shitubi, 2012). We dance "to improve the quality of life for all citizens" as promised by the *Constitution* (Republic of South Africa [RSA], 1996). In contemporary South Africa, dance has communal, cultural, public and political connotations, which informed my decision to explore the potential of dance education to promote social cohesion in a culturally and politically diverse post-apartheid South Africa.

Socio-political Context

In South Africa, 1994 marked the official end of apartheid, a political system that enforced racial segregation and discrimination against so-called "non-whites" with respect to rights, mobility, education, housing, land, and work opportunities (Struwig et al., 2012). The new *Constitution* (RSA, 1996) heralded the beginning of an era when all South African citizens would be regarded as equal; however, apartheid left behind a scarred and divided nation stained by divisions of race and class. Two decades later, pain and humiliation continue to mark the life stories of the many wounded, who transmit these to the next generation. The formerly "oppressed" and "oppressors" alike struggle with anger, shame, guilt, injustice, inferiority, superiority, anxiety, and fear (Adams, Van de Vijver, De Bruin, & Bueno Torres, 2014;

M. Marx (✉)
Nelson Mandela Metropolitan University, Port Elizabeth, South Africa

K. Bond (ed.), *Dance and the Quality of Life*, Social Indicators Research Series 73,
https://doi.org/10.1007/978-3-319-95699-2_22

Costandius & Bitzer, 2014; Delport, 2009; Hofstede, Hofstede, & Minkov, 2010; Nkomo, Webster, & Amsterdam, 2009; Soudien, 2012). Apartheid segregation policies also disrupted family structures as evidenced in the widespread absence of parents and in domestic violence, alcohol and drug abuse and high crime rates – the "social ills" that fuel distrust, stereotyping and fear of the other (Barolsky, 2012; Struwig et al., 2012).

South Africa is in dire need of strategies to "heal the divisions of the past" (RSA, 1996, p. 1243), to establish equality and social justice so that formerly separated groups can live together in "harmony" (Mandela, 2002, p. ix). This chapter reports on a study investigating the potential of a higher education dance education course to promote social cohesion in a culturally and politically diverse and divided post-conflict South Africa. A premise of the study is that social cohesion within the South African context requires a delicate balance between celebrating the uniqueness of each ethno-cultural group and establishing a sense of unity and harmony within the multicultural community (RSA, 1996).

Social Cohesion

Conceptualization of social cohesion as it pertains to South Africa has been neglected in South African scholarly literature. It is a complex subject, since the country's multiple ethno-cultural groups subscribe to diverse heritages of thought. Unlike mono-cultural nations, South African citizens are not united by a distinctive ethnicity, culture, or language, but by shared constitutional values such as human dignity, equality, respect, diversity, non-discrimination and social justice (Chipkin & Ngqulunga, 2008; Fleetwood, 2012; National Development Plan [NDP], 2011; RSA, 1996). South Africa's motto of "unity in diversity" represents an ideology in which each ethno-cultural identity is valuable, significant, and acknowledged in societal structure (RSA, 1996). When signing the country's post-apartheid *Constitution* in 1996, the late Nelson Mandela urged South Africans to "nurture our national unity by recognising, with respect and joy, the languages, cultures and religions of South Africa in all their diversity" (DoE, 2006, p. 15).

Social cohesion in South Africa is further seen to depend on individual agency and personal commitment to basic human rights for *all* citizens [emphasis added] (NDP, 2011). African, Western, and Asian worldviews correspond on this value in holding that the degree of cohesion and unity within a society depends on the extent and nature of interaction between individuals (Hacker, 2006; King, Samii, & Snilstveit, 2010; Masolo, 2006; Meena, 2005; Prinsloo, 1998; Struwig et al., 2012; Teffo, 1996). To these ends, South African social cohesion discourse endorses the African philosophy of *Ubuntu,* a way of thinking about life, self, and society that foregrounds individual moral responsibility for the wellbeing of others. Accordingly, the practice of care is integral to cohesion in South African society (Bennett, 2011; Soudien, 2012; Tutu, 2004; Venter, 2004).

This study is grounded in contemporary South African socio-political ideology and the African philosophy of *Ubuntu*. *Ubuntu* belief is that each person's character (sense of self and conduct towards others) is cultivated, nurtured, and shaped by being in community. A proposition of the study is that dance education is a unique platform for community interaction, an embodied space where a person can become consciously aware of self and other/s, develop positive attitudes and behaviour towards self and others, and ultimately support social cohesion in a culturally and politically diverse South Africa.

Research Methodology

As a teacher-researcher, I designed and implemented a qualitative study with first-year primary school student teachers who participated in a compulsory dance education course during their general education programme. The guiding research question was: *How did a culturally and politically diverse group of first year student teachers in a South African teacher education institution experience a compulsory first year dance education course?*

I offered the dance education module in seven 75-min sessions to seven groups of approximately 35 students over 7 weeks; 240 students completed the course, of which 76 volunteered to participate in the research. Seven African (six Xhosa (X), one Zulu (Z)), ten Coloured (C), three Indian (I), 26 white Afrikaner (A), and 30 white English-speaking students (EW), ranging from 18 to 32 years of age, participated in the study. Of these, ten were male and 66 were female. Participants were not evenly spread across groups or meticulously selected for cultural or gender affiliation – anyone who wanted to participate was welcome. This lack of demographic control can be viewed as a limitation of the study; however, the above cultural and gender profile approaches the typical demography of the B. Ed. classroom at the time of data collection, and is therefore a reasonably representative sample. In this regard, the lack of gender and cultural equality in South African teacher education was remnant of white privilege and decades of unequal education (and subsequent poverty) of our apartheid past. 2018 marks the first year of government subsidised tertiary education in South Africa, subsequently altering the demography of the current B.Ed classroom, considerably.

The study seeks meanings and locations of social cohesion as evidenced in students' accounts of experiences in the course titled "Arts and Culture: Dance Education." I combined participatory and interpretive research methods to examine the possible value of dance education in the promotion of social cohesion in South Africa. Epistemologically, the interpretive paradigm acknowledges all human communication and expression as grounded within and influenced by particular cultural and societal structures, which include subscribed meaning-making systems, prior socialization and historical pre-conceptions (Higgs & Smith, 2002; Usher, 1996). Ontologically, each interpretation is viewed as one perspective of a particular reality.

Qualitative data collection strategies often include interviews, journal reflections and observations.

The participatory paradigm views propositional knowledge as existing alongside other kinds of knowledge (Brennan, Voros, & Brady, 2011; Heron & Reason, 1997). Experience, for example, is regarded as a form of knowledge in its own right, even without any theoretical knowledge to sustain it. Heron and Reason (1997) describe experiential knowing as "feeling and imaging the presence of" something in reality through an "inner resonance with what there is" (pp. 280–281). In the present study, experiential knowledge is particularly relevant, since I explore the impact of dance education through participants' actual experiences of specific dance activities. Additionally, participants gained experiential knowledge of culturally diverse persons – their ways of moving, dance-making, negotiating, and participating. These experiences contributed to their knowledge of a multicultural environment, ethnocultural differences, interactions with others, intercultural communication, inclusion or exclusion and potentially, social cohesion.

After Yin (2009), I present the project as a case study, that is, an in-depth inquiry situated in a particular real-life environment and oriented by a specific proposition. As introduced earlier, this inquiry was framed in the following proposition: Dance education has the potential to promote social cohesion in post-apartheid South Africa. Participants were not informed of the proposition, since I aimed to access their authentic experiential reflections. As introduced above, the study focuses on students' experiences of a particular dance education course module offered in the first year of teacher education at the Faculty of Education, Nelson Mandela Metropolitan University, Port Elizabeth, South Africa.

The 76 volunteer participants were divided randomly into three groups for collection of qualitative data. Group A members (29 White females: nine EW, 20 A) reflected on two writing prompts at the end of their course in the form of open-ended questions:

1. Reflect on the past 7 weeks of dance education sessions and describe a meaningful experience.
2. Why was the experience meaningful?

Group B members (20 students: 2A; 2X, 5C, 11EW/6 male, 14 female) were asked to write reflections in a journal after each session, providing access and insight into the chronological narratives of their experience. Three prompts were provided: Today I felt...; Today I thought…; Today I noticed... Students submitted their reflective journals after completion of the course. Group C (27 students: 1Z, 3I, 4X, 4A, 5C, 10EW/4 male, 23 female) participated in focus group interviews. Focus group interviews enabled me to facilitate participants' exploration of their experiences. I conducted six focus group interviews with small groups of three to six participants each. I asked students to reflect on a meaningful experience they had during the dance education sessions. At the onset of each interview, I explained the purpose of the study as an inquiry into their dance education experiences. I prompted reflection through open and general questions, purposefully avoiding leading questions related to social cohesion (for example, references to "the other," inclusion, belonging, and ethno-cultural difference).

This study employed two independent data coders to strengthen research findings. Each coder worked separately to analyze, code and interpret the same data, over the same period of time. After Punch (2009), we chose open coding as the data analysis method. We first identified code concepts – issues and phenomena that emerged from the data themselves. Thereafter, we grouped codes under distinctive umbrella categories, and then recombined them in various logical ways to gain thematic insight into the data (De Vos, Strydom, Fouche, & Delport, 2011). Each independent coder analyzed the three data sets independently, making it possible to triangulate them in a manner that contributed to credibility of research findings. Finally, we amalgamated categories and themes of the three data sets for presentation and discussion purposes. Each coder presented their analysis and interpretation of findings at a meeting where consensus was reached.

Limitations of the Study

My dual role as teacher-researcher could have created potential bias in data analysis and interpretation. Conscious of this, I carefully navigated the "hermeneutic circle" during data interpretation (Higgs & Smith, 2002; Usher, 1996). I continuously referred back to my prior knowledge (experiential and theoretical) in order to make sense of new information from the data, whilst reflecting on how the new information relates to prior knowledge. Also, I interpreted the data while teaching the dance education module to further groups of students, enabling me to continuously reflect on and question my interpretation of participants' experiences during analysis. I also convened a consensus meeting with the two independent coders in order to identify and discuss final categories and themes. In retrospect, aspirations of consensus seemed to have been a limitation to this study, since inconsistencies could have provided a deeper analysis. Also, if I were to do a similar study in the future, I would include observational accounts of the teacher-researcher and a neutral outsider (for example, a psychologist or psychotherapist) to add further depth to findings.

Finally, the absence of critical prompts could be considered a limitation of the study. The magnitude of participants' positive accounts, while salient to theorizing productive associations between creative dance experiences and quality of life indicators, could have camouflaged students' experienced undisclosed challenges in "Dance Education." In this regard, almost 30% of participants noted initial discomfort incidentally: "In the beginning... it was very nerve-wrecking" (FG4:1.C-f), "I was scared at first, and little bit fat and a little bit old" (FG2:3.X-f) and "I was afraid to dance in front of the class (afraid that they will judge me and laugh at me)" (J4.C-f). Six white students (five female and one male) mentioned annoyance with fellow students for their "bad attitude." Investigation into subtle power relations and other challenges experienced during participation in a culturally and politically diverse dance education classroom would be meaningful future research. Three participants were excluded in the analysis below: two who reported on prior dance-training and musical theatre experiences and not on this dance education course, and one who only expressed how she hated her lecturer, because "she took my phone away."

Course Design

The purpose of "Dance Education" was to equip participants with basic knowledge to facilitate dance education in South African primary schools. The primary content of the programme (90% of each session) was active involvement in creative movement, an improvisational form of dance. I conceptualize creative movement as a vehicle for all students, regardless of ethno-cultural affiliation or prior dance experience, to explore natural play movements as they experiment with new ways of expression, also acquiring experiential understanding of the elements of dance. Creative movement activities occurred in small groups of five students each. Students participated in two to three different working groups per session, changing groups for each activity. In-class groups were designed to ensure ethno-cultural diversity.

Each session included two to three creative movement activities. At the onset of each activity, specific prompts guided the collaborative design of a dance. These included observations of how objects move (e.g., cars, animals, water, wind); experimentation with words and movement; and solving movement problems, for example: "Design six movements that occupy three levels simultaneously. Structure these movements to enable continuous flow." Activities were structured to involve analytic thinking and imagination simultaneously. Students spent approximately 15 min on collaborative dance-making and rehearsal. Thereafter, they performed their dances for each other, followed by my informal verbal feedback based on the aesthetic elements of dance, including choice of movements, use of space and levels, repetition, flow, quality of movement, togetherness and attention to detail. My aim was for students to cultivate a sense of quality criteria for evaluation of dance-making in the dance education classroom. Sessions also included learning an ethno-cultural dance, ranging from traditional South African dances associated with Zulu, Afrikaner, and Xhosa cultures, to more recent dances associated with particular communities, such as the *Kaapse Klopse* – an integrated dance and music style of the Cape Malay, and the township jive, a social dance originating in the 1950s in Soweto. I also included ethno-cultural dances from Greece and Spain that are familiar to me. In total, seven ethno-cultural dances were included in the module.

I want to emphasize that I did not teach this dance education course with the intentional aim to promote social justice or facilitate social cohesion. The aim was to equip student teachers to become dance education facilitators in South African primary schools. We did not explore issues of social cohesion, social justice, or ethnocentricity directly. Themes connected to movement explorations were ones that might be employed with primary school children, for example, animals, emotions, sport actions, and objects. Further, I did not assign readings on social-political topics. I reasoned that the absence of theoretical resources and discussion would allow me to isolate students' dance education experiences for analysis of direct social meanings.

Research Findings and Discussion

Qualitative analysis of student questionnaires, journals, and focus group interviews indicate that active bodily engagement in creative movement-based dance education provided spaces where student teachers' awareness of themselves and others was sharpened, and that these spaces were conducive to positive social interaction. Specifically, dance education supported awareness of self, awareness of self *in relation to* others, and interactive spaces for social cohesion.

In the remainder of the chapter, references to dance education relate to the specific dance education course at Nelson Mandela Metropolitan University titled "Arts and Culture: Dance Education." Data presented to illustrate findings are identified by source codes Q (exit questions), J (journal) and FG (focus group) followed by either an allocated student number (e.g. Q1, J1) or the interview number and student number (FG1:1). Ethnicity is indicated by acronyms: A (Afrikaner:White), C (Coloured), EW (English-speaking:White), I (Indian), Z (Zulu) and X (Xhosa). Gender is indicated by -f (female) and -m (male).

Dance Education Supports Self-Awareness and Expression

> Dance is an individual's way of expressing themselves, their thoughts, their emotions and their culture. (Q18.A-f)
>
> Dance made it easier for me to be open and express myself. (FG4:1.C-f, FG1.5.EW-f, FG5.1.C-f, FG5.2.EW-f, Q15.A-f)

Students variously described dance education as a non-judgemental, non-conforming, or safe space that enabled freedom of expression of individual difference and without fear of condemnation or rejection (J4.C-f, FG1.1.A-m, FG2.2.X-m, Q1.WE-f, Q23.A-f, Q26.A-f). Student J19.X reflected that sessions "allowed us to let go of fear and social awkwardness." Student FG4:4.C-f shared, "I was different in our class than in other lectures. It was like... something came off of me... and I could be more myself, and just let go." Similarly, FG2.3.X-f, FG3.1.X-f, FG4.5.X-f, FG5.1.C-f and J12.EW-f experienced the freedom to just "loosen up" and "be yourself."

Self-Esteem, Confidence and Self-Worth Many students (including FG6.4.C-m, J16EW-f, Q2.A-f and Q16.A-f) reported that involvement in dance education supported self-valuing in terms of confidence and self-esteem. Some overcame personal reservations, inhibitions and reticence. A Xhosa male, 32 years of age, for example, offers a developmental perspective in his personal journal (J10.X-m):

Week 1: Today I felt bad dancing with a partner...which made me interested to know dancing.

Week 5: My confidence grows more and more and I think this will eventually help me in the classroom as well as in church. Before these dance lessons I could not express myself the way I wanted. Many times, I thought about something but was unable to say it. These lessons have increased my confidence.

Week 6: Today we were given an opportunity to teach our dance movements, which has increased my belief that I can stand in front of many people.

Week 7: Group work has increased my communication skills. Also the ability to interact with others. My overall impression of the lessons is that they were exciting, morale boosting, also building up my self-esteem.

In dance education, this Xhosa student experienced agency and perceived his potential as a human being; he was able to transcend "bad" feelings. By the end of the course, he concludes that the class improved his communication skills and built his self-esteem. Dance education experiences facilitated the release of his potential as a valuable contributor to society. His journal projects a sense of developing dignity and quality of life.

Other students described feelings of self-worth in dance education as well:

I feel worthy and useful during the creative movement activities. (FG3:2.EW-f)

Today I felt that I mattered in dance class. (J4.C-f)

Student J2.C-m elaborates, "It makes each individual feel special." This finding supports Mans's (1994) premise that dancing increases experienced self-worth. In the present study participants reported feeling valuable ("I mattered"), "useful," and "special" in a context of ethno-cultural difference. Students' perspectives on dance education as a space of self-transformation are meaningful in post-conflict, post-apartheid South Africa where the majority of citizens were brought up in a political dispensation that reinforced the idea that some individuals and groups have less value than others (Hofstede et al., 2010; Soudien, 2012).

Ethno-Cultural Identity Scholars have theorized that an individual's self-acceptance as an authentic member of society is ultimately embedded in and influenced by their ethno-cultural identity (Kidd, 2002). Some dance education students revealed conscious positive awareness of their ethno-cultural identity. Performance of ethno-cultural dances supported students to engage with and embrace their ethno-cultural identities, regardless of their particular group's association with the political history of the country.

In a society formerly segregated on grounds of ethnicity, student responses point to the possibility of healing the dignity of both "oppressors" and "oppressed" through dance education experiences (RSA, 1996).

> Ja... we did the gumboots one. That was fun because that one I'm familiar with. In my culture we do it. So it was like my culture came in. I was not only being exposed to different cultures ... also something that I know. I got to express myself in it. (FG2:1.Z-f)

This reflection exemplifies how collective participation in ethno-cultural dances can affirm a particular ethno-cultural identity, even when fellow dancers do not share the same ethno-culture. Specifically, in the multicultural dance classroom, the co-participation of diverse individuals may encourage a person to reaffirm and take pride in their own ethno-cultural identity.

An Afrikaner student wrote that it "meant a lot" that all her classmates participated in *Afrikaners is plesierig*, a *volkspele* dance associated with Afrikaner culture (J8.A-f). Another Afrikaner participant wrote that dancing *Afrikaners is plesierig* reinforced her sense of affiliation, identification with, and pride in her ethno-culture:

> I really loved to do that ... it was meaningful because I'm Afrikaans and I didn't know how to dance it and thought it was a thing...that did not exist anymore, but I was wrong. I learnt something about my culture. (Q3.A-f)

While this student appreciated the course's acknowledgement of her ethno-cultural identity, she had thought the folk dance was "out of fashion," an assumption that needs further discussion. In contemporary South Africa, any reinforcement of Afrikaner identity within a multicultural environment is contentious, since Afrikaans was used as a "tool of oppression" during apartheid (Oppenheim, 2015, p. 3). Reinforcing Afrikaner identity could thus be frowned upon and interpreted as hegemonic reinforcement of the unequal power relations associated with the previous regime. The dance education classroom provided opportunities for students to celebrate their ethno-cultural identity alongside ethno-cultural others.

In retrospect, I wonder whether such experiences might help to ameliorate feelings of internalized guilt or shame, that is, by performing one's own traditional dances with ethno-cultural others who participate as well. As a white Afrikaner dance educator, I hoped that no students would take offense at being required to perform an ethno-cultural dance of the other. I did not observe negativity in the student group, which corresponds with previous studies showing that students in higher education are interested in exploring and understanding difference (Bond & Etwaroo, 2005; Bond & Gerdes, 2012). Students in my class were expected to participate in a variety of ethno-cultural dances, and one student reflected, "The traditional dancing was fun and I felt it added value to any race group" (J17.EW-f).

Dance Education Promotes Awareness of Self in Relation *to Others*

Student responses illuminate that dance education spaces provided bodily experiences of sameness and difference between self and others. I first present participant perceptions from the sameness end of the "recognition continuum" (Lash & Featherstone, 2001).

Sameness and Similarity Some students noted a common humanity with their peers in dance education. While anthropologists and cultural studies scholars have critiqued the premise that dance is a "universal language" (Bakare & Mans, 2003; Hanna, 1979; Royce, 1977), these students' perceptions align experientially with researchers who theorize dance as a fundamentally shared form of human communication that is not entirely based on culture (Bond, 2017; Bond & Etwaroo, 2005; Fraleigh, 2004; Kauffman & Ellis, 2007; Sheets-Johnstone, 2015).

> Dance is just like those universal languages that everyone…no matter what culture...can interpret as some form of expression or some sort of reflection of who we are. (FG6:2.A-f)
>
> It was so amazing to see and made me realise that everyone is just human… we are all similar in one way or another. (Q22.A-f)

Dance education experiences inspired some students' sense of South Africanness, or pride in a collective national identity, regardless of ethno-cultural boundaries and social identities: "I felt truly and proudly South African" (J15.EW-f). An Afrikaner student regarded African dances like the gumboot dance as part of her own identity, mentioning her pride when "people overseas talk about African dancing" since it represents "our identity" (FG1:3.A-f). Another White student shared,

> It's learning stuff that you would never otherwise have the opportunity to learn and experience. Like…I loved the gumboot dancing. It's not necessarily my culture, but it's South African culture. I mean, I don't normally get to gumboot dance. You get to experience a part of your culture, which is cool. (FG3:3.EW-f)

In focus groups, students expressed that dance education enabled them to experience a multi-cultural identity – a sense of belonging to a cohesive nation. It is important, however, that a particular ethno-cultural dance not be used to construct an *imagined* national identity [emphasis added] (Anderson, 1991). In South Africa, such a development could disenfranchise some ethno-cultural groups and their associated dance practices (see Rowe, Buck, & Martin, 2015). In this study, participation in a variety of ethno-cultural dances nurtured, for some students, a sense of belonging to a multicultural South African society. Opportunities to identify with others as members of the same broader society can disrupt the notion of "othering," which valorizes sameness (Rockefeller, 1994; Taylor, 1994). Students' experiences of dance education supported a conscious awareness of sameness in diversity.

Difference Through performing diverse ethno-cultural dances, students embodied difference. Several participants noted that bodily involvement in dances of others allowed them to "experience something that's not yours, it's not what you usually do" (FG3:4.A-f), expanding boundaries: "You don't always know what other cultures do, because you are used to your own" (FG5:4.EW-f, Q8.EW-f, Q25.A-f). One student articulated her experience in more colloquial terms: "It's so cool because you've got sort of that knowledge of this thing" (FG4:2.EW-f). A Zulu student got "in touch with other cultures and how things are done, how they dance. It was really a good experience and I enjoyed it" (FG2:1.Z-f).

Moreover, students expressed that ethno-cultural dances instilled appreciation and respect for other South African ethno-cultures. An Afrikaner student wrote, "I found respect for gumboot dancers because it's rather difficult and they do it so well… I found it so much fun and interesting that I went to watch video clips of gumboot dances" (Q7.A-f, J3.EW-m, J20.A-f). Another White student observed, "I became aware of all the traditional dances. I really liked the gumboot dance. Dance is so much deeper than we think" (Q9.A-f; J7.C-f). Similarly, a Zulu student identified Afrikaner traditional *volkspele* dance as her favourite dance; she had seen it on television "but actually to do it, was wonderful" (FG2:1.Z-f). Active involvement in ethno-cultural dances of others nurtured appreciation and respect, which according to Rockefeller (1994), enables recognition. Taylor (1994) argues that when the other acknowledges a particular ethno-cultural group as significant, this restores the particular group's dignity, also enabling experiences of equality—dignity and equality being core conditions required for social cohesion (Chipkin & Ngqulunga, 2008). Or, as student J17.EW said: "it added value to any racial group."

Some appreciated being allowed into the "inner circle" of the other: "You get to feel that culture," student FG4:2.EW-f reflected. "You get to experience and feel: This is what it's actually like!" (FG3.2.EW-f). A White student wrote, "I could connect with the gumboot dance… typically me!" (J9.EW-f), playfully mocking the irony of her experiencing emotional resonance to a dance of the other. Another White student wrote,

> I really enjoyed today's gumboot dancing. Although we only learnt basic steps, I found it interesting and fun! It made me think about what the original mine workers felt like, when they resorted to using gumboot dancing as a means of communicating. (J13.EW-f)

Gumboot dancing enabled this student to imagine what it would be like to be, as Wiredu (1998) described, "in the skin of the other" (p. 310), potentially cultivating empathyand compassion (Bond, 2017; Bond & Etwaroo, 2005; Greene, 1995; Nussbaum, 1997; Tropp, 2011). Empathy and compassion for fellow community members are elements of cohesion in *ubuntu* (Bell, 2002; Broodryk, 2010; Gyekye, 1998; Prinsloo, 1998).

Another student suggested that increased knowledge of diverse ethno-cultural groups through active involvement enhances understanding:

> Cultural dances bring in cultural understanding because…if you're born in a culture, you don't really understand other people's culture but if you can use that dance, it is a link. We can start bridging gaps between cultures and religions. Bridging the gap is not like you must accept everyone...that's not forced on you... You get to feel that culture and get into it. That's important especially in S.A. In our curriculum, we've got to keep it in mind. (FG4:2.EW-f)

This student mirrors Adinku's (2004) belief that study of others' dances facilitates insight and understanding. Intercultural understanding can moderate ethnocentrism and misinterpretation between diverse people, creating spaces for social cohesion. These reflections exemplify students' tangible willingness to cross boundaries and bridge difference towards social cohesion (Bond & Etwaroo, 2005).

Students in "Dance Education" became more aware that individuals and ethno-cultural groups have different movement vocabulary and styles (Bond & Etwaroo, 2005; Hanna, 2008; Royce, 1977): "You learn about different people and their ways of dancing" (Q21.A-f; FG2.3.X-f). This aspect acquires a humorous tone in the following description (FG4:2.EW-f):

Student:	This Coloured girl is like, "Do this," and we're like, "we can't do that, we Whities can't move like that. And it's just cool with these different personalities.
Interviewer:	Did you do it?
Student:	No, we cut it from the dance…there are parts of me that don't shake.
Interviewer:	How did she respond?
Student:	She laughed…she thought it was so funny. She watched us and said, don't worry about it—it's okay. It was just nice to see the different personalities… how they interpret a piece of music, a move.

According to participating students, dance education supported conscious personal awareness and appreciation of self in relation to other, also offering insights into the ethno-cultures of others. Dance education's capacity to facilitate awareness of sameness and difference supports South Africa's social cohesion vision, specifically, its valuing of *unity in diversity* [emphasis added] (RSA, 1996).

Social Conduct Many students reported that dance education promoted good social conduct, for example, "how to treat each other" (FG6:2.A-f), "how to conduct yourself…to interact with other people…get along with others, how to consider people" (FG3:4.A-f), and "what's socially acceptable, what's not acceptable" (FG4:4.C-f). Student J14.EW-m reflected: "I must learn to be more patient with others." Student FG4:2.EW-f noted that people have "different points of view, and you've got to learn to work with each other and compromise." An Indian student summed up a number of positive social values cultivated in dance education:

> …treating people with kindness, with everything...that is good in the world, something like that. It's weird…it gets you engaged, involved, talking, moving, exercising, dancing. It's an expression that everyone can benefit from. (FG6:1.I-f)

Another student reflects on the connection between self-respect and respect for others: "Because you respect yourself – you're not gonna want to make anybody else feel uncomfortable" (FG4:4.C-f).

Through the lens of *ubuntu,* student responses exemplify "personhood" (Bell, 2002; Gyekye, 1998; Venter, 2004; Wiredu, 1998). Interactions between students enabled them to experience kindness, compassion, and virtuous social conduct – nurturing *ubuntu* within persons. Further, creative movement offered opportunities "to help others" as well as "being helped" (FG3:4.A-f). Student J17.EW wrote, "During today's lesson it occurred to me that our class is pretty supportive of each other," a reflection that provides a segue to the theme of social cohesion.

Dance Education Provided Interactive Spaces for Social Cohesion

Participant responses suggest that dance education provided spaces conducive to social cohesion. Students could "bond" (FG3:4.A-f) and "connect" (Q26.A-f, FG1:4.EW-m, FG4:2.EW-f) as they "got to know" each other (J18.EW-f, Q9.A-f, Q13.A-f, Q14.A-f, Q17.A-f). They created friendships: "Everyone got along and some even became friends" (Q27.EW-f, FG1.5.EW-f, Q29.EW-f). Students engaged socially and emotionally with others to "form that relationship" (FG1.1.A-m) and discover "who they can connect with" (FG1:4.EW-m). Some described a sense of togetherness with a different "kind" (FG3:4.A-f) of person: "I connected to people I never talked to before" (Q26.A-f); "you make relationships with people you've never spoken to…in a multicultural inclusive environment" (FG6:1.Indian-f). While indirect, the various statements about "people we would not normally speak to," "different people," "different social classes" and "different backgrounds" may be interpreted as references to ethno-cultural differences in the classroom (Q26.A-f, FG3:4.A-f, FG4:2.EW-f, FG4:3.EW-f, FG6:1.I-f).

Dance education experiences afforded regular opportunities for students to engage with each other across social boundaries. One could say that involvement in the course cultivated an "affective bond between citizens," an indicator of social cohesion (Chipkin & Ngqulunga, 2008, p. 61): "It made us feel very involved" (FG5.1.C-f; FG1.6.EW-f) and "part of something" (Q20.EW-f). This resonates with *Ubuntu* philosophy where community wellbeing depends on "fellow-feeling" (Gbadegesin, 1998, p. 295), that is, the nature of social relationships within the community (Masolo, 2006; Prinsloo, 1998; Teffo, 1996).

Moreover, where connections are formed across social and ethno-cultural boundaries, one could surmise that fear of the other is being diminished. According to Tropp (2011), knowledge of the other potentially eliminates fear of the other. In South African society apartheid ideology was rooted in justifications for the fear of the other, causing major division in society (Barolsky, 2012; Struwig et al., 2012). When fear of the other is reduced, perspective transformations might be enabled that ultimately erode social division and racial prejudice. Tropp (2011) argues that the mere observation of intercultural friendship can reduce racial prejudice. It stands to reason, then, that interactions where intercultural friendships are cultivated might promote social cohesion (NDP, 2011).

Further, Blum (2014) holds that cultivation of connections across social and ethno-cultural boundaries enables individuals to recognise their duties towards others as members of the same nation. This resonates with African thought where realisation of obligations towards others provides evidence of community and thus of *ubuntu* (Bell, 2002; Gyekye, 1998; Wiredu, 1998). Interactions involving inclusion and mutual responsibility promote social cohesion (Jenson, 1998). Ultimately, social cohesion is predicated on interdependency, where citizens are obligated to grant dignity, equality, respect, and care for each other (NDP, 2011; RSA, 1996; Soudien, 2012). In this study, students' responses indicate that dance education supported connections, including friendships, across social and cultural boundaries, fostering social cohesion in the classroom.

Finally, this study suggests that dance education provided interactive spaces for social cohesion. One student stated that the class became "a little kind of community" (FG4:1.C-f). Students rehearsed intercultural interactions, explored togetherness with others who are different to themselves, and practiced citizenship in the form of active participation and cooperation.

> In the other modules we have done all year, all day it's multiculturalism, uh, inclusivity… and how to try to teach in that way... This is the only class where it is actually being practised. It makes this class much more, I don't know, rewarding. You get something out of this class. (FG6:1.I-f)

Through multicultural praxis, students experienced social integration:

> We were all holding hands. We had fun in this class in a multicultural, inclusive environment all the time…you make relationships with people you have never spoken to...even though you are in the same class. (FG6:1.I-f)

This Indian student suggested also that dance education countered cultural segregation in the classroom. During the same focus group, an Afrikaner student emphasized that dance education created a space for practicing citizenship:

> A lot of students struggle with citizenship. I think this class is one of those classes that you can actually practise strategies. A lot of people struggle because they can't bridge theory and practice and that's why a lot of students struggle with citizenship. (FG6:2.A-f)

Active participation in dance education enabled participants to practice intercultural negotiations, acceptance, and knowledge of the other in an inclusive environment for working through fear of the unfamiliar to a place of "understanding":

> It helps you with so many things, like talking to other people, engaging in other people's cultures. So you know what? I'm Muslim, she's Catholic…so maybe we do some sort of dance... We have to find out about each other's cultures. Now I know…oh, you weren't a weirdo after all, this is just what you do...because people are scared of things they don't understand. It's uncomfortable. If you learn about it, you engage, work with it, work with each other and you come past that. (FG6:1.I-f)

For this student, dance education provided a safe space to cross boundaries and confront preconceived ideas through active, bodily engagement: "maybe we do some sort of dance."

Collaborative problem solving in small groups enabled intercultural negotiations and ultimately, social cohesion; students had to seek ways to perform together as a unified entity, exploring active participation, inclusion, cooperation, conflict negotiation, and interdependency.

> It's that! How do you work as a society? You figure out...that you need to rely on every single person, or it's going to be a stuff-up. So, that whole dancing-together-thing...really does work in terms of getting us ready for society. What is your role going to be? Can you be dependable? … It's a nation-building exercise…that would be a nice way to put it. (FG6:3.I-f)

Kidd (2002) argues that in order to become integrated within a community one must develop positive social skills, which can be acquired through practice. In this study dance education invited students to practise social interactions with ethno-cultural others. And again, according to *Ubuntu*, a person attains the status of *ubuntu* (personhood) once they have fostered virtuous social skills. *Ubuntu* (personhood) within individuals is essential for cultivation of *ubuntu* (unity) as the feeling of togetherness within a community (Praeg, 2014).

Nineteen students across ethno-cultural groups showed awareness of the cohesive, unifying qualities of dance education. Responses suggested that noble interpersonal skills were being practised, including a sense of obligation towards others (interdependency). Various individuals said that dance experiences enhanced togetherness: "brings us together" (Q17.A-f); "brings people together" (J1.EW-f); "brought the class together" (Q27.EW-f); "helped to bring all of us students together, to create in my opinion a stronger unit" (Q12.EW-f). Student J15.EW-f noted, "there was a sense of unity amongst the class, when we all danced in a circle together." A Xhosa female student wrote, "It didn't matter if we were born dancers. What mattered was that we learnt something new together and the new knowledge united us as a class" (J19.X-f). Students Q28.EW-f and FG5.3.I-f noticed that the dance activities "made us work together as a team." Student FG4:2.EW-f reflected,

> It made the class come together because you work in a group and you don't know the people in your first year. You all come from different high schools, backgrounds ... you've all got ideas about people... But when you're in this little group and you have to work with them, you can see that she's just being as silly as I am and it's nice. The class sort of get together, laugh at each other.

And again, the dance education class became "a little kind of community" (FG4:1.C-f).

Concluding Remarks

If social cohesion can be understood as "the forces that bind society together" (Green, Janmaat, & Han, 2009, p. 1), students in dance education experienced cohesion in a culturally and politically diverse classroom. They shared feelings of both individual agency and togetherness, and they acted on these feelings (Chipkin & Ngqulunga, 2008). As such, dance education supported exploration of collective identity; mirroring South Africa's motto, students became "united in diversity." I conclude that, in alignment with *Ubuntu*, dance education provided interactive spaces where individuals could practice "becoming fully human," treating others with humanity while building community. This chapter has illustrated that dance education can contribute meaningfully to contemporary strategies aimed at bridging divides, promoting social cohesion, and enhancing quality of life in post-conflict societies such as South Africa.

References

Adams, B. G., Van de Vijver, F. J. R., De Bruin, G. P., & Bueno Torres, C. (2014). Identity in descriptions of others across ethnic groups in South Africa. *Journal of Cross-Cultural Psychology, 45*(9), 1411–1433.

Adinku, O. (2004). Cultural education in Ghana: A case study of dance development in the university system. *Dance Chronicle, 27*(1), 49–66.

Anderson, B. (1991). *Imagined communities: Reflections on the origin and spread of nationalism*. London: Verso.

Bakare, O. R., & Mans, M. (2003). Dance philosophies and vocabularies. In A. Herbst, M. Nzewi, & K. Agawu (Eds.), *Musical arts in Africa: Theory, practice and education* (pp. 215–135). Pretoria, South Africa: UNISA Press.

Barolsky, V. (2012). "A better life for all": Social cohesion and the governance of life in post-apartheid South Africa. *Social Dynamics: A Journal of African Studies, 38*(1), 134–151.

Bell, R. H. (2002). *Understanding African philosophy: A cross-cultural approach to classical and contemporary issues*. New York: Routledge.

Bennett, T. W. (2011). Ubuntu: An African equity. In F. Diedrich (Ed.), *Ubuntu, good faith and equity: Flexible legal principles in developing a contemporary jurisprudence* (pp. 3–23). Claremont, CA: JUTA.

Blum, L. (2014). Three educational values for a multicultural society: Difference recognition, national cohesion and equality. *Journal of Moral Education, 43*(3), 332–344.

Bond, K. E. (2017). "Boys are morons" … "Girls are Gross:" Let's dance! In W. Oliver & D. Risner (Eds.), *Dance and gender: An evidence-based approach* (pp. 135–157). Gainesville: University Press of Florida.

Bond, K. E., & Etwaroo, I. (2005). "If I really see you…" Students' experiences of identity and difference in a higher education setting. In M.-C. Powell & V. Marcow-Speiser (Eds.), *The arts, education, and social change: Little signs of hope* (pp. 87–100). Cambridge, MA: Peter Lang.

Bond, K. E., & Gerdes, E. (2012). Student performance in a dance-based humanities course at "Diversity U". In S. W. Stinson, Shu-Ying Liu, & C. S. Nielsen (Eds.), *Dance, young people and change – Proceedings of the World Dance Alliance/Dance and the Child International conference*. Retrieved from http://www.worlddancealliance.net/Publications.html

Brennan, L., Voros, J., & Brady, E. (2011). Paradigms at play and implications for validity in social marketing research. *Journal of Social Marketing, 1*(2), 100–119.

Broodryk, J. (2010). *Understanding South Africa: The Ubuntu way of living*. Waterkloof, South Africa: Ubuntu School of Philosophy.

Chipkin, I., & Ngqulunga, B. (2008). Friends and family: Social cohesion in South Africa. *Journal of Southern African Studies, 34*(1), 61–76.

Costandius, E., & Bitzer, E. (2014). Opening up spaces for social transformation: Critical citizenship education in a post-conflict South African university context. *Education, Citizenship and Social Justice, 9*(2), 128–139.

De Vos, A. S., Strydom, H., Fouche, C. B., & Delport, C. S. L. (2011). *Research at grass roots: For the social sciences and human service professions*. Pretoria, South Africa: Van Schaik.

Delport, A. C. (2009). *Emotions, social transformation and education*. Pretoria, South Africa: UNISA.

Department of Education (DOE), South Africa. (2006). *My country South Africa: Celebrating our national symbols and heritage* (2nd ed.). Retrieved from http://www.education.gov.za/Portals/0/Documents/Publications/My%20Country%20SA.pdf

Edwards, S. D. (2010). Dance for health: A disclosure. *African Journal for Physical Health Education, Recreation and Dance* (AJPHERD), *16*(1), 129–146.

Fleetwood, T. (2012). *Post-apartheid education and building 'unity in diversity': Voices of South African youth* (Doctoral thesis). Retrieved from http://etheses.dur.ac.uk/5934/

Fraleigh, S. H. (2004). *Dancing identity: Metaphysics in motion*. Pittsburgh, PA: University of Pittsburgh Press.

Gbadegesin, S. (1998). Individuality, community, and the moral order. In P. H. Coetzee & A. P. J. Roux (Eds.), *The African philosophy reader* (pp. 292–305). London: Routledge.
Glasser, S. (2000). Is dance political movement? In D. Williams (Ed.), *Anthropology and human movement: Searching for origins* (pp. 19–38). Lanham, MD: Scarecrow.
Green, A., Janmaat, J. G., & Han, C. (2009). *Regimes of social cohesion*. London: University of London Press.
Greene, M. (1995). *Releasing the imagination: Essays on education, the arts, and social change*. San Francisco: Jossey-Bass.
Gyekye, K. (1998). Person and community in African thought. In P. H. Coetzee & A. P. J. Roux (Eds.), *The African philosophy reader* (pp. 317–336). London: Routledge.
Hacker, P. (2006). Dharma in Hinduism. *Journal of Indian Philosophy, 34*, 479–496.
Hanna, J. L. (1979). *To dance is human: A theory of nonverbal communication*. Austin: University of Texas Press.
Hanna, J. L. (2008). A nonverbal language for imagining and learning: Dance education in K-12 curriculum. *Educational Researcher, 37*(8), 491–506.
Heron, J., & Reason, P. (1997). A participatory inquiry paradigm. *Qualitative Inquiry, 3*(3), 274–294.
Higgs, P., & Smith, J. (2002). *Rethinking truth*. Capetown, South Africa: JUTA.
Hofstede, G., Hofstede, J. H., & Minkov, M. (2010). *Cultures and organizations: Software of the mind: Intercultural cooperation and its importance for survival*. New York: McGraw-Hill.
Jenson, J. (1998). *Mapping social cohesion: The state of Canadian research* (CPRN Study No. F|03). Ottawa, ON: Canadian Policy Research Networks.
Kaufmann, K., & Ellis, B. (2007). Preparing pre-service generalist teachers to use creative movement in K-6. *Journal of Dance Education, 7*(1), 7–13.
Kidd, W. (2002). *Culture and identity: Skills based sociology*. New York: Palgrave.
King, E., Samii, C., & Snilstveit, B. (2010). Interventions to promote social cohesion in sub-Saharan Africa. *Journal of Development Effectiveness, 2*(3), 336–370.
Kothari, S. (2006). Dance as soft power for cultural diplomacy. *Dance/diversity/dialogue: Bridging communities and cultures – Proceedings of the 2006 World Dance Alliance Global Assembly* (pp. 260–262). Retrieved from http://www.wda-americas.net/wp-content/uploads/2014/01/WDA-2006-Global-Proceedings.pdf
Lash, S., & Featherstone, M. (2001). Recognition and difference: Politics, identity, multiculture. *Theory Culture Society, 18*(1), 1–19.
Mandela, N. (2002). Foreword. In K. Asmal & W. James (Eds.), *Spirit of the nation: Reflections on South Africa's education ethos* (pp. ix–ix). Claremont, CA: HSRC Press.
Mans, M. E. (1994). The co-supportive roles of music and dance in Namibian arts education. In H. Lees (Ed.), *Musical connections: Tradition and change* (pp. 60–69). Auckland, New Zealand: International Society for Music Education.
Masolo, D. A. (2006). Western and African communitarianism: A comparison. In K. Wiredu (Ed.), *A companion to African philosophy* (pp. 483–498). Malden, MA: Blackwell.
Meena, S. L. (2005). Relationship between state and dharma in Manusmriti. *The Indian Journal of Political Science, 66*(3), 575–588.
National Development Plan. (2011). *Vision for 2030*. Retrieved from http://www.npconline.co.za/pebble.asp?relid=25
Nkomo, M., Weber, E., & Amsterdam, C. (2009). Editorial: Is education making a difference in the creation of equitable societies? *Perspectives in Education, 27*(4), 331–340.
Nussbaum, M. C. (1997). *Cultivating humanity: A classical defense of reform in liberal education*. Cambridge, MA: Harvard University Press.
Onyeji, C. (2004). Igbo rural women in Africa as creative personalities. *Journal of the Musical Arts in Africa, 1*, 84–101.
Oppenheim, Z. (2015). *Tracks and reconciliation: Afrikaner identity through alternative music*. Unpublished manuscript, Department of Ethnomusicology, University

of Washington, Seattle, WA. Retrieved from https://www.academia.edu/13355372/Tracks_and_Reconciliation_Afrikaner_Identity_through_Alternative_Music

Praeg, L. (2014). From Ubuntu to Ubuntu: Four historic a prioris. In L. Praeg & S. Magadla (Eds.), *Ubuntu: Curating the archive* (pp. 96–120). Pietermaritzburg, South Africa: UKZN Press.

Prinsloo, E. D. (1998). Ubuntu culture and participatory management. In P. H. Coetzee & A. P. J. Roux (Eds.), *The African philosophy reader* (pp. 41–51). London: Routledge.

Punch, K. F. (2009). *Introduction to research methods in education*. London: Sage.

Republic of South Africa. (1996). *Constitution of the Republic of South Africa*. Retrieved from http://www1.chr.up.ac.za/chr_old/indigenous/documents/South%20Africa/Legislation/Constitution%20of%20South%20Africa%201993.pdf

Rockefeller, C. (1994). Comment. In A. Gutman (Ed.), *Multiculturalism*. Princeton, NJ: Princeton University Press.

Rowe, N., Buck, R., & Martin, R. (2015). The gaze or the groove? Emerging themes from the new meanings and pathways: Community dance and dance education symposium in Beijing. *Research in Dance Education, 16*(2), 184–197.

Royce, A. P. (1977). *The anthropology of dance*. Bloomington: Indiana University Press.

Sheets-Johnstone, M. (2015). *The phenomenology of dance* (50th anniversary ed.). Philadelphia, PA: Temple University Press.

Soudien, C. (2012). *Realising the dream: Unlearning the logic of race in the South African school*. Cape Town, South Africa: HSRC Press.

Struwig, J., Davids, Y. D., Roberts, B., Sithole, M., Tilley, V., Weir-Smith, G., & Mokhele, T. (2012). *Towards a social cohesion barometer for South Africa: Research paper*. Retrieved from http://policyresearch.limpopo.gov.za/bitstream/handle/123456789/750/Towards%20a%20Social%20Cohesion%20Barometer%20for%20South%20Africa.pdf?sequence=1

Taylor, C. (1994). The politics of recognition. In A. Gutman (Ed.), *Multiculturalism* (pp. 25–74). Princeton, NJ: Princeton University Press.

Teffo, L. J. (1996). The other in African experience. *South African Journal of Philosophy, 15*(3), 101–105.

Tropp, L. R. (2011). *A summary of research findings on the effects of intergroup contact*. Retrieved from http://www.school-diversity.org/pdf/Tropp_Minnesota_testimony_12-20-11.pdf

Tutu, D. (2004). *The second Nelson Mandela annual lecture*. [Address]. Johannesburg, South Africa.

Usher, R. (1996). A critique of the neglected epistemological assumptions of educational research. In D. Scott & R. Usher (Eds.), *Understanding educational research* (pp. 9–32). London: Routledge.

Venter, E. (2004). The notion of *ubuntu* and communalism in African educational discourse. *Studies in Philosophy and Education, 23*, 149–160.

Wanyama, M. N., & Shitubi, I. W. (2012). Emergent issues regarding 'African traditional dance' and 'African contemporary dance': A discourse on the current theory and practice of 'African dance' criticism and choreography. *Journal of Emerging Trends in Educational Research and Policy Studies* (JETERAPS), *3*(4), 433–437.

Wiredu, K. (1998). The moral foundations of an African culture. In P. H. Coetzee & A. P. J. Roux (Eds.), *The African philosophy reader* (pp. 306–316). London: Routledge.

Yin, R. K. (2009). *Case study research: Design and methods* (4th ed.). London: Sage.

Chapter 23
Quality of Working Life for Higher Education Dance Educators: Embodiment, Complexity, Transformation

Alba Pedreira Vieira

Quality of life is intimately related to quality of working life, which has many nuances, including one's desire to perform their work with excellence. This chapter approaches quality of life through a phenomenological study of pedagogical quality as found in 35 teachers' written stories about significant teaching memories in higher dance education. I bring to the study 20 years of teaching dance in higher education in Brazil, where the educational theories of Brazilian philosopher Paulo Freire have been highly influential. In his most famous text, *Pedagogy of the Oppressed,* Freire (1968/2018) is concerned in particular with quality of teaching. In Freire's critical pedagogical framework, the teacher is often depicted as the student's oppressor.

What does it mean to teach well? Even higher education teachers with preparation in professional certification programs, including myself, can feel gaps in their praxis that obscure understanding of deep meanings of teaching. Drawing on Max van Manen's (1991, 1997) phenomenological pedagogy, I suggest that one can strengthen the relation between knowledge and action by foregrounding lived experience itself as a valid basis for both practical action and theorizing. As van Manen (1991) affirms, "The stories that teachers tell may be treated as recommendations for acting. In our theorizing, in bringing life to speech, we are in a manner recommending a certain way of standing in the world" (p. 170). Accordingly, I build educational theory grounded in experience.

One of this study's aspirations is to help change the educational dance world in positive ways through illumination of teachers' meanings of "quality." My aim, however, is not to produce dogmatic prescriptions for teaching, but like van Manen (1997), to elucidate:

> the various ranges of human experiences possible, what worlds people inhabit, how these experiences may be described, and how language (if we give it its full value) has powers to disclose the worlds in which we dwell as fathers, mothers, teachers, students, and so forth. (p. 45)

A. P. Vieira (✉)
Federal University of Vicosa, Viçosa, Brazil

K. Bond (ed.), *Dance and the Quality of Life*, Social Indicators Research Series 73,
https://doi.org/10.1007/978-3-319-95699-2_23

Research Pathways

I adopt a qualitative approach to dance inquiry, as qualitative methods have such excellent potential to elucidate meanings. Denzin and Lincoln (2005) describe qualitative research as *bricolage*, a metaphor I embrace for connecting the webs of meaning in this study. The researcher selects from diverse frameworks and tools to produce "a complex, dense, reflexive, collage-like creation that represents the researcher's image, understandings, and interpretations of the…phenomenon under analysis" (p. 4). Hence, my aim is not to develop a theory of "model teaching," but rather to examine the "lifeworld" of teaching – the "world-as-lived" (Heidegger, 2005) by dance teachers in higher education.

Similar to German modern dance artist Pina Bausch (1940–2009), who often created choreography from the fragments of her individual dancers' stories and creativity, I attempt to assemble a collage from the fragments of dance educators' stories, depicting a dynamic dialogue between me, the choreographer-researcher, the dancers-participants, and the readers-audience, so that my text becomes coherent to the reader through bricolaging pedagogical quality of life with quality of life as a whole.

The study was guided, via Bond (2003), by Max van Manen's (1997) hermeneutic phenomenology. Put simply, hermeneutic phenomenology combines description of lived experience with interpretation of meanings; however, van Manen emphasizes that the method of this path is that there is no method or "recipe;" instead there is a tradition, a body of knowledge and history of thinkers and writers, who together cultivate a methodological ground for research. In this study, I strive to draw on the human capacities for interpretive sensitivity, multi-sensory cognition, imagination, logic, intuition, and artistic sensibility – all resources for human meaning making (Bond, 2003).

van Manen (1997) reminds us that we "have to understand the 'good' in order to give content to the meaning of competence when we speak of an adult as a 'good' teacher" (p. 157). While appreciating this premise, I also seek meanings and living examples from the full range of participants' self-perceptions of teaching in higher dance education, "good," "bad," and between. At the same time I agree with van Manen (1991) that it is more helpful to give a good example than to criticize examples of others; by neglecting meanings of quality teaching, dance educators could come to forget their true being. For their possibility to evoke participants' visceral memories of particularly strong teaching moments, I used *good* and *bad* in the provisional research title presented to participants: "Dance Teaching, Good and Bad: Stories from Higher Education."

I accessed potential participants via web search engines such as Google®. I found 30 American college/university websites that offer a minor or major degree in dance. From each university, I contacted all listed dance professors by sending them an invitational announcement. I also sought authorizations to seek participants from relevant professional associations, including the National Dance Education Organization (NDEO) and Dance and the Child: International (daCi). Both organizations posted my call for participants on their member listservs. Beyond this initial search, I did some active recruiting by emailing colleagues in different countries who in turn provided me with other teachers' email addresses, creating a snowball effect (used often in qualitative research) (Miles & Huberman, 1994).

Thirty-five teachers in six countries participated in the study (Brazil, Canada, Jamaica, Portugal, Turkey and the United States), the majority of whom were at an advanced stage of their careers. Each individual contributed two written stories via email about contrasting dance teaching experiences at the college level, one in which they felt effective and another in which they felt ineffective. Seventy anecdotes were collected from the 35 participants (33 female and two male) of varying ethnic backgrounds, all of whom had taught or were currently teaching in higher education dance. Their ages ranged from 20 to 70 years.

As per van Manen's (1997) guidelines for capturing lived experience description, I invited teachers to recount tactile sensations, mood, emotions, and other bodily experiences in order to vivify their memories of selected teaching episodes. I acknowledge that the quest for meanings through memories and stories is not straightforward and can be elusive, with ambiguity and contradictions (Denzin, 1989/2002). The discipline of bracketing, that is, the suspension of predispositions and theories about the phenomenon of inquiry (van Manen, 1997), helped me avoid premature closure or ungrounded interpretive leaps in data analysis (Bond, 2003). In my case, theoretical pre-dispositions were likely those gained through extended affiliation with post-colonial and post-structuralist thinking – the work of Paulo Freire in particular.

I created poetic composites from words and phrases that clustered initially into descriptive categories (Bond & Stinson, 2000/2001). Once I identified categories and distilled these to themes, my aims were to engage with "multiple, emerging, and conflicting meanings" (p. 56) and to be open to unexpected results. I sought to maintain a concept of an emergent research design that acknowledges scholarly endeavor as a creative process (see Bond, 2017).

Poetics of Teaching Dance in Higher Education

This section presents a descriptive analysis of participants' perceptions of teaching in the form of research poems based on five categories of description identified in the data. The first three categories: *body awareness, emotions and feelings*, and *metaphysical and naturalistic phenomena* relate to felt personal or inner states. The fourth category, *interactions with students and colleagues*, describes participants' significant interpersonal encounters, and the fifth "meta-category," *self-assessment*, contains participants' evaluative meanings of their selected teaching events. Collectively, the following poetic composites illustrate the range of participants' experiential language appearing in the writings.

Body ("Good"): I Jump
I am invigorated, really energized.
My energy is so alive.
I feel bubbly inside.
I tingle.

An organic feeling.
My body responds intensively, each organ separately.
I take a deep breath. My breath is flowing.
My chest expands.

My muscles and breath change and relax--no tension.
Immediately I feel relieved.
A sensation of lightness.
Free flow

I jump.

I see more clearly.
I can actually hear students' brains working.
Happy faces, alive bodies

I hear laughter…so much fun.

Body ("Bad"): It's Kind of a Strain
My breath is not in unison with my body.
Respiration is heavy.
Muscles are tight.
I'm tense.
It's kind of a strain.
I feel very stressed.

My physical fatigue is strong.
Walking a tightrope, lethargic and exhausted

I feel hot.
My blood, all of a sudden, starts to boil in my veins.

I am cold…extremely cold.
I can't feel my body.
My feet are disconnected from the floor.
I can't hear my own voice.
I am feeling smaller and smaller.

I hear my voice becoming sterner, the volume increases.
I look around and see drooping eyelids.
Yes, they stare at me!

I taste disappointment.
My chest contracts.

Emotions and Feelings: Inside, My Heart is Singing
A sense of joy comes over me

I feel joyous…I feel joy!
I am elated!
I feel euphoric.
I feel high.

I am happy.
Satisfied.
Alert
Surprised and rewarded
I am touched.

A warm sensation
A nice feeling
Hues
Love
My heart opens.

I am delighted.
Hooray!

Full of enthusiasm
I feel so excited.
I feel very good.
Refreshed and inspired

From somewhere – an unanticipated inner calm
I feel very comfortable in this classroom.

Emotions and Feelings: Teaching can be Hard!
I don't feel motivated.
I am not enthusiastic.
No high or low feelings – a monotone

I feel agitated and nervous.
I become anxious.
I feel upset and my anger is rising.
Frustration, disappointment

Anguish!
I cry and feel sad.
I feel guilty.
I feel not hooray.
Paranoia
I want to scream.

Disheartened
Fearful, insecure
Intimidated
I am desperate to find something that works.

Embarrassed, flabbergasted, and humiliated
I don't know how to handle the situation.
I want to not lose control.

A mixture of feelings: shock, surprise, shame, denial and confusion
A nightmare!

I feel tight, stifled, and trapped.
Empty and deflated

I feel smaller and smaller.
I want to disappear.

Metaphysical and Naturalistic Perceptions: Wind and Crickets
Space is alive.
Time is fast, fleeting, and uneven.

Space becomes a blur.
Time stands still.

A good teaching experience lifts my spirit.

The class has magic.
Their training wheels magically disappear.

A beautiful synthesis
Creativity, learning, play and experimentation

There is a chemistry in this class. A synchrony.

From somewhere, an inner voice. An unanticipated calm.
'Aha' moments – insights
I feel abundantly blessed.
Amen!

I hear myself speak as though a second voice.

There is a primal, ritual feeling…mysterious.
A meditative quality.

Wind and crickets.

Interactions with Students: Connectivity!
The energy in the room is like popcorn, popping.
The atmosphere is quiet, still, charged.
The energy is great, soothing, powerful, and welcoming.
The atmosphere is intense, purposeful.

Encounters…

A sensation of lightness towards others.
Ready for openness
Body contact
It feels good dancing together.
Our bodies linger…close to each other.
We move in synchrony as a unit.
I am being moved by them.

Intimacy…
A feeling of community and support
I feel on top of it, not in terms of power,
but in my connection to students.
There are multiple artists in the class, and no hierarchy.

I integrate with students,
we complete each other.
New possibilities…we overcome limitations.

I ask students' input
I take them very seriously
I feel included and respected.
Connectiveness!

Interactions with Students: I Lose Connection
Not one student acknowledges my presence.
I'm confused.
I ignore them and don't say a word.
I give them my back!!

Students criticize my class.
A student throws me questions.
It's a power play.
I feel intimidated and let them "undo" me.

I want to mix with students and break the ice.
But they turn their backs to me.
The class atmosphere is unbearable.

I use my authority to control the situation.
I raise my voice.
Tensions are high and my comments are peppered with "you should."
I refuse to accommodate students' desires.

I'm quiet…unable to say anything.
I lose connection.

Interactions with Colleagues: My Colleague is There
My colleague is there.
Watching my class, smiling encouragingly
Connectiveness: she gets caught up in the discussion.
This connection is thrilling.

Synchrony with my musician

Interactions with Colleagues: Less than Hospitable
A young female dance professor with three "old boys"
A less-than-hospitable ground
I feel I have to teach this course.

I resent my accompanist who is late.

I want the students to look good so that I look good.
But I am sure faculty are whispering.

I shouldn't have to teach this class.
I feel frustrated, annoyed, resentful.
This course should be rotated among the faculty.

Departmental dynamics…I'm fatigued.
I question my abilities as a teacher.

Self-Assessment: I Am a Teacher
I teach carefully and systematically.
I am thorough.
I know what I'm doing.

My teaching becomes easy, competent, inspired, embodied, creative, attentive, committed.

I am confident about the material, extremely secure and pumped up in my ego.
I say things in an integrated way.
A pivotal time of growth
I feel my reward.
I walk on clouds.
A highlight in my career that keeps me going

I trust in my insights.
I grow.

Students make connections.
I am satisfied I have done my job.
I feel the power of mastery.
I smile and make jokes—I have so much fun!
I let go my critical voice of authority and improvise with them.
I have their complete engagement.
They ask many questions and make comments.

My teaching is gratifying…it is my gift to students.
I feel fulfilled.
I feel good and whole.
A sense of accomplishment and completion

I am in the right field.
I have something to offer.
I'm smart!
Yes, I am an artist.
I am a teacher.

Self-Assessment: Talk about a Meltdown!
Students criticized me.
I did what I'd NEVER EVER done in my life—I gave them my back!!!!!
I let the students down.

I am tired, I feel uncertain.
I am not inspired to teach.

I am disappointed with myself.
Out of my depth, off center
I feel like a phony, a liar trying to cover up tracks.

I was not on the right wave length.
I didn't give myself to the experience, to the instant, to the students.
I'm not a good teacher!

Very bad memories
Embarrassment and nausea

My memory gave out.
Students stared at me blankly.
I wanted to stop and leave.
I didn't want to try other ways.

I felt like a failure…completely inadequate.
All washed out

I lost credibility. I didn't know what to do.
I made a wrong turn on a journey.
I hit a roadblock.
I spoilt the culmination of the semester work.

I was clueless about student dissatisfaction.
I questioned my role and competency.
My efforts were useless.

Disembodied
Discouraged
Unfulfilled
Confused

I cried.
I blew up.

Nightmare
Train wreck
Talk about a meltdown!

Experiential Themes: Embodiment, Complexity, Transformation

> I have lived on the lip of insanity, wanting to know reasons, knocking on a door. It opens. I've been knocking from the inside. (Jalal al-Din Rumi, 2004, p. 36)

This section presents a synthesis of findings through inter-subjective, hermeneutic engagement with three inter-related themes that emerged from descriptive analysis of dance teaching stories from higher education. I move now from phenomenological reduction towards inductive thinking and interpretation. Analysis of 70 teaching stories (two from each of 35 participants) identified three interrelated themes about teaching in higher education dance: *embodiment, complexity,* and *transformation.* I discuss each theme in reference to the descriptive analysis, using either pseudonyms or teacher (T) numerical codes (T1-T35) to identify exemplary texts and scope of lived experience descriptions, respectively.

Theme 1: Embodiment

I found two key dynamics of embodiment described by participants: the embodied self that teachers bring to the lifeworld, and the intersubjective embodiment of meanings in the teaching moment. At first, what drew my own bodily attention in the data was the connection between intra and inter-relationality and self-assessment. So, what I initially called "within body" and "between bodies," were each a way of perceiving. I perceived an association between embodied self-awareness and positive interpersonal connection with "effective" teaching qualities, and vice versa. In the midst of her anxiety, Duygu, for example, shifts her breathing and emotions to a balanced, relaxed state as she establishes connections of support and engagement with her students. She "smiles and makes jokes." Likewise, Darla lets go of her agenda to become a calm being who puts into practice her belief that a student "deserves to be guided toward clarification before we proceed." Janie also embodies a being who is "open to and present with students" and as a group they experience "connectedness." Stella opens her heart to students and feels "warm hues" as they interact with each other. She feels accomplished in connecting with her own self as creative and competent.

In terms of negative embodied experiences, I found an association between painful emotions and negative self-assessment. Mary Ann, for example, felt anxious and annoyed when she perceived her students' disrespect, disinterest, and disgust. She immediately embodies a critical perspective on students' performance, feeling frustrated by anything short of excellence. She feels "judged," as well as "embarrassed, overwhelmed, insecure…angry and hot." This was "a low point in my 35-year professional career." Afterwards Mary Ann berated herself for the "meltdown." To this day, she is not sure whether she misjudged the situation, yet the painful emotions live on. In Angela's story, her students feel like a threat when they criticize her course. She turns away, refusing to look at them; the "atmosphere could not have been worse." Her resistance to students makes her feel "disembodied." She is critical of her own dance knowledge.

My multi-sensory reading of participants' writings (Bond, 2003) deepened my recognition of their embodiment. This "chemistry" (T5) enabled me to infer that teachers' descriptions reveal engagement of their entire being through:

- *body awareness* (T1 feels light and energized, T23 feels bubbly inside, T26 feels refreshed, T28's muscles are relaxed),
- *feelings and emotions* (T3's joy, T3's and T9's "highs," T8's happiness, T12's elation, T17's enthusiasm, and T23's euphoria),
- *metaphysical connections* (T10's spirit, T22's synchrony, T25's primal feeling, and T26's inner voice),
- *connection to others* (T5's connectedness to the class and a colleague, T6's and T7's sense of community, T17's and T35's intimacy with students, and T22's moving as a unity with students,), and.
- *thought-full being,* a term I coined to represent experience that is *full of thought*, a holistic category that subsumes *self-assessment.* Teachers' self-assessments are embodied ones, *'full of thought'* as well as body, emotions, relations, and so forth (T1's accomplishment, T8's fulfillment, T12's mindfulness, and T26's empowerment). T8 sums it up, depicting her embodied teaching as follows: "I feel whole, bodily, and complete."

At various stages of data analysis my own teaching experiences allowed me to connect on a human level to each participant, many of whom I have never met. Their sensuous stories permit me to inhabit their experiences in time and space – I dance in their shoes, as if I were there. The transparency of participants' writing became an invitation between human beings who move through the dialectics and ambiguities of pedagogical existence. Like T12's "magic" experience, the "nakedness" of their writing enabled me to open my heart, to their "anguish" (T26) and their "warm hues" (T9). Their shifting self-assessments ("Now I feel competent…now I feel a failure"), sometimes in the same course, suggest that embodiment is the ground of pedagogical quality and that teaching is a process of becoming. Likewise, I propose that embodiment is the ground of quality of life and that living is a process of becoming (Carlisle, 2005).

Teachers' embodiment, as reflected in participants' writing, fuses past and present in the lived moment (van Manen, 1997). This brings me to the other side of embodiment illuminated in this study – the process through which new meanings become corporealized. It appears that as teachers self-reflect, recall and write their experiences, pedagogical meanings are embodied more deeply, becoming part of the developing self. Let me illustrate this point with examples. Many participants (T1-T5, T8-T12, T16, T18, T22, T23, T26, T31, T35) relate their selected experience of "effective" teaching to communication of who they are or would like to be. T35's embodied meaning of effectiveness is her "availability" to students, and her ability to give up her plan in favor of their expressed needs; T18's embodied meaning of "a nice class" is her flexibility with students. She does not "compromise to any kind of righteousness" and allows herself to dance with students freely.

Participants' embodied pedagogies are revealed also in instances when they translate values and philosophical orientation into action, including the way they orally, bodily and emotionally communicate with students. T1, for example, feels "joyous, light and energized" to embody the "good teacher" who "knows what I am doing." T8 is happy that she does what she believes in and fights for – to teach dance by dancing. At the same time, both of their "ineffective teaching" stories suggest bodily dis-ease. T1 was unable to let go of anger and disappointment and T8 did "what I never ever have done." Thus, embodied self-assessment might be oriented to who one wants or does not want to be. I consider that this study opens up discourse on the nature of *pedagogical ineffectiveness*. T5 likely speaks for many when she acknowledges: "I was basically flabbergasted and really did not know how to handle the situation."

As participants' stories became bodily-felt – for me – I began to overcome barriers; I came to appreciate participants' multiple ways of expression and the diverse meanings to which they flow. Before this turning point, I had been "living on the lip of insanity" (Rumi, 2004, p. 37), struggling with a mental puzzle that was taking me nowhere. It was too hard (or perhaps impossible?) to "get there" when I persistently, albeit unconsciously, looked for meanings using my critical theoretical perspective. My commitment to embodied presence for teachers' stories, or "knocking from within" (p. 37), taught me that if I strive to use all my multiple ways of perceiving – making connections, merging their paths – I might find relevant meanings that cohere in useful ways. Further, this kind of embodiment could be helpful to knowing self and world in unique particularities and full-blossoming wholeness.

Theme 2: Complexity of Teaching

Teachers' stories project a sense of dance education as a complex domain of doing, sensing, feeling, thinking, making, and relationality. Participants illustrate teaching as a continuous and dynamic "dance of possibility" (similar to life itself). Participants describe a wide range of bodily sensations, emotions, metaphysical perceptions, interpersonal interactions and self-assessments. The richness, depth, and vulnerability of pedagogical life is revealed by the intensity and volume of meanings articulated.

Speaking to complexity as an overarching theme, I found that the combination of positive emotions, pleasurable body sensations, productive interactions with students and colleagues, and spiritual meaning was often associated with positive self-assessment, or effectiveness. Sometimes a momentary awareness, event, or insight comes as an unexpected visitor, and participants welcome and entertain the newcomer. These factors might be fundamental not only in teaching, but also in the endless quest for meaning and quality of life (Bond & Stinson, 2000/2001). On the other hand, the mix of negative emotions, uncomfortable sensations, and difficult social interactions was often associated with negative self-assessment. In such cases teachers often described failure to deal successfully with or welcome the unexpected. According to Damasio, Melo, and Silva (2013), teachers' levels of well-being and quality of life have dropped in the face of adverse conditions of teaching.

Dance teachers' perceptions of effectiveness are holistic, not based solely on intellectual reasoning or moral superiority. Indeed, all the descriptions of experienced rigidity were full of self-doubt and emotional confusion. This might sound like a commonsense reflection or quite familiar for a reader who teaches dance in higher education. As Hegel observed, however, "the familiar just because it is *familiar*, is not comprehended [*erkannt*]" (as cited in Burch, 1989, p. 193). In this study, teaching revealed itself in all its affective complexity and sensuousness. Notably, Damasio et al. (2013) remind us that teachers are "a professional group that generally displays high levels of emotional exhaustion" (p. 74).

The similarities in participants' effective teaching accounts relate to being flexible, present, and open to the unexpected. There is a need to address all aspects of the teaching experience, particularly the dynamics of body senses and emotions that are intrinsic to dance teaching, making it a uniquely challenging area of pedagogy. Although there are no easy solutions to the affective challenges and dilemmas faced by dance teachers, a fundamental value associated with teachers' self-assessment is adaptability – an ability to meet the unpredictable challenge or novel opportunity.

Teachers who improvise might experience the reward of their flexibility. Within the complex teaching situation, they might feel effective. On the other hand, teachers' lack of flexibility can take the form of restrictive inner monologues, anger, and defensiveness. The unexpectedness of the memorable teaching moment – an element in all the "effective teaching" stories, reminds me to question assumptions that teaching in higher education (in general and in dance) is simple and predictable, as some theorists seem to suggest (Filene, 2005; Fortin, 1993; Hudson, 2006; Rogers, 2002).

Dance teachers' stories convey that effective encounters with the unexpected require self-awareness, the lack of which can decrease the ability to adjust to a novel situation (for example, when T8 felt disembodied, T9 and T17 felt hot, T19 and T22 became confused, and T28 experienced restricted breathing). T1, T8, and T13 wrote regretful wishes to have handled the challenging situation with less frustration and anger. As noted by Wats and Robertson (2011), "Teacher stress potentially impairs personal and professional competence" (p 33). On reflection, this could be a point of intersection between dance teaching in higher education and dance teachers' quality of life: an adaptable or improvisational attitude toward the unpredictable can unfold into "magic" experiences (P11) of growth and transformation.

Theme 3: Transformation

Participant stories often describe meaningful personal or social change, as evidenced in language like "turning point" (T5), "learning" (T6, T22), "high points" (T11) "pivotal," (T15, T26), "highlights of my career" (T22), and "growth" (T26). I was intrigued reading these experiences, as my writing prompts did not mention or request descriptions of change, nor of metaphysical experience or language, which were often companion to transformational teaching moments (T6, T15, T22, T26). Darla, for example, spoke in an integrated way, "as through a second voice." Her transformation or "pivotal" experience left strong traces, changing her "beingness" as a teacher. She can evoke pleasurable feelings by just thinking about this class.

Indeed, associated meanings of transformation leave positive memories, including physical and emotional ones. T8's transformational teaching brought her "excitement" and "energy" as she wrote about it, and T20 still feels the experience "close to her heart." These participants represent the human potential for transformative intersubjectivity, which in this study is illuminated as an embodied, emotional connection to the other. I believe that from this inner, yet transcendent source of life and existence, teaching transforms.

For some teachers, the context of transformation seems to be the "good" teaching experience (T2, T6, T8, T11, T20, T26–27). The self-discoveries that emerge from positive situations are, for me, evidence that pedagogical transformation is an essential constituent of the teaching life. Transformational qualities increase participants' options for *being*, *acting*, and *interacting*. Being oneself is mentioned by T9, who affirms herself to be a teacher and an artist, by T12 who finds evidence in her teaching that she is an artist and actually smart, and by T17 who allows herself to be spontaneous. T5 experiences "chemistry" in her "connectedness" to students and T12 feels elated in her new connection to students. T8 feels so excited about her teaching that, out of the blue, she decides to compose a dance in her technique class. It seems that what is always there, inside, from a deep place, gets permission to come out. It is like a dam is broken, releasing waves to come out of the sea.

Some participants describe their transformational experiences as an intense and unexpected moment in which inner and outer connection, perceptions of time and space are beyond what they normally experience. Qualities of transformation in dance teaching described by participants can be summarized as follows:

- metaphysical intervention or involvement of a higher power
- intense emotions, bodily sensations and/or spiritual connection
- integration with nature
- realization of something that was not realized before
- difficulty indescribing the experience
- a feeling that the transformation experience fed them
- a meditative state brought by engagement
- a sense that the experience allows them to be who they are/want to be
- a feeling that time seems different
- perception of a collective transformation

Bond and Stinson (2000/2001) found similar phenomena in their qualitative meta-analysis of young people's meanings of dance (600 dancers and dance students, ages 3–18), sourced by interviews, captioned drawings about dancing, and observations from a number of countries, again without prompts for such meanings. Such evidence supports Paul Crowther's premise that "the entire aesthetic realm is driven by the human need for transformation" (as cited in Bond, 2001, p. 49).

Although teachers in higher education dance often work in contexts that stress productivity and mastery, many of participants' stories emphasize transformation. In living their daily lives, inside and outside of university "walls," a dance educator might dynamically and continuously dance through anxiety and calm, high energy and exhaustion, pleasure and pain. Fortunately, similar to T2, T8, and T11, the "mysterious" and "magic" moments of "ah-ha" can keep us moving forward.

Research findings can be interpreted, then, in a heuristic and broad sense that affords insight into both teaching and everyday situations. There can be times, for example, when one engages in critical self-reflection based on embodied biases as a teacher and in life, including tendencies toward "isms" of authority and judgment, often projected through abstractions and intellectualization. But if we can let this kind of thinking subside, revelations might occur; with an open mind, body and heart, out of the blue, one can create a new understanding about teaching and about life. One can become more aware and connected to their body signs and learn to honor multiple ways of knowing, which have always been there, inside of a person, part of our human possibility.

Becoming Possibility

This study identifies embodied flexibility, openness, and creativity as elements of quality teaching. I propose that these aspects are key to quality of life as well. The importance of embodiment in perceiving, knowing, and meaning making poses a challenge to the traditional focus on abstract, intellectual knowledge in higher education. It also invites us to rethink the nature of interaction between teachers and adult learners as being solely based on verbal communication. The descriptive poetics illuminating the theme of embodiment suggest that dance teacher self and dance teacher body are a relational unity, living constant inner and outer connection and becoming. This study also elucidates qualities and nuances of pedagogical interaction between teachers and students including affective and ethical relationships, bodily contact, and communications that develop as an exchange of gifts, spreading delight of mutual learning and transcending prescribed boundaries and roles.

Further, in researching teachers' experiential meanings, the study acknowledges "knowledge mostly ignored or formally discounted by the extremes of logical positivism" (Brady, 2005, p. 983). As Rodgers and Raider-Roth (2006) explain, much research on teaching is embedded in an objectivist view, emulating values of efficiency originating in industrial management. Such approaches ignore teachers' meanings of their work as well as their personal practical knowledge. Freire (1968/2014) stresses the importance of ethical education, which is more than technical training, and that teaching of any specific content cannot happen apart from students' moral preparation. van Manen (1995) also speaks about "good" teaching as a moral concern for the good of the other.

Data related to interaction indicate that teachers fostered relationship with students through holistic care and respect, especially in their effective teaching experiences (for example, T3, T8, T25). Some stories of effective teaching, however, focus on students' technical training and academic knowledge. Does this imply that some dance teachers in this study fail to understand education beyond modernist values of technical training and academics? I bracket this question for now, as it sounds connected to critical theory interests rather than to participants' phenomenological meanings found in their lived experience descriptions.

Freire (1996/2016) reminds educators, "o ensino dos conteúdos implica o testemunho ético do professor" ("the teaching of content implies the professor's ethical testimony") (p. 95). His statement takes me back to P1, who felt ashamed and disappointed with herself for not being able to have a positive interaction with her students. For Freire (1993/2014), a positive student-teacher relation is a "dialogical" relation involving shared critique of socially constructed reality. This concept is crucial to Freire's notion of liberatory or emancipatory education where the aim is to provoke changes in students' worldview and engagement. The theme of *transformation* is grounded in teachers' descriptions that use language like "freedom," "growth," and "release."

Freire explains dialogue as "the encounter between men [and women]...who are attempting, together, to learn more than they now know" (pp. 62–63). Data on interaction suggest the importance of dialogical relationship in participants' working lives. Dialogue was often present in dance teachers' experiences they remembered as effective. Further, teachers' bodily and affective dialogue was as important as oral dialogue with students, as evidenced in their descriptions of embodiment. Accordingly, Parini (2005) notes that dialogue goes far beyond "talk," for a good deal of what is taught is transmitted almost unconsciously in the embodied interchange between teacher and student.

Many oppositions co-exist in current discourse on effective teaching such as students' evaluation of teaching versus teachers' self-assessment, reflection-in-action versus reflection-on-action, simplicity versus complexity, teaching versus mentoring, and of course, effective versus ineffective. By 1938, John Dewey (1976) had noted how education usually divides into two camps. He opened his book *Experience and Education* with the statement that, "Mankind (sic) likes to think in terms of extreme opposites" (p. 17). My analysis of teaching stories suggests that even when we are asked to think in binary terms, our lived experiences are full of nuances that continuously move between and around poles.

I want to emphasize that I am not denying the importance of keeping current in the field, or of commitment to students' learning of standards, or becoming knowledgeable in the didactic dimension of teaching. Further, I understand that despite efforts to defy binary thinking, most scholars are already implicated in the traditional dichotomous values they seek to oppose in research (see Burt, 2004). Arguably, dualistic thinking and writing are tools in a person's navigation and problem solving throughout life, as evidenced in our early binary utterances of "yes" and "no." At the same time, I do not want to neglect what van Manen (1995) discusses as crucial in the lived moment of teaching: being fully present. My intention is to develop a discussion that does not reinforce opposition between content excellence and teacher and student wellbeing. It seems clear that the nature of effective teaching, as depicted by this study's participants, goes beyond what teachers *must do* in relation to social-cultural norms and prescriptions.

Some participants are doctoral or master's students in dance who also teach and some are professors in graduate programs, but all of them are teachers in higher education. This suggests that they might be informed on new research and knowledge in the dance field. Some stated clearly their concern for students' learning, and some explicitly or implicitly shared their knowledge of standards, educational theories, and didactic methods, with some actually teaching these subjects – yet they still experienced times and spaces of ineffective teaching. van Manen (1991) writes, "What are the makings of a good educator? A person may have learned all curriculummethods and all the techniques of instruction and yet be a poor teacher" (p. xi). In their stories, participating teachers mediate the integrity of teaching, the curriculum, and the process of learning through their being, which includes but is not solely reduced to their academic knowledge.

Participants (T14, T20, T23–24) also describe overload in workloads outside of teaching, including administration, service, research, and publication. Susan Stinson (1993) described what many in higher education are still attempting:

> We support efforts to try to make the existing structure work by adding more competencies to our list, and expecting ourselves and our graduates to do more and more within the existing and shrinking confines of time, space and funds. … I believe that we err when we blame students and teachers for ineffective schools and look to national standards and more competencies to fix them. (p. 47)

Stinson notes that we "should" care for our students, while admitting how difficult this becomes in large classes. She reflects, "it takes time to provide care…time we do not have when we take on too much" (p. 46). T11 and T23 described students complaining about their lack of care, both writing, "I felt guilty."

I wonder whether guilt, or pedagogical regret, might also be a form of caring; that is, the feeling of guilt from a "negative" teaching experience can be a turning point, as it was for T6:

> I was stern with corrections and grudging with positive comments. I was so enmeshed in my sense that what I was teaching was the "right" thing. For me, while this was an ineffective teaching experience, it was one of my most effective learning experiences. This class was a huge turning point in my development as an educator and as an individual.

Acknowledging that we cannot have everything we want, Stinson poses existential questions: "What kind of lives do we want to live? What do we value most in our lives?" (p. 47). Along the same lines, Denton and Ashton (2004) suggest that we have the potential to come to something existentially, surpassing or transcending cultures. I agree with Stinson (1993) that being "superteachers" will not answer the problems we face today on any educational level, but rather prevent us from examining power structures in education and "from living full lives" (p. 47).

Participants wrote about classic existential dilemmas: wanting to feel included (T1, T4–5, T8) and appreciated (T4, T8, T17, T23), wanting to look good (T24), and to know and live up to who they are (T1, T8–9, T25). They experience questions in the teaching moment such as "What now?" and "What's next?" In moments of uncertainty, participants might feel "trapped" (T2) in the impasse of "What is the right action?" or "Am I going to do this well enough?" Are teachers' struggles existential, cultural, or both? In terms of lived experience, this study finds that teaching well involves integration of bodily, emotional, social, spiritual and thought-full (including cognitive, critical) being. Further, dance teachers are, first, human beings who do not know everything about the content they are teaching (T15, T22) and might have a tendency to prefer certain topics (T9, T17–18). They also deal with conflicts such as greater empathy towards some students than others (T13, T28). A dance teacher can unintentionally misjudge students (T1, T4, T28).

Moreover, similar to Åkerlind 's (2007) findings, excessive focus on learning outcomes is often companion to nervousness and anxiety – qualities most felt in selected episodes of ineffective teaching (T1, T4–6, T9, T13, T17, T23). Akin to this is Bond and Richard's (2005) study, which found that a dance teacher's goal to develop a collaborative approach to dance curriculum sits uncomfortably with her desire to fulfill the current arts education agenda that seeks to validate dance education on the grounds that it improves student performance in academic subject areas. (p. 116).

On the other hand, stories teachers wrote about their "effective teaching" are similar to those described in Bond and Etwaroo (2005), Bond and Richard (2005), Paris and Combs (2006), and Wu (2005), which, in terms of teacher-student interactions, include sharing of dance work and ideas, respect for each student's uniqueness within a community of learning, and appreciation for students' performances. These findings point to the value of teachers' and students' collective construction of knowledge. Indeed, these studies explore the possibilities for collaboration as inherent to quality teaching.

Closing Reflections

Findings of this study on dance teachers' experiences of pedagogical quality in higher education concur with theorists who have discussed effective teaching in education generally (Freire, 1993/2014; Jay, 2003; Shapiro & Stefkovich, 2001; van Manen, 2002). Overall, these theorists emphasize the importance of careful teaching along with openness, flexibility, creativity, and presence. I reflect,

> What if effective teaching *in dance* is the same as effective teaching in any field of knowledge? Should I be surprised? Does this have anything to say about dance as a body of *physical* knowledge, for so long considered to be unlike intellectual knowledge?

Dialoguing with literature, I faced a challenge. Much of the discourse is abstract, removed from the lifeworld of teachers. This study, in contrast, is not theoretically driven; the focus is on lived experience of teachers themselves, and the findings unveil aspects of pedagogical being that are not well understood. In particular, bodily, emotional, and metaphysical dimensions of teaching – all related to quality of life – are under-theorized. Participants' stories give a clear message that to live teaching involves more than subject knowledge and techniques.

An important finding of this study relates to the importance of body knowledge in quality teaching in dance higher education. Like Stinson (1995), I consider body knowledge crucial to dance educators' quality of life. Consciousness, world, and bodies as perceiving entities are intricately intertwined and mutually *engaged*. The phenomenal "thing" is not the unchanging object of the natural sciences, but a correlate of our bodily and sensory functions. Taking the study of perception as his point of departure, Merleau-Ponty came to recognize that one's own body is not only a thing, a potential object of study for science, but a permanent condition of experience, a constituent of our perceptual openness to the world (Baldwin, 2004). Influenced by Merleau-Ponty, Bond (2003, 2018) highlights a working assumption of experiential inquiry that I believe is essential to dance teaching and dance teachers' quality of life: that the lived body cannot be denied in knowing.

Future research is needed on teacher professional development (for example, differentiated learning, class size, gender issues in dance education, teacher inquiry), an important resource for dance teachers' quality of working life. Teachers' quality of life is also about their voices being heard and recognized. Keeping my commitment to lived experience, I advocate with Bond and Richard (2005) for a "return to the voices of students and teacher, whose meanings extend previous curriculum research and resonate with possibilities for the future" (p. 85). This statement suggests that teacher/student satisfaction "lives" closer to immediate experience in the classroom than to mandated curricular standards.

Teachers strive to perform educational work at their best. From a phenomenological viewpoint, the quest for "doing our best" can be considered part of human nature (Van den Berg, 2002) and therefore associated with quality of life. This seems quite pertinent for dance educators who aspire to teach dance at a high-quality level and to enjoy quality of life by doing our best at what we love to do.

I hope this study might have shown how blurred the lines can be between teaching and living, being and teaching, living and becoming. For future research in dance teachers' quality of life, I suggest phenomenological inquiry as the method of choice, since it promotes self-reflection, teacher-by-teacher. Husserl (1988) describes phenomenological reduction as "a piece of pure self- reflection…" (p. 419). Moreover, phenomenological writing speaks logically, kinesthetically, and poetically to the embodied mind. For both authors and readers, such texts can evoke reflective insights into lived experience. Phenomenological reflection also invites accountability and can thus lead to new perspectives and self-understandings, including changes in practice and, possibly, in Being.

> There is always danger for those who are afraid of it; let the inmates, your dreams, creativity and imagination, free the guards. Being is enough. (Villarreal, personal communication, January 20, 2007)

Quality teaching is an inner and outer connection to be created, not a prize to be won. For the higher education dance teachers involved in this study, teaching well is about personal fulfillment and living through transformational moments that go beyond daily academic life. It is about living and quality of life.

References

Åkerlind, G. S. (2007). Constraints on academics' potential for developing as a teacher. *Studies in Higher Education, 32*(1), 21–37.

Baldwin, T. (Ed.). (2004). *Maurice Merleau-Ponty: Basic writings*. London: Routledge.

Bond, K. (2001). "I'm not an eagle, I'm a chicken": Young children's perceptions of creative dance. *Early Childhood Connections, 7*(4), 41–51.

Bond, K. (2003). *Meaning in dance*. Doctoral seminar, Temple University, Philadelphia.

Bond, K. (2017). "Boys are morons … Girls are gross:" Let's dance! In W. Oliver & D. Risner (Eds.), *Dance and gender: An evidence-based approach* (pp. 135–157). Gainesville, FL: University Press of Florida.

Bond, K. (2018). "Me, a tree": Young children as natural phenomenologists. In S. Fraleigh (Ed.), *Back to the dance itself: Phenomenologies of the body in performance* (pp. 205–232). Urbana: University of Illinois Press.

Bond, K., & Etwaroo, I. (2005). "If I really see you": Students' experiences of identity and difference in a higher education setting. In M.-C. Powell & V. Marcow-Speiser (Eds.), *The arts, education, and social change: Little signs of hope* (pp. 87–100). Cambridge, MA: Peter Lang.

Bond, K. E., & Richard, B. (2005). "Ladies and gentlemen: What do you see? What do you feel?" A story of connected curriculum in a third grade dance education setting. In L. Y. Overby & B. Lepczyk (Eds.), *Dance: Current selected research* (Vol. 5, pp. 85–133). New York: AMS.

Bond, K. E., & Stinson, S. W. (2000/01). "I feel like I'm going to take off!": Young people's experiences of the superordinary in dance. *Dance Research Journal, 32*(2), 52–87.

Brady, I. (2005). Poetics for a planet: Discourse on some problems of being-in-place. In N. K. Denzin & Y. S. Lincoln (Eds.), *The sage handbook of qualitative research* (3rd ed., pp. 979–1026). Thousand Oaks, CA: Sage.

Burch, R. (1989). On phenomenology and its practice. *Phenomenology & Pedagogy, 7*, 187–217.

Burt, R. (2004). Genealogy and dance history: Foucault, Rainer, Bausch, and DeKeersmaeker. In A. Lepecki (Ed.), *Of the presence of the body: Essays on dance and performance theory* (pp. 29–46). Middletown, CT: Wesleyan University Press.

Carlisle, C. (2005). *Kierkegaard's philosophy of becoming: Movement and positions*. Albany, NY: SUNY Press.

Damasio, B. F., Melo, R. L. P., & Silva, J. P. (2013). Meaning in life, psychological well-being and quality of life in teachers. *Paidéia, 23*(54), 73–82.

Denton, D., & Ashton, W. (Eds.). (2004). *Spirituality, action, and pedagogy: Teaching from the heart*. New York: Peter Lang.

Denzin, N. K. (2002). *Interpretive interactionism* (2nd ed.). London: Sage. (Original work published 1989).

Denzin, N. K., & Lincoln, Y. S. (Eds.). (2005). *Handbook of qualitative research* (3rd ed.). Thousand Oaks, CA: Sage.

Dewey, J. (1976). *Experience and education* (19th ed.). New York: Macmillan. (Original work published 1938).

Filene, P. (2005). *The joy of teaching: A practical guide for new college instructors*. Chapel Hill, NC: University of North Carolina Press.

Fortin, S. (1993). The knowledge base for competent dance teaching. *Journal of Physical Education, Recreation & Dance, 64*(9), 34–38.

Freire, P. (2016). *Pedagogia da autonomia: Saberes necessários à prática educativa* (53rd ed.). [Pedagogy of liberation: Essential principles to the educative practice]. São Paulo, Brasil: Paz e Terra. (Original work published 1996).

Freire, P. (2018). *Pedagogy of the oppressed* (50th anniversary ed.) (M. Bergman Ramos, Trans.). London: Bloomsbury. (Original work published 1968).

Heidegger, M. (2005). *Introduction to phenomenological research*. Bloomington, IN: Indiana University Press.

Hudson, P. (2006). Examining mentors' personal attributes. In P. L. Jeffery (Ed.), *Proceedings of the 2005 AARE – Australian Association for Research in Education*. Parramatta, NSW: AARE.

Husserl, E. (1988). *Cartesian meditations: An introduction to phenomenology*. Boston: Martinus Nijhoff.

Jay, J. K. (2003). *Quality teaching: Reflection as the heart of practice*. Lanham, MD: Scarecrow.

Miles, M. B., & Huberman, M. A. (1994). *Qualitative data analysis: An expanded sourcebook*. Thousand Oaks: Sage Publications.

Parini, J. (2005). *The art of teaching*. New York: Oxford University Press.

Paris, C., & Combs, B. (2006). Lived meanings: What teachers mean when they say they are learner-centered. *Teachers & Teaching, 2*(5), 571–592.

Rodgers, C. R., & Raider-Roth, M. B. (2006). *Teachers and Teaching: Theory and Practice, 12*(3), 265–287.

Rogers, A. (2002). *Teaching adults* (3rd ed.). Buckingham, UK: Open University Press.

Rumi, J. al-Din. (2004). *The Masnavi* (book one). New York: Oxford University Press.

Shapiro, J. P., & Stefkovich, J. A. (2001). *Ethical leadership and decision making in education: Applying theoretical perspectives to complex dilemmas*. Hillsdale, NJ: Lawrence Erlbaum Associates.

Stinson, S. W. (1993). Realities, myths, and priorities: Teacher competencies in dance. *Journal of Physical Education, Recreation & Dance, 64*(9), 45–50.

Stinson, S. W. (1995). Bodies of knowledge. *Educational Theory, 45*(1), 43–54.

Van den Berg, R. (2002). Teachers' meanings regarding educational practice. *Review of Educational Research, 72*, 577–625.

van Manen, M. (1991). *The tact of teaching: The meaning of pedagogical thoughtfulness*. London: Althouse Press.

van Manen, M. (1995). On the epistemology of reflective practice. *Teachers and Teaching: Theory and Practice, 1*(1), 33–50.

van Manen, M. (1997). *Researching lived experience: Human science for an action sensitive pedagogy* (2nd ed.). Toronto, ON: Transcontinental. (Original work published 1990).

van Manen, M. (2002). *The tone of teaching*. London: Althouse.

Watts, J., & Robertson, N. (2011). Burnout in university teaching staff: A systematic literature review. *Educational Research, 53*(1), 33–50.

Wu, Y-J. (2005). *Dancing with little spirits: A journey towards enhancement of pedagogical relationship and intersubjectivity in a third grade dance education setting in Taiwan*. Doctoral dissertation, Temple University, Philadelphia.

Part VII
Identity, Change, Restoration

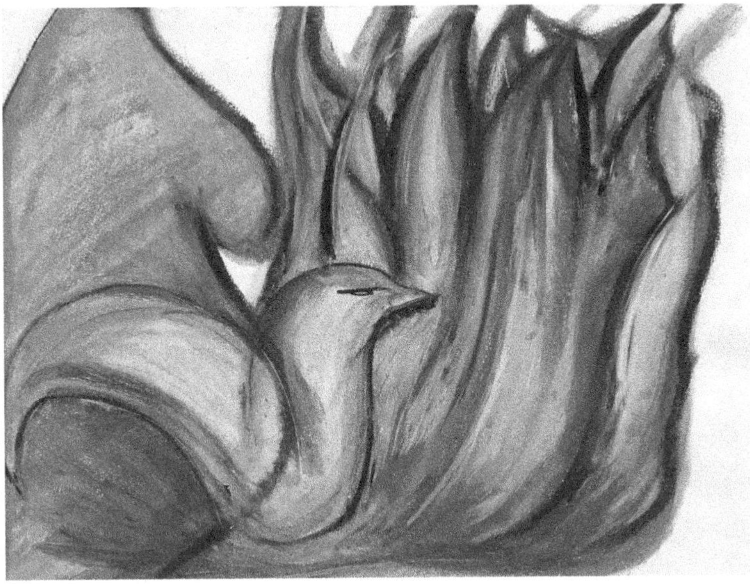

V Bird, Flames, Belly (M. Shanahan)

Chapter 24
Women Span Personal to Political in an Israeli Belly Dance Setting

Ephrat Huss and Karen Bond

Belly dance has been called "a global phenomenon" (World Dance Heritage, 2014, n.p.). This study highlights meanings of belly dancing in a multi-generational, intercultural group of women citizens of the state of Israel. As discussed initially in Huss and Haimovich (2011), 22 women, ages 25–60, participated in a 6-week series of once-weekly, 90 min belly dancing sessions run by the Women's Forum at Ben Gurion University (BGU). This chapter revisits the original study to extend its "site specific" personal-to-political analysis in dialogue with the growing body of literature on belly dance's global status as a mode of "empowerment" across genders (Hobin, 2015; Sellers-Young, 2016a, 2016b).

BGU is located in Beer-Sheva, a small university town in the Negev Desert of southern Israel with a largely Sephardic (Arab) and immigrant population. Like most Israeli universities, BGU has a mostly female administrative staff and a predominantly male academic profile (Hazan, 2008). Ashkenazi (European) students outnumber Sephardic by about three to one (Meir, 2005). Approximately half of the 22 participants in the study were Jews of Ashkenazi origin while the rest were Sephardic Jews and one Arab Muslim woman. Participants, most of whom were mothers, presented a range of body sizes and levels of fitness.

In Israel, as elsewhere, belly dance is often practiced as a leisure dance form in sports clubs and extra-curricular settings, with enough interest to support an annual competition in Tel Aviv (www.youtube.com/watch?v=ueZPtZLwMiI). Aligning with historical and contemporary literature on the functions and effects of belly dance for women, participants in the present study described experiences that move beyond belly dance's recreational and commercial value, touching on areas of

E. Huss (✉)
Ben-Gurion University of the Negev, Beersheba, Israel
e-mail: ehuss@bgu.ac.il

K. Bond
Department of Dance, Temple University, Philadelphia, PA, USA
e-mail: kbond003@temple.edu

K. Bond (ed.), *Dance and the Quality of Life*, Social Indicators Research Series 73,
https://doi.org/10.1007/978-3-319-95699-2_24

subjective knowing (bodily-affective experiences, memories of childhood), inter-subjective and intercultural meanings, and political agency.

For Eastern women in Israel, belly dancing is sometimes practiced at family celebrations (Holmes, 2003), but in terms of Zionist culture, with its largely Ashkenazi (European) values, belly dance has been marginalized as part of a denied cultural reality. For participants who were European immigrants and Ashkenazi Israelis, the BGU workshop was their first encounter with belly dance. Tovi Fenster (2014) notes that in recent years, Israeli-Jewish women have been showing increasing interest in belly dance, with schools opening in Jerusalem, "all in the Western, Jewish side of the city" (p. 191). The present study, with its multi-cultural group of participants (Arab-Muslim, Eastern Jewish, and Western Jewish), suggests that belly dance can be a meaningful component of women's quality of personal, social and cultural life within a divided society such as Israel.

Belly Dance: A Concise Overview

While the roots of belly dance are elusive, its origins have been widely associated with fertility and initiation rituals performed by and for women in indigenous cultures in the Far and Middle East, perhaps as far back as the Paleolithic Era (Helland, 2001) – over 11,000 years ago. Scholars continue to debate its beginnings, including some who suggest that belly dance has always been performed for entertainment, a premise contested by those who emphasize spiritual, religious, or since the 1960s, certain feminist constructions (Fenster, 2014). In any case, there seems to be little dispute that a significant tradition of belly dance developed as an expression of women's sexuality, fertility and emotional states in private female settings (Al-Rawi, 1999; Deagon, 2005; Harris, 2014; Stewart, 2000; Sellers-Young, 2016a), a practice that continues perhaps millennia later. Reneé Lyons (2012) asserts,

> Raqs Sharqi is certainly a dance by women for women. A famous Egyptian belly dancer of the 20th century, Armen Ohanian, called the dance 'our poem of the mystery and pain of motherhood.' (p. 124)

While the two major forms of belly dance, *Baladi* and *Sharqi* (or *Sharki*), can be differentiated by distinct histories, aesthetics, and movement vocabularies (Buonaventura, 1994; McDonald & Sellers-Young, 2013; Mishkin & Shill, 1973), they have mixed and morphed over time and context. The earlier "folk" form of *Baladi* emphasizes rotations of thighs and pelvis while the dancer remains stationary. *Sharqi,* a hybrid style emerging in Egypt in the early twentieth century, is considered a higher art than *Baladi* and includes dance movements from classical ballet and jazz (Buonaventura, 1994; Richards, 2000; Sellers-Young, 1992).

Fenster (2014) reports that belly dance instructors in western Jerusalem teach from an eclectic training base rather than specializing in a specific traditional style; she quotes her own teacher who "put all I've learned over the years including classic ballet, Israeli folkdance, etc." into her own style of belly dance (p. 194). Randy

Martin's (1998) notion of "composite body" seems salient, although as a variation that accommodates the existential, or phenomenological, as well as the culturally "composed." Fenster (2014) points out that the term *belly dance* is a misnomer – a western construction in fact, since all parts of the body are involved. Some dancers and teachers prefer to use the generic term *Middle Eastern dance,* which seems equally inadequate, as the latter encompasses much more than belly dance.

Like the classes described by Fenster (2014) in West Jerusalem, the belly dance workshop at BGU was a general introduction, reaching out to a "composite body" as one who dances differences of age, ability, body size, profession, lifestyle, *and* culture (authors' emphasis). Both Huss and Haimovich (2011) and Fenster (2014) conclude that belly dance reaches across boundaries of, in Fenster's terms, "age, class, level of education, and ethnicity," offering women a "language of performativity that investigates social and power relations with other means than words and texts" (p. 205).

Belly Dance: East and West, North and South

As theorized by Palestinian cultural theorist Edward Said (1978), 18th and nineteenth century Romanticism's "Orientalist gaze" contributed to a sexualized meme of Arab women that played on the image of the Oriental feminine as a mysterious being – covered in public while dancing seductively in the private sphere of harem culture (Deaver, 1978; Lazreg, 1994/2014; Macmaster & Lewis, 1998; Sellers-Young, 1992, 2016a). Early Israeli films portrayed Sephardic women as silent "exotics" with *bindi* and veils, combining the different stereotypes of "oriental" culture (Dahan-Kalev, 1997; Shay & Sellers-Young, 2005; Shohat, 1989/2010) and creating a group of well-known dancers who began to perform publicly (Sellers-Young, 1992). Belly dance became associated with "sexy" and "low" entertainment, which in "the East" implies immodesty if not "impurity." For fundamentalist Islamics in the Middle East, both music and dance are "sinful and unlawful," as evidenced when belly dancers were murdered in Iraq after the fall of Saddam Hussein in 2003 for having been part of an "impure profession" (Lyons, 2012, p. 131). Under "Censorship and the Status Quo," folk dance encyclopedist Mary Ellen Snodgrass (2016) writes that in 2014 belly dancers in Egypt were being threatened with flogging by the Muslim Brotherhood for "debasing sexual mores" (p. 47).

In the West, the sexualizing of belly dance became associated with the sex industry as "exotic dancing," burlesque, and stripping, constructions that spread globally during the first half of the twentieth century (Donalee, 2006; Dox, 2006; Hanna, 2010; Keft-Kennedy, 2005; Kraus, 2010; Regehr & Temperley, 2017; Shay, 2008; Shay & Sellers-Young, 2005). Today, strippers who belly dance or wear its "exotic" costuming receive backlash from professional belly dancers, while the latter have been accused of "same sex sexism" (Regehr & Temperley, 2017, p. 82). Challenging superficial treatments of belly dance as a form of male entertainment, scholars have discussed the homosocial potential and practice of the dance by both females and males, as well as a global culture of trans-gender and cross-gender belly dancers (Karayanni, 2004; Sellers-Young, 2016b; Shay & Sellers-Young, 2016).

A "wholesome" revival of belly dancing occurred in the 1960s when an interest in Eastern cultures within the women's movement inspired wide-spread participation as a way to support female sexuality and liberation (Al-Rawi, 1999; Fenster, 2014; Lyons, 2012; Maira, 2008; Stacey & Stickley, 2008). Within the middle classes, belly dance's sexual connotations were appropriated for what might be considered quality of life purposes – to legitimize the sexuality of suburban mothers. For example, in their instructional manual, *The Compleat Belly Dancer,* Julie Mishkin and Marta Shill (1973) proposed: "Housewives who want to get away from hot stoves and…put on a home-made fringed bra and harem pants…can start with the exercises outlined" (p. 3). Moreover, belly dance became a feminist tool for countering media images of "thin" femininity, and was (and continues to be) included in women's body image workshops (Carlton, 1995; Sellers-Young, 2016a).

The idea of belly dance as a feminist endeavor developed further with the advent of "new age" spirituality in the 1970s (Keft-Kennedy, 2005, 2013), although feminist academics protested belly dance's objectification of women's bodies as a form of sexual commodification (Maira, 2008). Amira Jarmakani (2013) asserts that rehabilitations of belly dancing, which continue today, "borrow from essentialist iterations of feminist thought, which privilege femininity (as naturally connected to womanhood) as a means of speaking back to patriarchy" (p. 136), while Victoria Keft-Kennedy (2013), views the 1970s' proliferation of belly dancing "self-help" manuals with their empowerment narratives of inclusion and freedom as a positive resource for women, who indeed carry the "essential" function of childbearing. Jarmakani (2013) asserts, however, that such popular constructions of belly dance exist "at the expense of any sustained consideration of systemic freedoms" (p. 139), arguing that the exploitive belly dance performance industry is mainly a "vehicle for white, male, heterosexual, American freedom" (p. 147) of the male gaze and the capitalist entrepreneur.

Barbara Sellers-Young (1992) cited media statistics that by the end of the 1970s at least one million women were practicing belly dance in the United States. Without knowing they were part of this statistical demographic at the time, Karen Bond and her young daughter, Deanna, were dancing with a bare-footed "tribal" group in San Francisco in 1979, a place where participation in belly dance remains strong, across genders (Sellers-Young, 2016b). In contrast to the "individualist" orientation of the "American belly dance performer" described in feminist cultural critiques (Alsultany & Shohat, 2013; Jarmakani, 2013), the Bonds recall their neighborhood studio experience in Clement Street as affording a sense of community through circle and serpentine dancing, the inclusion of children, and learning to play the *zils* (middle eastern finger cymbals) to accompany "ourselves and each other," as the teacher put it.

Since the 1970s, high levels of participation globally (World Dance Heritage, 2014, n.p.) have likely contributed to the growth of research on the health benefits of belly dancing, which go beyond fitness measures. In Brazil, Villela, Jones,

Natour, and Baptista (2012) found that belly dancing (twice a week for 16 weeks) was effective in treating individuals with fibromyalgia to reduce pain and improve function, quality of life, and self-image. Researchers in Hungary found that belly dance complimented standard medical care in women's rehabilitation after cancer treatment (Levay, Szirmai, Papp, Prémusz, Bódis, and Szalai, 2015), including improvement in health-related quality of life. In South Korea, results of a belly dance intervention suggested that a "dance program focusing on pelvic exercise can be used to prevent and relieve the symptoms of urinary incontinence as a non-surgical treatment" (An, Kim, & Han, 2017, p. 384).

Within the new age movement, the discourse of female transformation through belly dance continues to evolve. Various forms of indigenous, "tribal," and "goddess" dance have been combined with belly dance to create forms of spirituality that reify the value and power of women (Buonaventura, 1994; Carlton, 1995; Crosby, 2000; Keft-Kennedy, 2005; Jorgensen, 2012; Kraus, 2017; Maira, 2008; McDonald & Sellers-Young, 2013; Sellers-Young, 1992, 2016a; Stewart, 2000). The connection between belly dance and spirituality has been studied empirically. In a survey of 77 dancers (including three males) who practice belly dance as a leisure activity, sociologist Rachel Kraus (2009) found that 75% considered belly dancing a spiritual experience.

The above described renaissance of belly dance in popular culture has not extended readily to higher education, although the number of belly dance clubs and short courses found in American university settings has burgeoned in the past decade, including in "top tier" research university settings such as Columbia, Harvard, Stanford and Yale (www.google.com). The devaluing of traditional female crafts and "folk" forms of expression as a way to keep women out of the dominant art world canon continues to be critiqued from a feminist viewpoint (Mann, 2006).

Belly dance has been examined in both performance and therapeutic settings for its potential benefits to women's self-esteem. Numerous studies (both quantitative and qualitative) show that belly dancing can help bring about improvements in body image (Downey, Reel, SooHoo, & Zerbib, 2010; Huss & Haimovich, 2011; Lewis & Scannel, 1995; Moe, 2011; Reel, 2013; Tiggemann, Coutts, & Clark, 2014); in contrast, ballet dancing has been associated with body image pathologies such as anorexia nervosa (Akard, Henderson, & Wonderlich, 2004; Barr & Oliver, 2016). Performers report less desire for bodily change than counterparts in modern dance and ballet. In an entry titled "Dancers," for the volume *Eating Disorders: An Encyclopedia of Causes, Treatment, and Prevention,* Justine Reel (2013) elaborates:

> Only 18 percent of female belly dance participants were dissatisfied with their bodies in one study. This percentage is considerably lower than dancer or non-dancer populations of females. Likewise, belly dancers did not experience the same types of weight pressures (e.g., choreographer, other dancers, performance advantage) reported by modern dancers. Audience scrutiny (40%) was the sole pressure reported by belly dancers who as a whole described a supportive, body-accepting community of dancers. Curves were celebrated and belly dance seemed to play a positive role in promoting positive body image and health. (pp. 122–123)

Downey et al. (2010) associate the high level of body satisfaction (92%) found in their survey of 103 women belly dancers in Salt Lake City, Utah, in part, with the "free space provided by a gender segregated activity" (p. 377), a phenomenon found in Fenster's (2014) study in West Jerusalem:

> The studio is a safe female space. Men are not allowed to enter… Even male maintenance workers do not enter the studio area during classes. This is why religious women and even ultra-religious women are able to wander around the studio area dressed freely in traditional belly dance clothes and perform bodily gestures that are seen as immodest and forbidden in their daily lives. (p. 202)

Fenster describes the women's belly dance studio as a "third space…free of cultural and religious norms" (p. 202). A number of women in her study use the word "liberated" to describe the experience of belly dancing, and in a class exercise, dancers generated the following collection of word associations (italics indicate language or inferred meanings also found in Huss & Haimovich, 2011):

> *femininity; beauty*; Jerusalem; to *connect* to *body and soul*; soul; *freedom*; arabesque; *happiness*; growing; eternity; *body control*; *sensuality*; *knowledge of oneself*; *holiday*; investment; *love*; *women*; Yael and Dorit (teachers). (p. 194)

A Short Story of Belly Dancing at an Israeli University

We begin this account with brief commentary on the socio-political context of the belly dance activism recounted in this "short story." In terms of society as a whole, discourses and institutions of Israel have been gradually shifting from a "melting pot" ideology to a "multi-cultural" one that seeks to provide each cultural group in Israel with a distinct voice and agency (Kacen & Lev-Wiesel, 2002). International Studies professor Jonathan Adelman (2017) notes, however, that Israeli Arabs continue to have significant cause for unrest, including, "job discrimination, racism, an alien national anthem, lack of benefits given to army veterans, minimal state funding for education and social services, low income, limited elite employment…" (n.p.). Huss and Haimovich (2011) state that differences and inequalities between Israeli Jews and Israeli Arabs are embedded in a political reality characterized by tension with and rejection of Arabic cultural elements within Israel.

In spite of such conditions, recent polls show that 77% of Israeli Arabs prefer to live in Israel than in other parts of the middle east, with two-thirds reporting that "Israel is a good place to live" (Adelman, 2017, n.p.). Adelman (2017) lists a number of reasons, all related to quality of life: Arab population growth, beach, café and high tech lifestyle, relative peace, educational levels (compared, for example, to China and India), political and religious freedoms, equal rights for women and gays, income (relative to Gaza and the West Bank), relatively low government corruption, and universal healthcare. Nevertheless, after only 6 weeks, the predominantly male administration of an Israeli university refused to continue sponsoring a belly dance workshop for its multi-cultural population of female students and employees.

Belly Dance and Quality of Life Activism

The story began when Ephrat Huss and Shelly Haimovich (2011) employed preliminary biographical questionnaires, participant observation, group discussions, and individual post-workshop interviews with volunteer participants to collect qualitative data on women's experiences and meanings of belly dancing in a 6-week workshop at Ben Gurion University of the Negev. The study was approved by BGU's Human Subjects Research Committee. Qualitative analysis emphasized the therapeutic benefits of belly dance for participants in terms of body image and control, sexual self-esteem, and transformation, situating these findings in post-colonial feminist discourse related to resistance and power (Abu-Lughod, 1998; Spivak, 1993/2013). This chapter revisits the study, including now an external discussant as second author, to re-enact a personal-to-political analysis highlighting dance and quality of life. For this article, we reverse the meme, examining the BGU study from "political-to-personal."

Belly dancing took place in a university hall, and the only male observer was David Ben Gurion, the University's namesake, who gazed down from his portrait high on the wall. A founding father of Israel, Ben Gurion advocated the melting pot vision adopted by the university, which includes "melting away" differences between men and women. Some argue that within the institution, equality, or denial of sexual difference, is a strategy to inhibit women's advancement and thus their power (Hazan, 2008). For example, affirmative action is not available to women for the extra time it takes them to raise children and therefore to achieve promotion. Such a strategy preserves the status quo in which women do not progress beyond lower level administrative and academic ranks (Hazan, 2008; Motzafi-Haller, 2001).

Recognizing that people with a range of gender identifications are increasingly partaking, belly dancing continues to valorize difference in gender roles, and thus to resist the repression of difference. Twenty years ago, feminist anthropologist Lila Abu-Lughod (1998) suggested, "…even today, young Bedouin women in Egypt try to resist their elders and the kin-based forms of domination they represent by embracing aspects of a commoditized sexuality" (p. 13) (see Chakraborty (2015) for a contemporary analogy with Bollywood in India). Likewise, female belly dancers' expressions of sexuality, ostensibly for the pleasure of men, can become resistance to strategies used by the institution to ignore the different needs of men and women. This legitimized expression of female agency and gender difference in the symbolic space of the dance is captured in the following anecdotes from women in the BGU workshop.

> I get into this Arab film thing that was a central influence in my childhood, the movies about strong Arab women with a lot of drama and manipulation…things that aren't legitimate in our culture.

> I get out of my usual university self where I am very organized and no different from men.

Women carried this agency beyond the dance space:

> It's great to bump into people on the campus from the belly dancing workshop—it's like a secret club. It creates a network of women within the university.

As introduced in Huss and Haimovich (2011), an unanticipated development arose when participants organized to resist the university's reluctance to fund an ongoing belly dancing program. As the 6-week workshop drew to a close, group members sent letters that reached the university president asking that the program be continued. The university refused, stating that the content was inappropriate for a university leisure activity, even though the group's desire to continue showed its importance to participants, as evidenced in the following comments from group discussions:

> We want to continue dancing. It empowers us and creates a network.
> It's a shame they didn't come to see us…we invited them.
> Bezek (the phone company) has such courses. It's pretty common practice—it unites women working in an institution.
> Maybe if we define it as Mizrachi folk dancing rather than belly dancing it will be more acceptable.
> My letter shows how it is part of a tradition.

University opposition suggests that belly dancing was viewed by administration as a threat, although in their attempt to open up new agency and freedoms at the university, the women employed strategies that did not overtly or aggressively jostle the status quo, for example, appeals to tradition. Cultural theorists have described such approaches as characteristic of feminism in developing countries (Bhabha, 1994/2004; Lazreg, 1994/2014; Spivak, 1993/2013). Unfortunately, the BGU women's "polite," or "politic," advocacy was not successful, and the belly dancing group has not been reconvened on the Ben Gurion campus, even as such groups proliferate on university campuses in many countries…North, South, East and West. Perhaps Israel is not as "westernized" as generally thought.

Dancing the Personal and Social, the Cultural and Political

> Phenomenology is a philosophy or theory of the unique…the nonreplaceable practiced with awareness of the evasive character of…other, the whole, the communal, or the social. (van Manen, 1990, p. 5)

Despair as one might about the many examples of prohibitions to dancing across times and places (see Chaps. 1, 7, and 8), we can nevertheless acknowledge the particular, the "site specific" manifestations of dance that have likely enhanced quality of animate life since we know not when. We now revisit the phenomenological meanings of dance depicted by women in the BGU workshop, experiences that might be "nonreplaceable" in women's memories, like the Bonds' from almost four decades ago. Through the women's own descriptions, we endeavor to illuminate their desire to continue belly dancing through the Women's Forum at BGU.

Body Acceptance and Satisfaction Congruent with recent studies noted earlier (Downey et al., 2010; Reel, 2013; Tiggemann et al., 2014), women in the workshop described positive shifts in bodily satisfaction and acceptance while belly dancing.

> The whole process made me feel differently about my body, which is too fat, but when I danced, I felt fine.
> I like my body except my stomach…when I dance I also like my stomach.
> It helped me to feel that my body was not a bag of milk to feed a baby.
> I had difficulty…, but now, when I dance…I enjoy my body.
> The dancing helped me with depression after childbirth. It helped me accept my body.
> The cherry on the cake of dance is the joy of accepting my body as it is.
> I released my body to the roundness of the movements.

A number of women experienced body acceptance in relation to their sexuality.

> I felt like the sexiest woman alive.
> My body was…sexy and fun.
> I decided to be a gorgeous, sexy lady at age fifty…the dancing connected me to this wish.
> I liked…staring at people, forcing them to see me and to look at them—the eye contact is very strong, very sexual.

One of the older members reflected that belly dancing prompted her to "think of how to be a mother, an older lady, and still define my femininity as sexual."

Women in Fenster's (2014) study in West Jerusalem recounted similar bodily-affective changes in belly dancing. A 70-year old participant conveyed in interview that "the dancing does something good to her body. She feels very feminine and sexy when she dances. … She even grew out her hair because of the belly dancing. She likes the body gestures she uses while dancing" (p. 200). In addition to fitness and other bodily enhancements, "Diane" liked how her participation in belly dance challenges age stereotypes. "Leah" (age 38) "doesn't criticize her body anymore… She likes to look at herself in the studio mirror" and "associates specific body gestures with resistance…the movement of her shoulders and breasts" (p. 200). "Esther" (age 52), the only religious Jew of Fenster's three interviewees, "feels very much connected to her body…control of her body: 'I sit straight now'" (p. 201). She dresses modestly according to religious codes, but doesn't feel this diminishes her "deep connection to belly dance because it's the dancing of the body and not the showing off of the body that matters" (p. 201).

Such descriptions highlight women's experiences of belly dance as a form of holistic, integrated knowledge (body, thought, emotions), a human existential capacity that has been related to quality of living (Bond, 2014; Williamson, Batson, Whatley, & Weber, 2014). The following reflections describe integrated feeling states that participants recalled experiencing while belly dancing.

> I felt sad that my body is limited by age, but on the other hand I really enjoyed it.
> I have suffered from a medical disorder from an early age and can't dance, but I enjoyed what movements I could do. I felt happy and sad at the same time.
> When I dance, I become extroverted. I feel a huge smile, and my troubles disappear. I enter another zone.
> I did not have to care how I looked…I played and had fun.
> I laughed—the flexibility in body and soul, the movement in space—things you can lose as an adult.

> I can control my body, and it all comes together into a feeling of wholeness. Then I paradoxically dance more spontaneously and that is a great feeling.

Some women experienced their bodies and movement as part of a "real self."

> The dance connected me to myself—my wishes and wants, my vitality.
> I stand up straight. I feel my power.
> I don't hide my femininity.
> The dance is a chance not to think, to let my body express itself, to give place to its energy, to a big release.
> I always felt that words don't express me fully, but when I move, it's real.
> This returned me to something basic, authentic.

Some described imaginative metamorphoses in the workshop:

> I can be anything I want—delicate, classic, poetic. I can reach extreme places that are different parts of myself. In the dance, I'm part of these things that I'm not in real life.
>
> I got this feeling of someone entering my body, being totally someone else. The character enters me through my feet, my thighs…

Bridging Subjectivities: Personal-to-Social Belly dancing afforded inter-subjective experiences for this ethnically diverse, inter-generational, mixed-ability group of Israeli women.

> It's pleasant being in the group—it gives me a feeling of acceptance. We all dance at different levels and that's okay.
>
> I was surprised that my partner stated that she couldn't dance. It looked like she really knew how to dance, and this made me realize that the way you look and the way you feel aren't always the same thing.
>
> I got pulled in and it was great.
>
> I met her in the corridor and she wriggled her breasts at me – it was so funny.

One workshop process involved women taking turns to dance in the center of the circle for a set time while the group mirrored each one's movements. One participant noted that claiming individual space within the circle became more meaningful over time: "In the beginning, it was hard to enter the circle and take the space. By the end, I couldn't get enough of the center." She also talked about releasing her 'comparing mind' to experience inter-subjective meanings: "Most were younger than me, but instead of comparing how they looked compared to me, I found the special movement of each woman more interesting." In the final session, three women arrived in costumes and presented a belly dance trio while the other women observed, their clapping and gazes affirming the extended performances in the center.

Bridging Ethnicities: Personal-to-Cultural For participants of Eastern Jewish or Arab origin, the belly dancing workshop was a way to reconnect with hidden elements of their ethnic origins: "I denied my Eastern-Kurdish culture – it wasn't something to be proud of in Israel, but the belly dancing brought me closer to my roots. I loved that." Some women retrieved childhood memories of Eastern music and dance:

> My mother was from Morocco…but my father was Ashkenazi, and he didn't like that culture, so those friends and relatives only came when he wasn't there. Then we would put on Arab music and the house would be happy and full of laughter. This music reminds me of my childhood.
>
> I remember being ashamed of my aunts who would belly dance at weddings. Now, connecting to the music and movements feels like giving me back my childhood, my culture of origin.

The single Arab Muslim woman in the group described how her upper-class family did not allow her to do this "low-class" kind of dance; for her, too, belly dancing was a way of reclaiming her culture.

> Yes, I dance belly dancing. I am proud of it. The movements are intense, exaggerated, which make me seem less of a lady, but I want to be less of a lady. I am sick of dancing in a restrained way that makes me more high class than other Arab women.

Pointing to the tensions that might occur in an inter-cultural belly dancing workshop, she also expressed anger that "the Jewish culture took away this dancing from me—it's our dancing, not the Jewish women's dancing." Nevertheless, and in contrast to the women in Fenster's (2014) study in West Jerusalem, some Ashkenazi women described that belly dancing was a way to come closer to the Arabic elements of Israeli culture.

> Not just the dance, but the music, the language—a whole culture that stands around the dance, this raised my awareness. We live in the Middle East, and the Arab music speaks to me emotionally. It's not just the dance for me, it's what it represents.

Belly Dancing and Quality of Life

From women's descriptions, even their short program of belly dancing was rich with quality experiences, spanning personal-to-political and aligning with previous research (pre- and post- Huss & Haimovich, 2011). As a whole, the study portrays how belly dancing can confer a social context for silent or unheard aspects of experience (Cosgrove, 2000; Goldberger, Tarule, Clinchey, & Belenky, 1996). The arts, including belly dance (Moe, 2011), have often been vehicles for women to express resistance to oppressive structures (Meskimmon, 2003; Spivak, 1988). Three decades ago, Gayatri Chakravorty Spivak (1988) suggested that the voices of marginalized women are found in creative and aesthetic endeavors rather than in intellectual history, a male-dominated project traditionally. Discussing the role of dancing for women in the African diaspora, Marsha Meskimmon (2003) asserts,

> The fact that dance has been allied with the low, the corporeal, the feminine and the culturally marginal makes me take it all the more seriously. As in the case of performance art, such multi-sensory, boundary-crossing forms have the potential to disrupt fixed categories of knowledge and articulate embodied subjectivity in new and startling ways. (p. 37)

While participants in neither Huss and Haimovich's (2011) nor Fenster's (2014) study advance understanding of belly dance as a form of spiritual expression, both illuminate how metaphorical, creative bodily expression through belly dance can give space to identify and transcend elements of middle class reality in Israel. This chapter and the women's experiences it recounts, along with the abundance of current literature on the functions and meanings of belly dance, perhaps since ancient times, challenge rhetoric that reduces belly dance to a "low" or superficial mode of expression. Belly dancing can be a space for women to embody, create, and project meanings that bridge the bodily-affective and social, the cultural and political, in everyday life.

References

Abu-Lughod, L. (1998). *Re-making women: Feminism and modernity in the Middle East*. Princeton, NJ: Princeton University Press.

Adelman, J. (2017). The Israeli Arabs: Trailblazers of a better Middle East. *The World Post*. Retrieved from https://www.huffingtonpost.com/jonathan-adelman/the-israeli-arabs-trailbl_b_8010020.html

Akard, M., Henderson, B., & Wonderlich, D. (2004). The relationship between childhood dance training and adult distorted eating and related psychopathology. *Journal of Psychosomatic Research, 57*(5), 485–490.

Al-Rawi, R. (1999). *Grandmother's secrets: The ancient rituals and healing power of belly dancing*. New York: Interlink Books.

Alsultany, E., & Shohat, E. (Eds.). (2013). *Between the Middle East and the Americas: The cultural politics of diaspora*. Ann Arbor: University of Michigan Press.

An, S.-Y., Kim, S.-S., & Han, G. (2017). Effects of belly dancing on urinary incontinence-related muscles and vaginal pressure in middle-aged women. *Journal of Physical Therapy Science, 29*(3), 384–386.

Barr, S., & Oliver, W. (2016). Feminist pedagogy, body image, and the dance technique class. *Research in Dance Education, 17*(2), 97–112. https://doi.org/10.1080/14647893.2016.1177008.

Bhabha, H. (2004). *The location of culture*. London: Routledge. (Original work published 1994).

Bond, K. E. (2014). Dance and quality of life. In A. C. Michalos (Ed.), *Encyclopedia of quality of life and well-being research* (pp. 1419-1424). Dordrecht, The Netherlands: Springer.

Buonaventura, W. (1994). *Serpent of the Nile: Woman and dance in the Arab world*. New York: Interlink.

Carlton, D. (1995). *Looking for little Egypt*. Bloomington, IN: International Dance Discovery.

Chakraborty, K. (2015). *Young Muslim women in India: Bollywood, identity and changing youth culture*. New York: Routledge.

Cosgrove, L. (2000). Understanding women's lived distress as both lived experience and social construction. *Feminism & Psychology, 10*, 207.

Dahan-Kalev, H. (1997). Oppression of women by other women: Relations and struggles between Mizrachi and Ashkenazi women in Israel. *Israeli Social Science Research, 12*(1), 31-44.

Deagon, A. (2005). *In search of the origins of dance*. Retrieved from http://people.uncw.edu/deagona/raqs/origins.htm

Deaver, S. (1978). Concealment versus display: The modern Saudi woman. *Dance Research, 10*(2), 14–18.

Donalee, D. (2006). Dancing around orientalism. *TDR: The Drama Review, 50*(4), 51–71.

Downey, D., Reel, J., SooHoo, S., & Zerbib, S. (2010). Body image in belly dance: Integrating alternative norms into collective identity. *Journal of Gender Studies, 19*(4), 377–393.
Dox, D. (2006). Belly dancing in the West. *TDR: The Drama Review, 50*(4), 52–60.
Fenster, T. (2014). Belly dancing in Israel: Body, embodiment, religion and nationality. In A. Pine & O. Kuhlke (Eds.), *Geographies of dance: Body, movement, and corporeal negotiations* (pp. 191–205). Lanham, MD: Lexington.
Goldberger, N., Tarule, J., Clinchey, B., & Belenky, M. (Eds.). (1996). *Knowledge, difference, and power: Essays inspired by Women's ways of knowing*. New York: Basic Books.
Hanna, J. (2010). Many moves: Dance and sexuality. *The Journal of Sex Research, 47*(2–3), 212–241.
Harris, L. (2014). *The belly dance reader 2*. Fairfax, CA: Gilded Serpent.
Hazan, N. (2008, February 27). *Gendered politics within the university: Dilemmas and trends*. Conference on Women in Science: Challenges, Achievements, and Obstacles. Ben-Gurion University of the Negev, Beersheba, Israel.
Helland, S. (2001). The belly dance: Ancient ritual to cabaret performance. In A. Dils & A. C. Albright (Eds.), *Moving history/dancing cultures: A dance history reader* (pp. 128–135). Middletown, CN: Wesleyan University Press.
Hobin, T. (2015). *Belly dance for health, happiness and empowerment*. Hants, UK: Anyi Books.
Holmes, E. (2003). *Daughters of Tunis: Women, family and networks in a Muslim city*. Seattle: University of Washington Press.
Huss, E., & Haimovich, S. (2011). "The hips don't lie:" Dancing around gendered, ethnic and national identity in Israel. *Body, Movement and Dance in Psychotherapy, 6*(1), 3–16.
Jarmakani, A. (2013). They hate our freedom but they love our belly dance: The spectacle of the shimmy in contemporary US culture. In E. Shohat & E. Alsultany (Eds.), *Between the Middle East and the Americas: The cultural politics of diaspora* (pp. 130–152). Ann Arbor: University of Michigan Press.
Jorgensen, J. (2012). Dancing the numinous: Sacred and spiritual techniques of contemporary belly dancers. *Journal of Ethnology & Folkloristics, 6*, 3–28.
Kacen, L., & Lev-Wiesel, R. (2002). *Group work in a multicultural society*. Tel Aviv, Israel: Cherikover Publications (Hebrew).
Karayanni, S. (2004). *Dancing fear and desire: Race, sexuality, and imperial politics in Middle Eastern dance*. Waterloo, ON: Wilfred Laurier University Press.
Keft-Kennedy, V. (2005). *Representing the belly-dancing body: Feminism, orientialism, and the grotesque*. Doctoral dissertation, University of Wollongong, Wollongong, Australia. Retrieved from http://ro.uow.edu.au/theses/843/
Keft-Kennedy, V. (2013). 1970s belly dance and the "how to" phenomenon: Feminism, fitness and orientalism. In C. E. McDonald & B. Sellers-Young (Eds.), *Belly dance around the world: New communities, performance and identity* (pp. 68–92). Jefferson, NC: McFarland.
Kraus, R. (2009). Straddling the sacred and secular: Creating a spiritual experience through belly dance. *Sociological Spectrum, 29*(5), 598–625. https://doi.org/10.1080/02732170903051383.
Kraus, R. (2010). "We are not strippers:" How belly dancers manage a (soft) stigmatized serious leisure activity. *Symbolic Interaction, 33*(3), 435–455.
Kraus, R. (2017). *Gendered bodies and leisure: The practice and performance of American belly dance*. London: Routledge.
Lazreg, M. (2014). *The eloquence of silence: Algerian women in question*. New York: Routledge. (Original work published 1994).
Levay, B., Szirmai, A., Papp, I., Prémusz, V., Bódis, J., & Szalai, M. (2015). A clinical study to access the efficacy of belly dancing as a tool for rehabilitation in female patients with malignancies. *European Journal of Oncology Nursing, 19*(1), 60–65.
Lewis, K., & Scannel, E. (1995). Relationship between body image and creative dance movement. *Perceptual and Motor Skills, 81*, 155–170.
Lyons, R. (2012). The Orient's Raqs Sharqi (belly dance) faces trouble. In *The revival of banned dances: A worldwide study*. Jefferson, NC: MacFarland.

Macmaster, N., & Lewis, T. (1998). Orientalism: From unveiling, to hyperveiling. *The Journal of European Studies, 28*, 121–135.
Maira, S. (2008). Belly dancing: Arab-face, orientalist feminism, and US empire. *American Quarterly, 60*(2), 317–345.
Mann, B. (2006). *Woman's liberation and the sublime: Feminism, postmodernism, environment*. Oxford: Oxford University Press.
Martin, R. (1998). The composite body of dance: Re(w)rapping the multicultural nation. In *Critical moves: Dance studies in theory and politics* (pp. 107–150). Durham, NC: Duke University Press.
McDonald, C., & Sellers-Young, B. (Eds.). (2013). *Belly dance around the world: New communities, performance and identity*. Jefferson, NC: McFarland.
Meir, A. (2005). Bedouin, the Israeli state and insurgent planning: Globalization, localization or glocalization? *Cities, 22*, 3–8.
Meskimmon, M. (2003). *Women making art: History, subjectivity, aesthetics*. London: Routledge.
Mishkin, J., & Shill, M. (1973). *The compleat belly dancer*. New York: Doubleday Press.
Moe, A. M. (2011). Belly dancing mommas: Challenging cultural discourses in maternity. In C. Bobel & S. Kwan (Eds.), *Embodied resistance: Challenging the norms, breaking the rules* (pp. 88–98). Nashville, TN: Vanderbilt University Press.
Motzafi-Haller, P. (2001). Scholarship, identity, and power: Mizrachi women in Israel. *Signs, 26*(3), 697–734.
Reel, J. (Ed.) (2013). Dancers. *Eating disorders: An encyclopedia of causes, treatment, and prevention* (pp. 121–124). Santa Barbara, CA: ABC-CLIO.
Regehr, K., & Temperley, M. (2017). *The league of exotic dancers: Legends from American burlesque*. New York: Oxford University Press.
Richards, T. (2000). *The belly dance book: Rediscovering the oldest dance*. Concord, CA: Backbeat Press.
Said, E. (1978). *Orientalism*. London: Routledge.
Sellers-Young, B. (1992). Raks El Sharki: Transculturation of a folk form. *The Journal of Popular Culture, 26*(2), 141–152.
Sellers-Young, B. (2016a). Dancing the goddess in popular culture: Resistance, spirituality and empowerment. In *Belly dance, pilgrimage and identity* (pp. 41–64). London: Palgrave Macmillan.
Sellers-Young, B. (2016b). San Francisco and American tribal style. In *Belly dance, pilgrimage and identity* (pp. 65–90). London: Palgrave Macmillan.
Shay, A. (2008). *Dancing across borders: The American fascination with exotic dance forms*. Jefferson, NC: MacFarland.
Shay, A., & Sellers-Young, B. (Eds.). (2005). *Belly dance: Orientalism, transnationalism, and harem fantasy*. Costa Mesa, CA: Mazda.
Shay, A., & Sellers-Young, B. (Eds.). (2016). *Oxford handbook of dance and ethnicity*. Oxford: Oxford University Press.
Shohat, E. (2010). *Israeli cinema: East/west and the politics of representation*. Austin: University of Texas Press (Original work published 1989).
Snodgrass, M. (2016). *The encyclopedia of world folk dance*. Lanham, MD: Rowman & Littlefield.
Spivak, G. (1988). Can the subaltern speak? In C. Nelson & L. Grossberg (Eds.), *Marxism and the interpretation of culture* (pp. 271–313). Urbana, IL: University of Illinois Press.
Spivak, G. (2013). Interview with Spivak: "Subaltern talk – Concerning Sati." In D. Landry & G. Mclean (Eds.), *The Spivak reader* (pp. 287–308). New York: Routledge. (Original work published 1993).
Stacey, G., & Stickley, T. (2008). Dancing to keep young at heart. *Mental Health Practice, 11*(6), 34–38.
Stewart, I. (2000). *Sacred woman, sacred dance: Awakening spirituality through movement and ritual*. Rochester, VT: Inner Traditions.

Tiggemann, M., Coutts, E., & Clark, L. (2014). Belly dance as an embodying activity? A test of the embodiment model of positive body image. *Sex Roles, 71*(5–8), 197–207.

van Manen, M. (1990). *Researching lived experience: Human science for an action sensitive pedagogy*. Albany: SUNY Press.

Villela, A., Jones, A., Natour, J., & Baptista, A. (2012). Effectiveness of dance in patients with fibromyalgia: A randomized, single-blind, controlled study. *Clinical Experimental Rheumatology, 30*(6), 18–23.

Williamson, A., Batson, G., Whatley, S., & Weber, R. (Eds.). (2014). *Dance, somatics and spiritualities: Contemporary sacred narratives*. Bristol, UK: Intellect.

World Dance Heritage. (2014). *The issue of cultural appropriation and Egyptian belly dance*. Retrieved from http://www.worlddanceheritage.org/cultural-appropriation-egyptian-belly-dance/

Chapter 25
Life-Changing Life Journeys Through Artistic and Educational Inclusive Contemporary Dance Contexts

Tone Pernille Østern, Elen Øyen, and Philip Channells

Introduction

The three co-authors have been involved in inclusive contemporary dance contexts for several years in diverse roles of dance teacher, choreographer, and researcher (Tone), choreographer and dance teacher (Philip), and dancer (Elen). We perceive that this involvement has inspired significant life changes that have contributed to our quality of life. We come from and live in different parts of the globe (Finland, Australia and Norway) but have worked together in different constellations over years and know one another well. Tone and Elen danced together as choreographer-teacher and dancer in a community dance company in Norway (2005–2012), and since 2012 have freelanced as teaching partners in various settings. Tone has worked with arts education in higher education since 2009. Philip works with inclusive dance in Australia and worldwide, and led a four-week project in Norway in 2012 where we all met. Philip and Tone have presented together at international conferences.

As researchers and authors we have studied various aspects of inclusive dance: meaning-making among differently bodied dancers in an improvisation-based project (Østern, 2009); difference as a creative and critical force in teacher education (Østern & Øyen, 2014a); embodied transformative learning in improvisation with differently bodied dancers (Østern & Øyen, 2015); inclusive dance as an educational

T. P. Østern (✉)
Norwegian University of Science and Technology, Trondheim, Norway
e-mail: tone.pernille.ostern@ntnu.no

E. Øyen
Norwegian University of Science and Technology, Trondheim, Norway

The Dance Laboratory, Trondheim, Norway

P. Channells
The Dance Laboratory, Trondheim, Norway

K. Bond (ed.), *Dance and the Quality of Life*, Social Indicators Research Series 73,
https://doi.org/10.1007/978-3-319-95699-2_25

experience of plurality (Østern, 2015); the choreographer's reflections on creative process in an inclusive dance project (Channells, 2015); and deep learning and teaching as affordances in inclusive dance and arts education (Østern & Channells, 2016). In this chapter, we seek to understand how Elen's and Philip's experiences in inclusive dance contexts have contributed to their quality of life.

In an encyclopedia article on dance and the quality of life, Bond (2014) writes that systematic inquiry on dance and the quality of life is a recent development and that dance remains underrepresented in the literature relative to other arts. She surveys a range of scholarship related to dance and the quality of life, highlighting numerous associations including emotional wellbeing and optimism, experience of freedom, improvement in self-esteem, stress relief, promotion of community and solidarity, the ability to express the ineffable in dance, and the experience of transformation and change in dance, among others. She asks for more empirical research on the topic. In this chapter, we try to make a small, empirically-based contribution to the field through a case study approach.

Inclusive Contemporary Dance – A Brief Overview

In short, inclusive dance within contemporary dance contexts highlights, values and draws on cultural pluralism and diversity to experience and create dance (Albright, 1997; Benjamin, 2002; Channells, 2015; Kuppers, 2001, 2006, 2015; Østern, 2009, 2015; Østern & Øyen, 2014a, 2014b, 2015). In this chapter "inclusive contemporary dance context" refers to an artistic and/or educational dance community where differently bodied dancers, with and without disabilities, and with little or much previous experience of dance, participate in and contribute to creative dance processes, often ending up in performances on stage. The contexts we have been involved in are artistic and educational. Our work maintains a focus on dance as art and/or education and aims at examining what dance can mean in the meeting between different dancers where the intention is to meet, explore and create dance *as equals*. This supports a view that all participants, with their different abilities and disabilities, are active and creative contributors in dance.

Research Methodology

Designing this study, we turned to life story research (Goodson & Sikes, 2001; Pérez, 2006; Wigg, 2015) and narrative inquiry (Bullough & Pinnegar, 2001; Clandinin & Connelly, 2000). The experiences of change we illuminate happened slowly. Life story methodology seemed a plausible approach to address the following question: *How can participation in inclusive dance contexts contribute to quality of life?* Wigg (2015) characterises life story research as belonging to a larger methodological tradition often referred to as biographical. This approach suits well when researchers are interested in people's experiences in a longer-term perspective, as we are in this study. The aim with life story research is not to reveal what is 'true' about a person's life, but how the participant constructs meaning of and coherence in their life through telling, or as in our case, writing.

In this study, self-reflexive texts written by Elen and Philip are the focus of analysis; in other words, their life experiences create the basis for this chapter. In line with narrative inquiry (Clandinin & Connelly, 2000), we do not believe that Elen's and Philip's experiences of meaning in dance are only *articulated* through their writings, but also *created* through the narrative work they perform as they write. Tone stays on the outside and does not provide life stories. Instead, in this chapter, she contributes a more analytic perspective, meaning that she reads the stories produced by Elen and Philip with a more external eye, looking for what seems central to their participation in inclusive dance and its contribution to their quality of life. Within this collaboration, we seek to create a mix of nearness and distance to our research material.

Elen and Philip spent 3 weeks writing self-reflexively about the following theme: *How participation in inclusive dance contexts contributed to my life: examples and reflections.* As we were discussing how to analyse the material we turned to what Wigg (2015) calls *holistic* and *thematic* approaches to life story research, combined with a narrative inquiry approach. According to Wigg, holistic form analysis looks at a life story as a whole and tries to create an emplotment, like a dramaturgy of the life story. The primary question in a holistic life story analysis is how the research participant understands their self and organises their life story to create meaning. In our case, this holistic life story analysis is conducted mainly by Elen and Philip themselves. As they spent 3 weeks writing based on the prompt we formulated—Elen in Norway and Philip in Australia, they independently wrote about their lives in a chronological way. They both started with childhood, which was not something we had talked about but an independent choice by each of them. In writing, they each chose to emphasise certain aspects while allowing others to fall more in the background. They both sent their texts to the whole group and we all read and commented on them. From that reading and that discussion, Tone began to structure the chapter.

As Tone read the texts, being more on the outside from the personal experiences Philip and Elen wrote about, and with an eye for the research topic—*how participation in inclusive dance contexts contribute to quality of life*—she suggested what narrative theorists Bullough and Pinnegar (2001) call *nodal points*. Nodal points are aspects that seem central or pivotal to the story; the nodal points Tone suggested were all discussed with Elen and Philip. Gradually, Tone also began to identify themes in the stories. In this she aimed to condense the highlighted nodal points into individual themes that were then compared across Elen's and Philip's stories.

To sum up our collaborative work, Elen and Philip have been a driving force in writing their life journeys through inclusive dance contexts, whereas Tone has been a driving force in identifying nodal points, doing the thematic analysis, and structuring the chapter. Put simply, Elen and Philip contribute with nearness to their own lived experiences, whereas Tone contributes with a more analytical distance.

Ethical Considerations

In this case study, we move very close to Elen's and Philip's lives as dancer and choreographer-dance teacher, respectively. They become vulnerable and exposed. Ethical considerations have therefore been important throughout. The project was approved by the Norwegian Data Protection Official for Research. Elen and Philip, as participants contributing their life stories, have had equal influence and authority for the analysis—what to say, what to expose, and what to remove. We have all three read, commented, corrected, discussed, and approved all parts of the analyses and its resulting chapter. We have discussed all material between us by email, we have Skyped, and Tone and Elen (living in Norway) have met in person. In this way, we tried to implement a genuinely collaborative inquiry (Savin-Baden & Howell Major, 2013), although we live on opposite sides of Earth.

Theoretical Perspectives

Meetings in dance between differently bodied people with unique life experiences can set off a process of change among participants. Such meetings have the possibility to become a space for transformative learning and growth. We stress that deep learning and change are possibilities, not phenomena that occur in inclusive contemporary dance contexts automatically. As we have argued elsewhere (Østern & Channells, 2016) and in dialogue with Tochon (2010), the possibility for deep learning and change is present in inclusive contemporary dance contexts as these are places that reach to the whole person (participant-student and choreographer-teacher) and are characterised by difference and plurality.

Further, inquiry and creation in inclusive dance are fulfilled in action. The dance and the choreography incorporate participant experiences as material and the context is organised as a semi-structured physical and verbal dialogue around a theme being explored in dance (Anttila, 2013a, 2013b; Channells, 2015; Østern, 2015; Tochon, 2010). Improvisational and choreographic processes are relational and dialogic, with elements of risk-taking and challenge (Albright, 1997, 2003; Bozic & Olsson, 2013; Rustad, 2013). These characteristics of artistic and/or educational processes in inclusive contemporary dance contexts can serve as sparks for change.

Since we come from dance art and education, we interpret the experiences of change analysed in this chapter in terms of aesthetic transformation (Bond, 2008; Dewey, 1934/1980; Østern, 2008), transformative learning (Mezirow, 1991), experience-based transformation of the body-subject in dance and the importance of dance as a bodily art form (Fraleigh, 1987; Parviainen, 1998), difference and plurality in dance (Benjamin, 2002; Bond, 2017; Bond & Etwaroo, 2005; Channells, 2015; Kuppers, 2001, 2006; Østern & Øyen, 2014a, 2014b, 2015), and the choreographer-teacher's role (Buber, 1995; Stavik-Karlsen, 2014). We interweave these theoretical perspectives in this chapter.

Elen's Life Journey

Elen is 36 years old as this chapter is written. She has spina bifida, a neural tube defect resulting in incomplete development of the spinal cord (Mayo Clinic, 2016). Elen uses a wheelchair. In Fig. 25.1 she can be seen with members of The Dance Laboratory, the community dance company she belongs to in Norway. As we analyse Elen's story as a meaning-making emplotment, or dramaturgy, we highlight nodal points with bold font to indicate their specific relevance to how inclusive dance contributes to her quality of life.

Elen's life journey story starts before inclusive dance enters her life. She describes a time of confusion and **crisis**:

> 2005 changed my life in so many ways. The year started with losing my best friend. Apart from that, I was also in the middle of a life crisis, experiencing a moderate depression, and having no self-esteem whatsoever.

Elen was in need of change. An inclusive dance project existed in her town (later developing into a community dance company), and a friend invited her to try it out. Elen was hesitant, but this changed when she went with her friend to **see a performance** of the group.

> It really moved me, in a way I had never been moved by a dance performance. It was a kind of group and performance I had no idea existed. It was so full of quality and new ideas...a very contemporary expression. And it had differently bodied dancers. All kinds of people, with all kinds of bodies had access to that stage. Professionals, amateurs, people with disabilities, people without disabilities. That so many different people could create such a contemporary performance with such high quality really inspired me.

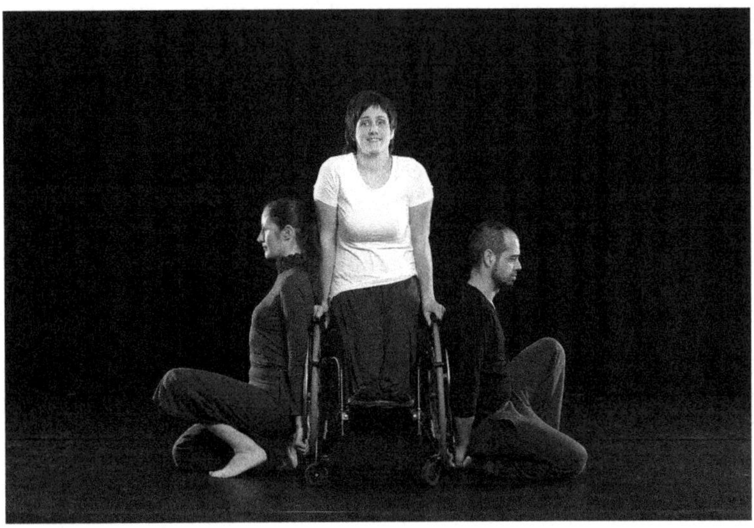

Fig. 25.1 Elen dancing with members of The Dance Laboratory. (Photo: Jøran Wærdahl/Klipp & Lim)

Even though seeing a performance motivated her to begin inclusive dance classes, Elen again experienced hesitation, which remained until the group started working on a new performance. Over time, the performance work and **performing itself** became a main motivation for her to go on with dance:

> We started working on a new performance. I still thought the others were better than me, but I felt a motivation working towards something specific. It took blood, sweat, and oh so many tears. But I made it to the first show. I even opened the show. With talking in front of the audience! And eleven years and so many milestones and powerful moments later, here I am.
>
> As the first performance took form, I truly felt I was a part of something important. It wasn't just about learning a few dance moves and showing it to a few people that I knew, just for fun. I had personally been a big part of the whole process towards the performance. I felt **ownership** for the choreography, because it was based on my improvisations. And **most importantly:** The performance was **high quality**. To show an audience true art of high quality did and still does do something for my self-confidence. It's really art!
>
> And after the performances I get a lot of feedback from the audience. People say this is nothing like they have seen before. That so many different people can share the same stage, that everyone is equally important. The fact that my ideas and movements can be a part of such an innovative performance makes me proud…of myself and of the group. Art gives something both to me and an audience. To be a part of the whole process from creating dance to learning it and finally performing it, feels empowering. It's my dance that I created and learned. I **give my dance to other people**, who are touched by it.

In Elen's dance company, the dancers work a lot with improvisation but they also create choreography through creative processes. In other words, they work with dance as an art form, emphasising both the creative process and the product created collaboratively in the group. This working towards something specific through creative processes was the key to open the world of dance for Elen. Improvising, composing, creating choreography, creating something specific and then communicating that to an audience, in other words **opening up dance as a full art form,** has been important for Elen's engagement in dance and how dance contributes to her quality of life.

In her writing Elen begins and ends with her mother. A life-thread of a strong mother and **the deep relation between mother and daughter** runs through her story. She emphasises that **she has changed** through participation in inclusive dance, but has also **come to value the life she has always lived**. In the inclusive dance context, she finds similar values as those of her mother:

> I have a mother who from the day I was born was set on giving me the same opportunities as everyone else…the tools to live an independent and complete life among "ordinary" people. Her idea of giving me quality of life was reminding me and everyone around me that despite my physical disability, there is a whole person inside of me with qualities like everyone else.
>
> Throughout my life, I have experienced many attempts by society to put me in the "disability box." People associating disability with something sad and assuming that I am this sad person who needs help with everything is the hardest part of having a disability. Not the

> disability in itself. My mother showed me from an early age that I am as ordinary and extraordinary as everyone else.
>
> My point of all this is this: with the inclusive community dance company, I found a whole group with the same idea that my mother had during my childhood. A diagnosis doesn't define a person, it's just a small part of that person. Difference is not a bad thing. It is a huge resource. In this case, this resource is used in creating art. With The Dance Laboratory I have a whole group of people behind me supporting the idea that difference is a resource, not a disadvantage. I have a whole group with me showing that people are people. Not disabled people. Not black or white people. Not thick or thin people. Not tall or small people. But people.

In the inclusive dance context, Elen's belief (attributed to her mother) that **different people cannot and should not be put into separate boxes**, is strengthened. Her experience of differences among people being a value and resource to creating dance art is liberating. In inclusive contemporary dance art and/or education, difference among dancers is seen as central and valuable, not additional (Bond, 2017; Bond & Etwaroo, 2005; Østern, 2009). Difference is not an ingredient that is being put on top of an already existing dance activity. Instead, inclusive dance starts from a genuine interest in difference and what that can give rise to in terms of aesthetic, artistic and pedagogical processes and products.

The meeting between diverse dancers is central for inclusive dance to become truly inclusive. Art educationalist A-L. Østern (2008) dialogues with John Dewey's (1934/1980) transformative aesthetic theory presented in *Art as Experience* as she writes about how transformation in art education or artistic experiences happens in the space between what I already know and the unknown. Such gaps become spaces for learning. Through aesthetic experiences in dance, dancers change both in bodily ways and in their "habits of mind" (Mezirow, 1991). In the words of dance phenomenologists Fraleigh (1987) and Parviainen (1998) an experience-based transformation of the body-subject takes place. In inclusive dance contexts, there is a strong aspect of the unknown, represented by the differences among dancers, bodies and experiences.

Another nodal point for how inclusive dance has contributed to quality of life in Elen's story is her experience of **being treated as anybody** in inclusive contemporary dance, in contrast with (as a wheelchair-user) often feeling underrated and treated like somebody in need of help in everyday situations. She writes, "Being told all the time that you are weaker than you are feels unfair, and so much of your day consists of telling people that you can do a lot more than people around you think." Elen describes how the experience of improvised duets with partners who have treated her as "anybody" has been ground breaking, giving her a **feeling of integrity**. Just the feeling of being treated like an ordinary adult, being trusted, being given body weight by a partner in dance, and not being treated carefully, has been liberating and strengthening (see also Østern & Øyen, 2015, p. 134).

> One moment in the dance company stands out as unforgettable when it comes to improvisation. The whole group would improvise. Suddenly I found myself dancing in dialogue with a dance artist I didn't know personally at the time. This woman I was confident with at first touch. She had a clear body and clear movements. Although she did not know me, she was

> not afraid to try things out with me. She leaned on me, laid on me, used her weight on me. Dragged me in different directions. At one point I was almost on my way out of the chair. She trusted that I could take her strength. She was not being careful with me. I felt I was given a lot of trust. And because of that, I trusted her as well. She had confidence that I was going to endure what she did. To her I was a full-fledged dance partner, not a person she had to be more careful with because I was in a wheelchair.
>
> In the duet with this non-disabled woman, for the first time in many years I had a feeling of being taken seriously by someone my age. She didn't look down on me like I expected she would, she treated me like an adult dancer like her. She treated me like an equal. Being a dancer in an inclusive dance group just wipes away the artificial line between "us and them."

Along with experiences of being treated as "anybody," Elen **builds integrity**. When she teaches student teachers about inclusive pedagogy alongside Tone, she often talks a lot about how participation in inclusive dance contexts gives her a feeling of integrity, which she understands as the feeling of being whole, of being respected and valued as she is, of having the feeling that her ideas and movements are welcome and important in the group, of being treated like an adult (which people using a wheelchair do not always experience, but rather might experience being underrated, treated like a child or helped "too much"):

> Although I have no education in dance, I am considered just as valuable a dancer as the trained dancers in the group. What I do is as important and good as what they do. For the first time in my life, I feel like I have integrity, and that is truly an amazing feeling.

Fraleigh (1987), Parviainen (1998), and Østern & Øyen (2015) write about how dance contributes to experience-based change of the body-subject precisely because of the movement experiences that dance offers. In the above-described duet, qualities of Elen and her partner's relationship developed through sharing full weight, a clear touch, and being stretched in different directions. Sensing and relating through weight sharing gave Elen a feeling of confidence, physical integrity as she was treated like "any*body*" and not like a fragile body, and social power. Elen is moving through change. As she is going through bodily, experience-based change, she finds herself creating a new space where she can take up more physical and psychological room, speak her mind, and set boundaries, becoming more open and integrated at the same time. Scholars have emphasized how improvisation has an important function in opening the individual to transformative learning and change, and that what happens in the dance studio influences life outside and vice versa (Albright & Gere, 2003; Benjamin, 2002).

Another important nodal point we locate in Elen's life story is the lived experience of dance. The kinds of **body contact and communication** she has found in inclusive dance contexts have made a huge impact on her. The meetings—the exchange of information and knowledge in dance, are primarily experienced through movement (Albright, 1997; Albright & Gere, 2003; Sheets-Johnstone, 2009). Bodily communication in dance improvisation often includes the exchange of touch. Touch engaged in dance improvisation is not *any* kind of touch, but a *specific* kind. Touch is engaged to allow the dancers to communicate through different body surfaces: through the skin, through the contours of the body, through taking and giving weight. Through touch, dancers may give and take information as they acknowledge each other, experience each other's bodies and construct each other. This skin-to-skin communication is very direct. Elen writes:

> I have gotten used to being in contact with many different bodies with different stories. We are very focused on contact improvisation in the dance company. In every dance class I learn something new about my own body. My boundaries. My strengths. My weaknesses. I learn to listen to my body. And also, to listen to other people's bodies, signals, boundaries. I feel enormously grateful for having learned that lesson.

In ending her story, Elen points to how her developed skills in and understanding of bodily communication brings quality to the relationship with her mother, who is now, 11 years later, seriously ill:

> My mother is seriously ill with Alzheimer's. She has almost no spoken language left. Every time I see her I feel so grateful that through inclusive dance I have learned to pick up bodily signals. And I am not afraid to touch her. I am not afraid to see her weak. Though it hurts to see my strong, secure mother disappear into the disease, I feel secure enough in my own body to take it. To be there for her. Even though it has become hard to have a conversation with her, I can still hold her hand. Mirror her when she smiles. Stroke her hand when she cries. Have a calm body language, a steady body no matter what. Seeing the value in music and movement when I'm with her. To have the ability to not get scared and run away from my mother's disease is something I have learned from dancing with so many different people. No body or situation is too scary to handle.

Through holistic life story analysis, we have tried to follow Elen on her life journey through inclusive dance contexts, lifting forwards so called nodal points that have had special value for the phenomenon of inquiry on Elen's journey. We looked at her life journey as a whole and identified nodal points and central themes. Table 25.1 presents the themes that best appear to illuminate the research question: *How has participation in inclusive dance contexts contributed to Elen's quality of life*? We turn next to Philip's life-journey through inclusive dance contexts, and will return to themes identified in Elen's story in later discussion (Fig. 25.2).

Philip's Life Journey

At this writing, Philip is 46 years old. He presents himself as a dance artist with a disability, but his disability is invisible and he is not met with the same societal prejudices as Elen, who uses a wheelchair. Philip's story starts from a point where dance was not part of his life.

> Who would've thought I'd become a dancer working in disability-inclusive dance? Certainly, not me. I grew up in a working class family who, like many white, privileged Australian families with a big back yard, were more interested in playing sports than in the performing arts and culture. In fact, dare I out myself on this detail about my childhood and youth, but apart from going to the movies and watching TV, I wasn't introduced to dance as an art form until I was in my late 20s.

Table 25.1 How Elen's participation in inclusive dance contexts has contributed to her quality of life

Nodal Points	Themes
Crisis	Embodied relations
Seeing a performance	Body contact and communication
Performing itself	
Giving my dance to other people	Dance as improvisation, choreography, performance and communication
Owning the dance created	
Experiencing our dance as a full art form of high quality	A valuing of difference among people
The deep relation between mother and daughter	Building integrity—Being treated as any *body* becoming herself
Moving through change	Transformative change
Coming to value the life she has always lived	
Different people cannot and should not be put into separate boxes.	
Being treated as any *body*	
Feeling of integrity	
Building integrity	
Body contact and communication	

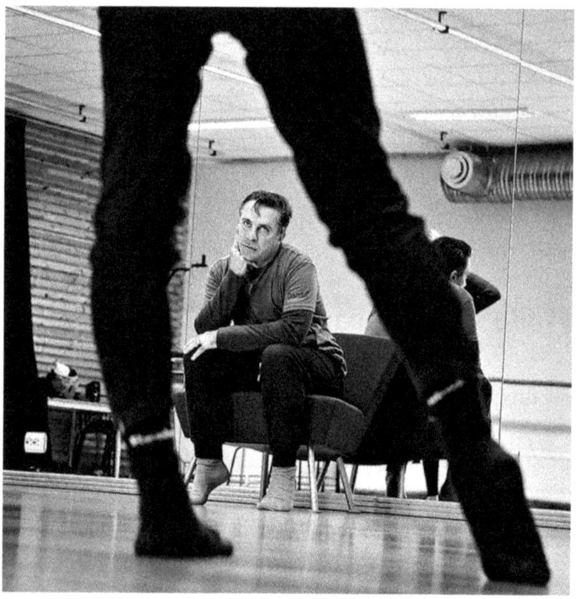

Fig. 25.2 Philip choreographing at MultiPlié Dance Festival in Trondheim, Norway (2012). (Photograph: Arne Hauge)

Leaving his family and home as he became an adult, travelling around the world, and then returning to Australia at the age of 26, Philip writes about how he was introduced to a dance class and discovered that he loved it. He prepared rapidly to audition to study dance in higher education, but ten days before his audition sustained a severe car accident, throwing him into a **life crisis**. A long period of recovery lay ahead, giving Philip time to think.

> I needed direction in my life, I needed purpose and a reason for living, which I hadn't discovered in my four years travelling abroad. Some say they go travelling to find themselves…I didn't. I guess I was not really looking for that. But I think I finally woke up and realized that I needed to dance.

After months of recovery, Philip finally reached a point where he could skip and then run along the beach again. During that time, he also came to the realisation that he needed dance to be part of his life. A men's dance group was about to start up in a nearby town, and Philip found himself dancing in a non-judgmental environment where he could feel safe to be expressive in the way he wanted. This was also the environment where he **found, or allowed, his own sexuality**—a turning point in his life. **Dance served as a catalyst for change** (Albright & Gere, 2003; Benjamin, 2002; Bond & Etwaroo, 2005; Fraleigh, 1987; Parviainen, 1998; Østern, 2009).

> I recall dancing with a guy and for the first time I felt the warmth of touch of another man. It was gentle and caring, strong and sensitive. This surprised me, I guess because I had not wished to acknowledge my tendencies to be attracted to men. I had probably spent a great proportion of my teen and adult life running from the possibility that I could love another man intimately. This dance made me realize it's absolutely possible, and it felt so right for me. I felt like I could be myself whilst at the same time it scared me—it was such a new experience. But none-the-less, it is another period of my life where dance was a catalyst to change.

In this dance context, Philip had the feeling of **being able to be himself** (a scary feeling).

Philip moved to a city and started his professional training as a dance artist. This is also the point where he first attended a dance class for people with and without disabilities. He describes this as an overwhelming experience of having "**found myself**" even though it took him two weeks to pick up the courage to try again.

> I realized dance was the unifying language and that no matter what our background, we all had something to say, something to offer, something to express, openly and without judgment. I remember finishing the class and running and skipping down the street so elated that I had "found myself"—found something that was meaningful in a place where I could just be me. It was dance that was neither wrong nor right. It was a place where everyone was valued, and I felt empowered by this. Without being able to put my finger on what it was exactly about the people I danced with that night that made me feel so alive, I can recall thinking, "this is it!" This is what life's all about.

Starting from discovering a fascination for **unique individual movements by uniquely bodied dancers** (Albright, 1997; Benjamin, 2002; Bond, 1994, 2008; Channells, 2015; Kuppers, 2006), Philip grew more and more into becoming a professional dance artist, also beginning his **choreographic journey** in the inclusive contemporary dance landscape, and with inspiration from inclusive dance artists like Adam Benjamin, Sally Chance, Ingrid Voorendt, and Kat Worth. A nodal point in his meaning-making life journey was when he started paying attention to **culture and politics** of disability on one hand and contemporary dance choreography on the other. Working in inclusive dance contexts often includes being politically engaged

(Albright & Brandstetter, 2015; Albright & Gere, 2003; Benjamin, 2002; Kuppers, 2001, 2006, 2015; Østern, 2009).

> The culture and politics of disability and the culture and politics of contemporary dance were equally complex and yet I felt there was potential for them to collide in a way that was positive and nurturing. I saw scope to provide other people an opportunity to challenge their own perceptions of difference and equality as I had done very early on in my career.

As an artistic space characterised by plurality, inclusive contemporary dance can open up a political space in a clear and loud way. Differently bodied dancers bring their unique life experiences right into the dance studio. The (im)possibilities that different dancers have had in life and dance, the expectations of viewers towards different people's body capacities (Bresnahan & Deckard, this volume; Whatley, 2007), and the tacitly different ways of relating to different people turn up and offer possibilities to change, expect and act differently. However, opening up a political space and acting differently is a possibility, not something that happens in inclusive dance automatically.

While political awareness can be manifested and investigated in the very choreographic work on the movement level (Albright, 1997, 2003; Albright & Brandstetter, 2015), democratic ways of acting need to have influence right into the choreographic process. During Philip's artistic journey, he continuously studied how creative processes could be developed in dialogue and through an investigating approach to movement together with different and unique dancers, resulting in performative "magic." He tells about his meeting with a choreographer in an inclusive dance context:

> I was impressed with her ability to harness the individual strengths and creative nuances of performers she had only just met. In a short period of time, she created what I thought was a masterpiece with a cast of adults with a wide range of skills and abilities, some who had never performed before. She performed magic. It was jaw dropping. I wanted that, **I wanted to learn** how to do that, how to be that patient, **how to look for that unique something about someone** and turn it into a performative gesture or phrase that gave meaning to dance. It wasn't the dance steps that were important, it was the connections the performers made to each other, to the music and to the audience that I found astonishing. I continue to **search for a process that gives meaning to the work from which a performer "owns" their creativity**.

The final nodal point we lift forward from Philip's story is how he, now as an experienced choreographer and dance teacher, discovered his own **compassion, vulnerability and intuition** as important in the creative processes of choreographing.

> I realized compassion and consideration is an important aspect of how I work and unless I am also willing to be honest enough to express my own vulnerability in the creative process, I am hardly qualified to expect this from the performers. More importantly, what I have learnt is that my intuition is finely tuned and this I know creates a deeper learning experience.

Educational philosopher Stavik-Karlsen (2014) describes a "pedagogy of vulnerability," building on his reading of existentialist philosopher Martin Buber. A meeting, Stavik-Karlesen argues, can only be a real meeting if it is open and not rigorously planned in advanced; in this lies the paradox of vulnerability (p. 166). The strength

Table 25.2 How Philip's participation in inclusive dance contexts has contributed to his quality of life

Nodal Points	Themes
Life crisis	Becoming himself
Finding, or allowing, his sexual identity	A valuing of difference among people
Dance was as a catalyst for change	Dance as improvisation, choreography and communication
Being able to be himself	Political engagement in society and in movement
Finding himself	A journey towards collaborative choreographic processes
Unique individual movements by uniquely bodied dancers	Development of compassion, vulnerability and intuition as choreographer/teacher
Choreographic journey	
Culture and politics of disability and dance	Transformative change
Choreographic work on the movement level	
Searching for a choreographic process that gives meaning to the work from which a performer "owns" their creativity	
Compassion, vulnerability, and intuition	

of a trustworthy choreographer/teacher resides in finding the courage needed to be vulnerable in meeting the dancer/pupil. The teacher needs to have courage to be open to investigating creative learning processes, and to partake in those him/herself, even if it means being personal and vulnerable.

Again, in Table 25.2, we condense the nodal points that we have lifted forward through holistic life story analysis of Philip's life journey through inclusive dance contexts into themes that best appear to answer the following research question: *How has participation in inclusive dance contexts contributed to Philip's quality of life*?

Elen and Philip make meaning through the stories they tell, and through life story analysis it is possible to see the importance of inclusive dance in their lives. Both stories show that inclusive contemporary dance contexts are pivotal spaces where quality of life has been nurtured. Elen's and Philip's journeys through inclusive dance are different and similar. In the next and final section of the chapter, we return to the individual themes identified through the analyses and discuss them across two life journeys.

Discussion and Conclusion

How Can Participation in Inclusive Dance Contexts Contribute to the Quality of Life?

As we zoom in to focus on the core of how participation in inclusive contemporary dance contexts can contribute to quality of life (diagramed in Table 25.3), we conclude that for Elen and Philip inclusive contemporary dance has inspired

Table 25.3 Themes describing how participation in inclusive dance contexts has contributed to Elen's and Philip's quality of life

Elen	Elen and Philip	Philip
Integrity – Being whole and treated as any *body*	Becoming oneself	Journey towards collaborative choreographic process
	Valuing of difference	
A new way of taking up personal and social space	The embodied experience of dance	Political engagement through movement
Body contact and communication	Dance as improvisation, choreography, and communication	Development of compassion, vulnerability and intuition as a choreographer-teacher
	Transformative change	

transformative change. Also from dance artistic (Albright, 1997, 2003; Benjamin, 2002; Kuppers, 2006; Østern, 2009) and dance phenomenological (Bond, 2017; Bond & Stinson, 2000/2001, 2007/2016; Fraleigh, 1987; Parviainen, 1998) perspectives, the experience-based transformation of body-subject in relational, artistic processes can contribute to quality of life. As Elen wrote, "I am becoming more of myself, or more the person I want to be."

Life story analysis suggested that three characteristics of context were perceived as important and salient to experienced quality of life by both Elen and Philip: contexts that (1) value difference, (2) offer the embodied, creative experiences that contemporary dance as an art form can offer; and (3) work toward choreography, performance and communication valued and not excluded on the basis of ableist stereotypes, the dance process is often pushed towards improvisational, open-ended working methods. Improvisation allows space for the untried, in and between different bodies (Albright, 1997, 2003; Benjamin, 2002; Bond, 2008). In dance improvisation, this experimenting with what is unseen and unknown in advance a kind of thinking in movement that is "motional through and through, at once spatial, temporal, dynamic" (Sheets-Johnstone, 2009, p. 30). The felt-sense of body is heightened through movement. This is what dance as an art form specifically can give: a heightened, felt sense of self relating to others through movement. This dance can be energizing—bodily, relationally and politically, both in collaborative choreographic processes and in culminating performances on stage. Deeply felt, relational moving experiences crystalize, as both Elen and Philip described in their self-reflexive texts.

As illustrated in Table 25.3, Elen and Philip have discrete themes reflecting where they come from and where they see themselves heading. Their stories also reveal some shared themes connecting with participation and quality of life. Elen, using a wheelchair, comes from a place where her personal space has been limited by the prejudice she bumps into in everyday life (Sandahl & Auslander, 2005). For her, the "integrity" she has built in inclusive dance contexts has been agentic and life-changing. For Philip, his singular themes reflect that he has been working towards becoming a choreographer-teacher and experienced personal vulnerability in this process (see Stavik-Karlsen, 2014). As a leader of inclusive contemporary dance contexts, he seeks to be able, artistically in movement and politically in society, to open the inclusive space for dance that Elen as a dancer experiences as so refreshing. Summing up, in different and similar ways, Elen's and Philip's life journeys through inclusive contemporary artistic and educational dance contexts have been transformative, contributing to their quality of life. In this chapter, we have tried to illuminate and communicate how.

Critical Perspectives

Reflecting on study design and analysis, one critique might be that the guiding question and therefore the findings are biased towards the positive, that is, lacking in criticality. Indeed, life story analyses illuminate Elen's and Philip's journeys through inclusive contemporary dance contexts specifically in regard to *enhanced* quality of life. In this particular study, the positively biased starting point was deliberate, allowing us to examine their perceptions of *how* enhancement happened, not *if* it happened. This is not to say that their life-journeys have been easy. Quite the contrary: they have been challenging with, as Elen put it, "blood, sweat, and oh so many tears." As numerous dancers have reported, challenge can be demanding and rewarding at the same time (Bond & Stinson, 2007/2016).

Further, from a scientific perspective, the study is not generalizable to a population. The case study of Elen and Philip does not prove that participation in inclusive contemporary dance contexts leads to increased quality of life. We have all three, during our time in the inclusive dance landscape, experienced artists who did not like what we were offering and dancers who stopped coming to class. Those who do not experience enhanced quality of life in inclusive dance contexts have not been our focus here, but hopefully will be another time, as there is much to learn from negative cases. For this study, we began with the personal experiential understanding that inclusive contemporary dance contributes to our own wellbeing, employing life history writing by two of us to document the lived experience of inclusive dance contexts. We hope this study will be valuable and interesting for others interested in questions of dance and the quality of life.

References

Albright, A. C. (1997). *Choreographing difference: The body and identity in contemporary dance*. Middletown, CT: Wesleyan University Press.

Albright, A. C. (2003). Dwelling in possibility. In A. C. Albright & D. Gere (Eds.), *Taken by surprise. A dance improvisation reader*. Middletown, CT: Wesleyan University Press.

Albright, A. C., & Brandstetter, G. (2015). The politics of a prefix. *Choreographic Practices, 6*(1), 3–7.

Albright, A. C., & Gere, D. (Eds.). (2003). *Taken by surprise. A dance improvisation reader*. Middletown, CT: Wesleyan University Press.

Anttila, E. (2013a). Dance pedagogy in the contemporary world. In A. K. Ståhle (Ed.), *Close encounters – Contemporary dance didactics: Exploration in theory and practice* (pp. 13–30). Stockholm, Sweden: Dans- och cirkushögskolan.

Anttila, E. (2013b). *Koko koulu tanssii! Kehollisen oppimisen mahdollisuuksia kouluyhteisössä* [The whole school dances! The possibilities with embodied learning in school.]. *Acta Scenica 37*. Helsinki, Finland: Teatterikorkeakoulu.

Benjamin, A. (2002). *Making an entrance. Theory and practice for disabled and non- disabled dancers*. London: Routledge.

Bond, K. (2008). The human nature of dance: Towards a theory of aesthetic community. In S. Malloch & C. Trevarthen (Eds.), *Communicative musicality: Exploring the basis of human companionship* (pp. 401–422). Oxford, UK: Oxford University Press.

Bond, K., & Etwaroo, I. (2005). "If I really see you …:" Experiences of identity and difference in a higher-education setting. In M.-C. Powell & V. Marcow-Speiser (Eds.), *The arts, education, and social change: Little signs of hope* (pp. 87–99). New York: Peter Lang.

Bond, K. E. (1994). Personal style as a mediator of engagement in dance: Watching Terpsichore rise. *Dance Research Journal, 26*(1), 15–26.

Bond, K. E. (2014). Dance and quality of life. In A. C. Michalos (Ed.), *Encyclopedia of quality of life and well-being research* (pp. 1419–1424). Dordrecht, The Netherlands: Springer.

Bond, K. E. (2017). "Boys are morons"…"Girls are gross"…Let's dance! In W. Oliver & D. Risner (Eds.), *Dance and gender: An evidence based approach* (pp. 37–57). Gainesville: University Press of Florida.

Bond, K. E., & Stinson, S. W. (2001). "I feel like I'm going to take off!" Young people's experiences of the superordinary in dance. *Dance Research Journal, 32*(2), 52–87.

Bond, K. E., & Stinson, S. W. (2016). "It's work, work, work, work:" young people's experiences of effort and engagement in dance. In S. W. Stinson (Ed.), *Embodied curriculum theory and research in arts education: A dance scholar's search for meaning* (pp. 269–295). Dordrecht, Eastern Cape: Springer (Original work published 2007).

Bozic, N., & Olsson, B. K. (2013). Culture for radical innovation: What can business learn from creative processes of contemporary dancers? *Organizational Aesthetics, 2*(1), 59–83.

Buber, M. (1995). *Det mellanmänskliga [The interhuman]*. Ludvika, Sweden: Dualis.

Bullough, R. V., Jr., & Pinnegar, S. (2001). Guidelines for quality in autobiographical forms of self-study research. *Educational Researcher, 30*(3), 13–21.

Channells, P. (2015). Perfect (im)perfections: The choreographer's reflections on the creative process. *Nordic Journal of Dance, 6*(1), 48–53.

Clandinin, D. J., & Connelly, F. M. (2000). *Narrative inquiry. Experience and story in qualitative research*. San Fransisco: Jossey-Bass.

Dewey, J. (1980). *Art as experience*. New York: Perigee Books (Original work published 1934).

Fraleigh, S. H. (1987). *Dance and the lived body. A descriptive aesthetics*. Pittsburgh, PA: University of Pittsburgh Press.

Goodson, I. F., & Sikes, P. J. (2001). *Life history research in educational settings: Learning from lives*. Buckingham, UK: Open University.

Kuppers, P. (2001). Deconstructing images: Performing disability. *Contemporary Theatre Review, 11*, 3–4.

Kuppers, P. (2006). Vibrant agencies: Dance, disability embodiment and phenomenology. *Discourses in Dance, 3*(2), 21–31.

Kuppers, P. (2015). Waltzing disability culture: Moving history with Raimund Hoghe. *Choreographic Practices, 6*(1), 41–57.

Mayo Clinic. (2016). *Diseases and conditions: Spina bifida*. Retrieved from http://www.mayoclinic.org/diseases-conditions/spina-bifida/basics/definition/con-20035356

Mezirow, J. (1991). *Transformative dimensions of adult learning*. San Francisco, CA: Jossey-Bass.

Østern, A.-L.. (2008). Pedagogisk teori for estetiske fag – om kunstneriske læringsprosesser og om å undervise på estetisk nivå [Pedagogical theory for art subjects – Artistic learning processes and teaching on an aesthetic level]. In T. Ørbæk Svee (Ed.), *Dans og didaktikk* [Dance teaching and learning] (pp. 19–37). Trondheim, Norway: Tapir akademisk forlag.

Østern, T. P. (2009). *Meaning-making in the dance laboratory. Exploring dance improvisation with differently bodied dancers* (Doctoral dissertation). Theatre Academy, Helsinki, Finland.

Østern, T. P. (2015). The dance project perfect (im)perfections as a deep educational experience of plurality. *Nordic Journal of Dance, 6*(1), 36–47.

Østern, T. P., & Channells, P. (2016). Deep learning and teaching as affordances of inclusive dance and arts education. In A. B. Sæbø (Ed.), *International yearbook for research in arts education* (pp. 123–131). Münster, Germany: Waxmann.

Østern, T. P., & Øyen, E. (2014a). Difference as a creative and critical force in teacher education: Reflective partners teaching in and out of the wheelchair. *Journal of Dance Education, 14*(3), 101–108.

Østern, T. P., & Øyen, E. (2014b). Ulikhet som impuls til nye oppdagelser i dans: Å tøye både muskler og meninger gjennom mangfold i Danselaboratoriet [Difference as an impulse to new discoveries in dance: To stretch muscles and minds through diversity in The Dance Laboratory]. InFormation (Nordic Journal of Art and Research), 3(2), 94–109.

Østern, T. P., & Øyen, E. (2015). Moving through change. *Choreographic Practices, 6*(1), 125–144.

Parviainen, J. (1998). *Bodies moving and moved: A phenomenological analysis of the dance subject and the cognitive and ethical values of dance art* (Doctoral dissertation). Tampere University, Tampere, Finland.

Pérez, P. (Ed.) (2006). *Erfarenhet, berättelse och identitet* [Experience, narration and identity]. Karlstad, Sweden: Karlstad University Press.

Rustad, H. (2013). *Dans etter egen pipe; En analyse av danseimprovisasjon og kontaktimprovisasjon – aom tradisjon, fortolkning og levd erfaring* [Dance as you wish: An analysis of dance improvisation and contact improvisation – As tradition, interpretation and lived experience]. Doctoral dissertation, Norwegian School of Sports Sciences, Oslo, Norway.

Sandahl, C., & Auslander, P. (Eds.). (2005). *Bodies in commotion: Disability and performance.* Ann Arbor: University of Michigan Press.

Savin-Baden, M., & Howell Major, C. (2013). *Qualitative research: The essential guide to theory and practice*. New York: Routledge.

Sheets-Johnstone, M. (2009). *The corporeal turn. An interdisciplinary reader*. Exeter, UK: Imprint Academic.

Stavik-Karlsen, G. (2014). Konturer av sårbarhetens pedagogikk [Contours of a pedagogy of vulnerability]. In A.-L. Østern (Ed.), *Dramaturgi i didaktisk kontekst* [Dramaturgy in educational contexts] (pp. 149–168). Trondheim, Norway: Fagbokforlaget.

Tochon, F. V. (2010). Deep education. *Journal for Educators, Teachers and Trainers, 1*, 1–12.

Whatley, S. (2007). Dance and disability: The dancer, the viewer and the presumption of difference. *Research in Dance Education, 8*(1), 5–25.

Wigg, U. J. (2015). Att analysera livsberättelser [To analyse life stories]. In A. Fejes & R. Thornberg (Eds.), *Handbok i kvalitativ analys* [Handbook of qualitative analysis] (pp. 238–255). Stockholm, Sweden: Liber.

Chapter 26
Young People's Experiences in Hip Hop Dance Participation

Jacinda Richards and Sally Gardner

Introduction

This essay discusses a qualitative study involving young people of recent migrant and refugee backgrounds living in the western suburbs of Melbourne, Australia and attending regular after-school hip hop dance activity there. The project, (initiated by one of the authors, Jacinda Richards [JR], who is the community artist conducting these activities), aimed to discover why the young people chose to learn and participate in hip hop dance activity and what they gained from it in the context of their transition into the broader Australian culture and society.

Individuals and groups newly arrived and seeking to live permanently in a country are usually seeking to "integrate" with the society of that country. Integration, here, is a question of the extent to which "people are able to participate in society, to feel they belong to both their own communities and to the new host communities in which they are now living" (Omar, 2011, p. 47). Wulfhorst, Rocha, and Morgan (2014) suggest that integration entails "transnational belonging" where migrants aim to "forge and sustain multi-stranded social relations that link together their societies of origin and settlement" (p. 1799). As far as young migrants or refugees are concerned, Mansouri (2009) writes that transnational experience "may or may not continue…during settlement, but the transnationalism literature strongly suggests that diasporic connections and multiple national loyalties are a key feature of the migration experience" (p. 26).

At the same time, in Australia, "newly arrived" individuals and groups, especially those of non-English speaking backgrounds and non-European appearance, can frequently be deemed outside of mainstream society and therefore not eligible to participate fully in the much touted Australian "way of life." Certainly, Australia has a racist history; and the advent of the official policy of multiculturalism, despite

J. Richards (✉) · S. Gardner
Deakin University, Geelong, VIC, Australia
e-mail: jacinda@l2r.com.au; sally.gardner@deakin.edu.au

K. Bond (ed.), *Dance and the Quality of Life*, Social Indicators Research Series 73,
https://doi.org/10.1007/978-3-319-95699-2_26

its successes, has eradicated neither institutionalised nor casual racism (see Australian Government, 2013). Hage (2012) calls multiculturalism in Australia a "white nation fantasy" (p. 126). The policies of recent Australian federal governments have also vilified refugees and asylum seekers. Aggressively seeking to prevent them from landing on Australian soil, they contravene international laws and covenants on human rights, while maintaining only a small planned "intake" of refugees who are "processed" in camps and transitional facilities far from our shores (http://www.aph.gov.au/About_Parliament/Parliamentary_Departments/Parliamentary_Library/pubs/rp/rp1415/RefugeeResettlement). In May, 2016, the Immigration Minister Peter Dutton was widely reported saying on radio during a discussion about how large or small Australia's refugee, or indeed migrant intake should be, that refugees were illiterate and innumerate, and that they would take jobs from Australian workers (Thomsen, 2016).

There is ample evidence that young people of migrant or refugee backgrounds, particularly those whose appearance is not white, Anglo-European can experience significant difficulties in establishing a sense of belonging within Australian society. Regular news items pinpoint the kinds of obstacles faced by young people who may be seeking to build or find a sense of belonging in their new country. Melbourne's *The Age* newspaper reported recently, for example:

> A manager of an Apple store in Highpoint shopping centre has apologised to a group of African students who were asked to leave the store because security guards feared they were going to shoplift. (Wells, 2015)

It was reported that an Apple staff member, apparently on behalf of the security guards, asked the year 10 students to leave the shop and that, subsequently, the principal of the boys' school accompanied his students to demand an apology. The journalist reported that, given this apology, the students felt that justice had been served, while Highpoint Centre manager, Ryan Ling said: "Melbourne's West is a multicultural area and we want to stress that Highpoint welcomes guests" (p. 3). Similarly, in Melbourne's *Maribyrnong Leader* newspaper, Byrne (2016) reported that two Sudanese men of refugee background were told that "black people aren't allowed in the hotel" and "only Australians are allowed here" (p. 8).

Daily encounters and experiences such as these can seriously challenge young people's sense of belonging. The students involved in the Highpoint incident are deemed to be African (not Australian) by the journalist; are assumed to be dishonest by shopkeepers; and are subsequently welcomed as "guests" by a manager, as though being granted permission to enter a place not fundamentally theirs. Such experiences often come on top of migrants having undergone serious trauma and dislocation *on their way* to Australia and simply through arriving in a completely different place. Yusuf Omar (2011) writes that whether people migrate voluntarily or are forced, migrating to a new country,

> …often entails severing relationships with family, friends, and the familiar milieu and ways of being in daily life. It also often involves emotional difficulties, psychological ambivalence, physical exhaustion and alienating experiences. For refugees and other forced migrants, these experiences are all the more traumatic as they often involve violence and

> traumatic loss… Resettlement in a new country is accompanied by many difficulties, including acquiring cultures, languages and life styles previously unknown. (pp. 4–5)

Young people of recent migrant or refugee backgrounds may also experience intergenerational problems as their parents can lose or appear to lose social status and respect in the new country. And "generation" need not only be understood in terms of age cohort; there is "heterogeneity within each migrant (so-called) 'generation'" (Skrbis, Baldassar, & Poynting, 2007, p. 264). Intergenerational differences, "in some cases, can develop into conflict and family destabilization. Thus, the 'whole life' of refugees can be consumed by experiences of relocation" and resettlement hardships (Oikonomidoy, as cited in Omar 2011, p. 4). In addition, young people can be caught between the values and behaviour of their parents and home culture and those of their young locally born peers (see, for example, https://www.youtube.com/watch?v=GhSv2E9BfwQ). Based on his study of Somali youth in Australia and the USA, Omar (2011) observes that all of these issues together:

> …can hamper refugees' participation in mainstream social activities, and delay their integration even further (Ali, 2003; Oikonomidoy, 2005). These challenges can be compounded by a lack of access to the facilities and services that are available, and a lack of well-designed programmes to support integration. (p. 6)

The newspaper story mentioned above, despite its own unconscious complicity in the racism on which it reports, also suggests, however, that there *are* resources to which such young people can turn, such as the school principal in that case and others via social media where they posted their story. Considering the need for resources to support migrants and refugees as they transition to living in and contributing effectively to Australian society, this study sought data on reasons that migrant and refugee youth attend hip hop dance activities, its positive and negative aspects as perceived by them, and the range of meanings they attribute to the hip hop dance experience. It must be noted that resources are also necessary to support development of non-racist attitudes and behaviour in the broader settled communities where refugees or migrants newly find themselves.

Hip Hop Dance

Review of the scholarly literature on hip hop culture in English reveals that the emphasis in studies of hip hop has tended to fall much less on the dance element than on its other elements of rap, dj-ing and graffiti practices (see Perkins, 1996; although for dance see Banes, 1994; Hassard-Donald, 1996). Numerous scholars have investigated young people's engagement in dance in the community more generally, which might include hip hop styles (Brabazon, 2002; Fensham & Gardner, 2005; Fensham, Gardner, & Komesaroff, 2008; (McCarren, 2012; Thomas, 1993), as well as the whole phenomenon and spread of hip hop culture worldwide (now more than three and a half decades old), including in Australia (see especially Mitchell, 1998, 2003, 2008).

The current study was considerably more limited than existing ethnographies of hip hop (sub-)cultures in particular regions or suburbs (see, for example, Maxwell, 2003). Here, we focused solely on attendance and participation of nine minors and young adults in hip hop dance classes and workshops that functioned also as the basis of rehearsal and performance activities of L2R, a not-for-profit organisation working with young people through the medium of hip hop dance. L2R was founded by co-author JR, who practises as a community artist with financial support from charitable trusts and local government agencies. According to Mitchell (1998), a community theatre orientation "conflicts with some … rappers' concept of hip hop" (p. 7). In Australia, however, hip hop practitioners who are well-respected in the hip hop milieu have often been engaged in community building activities or "community arts."

Notable aspects of hip hop culture include its global diversity and its ongoing vitality as a vehicle for individuals and groups—primarily youth from disadvantaged and marginalised sections of the community, to make their presence felt creatively in public space. Hip hop comes from "the street" and at a fundamental level has stayed there, despite the financial and recording success of some high-profile rap artists. In a broadcast interview for ABC Australia, L-Fresh the Lion (born in western Sydney as Sukhdeep Singh) explains hip hop's appeal to marginalised youth:

> Hip hop has never been shy. Hip-hop's always been in your face. And it's about telling you the message upfront and clearly. And in a way, that can sometimes be confrontational. (as cited in Schafter, 2015, n.p.)

He goes on to cite a line from one of his raps about racial prejudice in Australia: "They tell me to go home but I came from here" (n.p.). Indigenous hip hop artist Juanita Duncan (2015) tells other indigenous young people: "Don't be shame, be game" (n.p.).

According to Australian rapper Nick Bryant-Smith (aka Solo), hip hop is about "partying, celebrating who you are, celebrating the place that you come from, celebrating your identity, and also, you know, using your platform to, um, call things out, criticise things, point out things that aren't how they should be" (as cited in Schafter, 2015, n.p.). Hugues Bazin, author of *La Culture Hip-Hop* (1995) comments that hip hop has "gangsta" appeal and is associated with an ironic, visible consumption or bling style, a form of "self-commodification in the culture industry" (Silverstein, as cited in Durand 2002, p. 49). To others hip hop is an ethos and a set of forms giving voice and social visibility to "the concerns of ethnic minorities all over the world" (Mitchell, 1998, p. 2), particularly concerns made residual by the powerful.

According to Tricia Rose (1994), "hip hop culture emerged in the 1970s as a source of alternative identity formation and social status for youth in a South Bronx community whose older local support institutions had all but been demolished" (p. 78). A comparison might be made with refugee youth who find themselves bereft of their cultural coordinates in a new country and who have often been witness to the destruction of those co-ordinates in their country or region of birth. Rose notes that, in a post-industrial landscape, the crew is a local source of affiliation and support: "these crews are new kinds of families forged with intercultural bonds," providing "insulation and support in a complex and unyielding environment" (p. 78). Citing cinematographer Arthur Jafa, Rose also discusses aesthetic values across the forms of hip hop (dj-ing, graffiti, b-boying, and rap), namely a poetics of flow, layering and rupture, arguing, "These values suggest affirmative ways in which profound social dislocation and rupture can be managed and perhaps contested in the cultural arena" (p. 82). Practitioners are encouraged to:

> ...create sustaining narratives, accumulate them, layer, embellish and transform them. But also be prepared for rupture, find pleasure in it...When these ruptures occur, use them in creative ways which will prepare you for a future in which survival will demand a sudden shift in ground tactics. (p. 82)

Mention of these values raises the question of what defines hip hop dance. Its beginnings in the oppressed areas of the Bronx, New York in the 1970s was as breaking or b-boying. One of the art form's pioneers, Buddha Stretch of Elite Force says in an interview:

> Hip Hop is considered an umbrella and they like to stick all street dances under that umbrella, like popping, locking or b-boying, but those dances all have an entirely separate history. Hip Hop is again what I and my crew do, social dancing or what the B-boys call it Party dancing. But you take all the social dances and spontaneously mix them up and that's what Hip Hop is. (Stretch, 2009)

Stretch emphasises that many genres of street dance fall under the umbrella of hip hop. Breaking, or b-boying, is the original form of hip hop dance and is danced to a genre of music called break music. Other genres of hip hop such as locking, popping, and house were born out of breaking, but all have their own history, are danced to different styles of music, and embody hip hop's multi-cultural roots.

In a talk at Brown University, Stretch (2010) identified four grass roots pillars of hip hop: "peace, unity, love and having fun." He highlights the commercialisation of hip hop in the early 1980s, calling this period the "Beat Street era." He refers to the lengthy history of hip hop documentaries and the string of hip hop films that began with *Style Wars* (Silver, 1983) followed by *Wild Style* (Ahearn, 1983), which brought hip hop culture into the wider community. These films primarily explored the cultural politics of graffiti writing, but in 1984 three films were released: *Beat Street* (Lathan, 1984), *Breakin'* (Silberg, 1984), and *Breakin' 2-Electric Boogaloo* (Firstenberg, 1984), which focused on B-boying, the original form of hip hop dance. The last three decades have seen an abundance of hip hop films produced from grass roots community projects to Hollywood blockbusters such as *Save the Last Dance* (Carter, 2001) and *Step Up* (Fletcher, 2006).

Australian hip hop culture is part of the now global phenomenon of hip hop cultures. Arguing against seeing hip hop as a form of dominantly African-American popular culture, Mitchell (1998) has drawn out the multi-cultural roots of hip hop and writes that, with its spread worldwide, it has become "a way of signifying one's place in a subculture that is both local and global at the same time" (p. 4). Mitchell has also interviewed local New South Wales MCs, including Arab-Australian, MC Peacefender, who says:

> In the media, there's continuous reminders, the way the stories are structured. You see this, I see this, but what can we do? We are also Australian and we are here. We can't just pack up our bags and sell our citizenship and go back to 'wherever we came from.' (Peacefender & Mitchell, 2007)

He discusses how hip hop offers opportunities for artistic expression and for communicating experiences of struggle and alienation to the world-at-large. Clearly, migrant and refugee youth can use hip hop as a vehicle for self-expression and a means to carve identity and place in the broader community, especially where they struggle to express themselves verbally due to speaking English as second language.

Language barriers are common among newly arrived refugees who have often experienced disrupted formal education and schooling due to war, poverty or disadvantage experienced in their countries of origin. Hip hop dance may be attractive to these young people as it does not require them to speak English. Hughes Bazin notes that "dance was the training ground for most of the rappers in France… it was not yet conceivable to rap in French" (as cited in Durand, 2002, p. 99). Some of the youth in the current study met JR at Western English Language School (WELS) where they were learning English prior to joining the mainstream school system.

Research Methods

This study was undertaken as part of an Honours degree program at Deakin University in Melbourne and received ethics clearance from the university's Ethics Review Committee. It differs from some other studies where hip hop or other dance classes or physical activity have been provided to youth specifically for research purposes (see for example, Beaulac, Olavarria, & Kristjanssonl, 2010; Ransdell, Oakland, & Taylor, 2003). In this case, JR had already been working as a community dance practitioner with youth in Melbourne's West for some years. She was known to the families of study participants, and because of this relationship of trust the research was possible. Participants were recruited from the Phoenix Youth Centre in Footscray and the Flemington Community Centre and attend JR's after-school classes for free. Study participants ranged in age from 11 to 16 years and their family nationalities or ethnicities prior to arrival in Australia included Burmese, Karen, Chin, Vietnamese, Congolese, Sudanese, Ethiopian, Eritrean, Liberian and Iranian.

Two focus groups, lasting 50 min and 40 min respectively, were organized at accessible locations: Western English Language School (WELS) and Flemington Community Centre (FCC). These focus groups were conducted by Gardner with JR in attendance. Ten youth (three female and seven male) participated in the WELS focus group, while five young female adolescents (ages 11 and 12) still attending primary school participated at FCC. The focus groups acted as a way to familiarise participants with the idea of being invited to comment on or being questioned about their dance experiences. This was important in view of a significant number not having English as their first language, and the importance of presenting the attention focused on them (as study participants) as safe and supporting rather than critical or exploitative. We hoped to put the young people at their ease and tried to establish an atmosphere that would not suggest that they needed to give certain kinds of responses.

The two focus groups differed from each other in terms of the discussion that took place. One involved mainly high school-aged male participants expressing a degree of shyness, while the other had younger female participants only who had been in Australia for longer or had been born there of migrant or refugee parents, and who were more at ease with talking about why they danced. This group did not take up an opportunity offered to them to talk about gender issues. The in-depth interviews demonstrated not only different participants' personalities, but also their relative command of English and ability to express their thoughts in that language.

From the focus groups, questions for further inquiry were developed for individual semi-structured interviews conducted by JR. Interviews, which lasted for different lengths of time in each interviewee's case (from 8 to 30 min), were transcribed and analysed according to established qualitative techniques. We immersed ourselves in the data, reading and re-reading the interviews, while following the initial two phases of grounded theory coding: 1) "naming each word, line or segment of data" followed by 2) "a focused selective phase that uses the most significant or frequent initial codes to sort, synthesize, integrate and organize" the data. (Charmaz, 2006, p. 46).

By grounded theory we mean that a theory of what is going on for participants in a social practice is generated, provisionally, from out of the data that they provide, rather than is chosen or constructed beforehand. Thus, hypotheses are "'grounded' in the data themselves" (p.2; see also Halberg, 2006, p. 143). The relation to the data, however, is hermeneutic in view of the research question, in this case of what role participation in hip hop dance might play in migrant and refugee youth making a transition to Australian society. In other words, the grounded coding is also a response to or informed by this broad question. Hypotheses, thus generated, remain to be tested and re-tested through further research. We undertook an open coding process separately, and then discussed and identified themes. A third experienced researcher was invited to cross-check processes, encouraging further questioning of transcribed audio files and identification of themes.

Findings: Hip Hop Feels Right

Of the fifteen focus group members, nine young people who were attending school and living with immediate family members managed to proceed to the next phase of attending an interview. They included three young females who were in grade six primary school, and three females and three males who had graduated from WELS in the past 6 months and entered the mainstream school system in year seven (WELS is a school for newly arrived migrant and refugee students in their initial settlement period). Analysis of transcribed interviews produced three major themes that reflect participants' thoughts, feelings and experiences while taking part in hip hop dance classes and workshops, and in L2R: 1) building a sense of self, confidence and respect for self and others; 2) having a sense of belonging within the group and gaining wider social connections; and 3) hip hop as a form of communication and expression that feels right. In illustrating these themes below, we use participants' actual names, as they themselves were keen to be identified. We also identify their "ethnicity" but with awareness that, since the participants are newly arrived and are in a settlement phase they are now also Australian.

Themes

1. **Building a sense of self, confidence, and respect for self and others.** All the participants saw the dance activity as a vehicle for furthering self-respect, self-confidence and respect amongst peers and community. It provides them with a framework within which to have goals to strive for and to experience achievements in a pleasurable way. One participant discussed how she enjoyed seeing her skills develop through practice and effort, while performance opportunities and hip hop dance competitions helped her set personal goals: "Because it's like fun seeing yourself improve in dance if you are really good. If you come last you know that next year you have to step up" (Ayom, female, 11, Sudanese)! Another explains how he was able to share his achievement with family: "Yeah, my father knows about my dancing cause Lonowon and I won a comp and I brought the medal to him and he was really happy" (Rominglian, male, 15, Burmese). Another Burmese male participant noted:

> When you come, you learn routine and new friends and then on performance day.... Hmmmm I forget how to say... Um, you make it perfect!' (Van Biak Thang, male, 15, Burmese)

Confidence could be gained from hip hop dance and extend into other parts of life. One participant from Flemington who had recently transitioned from primary to secondary school claimed:

> Now I have a new confidence...I have always been one of the shy people. If I was in a group I would always be the one at the back. But now, I'm not scared of being at the front and everyone staring at me. (Jaklin, female, 11, Sudanese)

Another shared his personal confidence and faith in his crew: "Yeah good, we can smoke anyone, any B-boy. We are ready for them anytime" (Lonowon, male, age 15, Liberian). The following felt that hip hop dance was fun—something she enjoyed people watching her do—suggesting that it promoted a positive sense of self: "I feel like I can do something and people can watch it and it's challenging—it just makes my life" (Nastaran, female, 14, Iranian)!

Participants found that friends were supportive of their dancing. However, there could be a lack of support from parents: it was potentially a waste of time, not a suitable career choice compared to becoming a doctor or engineer, or interfered with family and household chores. When asked if his parents were happy with him dancing, Lonowon declared: "NO! No family, only friends. Cause they don't like dancers…I come home late." A female participant described family ambivalence, noting,

> Um yes, but not my mum and dad. Sometime they are happy about dancing and sometime not. They don't like me to dance. They just want me to dance for fun and not the future. (Nolly, female, 13, Burmese)

Van Biak said that his mother was supportive but also emphasized that the dancing was a serious commitment: "My mum told me, you go to class every week, so if you are going to keep this up in the future I am happy for you to go."

Jerry revealed that she did not practice at home, suggesting that she might attend classes for the social interaction, or alternatively, perhaps the home environment was not conducive to her feeling free to practice: "Actually, I don't practice when I go home. Every Thursday that's it. I never practice at home" (female, age 15, Ethiopian).

On the other hand, a young person's hip hop dance classes and dance achievements could create discussion amongst friends and family. It gave parents something to be proud of, while carving the child's identity within the family structure, even if some claimed to be embarrassed by their parents' boasting about them. Two female participants from Flemington explained:

> Like when you are with your family, the families show off to other people that my daughter is good (at dancing) or something like that. That's why it's kind of embarrassing. (Linda, female, age 12, Eritrean)

> If I dance in front of my mum, the next minute you hear her on the phone talking about it and it's embarrassing. The most embarrassing thing you do and straight away she is on the phone about it. (Jaklin, female, age 11, Sudanese)

When asked what hip hop dance and culture meant to them, participants identified strongly with it, such as Jaklin, who said, "It's everything to me, it's part of me!" Nastaran's reflections had an existential ring: "Hip hop means a lot to me, if hip hop wasn't like, if there was no hip hop I couldn't be alive cause hip hop means everything to me." Jaklin emphasised further that hip hop dancing was her "thing," suggesting that it contributed to her sense of identity. She was aware that different people have different "things and interests," however dancing gives her something to do and share:

> I feel different 'cause some of them can really sing and at least I have something to do in my spare time, and some just read books. I don't read books. I dance. They read books and some sing! At least we have our own thing. If I didn't have my own thing I would feel lonely. Nothing to do!

Lonowon highlighted his knowledge of the genres within hip hop dance discussing what he identified within hip hop, namely, the male-identified genre of breaking or b-boying, and thus with a form through which he could shape a confident masculine identity as a dancer: "original style and Flava…just breaking."

Female participants expressed awareness of the importance of dance as physical activity, a vehicle for staying fit and healthy and not becoming isolated. Jaklin reflected:

> Because it's exercise. It's better than sitting, it's better than do nothing. And exercise is really important in life because I don't want to grow up to be a fat person that doesn't walk. I want to be a person that is healthy and has a lot of confidence.

2. **Having a Sense of Belonging within the Group and Gaining wider Social Connections.** Most participants expressed a strong personal connection with their dance crew, relating to notions of family. Jaklin and Nastaran explained:

> J: I know everyone and they are like technically my family and we all get along well and we like each other and we share.
> N: Cause it's a good crew and it's like a family and you can learn different stuff here.

Rominglian described the dance environment as friendly and welcoming: "They are pretty good and they are friendly. They always welcome new people and I like that." Twelve-year-old Linda highlighted the level of trust among her crew, which gives her a sense of well-being. She also recounted that hip hop dance participation gave her opportunities to travel, which suggests that her social world has expanded through participation, supporting her to venture from her home community into the broader community:

> I feel happy … being with a group I can trust together, and like you see and you go to different places and lessons and see what they have been working on and stuff.

Hip hop dance classes gave these young people something positive to do with spare time, getting them out of the house while increasing opportunities and good experiences. Ayom explained:

> I'm normally just at home watching TV but hip hop gave me something good to do and now I have more things to do like perform and perform in places I thought I would never perform in.

Nastaran spoke about the classes at Footscray, disclosing, "I don't feel like I am sitting at home by myself and lonely. There are people here and I am happy and excited, YEAH!" Not only other members of the crew but also the community artists who teach and organise can become close relations. Rominglian shared:

> Yeah, Katsu and Nasa are important to me and the crew because they are really great. They support us, even if we don't want to train they say, "c'mon guys let's train." Motivate us! Especially Katsu tells us bits of his life and how he became a b-boy. So they are really important to us.

3. **Hip Hop as a Form of Communication and Expression that Feels Right.** Several participants discussed hip hop dance in relation to other activities that

could be available to them, or other activities they were aware of as being common and valued in Australian culture. To them hip hop dance compared favourably to those activities. For example, Linda noted, "In hip hop it doesn't hurt and you don't feel the pain or anything." Comparing soccer to hip hop, she explains,

> In soccer, you need to be really, really good... (In hip hop) if you have a new move you can show it to the teacher and she can do it in a dance. But in soccer it's like you have to listen to the captain and be good at everything.

Ayom compared different dance genres. She discussed how the slower movements and music typical of ballet could be challenging, although the strength required to perform power moves and floor work in break dancing were just as difficult. She expresses a level of experiential awareness:

> You have to make your moves more perfect [in ballet] … it's like slower and you do it slower going into it and you need more balance. Yeah, but sometimes in hip hop dancing, some things you have to do on the floor or if you want to learn how to do a back flip.

A majority of participants expressed that by doing hip hop dance they had something to share with others—that their dance skills could orient them towards others, both now and in the future. Linda explained:

> I really like going to hip hop because like in the future I want to be a dancer or a dance teacher in the group, so I need like a lot of practice. It just makes me feel happy! If you are sad and you come to hip hop it takes everything away. You just like go and dance and like sharing stuff that you did. Like if you have a dance move you can share with everybody.

Several participants believed it is important to share hip hop because it had helped them in difficult circumstances and has the potential to assist others. Nastaran said, "If they know about hip hop they can be dancers too and it can make them more better person." Fifteen-year-old Lonowon discussed his feelings about passing on his knowledge, assisting and teaching other students: "It makes me feel awesome, it makes me feel great!"

Some participants recognised the value of the dancing and music in uniting them across boundaries of language and culture. Ayom viewed hip hop as a universal language, explaining, "Everyone has different languages but with hip hop it's like one language and you can do it to different types of music. It doesn't have to be in English." Hip hop dance provided Rominglian with an avenue for him to represent his cultural origins as well as his new cultural experiences in Australia. He put it succinctly: "Yeah it's important for me because I want to represent my country and myself." Connections with hip hop culture were also discussed, specifically the music and lyrics of the songs, which spoke to participants' own feelings and experiences. Nolly reflected,

> It's like real in our life. Like the music comes and we dance and then the music, we feel dancing better and better. The music is like...I'm not sure how to say. Without music we cannot dance, but if it's with music we have a lot of energy and then our dancing is better with the music. So music keeps you interested in the dancing… Yeah, real life means like... the music, like some music has meaning and some of the words feel like real life.

Hip hop could be serious business, as noted by Rominglian: “Hip hop means to me, freedom. Like expressing your feelings no matter if you are angry or sad, happy. Just dance you know. That’s why I choose hip hop.” Jerry spoke of the hip hop dance activity as a structure that made certain demands on her, somewhat like school. She felt a responsibility to attend and to make the same sort of commitment as others: “I have to come. When I come to school I have to go every day. It’s the same as school. Because everyone is coming to teach us so we have to go.” Nastaran noted that hip hop could simply be “cool,” not requiring verbal explanation and giving the young person a “cool” identity amongst peers.

Discussion

Young people newly arrived, especially from non-Western countries, can experience difficulties in being and feeling accepted into the wider Australian community in which they find themselves. This experience can be related to both their mixed reception here and to the experiences of dislocation, sometimes of war and violence, that they have been through or carry with them through their parents’ experience. This study suggests that newly arrived migrant and refugee youth in the initial settlement stages can develop a sense of well-being, self-confidence, and social connectedness through hip hop dance class participation and membership in a dance crew.

For the young people who participated in our study, hip hop dance can be a medium for exploring and asserting their own worlds and identities in relation to those of their parents, on the one hand, and those of the often-disapproving mainstream culture, on the other. When they perform, or show what they can do in formal or informal situations, they can gain a positive view of themselves as well as the sense that they are viewed positively in the eyes or through the gaze of others in the society—their teachers, passers-by, the audience. While dancing, they can forget other concerns, such as anxieties to do with school and the future, and feel the exhilaration of being in motion (see Bond & Stinson, 2000/2001). At the same time, the lyrics of the music and the poetics of the dance itself, as Rose (1994) has explained, can express something of what “real life” feels like as they have experienced it.

It seems clear from our study that the hip hop dance can provide personal satisfaction while membership of a crew can be a source of positive feelings of sharing and belonging. Participation in dance allowed our young participants to feel they could help others, share something with them and contribute to something larger than themselves. Since most participants in this study speak English as a second language, they could employ dance as an inclusive vehicle for self-expression and sharing with others across differences in language and cultural background.

Hip hop has become a global phenomenon demonstrating an extraordinary capacity to maintain its relevance to youth from many different ways of life (see Chap. 16, this volume). This study illuminates that hip hop dance can act as a kind of bridge—a medium through which one can belong to a sub-culture, acquire a valued style or "cool," and through this sense of belonging and participation be able to assert one's presence more confidently within the sometimes-unwelcoming wider society. The roots and elements of hip hop culture and specifically hip hop dance can help to fill the void of stable cultural co-ordinates, giving youth an artistic outlet and basis for meaningful cultural dialogue in a voice that feels authentic to them.

It is worth considering that hip hop dance activities play a role in these young people's building what might be called a way of life—a quality life—in their new country of residence. The late Welsh cultural theorist, Raymond Williams, has been one of the key thinkers of this concept. For Williams (1977), a Marxist, culture is *ideally* democratic in that all members of a society might participate in the creation of meanings, contributing to the "common culture." For Williams, too, culture is always material, in process, and entwined in daily life; thus, for him culture, and experiences of the "superordinary" (Bond & Stinson, 2000/2001) that it can give access to, is "ordinary." Williams opposed thinking and practice that reified culture in institutions and static structures, concepts, and traditions as this effectively denies the role of people making and living culture in the present.

Obstacles to achievement of cultural democracy in Williams' time (early and mid-20th century) included increasing centralisation and corporatisation of the media, the rise of managerialism, and the ongoing effects of the class system and socio-economic disparity, especially in education and in the specifically so-called "cultural" domain of the arts. These issues have only intensified in the current neo-liberal and global era (see, for example, Glow and Minahan 2008). The community-based activities supporting these young people's involvement in hip hop dance are to some extent the legacy of Williams' influential approach to culture—even if these, too, can now be subject to processes of managerialisation. It seems valid to suggest that our young study participants gain a sense of being able to contribute their own meanings to the wider society as they put their moves dynamically on show.

For the young people in our study, participation in hip hop dance was not necessarily the only or even main axis of their identity in the new country. Similarly, these young people did not appear to want to live or remain as "outsiders." Unlike graffiti writing, hip hop dancing is not illegal, even when performed on the street. Furthermore, it is important to reiterate that, globally, hip hop culture can be commercialised and commodified, on the one hand, and exist as an authentic form of resistance on the other. In its multi-dimensionality hip hop dance potentially allows newly arrived young people to both express resistance to oppressive or exclusionary structures and be accepted and "integrated" as youth who embody the style or cool valued in mainstream youth culture.

At the same time, the hip hop dance activities in this study, available as they were in a community arts context, provided opportunities for vulnerable youth to both "stand up and be counted" as well as to be cared about and nurtured beyond the contexts of family and close friends. Indeed, hip hop dance was a way to separate or distinguish themselves from family or original community in a safe way, to move out into the sometimes-hostile wider world with the knowledge and felt sense of having personal achievements and local supports.

Our participants had a mixed response to the topic of their families' support for and knowledge of their hip hop dance participation. In some family households, a child's dancing fostered respect and was a topic of discussion amongst friends, family and community members, suggesting a sense of pride and achievement. Alternatively, some participants suggested their parents were not supportive because they felt the arts, and more specifically dance, were not suitable career choices for the future. Although participants expressed that they could see themselves dancing in the next year or two, many—particularly the older ones, were unclear about their future choices and career pathways (but see below). These issues speak to the intergenerational and transitional conflicts that can be intensified for newly arrived young people.

Clearly the young people participating in our study have found a way to include regular hip hop dance participation in their lives and schedules. Many of the young newly arrived, however, do not attend or continue to attend such activities due to their specific circumstances of local knowledge, language, community, and the dislocation and alienating experiences discussed at the beginning of this chapter. Unstable housing arrangements can be an issue while waiting on government assistance for permanent public housing. According to JR, from her experience it is also common for youth to live with other family members such as uncles and aunts whom they have never met before arriving in Australia. This can put stress on household relations and disrupt schooling patterns, affecting the young person's ability to maintain connections they may have made. These young people need support and encouragement to seek out resources that are relevant to their cross-cultural experience and their new lives in Australia.

To that end, it would be valuable to broaden this study to involve other Melbourne communities with high concentrations of newly arrived migrants and refugees such as those in Dandenong and Wyndham. This would generate statistical weight and potentially identify further important themes. It would also be illuminating to follow the current participants as they move on to high school and beyond, and to compare this group with another who have not been involved in this kind of activity.

Already the young people involved in our study are following diverse paths. Lonowon, Van Biak, Rominglian and Nolly have become youth ambassadors and emerging dance artists who represent L2R and their cultural communities. Lonowon and Van Biak now earn an income through busking in the streets of Melbourne, teaching dance at local dance schools and through other professional engagements. Nastaran's family moved away from the West soon after our study was completed but she continues to drop in occasionally for a visit to see the crew and enjoy some free dance time. Jerry is busy with her basketball training but continues to meet up with JR at local events and festivals. Linda, Jaklin and Ayom have transitioned into high school and currently do not practise or perform with L2R.

References

Ahearn, C. (Producer & Director). (1983). *Wild style* [Motion picture]. USA: First Run Features.
Australian Government, Department of Social Services. (2013). *The people of Australia: Australia's multicultural policy*. Retrieved from https://www.dss.gov.au/our-responsibilities/settlement-and-multicultural-affairs/publications/the-people-of-australia-australias-multicultural-policy
Banes, S. (1994). *Writing dancing in the age of postmodernism. Middletown, CT.* Wesleyan University Press.
Beaulac, J., Olavarria, M., & Kristjanssonl, E. (2010). A community-based hip-hop dance program for youth in a disadvantaged community in Ottowa: Implementation findings. *Health Promotion Practice, 11*(3), 61S–69S. https://doi.org/10.1177/1524839909353738.
Bond, K. E. & Stinson, S. W. (2000/2001). "'I feel like I'm going to take off!": Young people's experiences of the superordinary in dance. *Dance Research Journal*, 32(2), 52–87.
Brabazon, T. (2002). Dancing through the revolution: The political and social meaning of the rave. *Youth Studies Australia, 1*(1), 19–24.
Byrne, B. (2016, February 9). Our job to end racism. *Maribyrnong leader.* Retrieved from http://maribyrnongleader.localnewspapers.today/
Carter, T. (Director). (2001). *Save the last dance* [Motion picture]. USA: Paramount Pictures.
Charmaz, K. (2006). *Constructing grounded theory: A practical guide through qualitative analysis*. London: Sage.
Duncan, J. (2015). *Hot Brown Honey is unsticking stereotypes aimed at indigenous with hip hop*. Retrieved from http://www.sbs.com.au/nitv/article/2015/09/09/hot-brown-honey-unsticking-stereotypes-aimed-indigenous-hip-hop
Durand, A.-P. (2002). *Black, blanc, beur: Rap music and hip-hop culture in the francophone world*. Lanham, MD: Scarecrow.
Fensham, R., & Gardner, S. (2005). Dance classes, youth cultures and public health. *Youth Studies Australia, 24*(4), 14–20.
Fensham, R., Gardner, S., & Komesaroff, P. (2008). Dancing beyond exercise: Young people's experiences in dance classes. *Journal of Youth Studies, 11*(6), 701–709.
Firstenberg, S. (Director). (1984). *Breakin' 2: Electric boogaloo.* [Motion picture]. USA: TriStar, Cannon.
Fletcher, A. (Director). (2006). *Step up* [Motion picture]. USA: Walt Disney.
Glow, H., & Minahan, S. (2008). "I'm here to save you:" a case study of the arts and managerialism in Australia. *Journal of Workplace Rights, 13*(2), 133–145. https://doi.org/10.2190/WR.13.2.c.
Hage, G. (2012). *White nation: Fantasies of white supremacy in a multicultural society*. London: Routledge.
Halberg, L. (2006). The "core category" of grounded theory: Making constant comparisons. *International Journal of Qualitative Studies on Health and Well-being, 1*, 141–148.
Hassard-Donald, K. (1996). *Dance in hip hop culture. Droppin' science: Critical essays on rap music and hip hop culture* (pp. 220–235). Philadelphia: Temple University Press.
Lathan, S. (Director). (1984). *Beat Street* [Motion picture]. USA: Orion.
Mansouri, F. (Ed.). (2009). *Youth identity and migration: Culture values and social connectedness*. Altona, VIC: Common Ground.
Maxwell, I. (2003). *Phat beats and dope rhymes: Hip hop down under comin' upper. Middletown, CT.* Wesleyan University Press.
McCarren, F. (2012). *French moves: The cultural politics of le hip hop*. Oxford: Oxford University Press.
Mitchell, T. (1998). *Australian hip hop as a "glocal" subculture*. Paper for the Ultimo Series Seminar, University of Technology, Sydney. Retrieved from http://snarl.org/youth/tonym2.pdf
Mitchell, T. (2003). Local noise: Australian hip-hop as a subculture. *Youth Studies Australia, 22*(2), 2–13.

Mitchell, T. (2008). Australian hip hop's multi-cultural literacies: A subculture emerges into the light. In S. Homan & T. Mitchell (Eds.), *Sounds of then, sounds of now: Popular music in Australia* (pp. 231–252). Hobart: ACYS Retrieved from https://opus.lib.uts.edu.au/bitstream/10453/8171/1/2008002722.pdf.

Omar, Y. S. (2011). *Integration from youth perspectives: A comparative study of young Somali men in Melbourne and Minneapolis*. Unpublished doctoral thesis, La Trobe University, School of Social Sciences, Melbourne, Australia.

Peacefender, M. C., & Mitchell, T. (2007). *Hip hop from Auburn to Beirut*. Retrieved from http://peacefender.com/source/Media/Publications/4-Peacefender%20Hip%20hop%20from%20Auburn%20to%20Beirut%20UTS%202007.pdf

Perkins, W. E. (1996). *Droppin' science: Critical essays on rap and hip hop culture*. Philadelphia: Temple University Press.

Ransdell, L., Oakland, D., & Taylor, A. (2003). Increasing physical activity in girls and women: Lessons learned from the DAMET project. *Journal of Physical Education, Recreation and Dance, 74*(1), 37–44.

Rose, T. (1994). A style nobody can deal with: Politics, style and the postindustrial city in hip hop. In T. Rose & A. Ross (Eds.), *Microphone fiends: Youth music and youth culture* (pp. 71–88). New York: Routledge.

Schafter, M. (2015). *Hip hop's new wave tackles racism and what it means to be*. Australian Retrieved from http://www.abc.net.au/7.30/content/2015/s4327196.htm.

Silberg, J. (Director). (1984). *Breakin'* [Motion picture]. USA: MGM/UA.

Silver, T. (Director). (1983). *Style wars* [Motion picture]. USA: Public Art Films.

Skrbis, Z., Baldassar, L., & Poynting, S. (2007). Negotiating belonging: Migration and generations. *Journal of Intercultural Studies, 28*(3), 261–269.

Stretch, B. (2009). *Buddha Stretch (Elite Force) interview*. Retrieved from https://youtu.be/4if1XfMr78w

Stretch, B. (2010). Buddha Stretch interview - About hip hop (part 1) - March 6. Retrieved from http://www.youtube.com/watch?v=U3wPcDnLszk.

Stretch, B. (2012). *Buddha Stretch (Elite Force) interview*. Retrieved from http://www.youtube.com/watch?v=I7NJY0hK_mo

Thomas, H. (1993). An-other voice: Young women dancing and talking. In H. Thomas (Ed.), *Dance, gender and culture* (pp. 69–93). London: Macmillan.

Thomsen, S. (2016). *Immigration Minister Peter Dutton says refugees take Australian jobs*. Retrieved from http://www.businessinsider.com.au/immigration-minister-peter-dutton-says-refugees-take-australian-jobs-2016-5

Wells, R. (2015, November 12). Apple shop apologises for "racist" eviction. *The age*, News 3.

Williams, R. (1977). *Marxism and literature*. Oxford: Oxford University Press.

Wulfhorst, R., Rocha, C., & Morgan, G. (2014). Intimate multiculturalism: Transnationalism and belonging amongst capoeiristas in Australia. *Journal of Ethnic & Migration Studies, 40*(11), 1798–1816.

Chapter 27
Dancing it Out: Building Positive Peace

Erica Rose Jeffrey and Lesley J. Pruitt

Introduction

Interest in the potential for fostering peace through the arts continues to grow globally. This work recognizes that the arts—such as dance, music, theatre, written work, drawing painting, photography, and film—have historically been a component in building peace and addressing conflict (Dissanayake, 1988; Hanna, 1979). While there is an extant body of research on arts and peacebuilding broadly (Cohen, Gutiérrez Varea, & Walker, 2011), dance remains comparatively under-researched. This chapter discusses links between dance and peacebuilding and the key theme of this book, *quality of life,* drawing on research from a range of disciplines.

We undertake this exploration in two main ways: first, by identifying and mapping out some key ways dance is deployed in peacebuilding contexts; and second, by more deeply exploring an empirical case focusing on the dance experiences of peacebuilders in the southern Philippines. *Peacebuilders* are agents of social change, in this case community organizers engaged in activities aimed at preventing, reducing, or recovering from conflict. In considering both the broad picture and a specific case, we are able to make an argument for the prospects for "dancing toward peace," while also engaging with literature and lived experiences to acknowledge challenges and limitations of the claim.

The chapter begins with definitions of key terms. Next, we provide an overview of related literature to situate our work within scholarship on peacebuilding, dance, and connections between the two, noting the complexities identified in existing literature with regard to the practice of dance for peacebuilding. From there, we

E. R. Jeffrey (✉)
Queensland University of Technology, Brisbane, QLD, Australia

L. J. Pruitt
Monash University, Clayton, VIC, Australia
e-mail: lesley.pruitt@monash.edu

K. Bond (ed.), *Dance and the Quality of Life*, Social Indicators Research Series 73,
https://doi.org/10.1007/978-3-319-95699-2_27

introduce a preliminary typology of existing approaches to peacebuilding in the context of quality of life, identifying and analyzing six ways dance is being deployed for peacebuilding. For each approach, we describe content, settings and underlying theories. Having situated our work within this broad conceptual and practical environment, we shine a spotlight on practice, offering a critical, reflexive look at the practice of dance for peace in one particular context facilitated by a dancer trained in peacebuilding. The chapter concludes with a summary of main points and suggestions for future research.

Scope & Key Concepts

Our aim with this chapter is to stimulate discussion through identifying and analyzing relevant information and resources across areas of practice. We do not seek to be all-encompassing or definitive. Dance, peacebuilding, and quality of life are fluid in their definitions, interpretations, and cultural and social meanings. Likewise, their porous boundaries of interaction and limitation leave multiple directions for further development and investigation. Our scope provides a reading of the current field to suggest ways of mapping it, to identify areas of overlap, and to make current work more visible while prompting further discussion. As the arts continue to be applied in peacebuilding, it is important to continue to create shared language, theories, and approaches to implementation. To begin with, we discuss our use of key concepts and definitions, which include *dance*, *peacebuilding*, and *quality of life.*

In many cultures, dance is entwined with music. Coe and Strachan (2002) describe dance as multifaceted, "a multisensory experience that includes the visual, the spiritual, the kinesthetic, and the auditory" (p. 507). Here we rely initially on Judith Lynn Hanna's (1979) first definition of dance as "human behavior composed of purposeful, intentionally rhythmical, and culturally patterned sequences of nonverbal body movements other than ordinary motor actions," while recognizing that "dance serves a wide spectrum of purposes, often several simultaneously" (p. 35). We also note that many dance makers explore movement outside of intentional rhythm structures, emphasizing creative process. Bond (2014) notes that dance's "longevity and multiplicity of forms and functions" makes definition "elusive" (p. 1419).

Still, we assert that dance is based in everyday movement and that dancing is movement within space, time, shape and motion (Blumenfeld-Jones, 2004), making it culturally and socially situated. In this chapter, we are looking at dance as encompassing a range of forms from participatory community dance activities through to aesthetic dance performed by professional practitioners. Given the complexity and nuance of dance, we acknowledge that this chapter's format—the written word—cannot capture the full range of how dance has been and is currently being practiced in peacebuilding. We acknowledge that one of the inherent challenges of writing about dance is that doing so presents only one form of analysis or way of understanding.

By "peacebuilding," we refer to actions, initiatives, policies, and projects that aim to reduce, prevent, or aid in the recovery from conflict and violence of all types. This includes a spectrum of activities from individual or grassroots community-driven, bottom-up approaches through to high-level formalized international processes, such as post-conflict peace negotiations assisted by the United Nations or other multilateral organizations (Jeong, 2000). The spectrum also includes the activities and quality of life of peacebuilders or peace-workers themselves. We situate this range within our commitment to pursuing positive peace, which has been "conceptualized as working in a bottom-up rather than a top-down fashion… to ultimately change general cultural norms about dealing with violence" (Forcey & Murray, 1999). Likewise, in 1998 the UN General Assembly adopted Resolution 52/13 to establish its goal of peacebuilding through creating a culture of peace, which encompasses the activities analyzed in this chapter. Scholarship has also documented music and dance being used at various levels to inform, practice, and move toward peacebuilding (Bond, 2000; Lederach, 2005; Pruitt, 2011a; Schirch, 2005).

Quality of life encompasses multidimensional factors and aspects of subjective elements such as life satisfaction. For purposes of this chapter, we look at quality of life using the World Health Organization Quality of Life (WHOQOL) Group's (1995) definition as "individuals' perception of their position in life in the context of the culture and value systems in which they live and in relation to their goals, expectations, standards and concerns" (p. 1403). This definition recognizes quality of life as "a broad ranging concept affected in a complex way by the person's physical health, psychological state, level of independence, social relationships, personal beliefs and their relationship to salient features of their environment" (WHO, 1997, p. 1). Reflective practice around understandings of quality of life must also include the creation of meaning and formation of standards, such as understanding what "living well" means to people, what people value, and people's resiliency (Camfield, 2011, p. 400). These concepts intertwine, creating overlap and interaction with building positive peace.

Dance and Peacebuilding

Arts-based approaches to peacebuilding encompass a variety of multifaceted and multidisciplinary modes of expression. The range of forms include oral, written, dance, music, theatre, film, photography and digital arts. Scholarship suggests that arts can foster openings for creativity, symbolic transformation, greater emotional understanding, and empathetic connections (Francis, 2010; Schirch, 2005; Sklar, 2001). Using multilayered communication for transformation, arts offer creative approaches needed for peacebuilding (Lederach, 2005). The arts are seen to hone in on certain aspects of a conflict while providing opportunities to *reframe* familiar situations, encourage fresh thinking, and cultivate new perspectives. Researchers (see Pruitt 2011b, 2013; Shank & Schirch, 2008) highlight the ability of the performing arts to promote dialogue and underscore essential components for peacebuilding. Zelizer (2003) argues that through non-linear and creative means of expression, the arts can facilitate increased understanding and contribute to building relationships between groups in conflict; we have seen this potential in dance and creative movement in our own work and seek to explore these prospects further in this chapter. While research and interest in dance and peacebuilding are growing, many areas remain to be explored.

Dance has long (perhaps always) been a means of human communication—a kinesthetic, or felt, way of connecting non-verbally across cultures (Royce, 1977). Dance, or movement in rituals, can be seen as symbolic communication and transformation in a social space (Schirch, 2005; Sklar, 2001) offering new ways to shift conflict (LeBaron, MacLeod, & Acland, 2013). Dance also holds potential as a force for social change more broadly (Jackson & Shapiro-Phim, 2008). As Hanna (1979) suggests, dance has the ability to express messages of power, dominance and equality, and can provide a route to change. Accordingly, dance can be a mode of resistance and a means of healing. The arts can afford embodied agency and open spaces outside of habitual realities (Bond, 2008; Fraleigh, 2004).

In the context of conflict resolution, LeBaron et al. (2013) advocate for conflict resolution training to incorporate movement practices with potential benefits for affected parties as well as practitioners. They assert that dance develops new, embodied ways of knowing and being, along with an increased awareness of internal responses to conflict. They suggest further that nonverbal, embodied communication is an effective way to foster inter-group trust in conflict and post-conflict settings. Eddy (2009) investigated connections between dance/movement and violence prevention in six K-12 settings across the United States, and the topic has been addressed through a doctoral study at the University of Aberdeen, Scotland (Acarón, 2015). While research on dance for peacebuilding continues to evolve, it is important to acknowledge valuable related research in dance therapy, conflict resolution, violence prevention and human rights, all of which contribute to the overarching goals of peacebuilding.

We link these peacebuilding goals to the material, relational and subjective dimensions of quality of life. The material includes physical aspects, such as food, bodies and shelter. Relational involves social interactions, power and identity, and the rules and practices of distribution. Cultural values, ideologies and beliefs, as well as people's own perceptions of their situation are likewise connected to subjective quality of life (Camfield, 2011). Cohen (2015) outlines how arts-based peacebuilding approaches are used to strengthen campaigns of nonviolent resistance, afford opportunities for positive creative connections across difference, support rehumanizing of former enemies, encourage reconciliation, draw global attention to human rights abuses, and to restore identity, meaning and hope in the face of challenges, all of which relate clearly to quality of life.

Limitations and Prospects

We do not suggest that dance inherently leads to peacebuilding. As noted in Karen Bond's Introduction to this volume, performing arts can be used in ways that encourage peace or violence, freedom or oppression, inclusion or exclusion (Ayindo, 2008; Shank & Schirch, 2008; Zelizer, 2003). It is thus important to acknowledge limitations of dance as a tool for building peace. Stock (2001) cautions that while universal as a multi-sensory expression, dance is not a "universal language." Operating on multiple social, conceptual and artistic levels within and across cultures, dance opens the potential for transformation, but is subject to interpretation and has been used for political and ideological gain (Bond & Stinson, 2000/2001; Shay, 2002). Researchers working in diverse contexts including Israel, Palestine, Zimbabwe, and the Philippines have argued that dance can be appropriated (Rowe, 2011), or instrumentalised to further nationalism (Bond, 2016; Kaschl, 2003; Chap. 9, this volume), or used for control and coercive manipulation (Gonye, 2013; Chap. 1, this volume), with dance being used in some contexts as both punishment and rehabilitation (Williams, 2013).

Dance is not always accessible to all people. In some situations, dancing is banned or deemed inappropriate based on gender or religion, or may occur in separated gender groups (Jackson & Shapiro-Phim, 2008; Chap. 24, this volume). Dance is inherently about the body, and in activating embodied knowledge can present risks of traumatization (Thompson, 2013). At the same time, with the constant pressure to legitimize the arts, some arts-based practitioners might be less inclined to analyze or acknowledge the possibility of negative effects (2013); for example, men and women dancing together might be unacceptable in some peacebuilding contexts (Shay, 2008). Examining potential limitations of dance in peacebuilding, however, could also strengthen existing theory and praxis regarding arts-based peacebuilding approaches.

Finally, even where dance apparently fosters peacebuilding, connections might not be immediately visible or clear; change facilitated through the arts can be difficult to measure with traditional scientific methods (Hunter & Page, 2014; Chaps. 15 and 28, this volume). This makes it difficult to quantify success, certainly in the short term. The complexity of peacebuilding and the arts presents a challenge of attribution; when there are many personal and subjective variables, it can be hard to document and discern the contributors to change, suggesting the value of a plural approach to methodologies. Ongoing consideration of the material, relational, and subjective dimensions of quality of life in relation to peacebuilding helps to address these limitations and support optimal practice.

A Typology of Dancing for Peace

We now turn to a brief scoping of the field of practice when it comes to using dance for peace. As a first step, we offer a preliminary typology of the varied ways dance is used for peacebuilding. We do not claim that these categories are exhaustive or that it would necessarily be possible to identify every way dance is used for peace. We believe, however, that developing a starting point such as this is important to help map the field towards understanding how different kinds of dance work in different modes of peacebuilding and for different contributors to the peace process.

We present this typology with the caveat that our analysis is based on the activity or program's stated intent, which might at times differ from underlying ideas or assumptions held by participants or facilitators. Moreover, while we propose it is possible to delineate to some extent between the stated intentions of different approaches, we acknowledge that there is likely to be crossover and that many artists and their practices defy categorization. This does not preclude trying to deepen understandings of how and why arts practices work or how a practitioner's stated intent or focus can influence outcomes. Rather than as rigid frameworks, however, these categories are perhaps best understood as fluid and in flux themselves, with many practitioners simultaneously straddling several different approaches.

Finally, some initiatives might use similar practices with different underlying assumptions, or alternatively, similar underlying assumptions with widely varying practices. For now, we merely note this salient point, but future research could fruitfully explore such comparisons in analyzing and evaluating programs. Conceptual typologies are useful to this end, as they can aid in comparison and help highlight theoretical dimensions of a type; indeed, as Bailey (1994) argues, "a sound typology forms a solid foundation for both theorizing and empirical research" (p. 33).

Cohen (2015) and Zelizer (2013) developed categories of general arts-based peacebuilding, which Acarón (2015) extends to include dance/movement practices and the fluidity of boundaries between fields. We advance the discussion further to explore dance and peacebuilding in relation to the material, relational and subjective dimensions of quality of life, proposing a typology of six categories: (1) therapeutic, (2) artist led social change or protest, (3) community led social change or protest, (4) collective forms, (5) educational, and (6) diplomatic. As depicted in Fig. 27.1, we visualize these categories as overlapping circles. The goal is not to delineate static groupings, but to promote discussion, research, and development of the field. Fig. 27.1 also outlines notable programs, works, and practitioners in peacebuilding. The remainder of this section presents brief descriptions of each category.

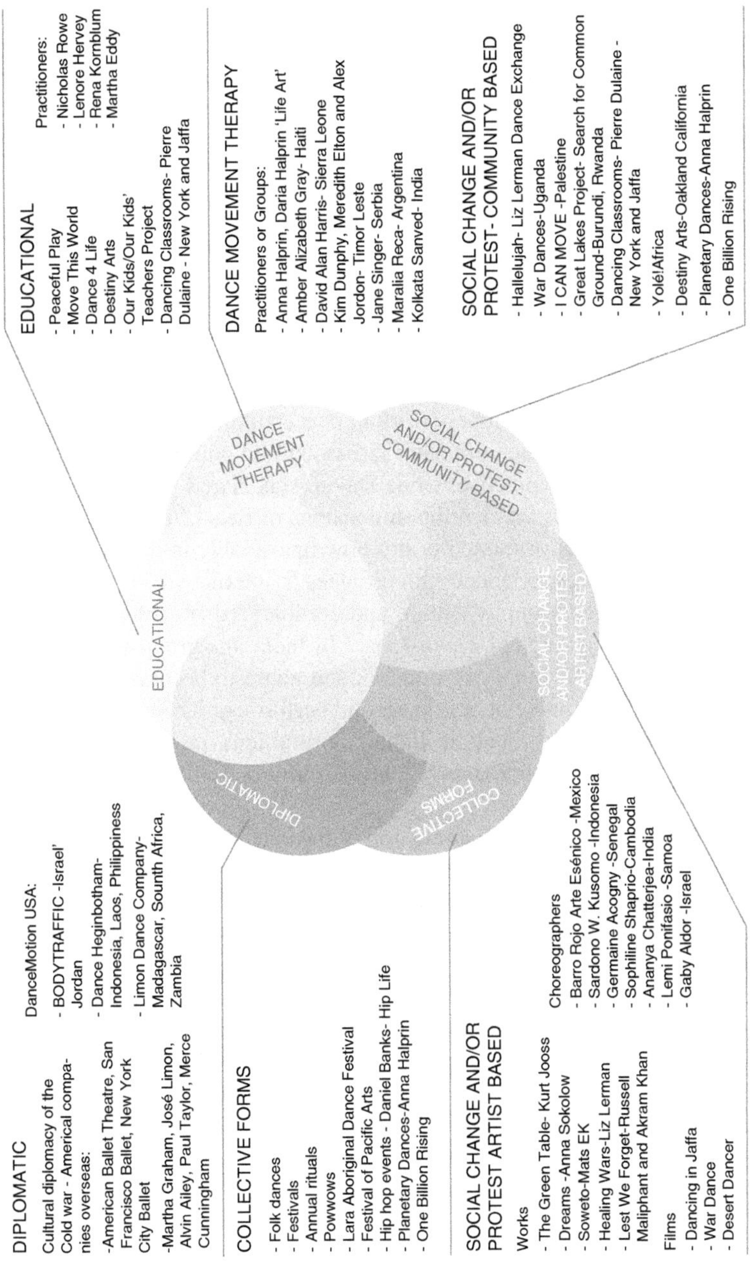

Fig. 27.1 Typology of Dancing for Peace

Therapeutic

Dance Movement Therapy (DMT) is defined by the American Dance Therapy Association as "the psychotherapeutic use of movement as a process which furthers the emotional, cognitive, physical, and social integration of the individual" (www.adta.org). In definitions and practice the field was conceptualized initially through a Western lens. Pioneers include Marian Chace, Katherine Dunham, Blanche Evan, Anna Halprin, and Mary Starks Whitehouse among others, with a growing body of practitioners today working in conflict, post-conflict and international development contexts (Reca, 2017; Singer, 2008). While there is some overlap between dance therapy and dance for peacebuilding, and a DMT practitioner can of course use dance in non-therapeutic contexts, classical DMT is grounded in the therapeutic relationship between practitioner and client (www.adta.org). As Acarón (2015) outlines, the contributions of somatic practitioners who might or might not define their work as dance are also important as embodied approaches.

Several notable DMT practitioners work in peacebuilding globally. Amber Gray (2008) focuses on post-conflict and natural disaster and considers Indigenous and Western frameworks in her practice, while David Alan Harris (2008) discusses the importance of the process of recreating dimensions of rites of passage that former male combatants might have missed or are now unavailable in their communities. Singer (2008) describes experiences with refugees or internally displaced people in post-conflict Serbia; and Dunphy, Elton, and Jordon (2014) explore using group DMT in post-conflict settings in Timor-Leste. In India, the group Kolkata Sanved prepare survivors of trafficking, exploitation, and abuse to become peer educators and advocates as well as movement trainers and performers. Their work is based on concepts of DMT applied through an Indian cultural lens, including Indian dance movements and their own approach of *sampoornata* or fulfillment (Chakraborty, 2010).

Within DMT literature there is discussion of the ebb and flow of personal versus group and the interrelation of concepts perceived as Western within international contexts. Some reflections consider how to reframe understandings of therapy in a community sense—to be more about building relationship, working in groups, and "finding possibilities for living" (Singer, 2008, p. 103), or for community forgiveness (Harris, 2008). Kolkata Sanved stands out as being developed by local practitioners to activate in their own communities and language. In addressing healing from an embodied perspective, DMT taps into the vast resources of often local cultural traditions and practices that hold the potential to offer a broader range of quality of life. Yet, like all peace and development work, there is a challenge to balance the potential value of outsider ideas with communities' needs for developing their own pathways and approaches.

Artist Led Social Change or Protest

This category of artists and projects is performance based, emphasizing refined, virtuoso artistic expression, inviting transformation from audiences who witness performances (Cohen, 2015). There are numerous examples of how dance has been used as a form of protest or advocacy by highly trained artists and groups. In such works, audiences act as witnesses and potential change agents. Jackson and Shapiro-Phim (2008) collate the work of multiple choreographers from a human rights perspective—such as Germaine Acogny, Liz Lerman and Lemi Ponifasio, while Morris and Giersdorf (2016) explore choreography in response to twenty-first century wars.

A broad treatment of the temporal, geographic and aesthetic diversity held in this category is beyond the scope of our chapter, but we include a few examples. Forsythe's (2005) *Human Writes* is a performative installation with dancers creating an embodied commentary on the human rights agenda. In *Archive,* Tel-Aviv based choreographer Zaides (2014) combines footage from the B'Tselem Video Archive of the Israeli Center for Human Rights in the Occupied Territories with physical manipulations and gestures to embody the images and change them in an attempt to alter the audience's perceptions. The *Table of Silence Project 9/11*, a collaboration between Buglisi and Vasta (2011), offers a multi-cultural performance for peace. These artist-led works focus on the power of aesthetic resonance to carry the meaning and exploration of ideas to those who witness the performances, rather than consciously engaging in a directed transformational process with communities.

Community Led Social Change or Protest

These are inclusive works, focused on a transformational process for those engaging in creating and performing the art (Cohen, 2015). Programs seek to connect people across difference, to cross borders—physical, political or representational, or to provide opportunities to marginalized communities. For example, in Pruitt's (2013) work on youth peacebuilding in Australia, the ways young people from different cultural backgrounds danced to communicate across difference, dispel stereotypes, and make space for peace in their local communities was documented and analyzed. Related documentation and analysis can be found in Mary Ann Hunter's (2011) contributions in *Acting Together: Performance and the Creative Transformation of Conflict*.

Nadia Arouri, founder of Youth, Art, & Levante and the I CAN MOVE community dance project in Ramallah in the West Bank, concentrates on the resilience of people and their opportunities for quality of life within her own community rather than engaging in cross cultural exchanges, which often leave Palestinian artists seeing no change in their situation. Yolé!Africa provides creative opportunities, dance classes, performances, and chances for integration for marginalized youth and former child soldiers in the Democratic Republic of Congo. Nicholas Rowe has worked in Israel and Palestine engaging in artistic, community, educational and research approaches. His work with young people in the Occupied Territories through the Our Kids program focused on sustaining existing community within a locality of ongoing trauma (Rowe, 2015). Overall, social change can happen within a community or across boundaries. Challenges to consider include defining expectations, creating sustainable programs, and avoiding reinforcement of inequalities of power or agency.

Collective Forms

Collective forms are generally participatory, with a focus on community affirmation or transformation (Cohen, 2015). In our typology, this category includes folk dance, social dance, rituals, communal dance forms, and other ways that groups dance to enact change. This can be about building a collective in peacebuilding, engaging groups often seen as at odds, or developing a sense of group consciousness. For example, Walker (2012) describes the process of ritual and ceremony as a means to connect Indigenous and Settler peoples, including powwows for Methow Indians and Settler descendants in the United States, and annual rituals between Australian Indigenous communities and descendants of Settlers. Alternatively, in Gezi Park in Turkey dancers in gas masks danced tango in the square in a response to violence. Through social media, this non-violent response inspired dance demonstrations around the world (Acarón, 2015).

Collective forms can also occur on a larger scale, at times even with global reach. For example, One Billion Rising, initiated in 2012 by Eve Ensler, aims at ending rape and violence against women and girls. It is implemented through multiple channels, including community performances and social media with new choreography being learned worldwide. This is a popular and growing global call to action with people around the world performing unison movements with their bodies (Gerdes & Sorge, 2015). At the same time, One Billion Rising blurs the boundaries of our typology, as it can be viewed as both a collective form—it is participatory and focuses on transformation of communities through ritual creation—and as artist or community led social change or protest (Acarón, 2015; Aston, 2016).

Educational

Educational approaches strategically use dance in ways that also provide or support other forms of learning; for example, dance can be a resource for teaching non-violence, conflict resolution, and social and emotional intelligence. Many educational approaches exist within school settings, but peace and development practitioners recognize the value for dance outside of school settings, such as Dance

4 Life's work against HIV/AIDS in Africa and Asia. Whether for self-exploration or as a means to grasp difficult concepts, dance is being turned to as a physical and creative medium.

Educational programs can be local, national, international or a combination of these. For example, Move This World (formerly Dance 4 Peace) was launched in Colombia in 2007 with a dance-focused program aimed at building social and emotional intelligence for school children. Operating as an international NGO, in 2013 it rebranded to include empathy education and other creatives arts. The majority of its work is in the United States, with hubs in Colombia and the Philippines, featuring programs that have evolved within their own cultural contexts. In a keynote address for Dance and the Child International (daCi), Bond (2000) noted that the children of Colombia have a history of peace advocacy, beginning with the Children's Peace Movement in the 1990s. Assisted by UNICEF, in 1996 2.7 million children voted for the Children's Mandate, a set of twelve human rights including the right to peace, also creating peace zones in schools and parks.

In the United States, Eddy (2009) created the Peaceful Play schools program, as well as completing a comprehensive study of diverse movement strategies within K-12 violence prevention education in the United States. As introduced earlier, she investigated six dance-based programs, finding that different aspects of dance address different non-violence educational goals, while also identifying consistent teaching elements. Similarly, Hervey and Kornblum (2006) created and evaluated a dance-based violence education program and found increases in self-regulation, communication, positive risk taking and greater interpersonal spatial awareness. In crossover with a therapeutic approach, other dance/movement therapists have created peace practices curricula for schools (Beardall et al., 2007). These blended approaches illustrate the porosity of boundaries between therapeutic and educational approaches.

Diplomatic

Cultural diplomacy is broadly applied within peacebuilding, and dance is incorporated in diplomacy in formal and informal ways that connect to ideas of quality of life. For example, throughout the world, folk dance, or national dances, have exported ideas of cultural identity and connected regions and countries. State-run dance companies across the globe have masked brutalities and shady politics with colorful costumes, exciting dances, and music in efforts to control local and international opinion. Often such companies claim to be ambassadors of peace and friendship, bringing joy into a world affected by conflict (Shay, 2002). Many peace programs and events hold a cultural night or showcase of local dances and music performed by professionals or program participants. While this is often included as a means of social connection and to show respect, there are challenges around how dance forms have been appropriated, repurposed, or misinterpreted (Foreman, 2013).

Moreover, during the Cold War, performances and arts tours were one of the few channels of communication that remained open between the United States and the Soviet Union. Through the 1970s many major American companies, such as American Ballet Theatre and Alvin Ailey American Dance Theater, were sent overseas (Croft, 2015; Prevots, 1998). In such instances dance serves a diplomatic purpose through embodiment of national identity; in both the dancing and the "everyday body," dancers as artists and nonpolitical entities (overtly speaking) can create commonalities across cultural difference (2015). After 9/11, the United States revived the dance tours through a dance exchange program, which evolved into DanceMotion USA in 2010 (Croft, 2013).

Differing from Cold War performance tours, there is now more community engagement through teaching, community workshops, and social media directed toward relational experiences within a global network (Croft, 2015). Overall, when considering diplomacy, a constant critical reflective attitude is required, one that recognizes the challenges of placing firm boundaries or overstating connections between positive peace and diplomacy. As proposed earlier, though, this critical perspective need not obscure possibilities for positive, peaceful change that might be enabled through this channel.

Spotlight on Practice

Having scoped the literature and started to map the practice field of dance for peacebuilding, we recognize this is only a starting point for discussion. As part of mapping the field further it is also important to understand how peacebuilders themselves experience dance interventions. Connected to quality of life, understanding what peacebuilders value—their own resiliency and perceptions of living well—is an important component of studying relationships between dance and peace. We now aim to deepen the discussion through a case study involving international peacebuilding practitioners. Using an example from Erica Rose Jeffrey's research in the southern Philippines, we consider the stories and experiences of peacebuilders and their interaction with creative dance workshops. This section reflects on how peacebuilders can incorporate dance not only in their work with fractured communities internationally but also potentially for and amongst themselves.

Methodology

This research was based in Mindanao, the southern island of the Philippines. Made up of over 7100 islands, the Philippines is home to over 95 million people. Mindanao holds a wide variety of people, languages, and religious groups—often divided into Lumads, the Moro group (Muslims), and Christians (settlers or migrants) (Montiel, Rodil, & Guzman, 2012). The long-standing conflicts in Mindanao, which can be traced to Spanish colonization in the sixteenth century ACE, are fueled by different perceptions, goals and histories influenced by both Spanish and American colonialism (Hernandez, 2017).

Here we discuss a qualitative research project investigating participants' experiences of creative dance classes in conjunction with peacebuilding training delivered through Peace in Mindanao (PM) (a pseudonym), while also considering how dance occurs in participants' communities more broadly. PM is a non-governmental organization providing peacebuilding trainings for the Philippines while serving as a resource within the broader Asia-Pacific Region. Established through the collective effort of the community to bring together peacebuilders of diverse cultures from the Asia-Pacific Region, PM draws on experiences of building peace in the Philippines itself. Here we report on data gathered in 2015 around a series of creative dance workshops offered in addition to the existing PM peacebuilding training curriculum. Standard PM program offerings include courses on conflict resolution, mediation, trauma, community-based approaches to peacebuilding, and nonviolent action.

For the creative dance workshops, data were collected through semi-structured interviews, reflective practice, and photo and video documentation. The Human Research Ethics Committee of the Queensland University of Technology approved the study and all participants provided informed consent. Five creative dance and movement workshops lasting 90–120 min each were offered to the participants of the PM training program in addition to their standard courses. Cultural evenings were held as part of the standard PM program, as well as presentations/performances to share learning. From participant feedback, the standard program was similar to other peacebuilding programs.

Dance workshop participants were diverse in age and cultural background. At the time of the study in 2015, participants were from over 20 countries. Twenty individuals from the dance workshops volunteered to participate in semi-structured interviews, which were conducted in English and focused on their experiences in the workshops as well as the role of dance in their home contexts. Interview participants ranged in age from 20 to early 60s and included 15 women and five men. Half of the interview participants were from the Philippines, with others coming from Myanmar, India, Cameroon, Liberia, Democratic Republic of Congo, Timor Leste, Indonesia, and Kenya. Participants disclosed a range of religions including Buddhist, Christian, Hindu and Muslim. All of them work as peacebuilders in a variety of aspects including human rights education and advocacy, reintegration of child soldiers, peace education, gender equity, working with non-state armed actors, and religious and government peace programs. Most interview participants did not have experience working with dance or the arts in peacebuilding prior to the dance workshops.

Jeffrey, PM facilitators, and members of the organizational team designed the workshops collaboratively with a focus on needs connected to the overall training. Presented as a creative dance and movement workshop for building peace, a variety of creative dance activities and exercises were offered. Activities included breathing and full body warm-ups to highlight body awareness; movement exploration using the elements of dance such as body, action, space, time, energy (see Reedy, 2015);

creative expression and movement improvisation; connecting with partners; and personal reflection through dialogue and drawing. Thematic content included dance concepts such as exploring pathways, as well as ideas drawn from peacebuilding such as movement explorations of power or reconciliation. Throughout the workshops, Jeffrey observed a high level of individual and group engagement, including a quality of enthusiastic and playful participation with willingness to try new experiences. Key themes identified in interviews and visual documentation were personal change, connection to others, opportunities for creativity, and prospects for peacebuilding.

Reflecting on the typology presented in Fig. 27.1, the PM creative dance and movement workshops fall under educational approaches in both aim and design. However, this case illustrates that outcomes can fall into different categories to the stated intentions. While designed and facilitated as a creative dance and movement experience, many participants described personal therapeutic benefits as well as a sense of building positive community. One of the most prominent themes to emerge from participant statements was positive personal change, which we link directly to improved sense of experienced quality of life. Participants described feeling both relaxed and energized, connecting with their own bodies, and valuing being able to do something for oneself while learning. In addition, they repeatedly used words such as "free," "light," and "flexible." Many noted that creative dance provided stress relief in a safe environment. Some individuals who "love to dance" expressed appreciation for the opportunity as they had previously felt too ungraceful to be a "dancer" or to even explore dance. One Muslim Filipina described her experience through a drawing of bamboo she created as part of the workshop.

> The class is like water. Bamboo is resilient—it is flexible, but then again it is stiff in a way and then after that…it's still a bamboo but the leaf of the bamboo is floating in the water… going with the movements being flexible, enjoying being.

Connection to others was another valued experience reported by participants. For many, the dance workshops afforded an opportunity to get to know individuals from other cultures and backgrounds for the first time. Even though they were all living in the same residence area, there were informal barriers to connecting, for example, English language proficiency and speaking styles (dialect). One male participant described working with a male from another country, noting how there were challenges in verbal communication, yet they found a way of understanding each other through movements of leading and following.

> There were times when he took the lead and times when I took the lead…I would just notice what he was doing and follow in the same moves and then he is leading…and when he notices that the movements are slightly changing, he knows that I want to take over and he just follows what I am doing. I think it was beautiful. There was that understanding, even when we stopped communicating with our words.

Similarly, some expressed that by focusing on themselves with a more embodied sense, they were able to connect better with others and to see different perspectives, something that they valued for their work as peacebuilders:

> I really appreciate the dance…that it…got me, personally, into myself…some of the moves were very simple, but they reached deep. … It built a certain type of confidence in me, and the ability…to rely on the leadership of another person, my partner, so…if I could rely on their leadership, then obviously, I was able to see from their perspective.

For several participants, connections from the dance workshops continued through the other trainings—they consciously and confidently called on dance elements as energizers throughout their other classes.

When asked about their experience, participants repeatedly mentioned feeling positive about having an opportunity for creative expression while also witnessing others' creativity. One example was creating and sharing short dance phrases based on individuals' names and how this revealed people's personalities as well as showing the range of possibilities for expression. The program director also reported a strong positive reaction to seeing creativity in motion; in response to a closing movement activity that involved passing an imaginary gift around the circle of participants, she reflected,

> I was just in awe of the creativity that emerged from the first time you passed your gift to the person next to you and then as the gift went around the circle, that was a very beautiful experience.

For some, the opportunity to move in the space gave a sense of expansiveness. As one male from Cameroon stated,

> At first, when we were standing in the circle, even though we had a big space inside…I felt limited from the size, but when we started moving, it felt free… like…the space grew bigger with every move.

These comments suggest that participants had an opportunity to express a deeper sense of self-understanding and embodiment, beyond instrumental outcomes. This seems significant, as peacebuilders themselves might benefit from enhancements to experienced quality of life, potentially strengthening them as facilitators; at the same time, dance can be a vehicle for peacebuilding more broadly.

Many participants drew connections between the dance workshops and other peacebuilding work or training. For some it was about the necessity of developing positive relationships with colleagues as well as tools to work with other groups. As one Filipina said, "I think it created some kind of invincible, invisible tie among those who attended… There [was] sort of a bonding, a relationship bonding." Building positive relationships, an important indicator of quality of life (Nussbaum, 2011), was echoed as a peacebuilding theme among many participants.

Alongside the experienced benefits of dance practice in peacebuilding, participants described challenges and limitations. Some reported discomfort participating in the "cultural exchange" performances that are often part of peacebuilding programs. For example, a woman from India discussed that while she appreciates dance, she is uncomfortable performing as a dancer in these exchanges. Yet, she enjoyed taking part in the creative dance workshops, which helped her feel more confident joining in cultural sharing events.

Dance performance discomfort might also relate to an unexpected theme that arose from participant feedback—that of body image. Both males and females repeatedly mentioned enjoying the "permission" to dance, as their previous experiences had been limited to watching dance and that they did not think they were good enough or had the right body type to dance. While participating in a mixed gender dance workshop was reportedly unproblematic, many mentioned the need at times for gender-segregated activities to address cultural or religious sensitivities.

Within the wider context of peacebuilding education and training, individual peacebuilders are inadvertently being called on to be performers and creators while training. Participant interviews confirmed that some feel uncomfortable or pressured into performing, such as dancing or singing, in contexts aimed at peacebuilding. Where such actions are compelled, directly or implicitly, they might erode the trust and freedom of participants rather than grow it. This is important to consider in the arts and peacebuilding. Still, overall, the dance element contributed to peacebuilding, as participants valued being able to practice in a safe space and enjoyed the opportunity for new experiences and chances to stretch their creativity in ways that afforded learning and relationships.

Conclusion

The personal, relational, and educational benefits that participants described from involvement in dance workshops show the possible intersections between processes of building positive peace and quality of life. Many peacebuilders in this study described shifts in their perception of their position in life, including physical health, mental health, social relationships, and the creation of meaning. By applying the lens of quality of life in relation to dance and peacebuilding, we see intersections in the categories described. For example, while the workshop approach was educational, experiences of participants throughout the training touched on social change: artist led, community led, and collective forms.

Whether for stress relief, creative expression, confidence building, connecting with peers, or a different perspective, dance can be and is practiced to support quality of life, in tandem with seeking and promoting positive peace. This is intentional in some cases, whereas in others it can be a side effect with both benefits and limitations. While we have started some important aspects of exploration here, additional research is needed. For example, we see a need to consider the politics, or power dynamics, involved in different approaches and how they might both enable and hinder alternative approaches.

In creating an initial typology, we hope this will be a jumping off place for further discussion and development of the field. Framing the discussion from a quality of life perspective provides deeper connections to parallel concepts in peacebuilding. In making dance and peacebuilding approaches more visible, including challenges and limitations, we see an opportunity to enrich peacebuilding approaches from an arts perspective, specifically, to study and question why and how dance practice can partner with peacebuilding.

References

Acarón, T. R. (2015). *The practitioner's body of knowledge: Dance/movement in training programmes that address violence, conflict and peace.* Doctoral dissertation, University of Aberdeen, Scotland.

Aston, E. (2016). Agitating for change: Theatre and a feminist "network of resistance". *Theatre Research International, 41*(1), 5–20.

Ayindo, B. (2008). Arts approaches to peace: Playing our way to transcendence? In B. Hart (Ed.), *Peacebuilding in traumatized societies* (pp. 185–204). Lanham, MD: University Press of America.

Bailey, K. D. (1994). *Typologies and taxonomies: An introduction to classification techniques.* Thousand Oaks, CA: Sage.

Beardall, N. G., Bergman, S. J., & Surrey, J. L. (2007). *Making connections: Building community and gender dialogue in secondary schools.* Cambridge, MA: Educators for Social Responsibility.

Blumenfeld-Jones, D. (2004). Bodily-kinesthetic intelligence and the democratic ideal. In J. L. Kincheloe (Ed.), *Multiple intelligences revisited* (pp. 119–131). New York: Peter Lang.

Bond, K. (2014). Dance and quality of life. In A. C. Michalos (Ed.), *Encyclopedia of quality of life and Well-being research* (pp. 1419–1424). Dordrecht, Eastern Cape: Springer.

Bond, K. E. (2000). Revisioning purpose: Children, dance and the culture of caring. In J. E. LeDrew & H. Ritenberg (Eds.), *Proceedings of the 8th dance and the child international conference – Extensions & extremities: Points of departure* (pp. 3–14). Regina, SK: University of Regina.

Bond, K. E. (2008). The human nature of dance: Towards a theory of aesthetic community. In S. Malloch & C. Trevarthan (Eds.), *Communicative musicality: Exploring the basis of human companionship.* Oxford: Oxford University Press.

Bond, K. E., & Dilodovico, A. (2016, November). *Romuold Iodko's (1939) Detskiy Khorovod (children's round dance): Migrations and in/appropriations.* Paper presented at the Joint Conference of the Congress on Research in Dance and the Society of Dance History Scholars, Pomona College, CA.

Bond, K. E., & Stinson, S. W. (2000/2001). 'It feels like I'm going to take off!' Young people's experiences of the superordinary in dance. *Dance Research Journal, 32*(2), 52–87.

Buglisi, J. & Vasta, R. (chor.). (2011). The table of silence project, dance performance., 11 Sep 2011. Lincoln Center, New York. Retrieved from https://www.tableofsilence.org/table-of-silence

Camfield, L. (2011). Quality of life in developing countries. In K. C. Land, A. C. Michalos, & J. Sirgy (Eds.), *Handbook of social indicators and quality of life research* (pp. 399–432). Dordrecht, Eastern Cape: Springer.

Chakraborty, S. (2010). *Dance matters: Performing India.* Abingdon, OX: Routledge.

Coe, D., & Strachan, J. M. (2002). Writing dance: Tensions in researching movement or aesthetic experiences. *International Journal of Qualitative Studies in Education, 15*(5), 497–511.

Cohen, C. (2015, Summer). Arts and building peace: Affirming the basics and envisioning the future. *Insight*, 5–7, 11. Retrieved from https://www.usip.org/sites/default/files/Insights_Summer-2015-Arts-Peacebuilding.pdf

Cohen, C., Gutiérrez Varea, R., & Walker, P. (Eds.). (2011). *Acting together: Performance and the creative transformation of conflict, vols. 1 and 2.* Oakland, CA: New Village.

Croft, C. (2013). Dance returns to American cultural diplomacy: The U. S. State Department's 2003 dance residency program and its after effects. *Dance Research Journal, 45*(1), 23–39.

Croft, C. (2015). *Dancers as diplomats: American choreography in cultural exchange.* New York: Oxford University Press.

Dissanayake, E. (1988). *What is art for?* Seattle: University of Washington Press.

Dunphy, K., Elton, M., & Jordan, A. (2014). Exploring dance/movement therapy in post-conflict Timor-Leste. *American Journal of Dance Therapy, 36*(2), 189–208.

Eddy, M. (2009). The role of dance in violence prevention programs for youth. In L. Overby & B. Lepczyk (Eds.), *Dance: Current selected research* (Vol. 7, pp. 93–143). New York: AMS.

Forcey, L. R., & Murray, H. I. (1999). *Peacebuilding for adolescents: Strategies for educators and community leaders*. New York: Peter Lang.

Foreman, K. (2013). Dancing on the endangered list: Aesthetics and politics of indigenous dance in the Philippines. In A. Dils & A. Albright (Eds.), *Moving history/dancing cultures: A dance history reader* (pp. 384–389). Middletown, CT: Wesleyan University Press.

Forsythe, W. (chor.). (2005). *Human writes, performance installation*, 23 Oct 2005. Schauspielhaus Zürich, Schiffbauhalle 1, Zurich. Retrieved from https://www.williamforsythe.com/installations.html?&no_cache=1&detail=1&uid=16

Fraleigh, S. (2004). *Dancing identity: Metaphysics in motion*. Pittsburgh, PA: University of Pittsburgh Press.

Francis, D. (2010). *From pacification to peacebuilding: A call to global transformation*. London: Pluto.

Gerdes, E. V. P., & Sorge, T. (2015). Building humans and dances: Exploring cultural relevancy as teaching artists. *Journal of Dance Education, 15*(2), 72–76.

Gonye, J. (2013). Mobilizing dance/traumatizing dance: Kongonya and the politics of Zimbabwe. *Dance Research Journal, 45*(1), 64–79.

Gray, A. E. (2008). Dancing in our blood: Dance/movement therapy with street children and victims of organized violence in Haiti. In N. M. Jackson & T. Shapiro-Phim (Eds.), *Dance, human rights, and social justice: Dignity in motion* (pp. 222–236). Lanham, MD: Scarecrow.

Hanna, J. L. (1979). *To dance is human*. Chicago: The University of Chicago Press.

Harris, D. A. (2008). Sudanese youth: Dance as mobilization in the aftermath of war. In N. M. Jackson & T. Shapiro-Phim (Eds.), *Dance, human rights, and social justice: Dignity in motion* (pp. 253–256). Lanham, MD: Scarcrow.

Hernandez, M. B. (2017). *The Philippines' Moro conflict: The problems and prospects in the quest for a sustainable peace* (Master's thesis). Georgetown University, Washington, DC.

Hervey, L., & Kornblum, R. (2006). An evaluation of Kornblum's body-based violence prevention curriculum for children. *The Arts in Psychotherapy, 33*(2), 113–129.

Hunter, M. A. (2011). Change the world as we know it: Peace, youth and performance in Australia. In C. Cohen, R. Gutiérrez Varea, & P. O. Walker (Eds.), *Acting together II: Performance and the creative transformation of conflict* (pp. 73–91). New York: New Village.

Hunter, M. A., & Page, L. (2014). What is "the good" of arts-based peacebuilding? Questions of value and evaluation in current practice. *Peace and Conflict Studies, 21*(2), 115–134.

Jackson, N. M., & Shapiro-Phim, T. (Eds.). (2008). *Dance, human rights and social justice: Dignity in motion*. Lanham, MD: Scarecrow.

Jeong, H. W. (2000). *Peace and conflict studies: An introduction*. Aldershot, UK: Ashgate.

Kaschl, E. (2003). *Dance and authenticity in Israel and Palestine*. Leiden: Brill.

LeBaron, M., MacLeod, C., & Acland, A. F. (2013). *The choreography of resolution: Conflict, movement, and neuroscience*. Chicago: American Bar Association.

Lederach, J. P. (2005). *The moral imagination: The art and soul of building peace*. Oxford: Oxford University Press.

Montiel, C. J., Rodil, R. B., & Guzman, J. M. (2012). The Moro struggle and the challenge to peace building in Mindanao, Southern Philippines. In D. Landis & R. Albert (Eds.), *Handbook of ethnic conflict* (pp. 71–89). Boston: Springer.

Morris, G., & Giersdorf, J. R. (Eds.). (2016). *Choreographies of 21st century wars*. New York: Oxford University Press.

Nussbaum, M. (2011). *Creating capabilities: The human development approach*. Cambridge, MA: Belknap.

Prevots, N. (1998). *Dance for export: Cultural diplomacy and the Cold War*. Middletown, CT: Wesleyan University Press.

Pruitt, L. J. (2011a). Music, youth, and peacebuilding in Northern Ireland. *Global Change, Peace & Security, 23*(2), 207–222.

Pruitt, L. J. (2011b). Creating a musical dialogue for peace. *International Journal of Peace Studies, 16*(2), 81–103.

Pruitt, L. J. (2013). *Youth peacebuilding: Music, gender and change*. New York: SUNY Press.
Reca, M. (2017). Reconstructing the world of survivors of torture for political reasons through dance/movement therapy. In V. Karkou, S. Oliver, & S. Lycouris (Eds.), *The Oxford handbook of dance and wellbeing* (pp. 647–660). Oxford: Oxford University Press.
Reedy, P. (2015). *Body, mind & spirit in action*. Berkeley, CA: Luna Dance Institute.
Rowe, N. (2011). Dance and political credibility: The appropriation of Dabkeh by Zionsim, Pan-Arabism, and Palestinian nationalism. *The Middle East Journal, 65*(3), 363–380.
Rowe, N. (2015). Dancing beyond the post-trauma paradigm: Community projects in the Occupied Palestinian territories. In C. S. Nielsen & S. Burridge (Eds.), *Dance education around the world: Perspectives on dance, young people and change*. New York: Routledge.
Royce, A. P. (1977). *The anthropology of dance*. Alton, UK: Dance Books.
Schirch, L. (2005). *Ritual and symbol in peacebuilding*. Bloomfield, IN: Kumarian Press.
Shank, M., & Schirch, L. (2008). Strategic arts-based peacebuilding. *Peace & Change, 33*(2), 217–242.
Shay, A. (2002). *Choreographic politics: State folk dance companies: Representation and power*. Middletown, CT: Wesleyan University Press.
Shay, A. (2008). Dance and human rights in the Middle East, North Africa, and Central Asia. In N. M. Jackson & T. Shapiro-Phim (Eds.), *Dance, human rights and social justice: Dignity in motion*. Lanham, MD: Scarecrow.
Singer, A. J. (2008). Hidden treasures, hidden voices: An ethonographic study into the use of movement and creativity in psychosocial work with war-affected refugee children in Serbia. In H. Payne (Ed.), *Dance movement therapy: Theory, research and practice*. New York: Routledge.
Sklar, D. (2001). Toward cross-cultural conversation on bodily knowledge. *Dance Research Journal, 33*(1), 91–92.
Stock, C. (2001). *Myth of a universal dance language: Tensions between globalisation and cultural difference*. Paper presented at the World Dance Alliance Asia Pacific Dance Bridge, Singapore, June 6–10.
Thompson, J. (2013). Questions on performances: In place of war. *Applied Theatre Research, 1*(2), 149–156.
Walker, P. O. (2012). *Ceremonies of dance and song in native American peacemaking*. Retrieved from https://www.brandeis.edu/ethics/peacebuildingarts/images/news_from_the_field/2012_11_Polly_Walker_NativeAmericanRenewalCeremonies.pdf
WHOQOL Group (World Health Organization Quality of Life Group). (1995). The World Health Organization quality of life assessment (WHOQOL): Position paper from the World Health Organization. *Social Science & Medicine, 41*(10), 1403–1409.
Williams, F. C. (2013). The embodiment of social dynamics: A phenomenon of Western pop dance within a Filipino prison. *Research in Dance Education, 14*(1), 39–56.
World Health Organization. (1997). *WHOQOL – Measuring quality of life*. Geneva, Switzerland: World Health Organization. Retrieved from http://www.who.int/iris/handle/10665/63482
Zaides, A. (2014). *Archive, dance performance*. France: Festival d'Avignon Retrieved from http://arkadizaides.com/archive.
Zelizer, C. (2003). The role of artistic processes in peacebuilding in Bosnia-Herezegovina. *Peace and Conflict Studies, 10*(2), 62–75.
Zelizer, C. (Ed.). (2013). *Integrated peacebuilding: Innovative approaches to transforming conflict*. Boulder, CO: Westview.

Chapter 28
Dance and Quality of Life for Indigenous Communities in Australia

Kim Dunphy and Vicki-Ann Ware

Introduction

This chapter focuses on dance for Indigenous people in Australia, exploring dance's relationship to Indigenous quality of life. We begin with a broad overview of diverse understandings of quality of life and associated phenomena such as health and wellbeing, and then hone in on the topic in relation to Indigenous people. We then explore the role of dance in Indigenous cultures past and present, complementing analysis of selected literature with two examples of dance practices contributing to quality of life for Indigenous Australians. In this article, we use the terms Indigenous, Aboriginal and Torres Strait Islander, and First Nations people interchangeably to refer to the Aboriginal and Torres Strait Islander peoples of Australia.

We preface the chapter by acknowledging that we, as Anglo-Australians, are sharing information about a culture that is not our own. Our writing is informed by backgrounds in cultural and community development in Australia and internationally, however, and we both have experience researching with Indigenous peoples in Australia and elsewhere, along with other cultures in South East Asia. We also bring a lifetime of enjoyment of art forms of dance (Dunphy) and music (Ware) that inspire us to continue learning about other cultures, particularly that of the first peoples of our own country. We would have preferred to develop this chapter with an Indigenous co-author, but in spite of a concerted effort, were not successful in locating a collaborator during our time frame. Nevertheless, we have been reflexive in the selection of dance examples and literature that foreground Indigenous perspectives and concerns.

K. Dunphy (✉)
University of Melbourne, Melbourne, Australia
e-mail: k.dunphy@unimelb.edu.au

V.-A. Ware
Deakin University, Geelong, Australia
e-mail: v.ware@deakin.edu.au

K. Bond (ed.), *Dance and the Quality of Life*, Social Indicators Research Series 73,
https://doi.org/10.1007/978-3-319-95699-2_28

Accordingly, we also wish to disclose our shared position that in spite of various and continuing efforts at decolonization over the last 50 years, there is a long way to go in achieving quality of life for Indigenous Australians (to be discussed further). Trust and satisfaction with government has been examined widely as a quality of life indicator, including in the first volume of *Social Indicators Research* (Møller, 1997). Historically recent events such as the 2007 "Northern Territory Emergency Response" (NTER), known as "the Intervention," a military exercise that entailed the suspension of the *Racial Discrimination Act 1975* and sudden passing of a *Northern Territory National Emergency Response Act* (NTNERA), for example, have seriously eroded Indigenous satisfaction with or trust in government (Scott & Heiss 2016).

In addition, despite notable Australian landmarks towards decolonisation which include: a 1967 referendum granting the Commonwealth authority to make special laws for its Indigenous population (for example, Native Title laws) and to include Indigenous citizens in population census statistics that determine government financial responsibilities; the *Racial Discrimination Act 1975*; and the 1992 Mabo decision, which for the first time recognized the legal doctrine of native title (Australian Institute of Aboriginal and Torres Strait Islander Studies [AIATSIS], 2015), the fact that Australia was already inhabited prior to the arrival of the British in 1788 is still not recognized in the Constitution of Australia.

Approach

This desk-based study was developed from a broad literature review about how dance can contribute to quality of life for Indigenous Australians. We searched primarily for peer-reviewed studies offering insight into Indigenous dance participation, particularly in promoting quality of life. This included an iterative search of social science and humanities databases such as EBSCO Host's meta-search facility, PAIS International and Google Scholar. Grey literature was also searched for self-published reports, along with websites of organisations known to conduct dance activities with Indigenous peoples. We employed reference snowballing techniques, scrutinising reference lists in journal articles and grey literature for relevant material. We also asked experts in academic and professional roles for referral to current studies.

We used two existing frameworks to analyze dance examples and literature: the domains of Aboriginal and Torres Strait Islander social and emotional wellbeing identified by Gee, Dudgeon, Schultz, Hart, and Kelly (2014) and Cultural Development Network's (CDN 2017) outcomes measures for cultural engagement. The latter were created to assist Australian cultural organisations and practitioners understand the impact of their work. These frameworks we selected are overlaid on approaches to outcome evaluation, whether formal or informal, taken by the authors. Processes of change and causal factors were also analysed, where they were identified by authors in their articles.

Introducing Quality of Life

To begin with, we document our findings about quality of life broadly, then in relation to Aboriginal and Torres Strait Islander peoples, and then as explored in scholarship on dance. Finally, we bring together all of these ideas to answer our major question, how dance can contribute to quality of life for Indigenous Australians.

A wide range of sometimes competing understandings and antecedent factors exists among quality of life researchers. Seeking a global theory, Ruta, Camfield, and Donaldson (2007) extend Amartya Sen's *capabilities approach* (Chaps. 16 and 19, this volume) to redefine quality of life as "the gap between what a person is actually capable of doing and being, and what they would like" to do or be (p. 409). The authors report that only Alex Michalos has measured quality of life "close" to the way they define it (p. 409). They also posit a causal relation between resources, capabilities, and quality of life (p. 397).

In spite of inherent definitional problems, there appears to be wide agreement that life satisfaction is a, perhaps *the*, vital element of quality of life (Bergland & Narum, 2007; Galloway, 2006). Galloway (2006) discusses how an individual's perception of being able to meet their needs and aspirations is crucial to satisfaction and wellbeing. Happiness, good health, and independence are other commonly measured factors (McKevitt, Redfern, La-Placa, & Wolfe, 2003), and increasingly, scholars are considering connections between dance, spirituality, and quality of life (LaMothe, 2015; Valenkamp & van der Walt, 2009; Chaps. 2, 5, 6, 7, 8, 13, 14, 17, 18, 20, and 23, this volume). The World Health Organization (WHO, 1995) continues to offer a broad view of quality of life as mental, social and cultural wellbeing, suggesting also that understandings of quality of life are influenced by individuals' culture and value systems.

Quality of Life for Indigenous Australians

Conceptions of quality of life for Aboriginal and Torres Strait Islander people, and methods for assessing these, that are predominantly shaped by Western cultural codes, can be problematic. Kite and Davy (2015) assert that mainstream understandings might not be appropriate for Indigenous people, as they do not give sufficient credence to value systems, cultural practices and ways of knowing and being that underpin a meaningful and good life for those communities. However, they do not offer alternatives, other than identifying factors that could be seen to affect both Indigenous and "mainstream" communities—complex relationships between people, their communities, their environment, and the natural and spiritual world.

Further, concepts of wellbeing, including social and emotional wellbeing considered culturally relevant for Indigenous Australians are being identified at organizational levels. The following definition offers a holistic construction of Indigenous health:

> Aboriginal health does not mean the physical wellbeing of an individual, but refers to the social, emotional, and cultural wellbeing of the whole community. For Aboriginal people this is seen in terms of the whole-life-view. Health care services should strive to achieve the state where every individual is able to achieve their full potential as human beings, and must bring about the total wellbeing of their communities. (Aboriginal Health and Medical Research Council of New South Wales, 1989, p. 5)

Australian Indigenous psychologist Graham Gee and colleagues identify seven domains of social and emotional wellbeing important for Indigenous people that resonate both with the preceding definition of health, and with Kite and Davy's (2015) ideas about quality of life. These domains include: connection to body, to mind and emotions, to family and kinship, to community, to culture, to country or land, and to spirit, spirituality and ancestors (Gee et al., 2014, p. 57). Loss or disruption of harmony between any of these domains is considered to result in negative health or social and emotional wellbeing (Dudgeon, Milroy, & Walker, 2014). These domains will be considered as quality of life parameters for the remainder of this chapter.

No matter how quality of life is defined, it is clear that ATSI people have more difficulties in experiencing good lives than other Australians (Australian Indigenous Health Infonet, 2015). Evidence of this includes much higher imprisonment (Australian Bureau of Statistics, 2015) and lower levels of attainment of mainstream educational milestones in all levels of schooling (Krakoeur, 2015) than the rest of the Australian population. These challenges are the result of multiple social, emotional, physical, cultural, and political abuses wrested on Indigenous Australians since the arrival of non-Indigenous people 250 years ago. Colonization and related policies included forced eviction of Indigenous people from their lands often through extreme violence. Practices of removing children from families seen to be "not coping" or using "inappropriate" (that is, non-Anglo-European) child rearing practices (Ryan, 2011; Secretariat of National Aboriginal and Islander Child Care [SNAICC], 2011; Ware, 2012)—including those who became known as the "stolen generations" (Commonwealth of Australia, 1997)—continue today. Significant negative effects have been reported, including a damaging disconnection from culture (Elder, 2003), trauma described as historical, intergenerational and cumulative, and cycles of disadvantage, discrimination, poverty, incarceration, and violence (Calma, 2008; Dudgeon et al., 2014; Garvey, 2008).

Indigenous Australians continue to be subjected to structural violence, that is, social structures that impede a group's ability to live a life of dignity or meet their own needs. Daily experiences of racism (both overt and more subtle forms) constitute a form of structural violence that reduces quality of life (National Aboriginal Community Controlled Health Organisation [NACCHO], 2014). Current author Ware witnessed an example of such racism during a visit to a remote Australian town. She observed a group of Indigenous people who were walking along the street and not apparently interfering with anyone else. When a police car drove by and noticed these people, the officers drove their vehicle over the curb onto the footpath, obstructing passage, and verbally interrogated the group for an extended period with aggressive body language displayed. A conversation with long-term local residents after this observation indicated that such experiences are common.

The Indigenous peoples of today's settler societies—for example, in Australia, Canada, USA, and New Zealand, have suffered historical narrowing of their identities to the point of dehumanization, resulting in displacement, and in earlier times, mass murder when Indigenous peoples were not officially recognized as human beings (Clark, 1995; Kiernan, 2007). This constriction of identities continues today in various types of systemic social exclusion. Sarah Maddison (2013) documents the negative effects of ongoing scrutiny of Indigenous identities by non-Indigenous Australians. She finds that "an imposed view of the 'authenticity' of Aboriginal people" constitutes a form of ongoing structural violence through others continually "insulting [their] identity needs" (pp. 289–90).

Amartya Sen's (1999) important work on human development points out the "terrible burden of narrowly defined identities, including those firmly based on communities and groups" (p. 8). Narrowed identities of "excluded," "dysfunctional," or "disconnected from one's heritage," Sen (1999) warns, can adversely affect wellbeing and quality of life in disadvantaged communities (p. 8). He suggests that such "unfreedoms" hamper people's ability to live "the kind of lives they value—and have reason to value" (p. 18), and thus reduce quality of life. On the other hand, he proposes that enhancement of people's *capabilities* to live the lives they value results in improved quality of life across physical, social, economic, political and cultural domains (Chaps. 16 and 19, this volume). Sen redefines concepts and criteria of human development and wellbeing as determined by community members themselves, rather than according to outsiders' definitions of a quality way of life. He offers recommendations for how the burdens and limitations of restricted identities can be addressed, suggesting that individuals can effectively shape their own destiny and help each other if they have "adequate social opportunities" (p. 11).

In this chapter, we propose that traditional and contemporary dance—and hybrid forms of the two—are cultural practices integral to formation of a healthy sense of self, community, and cultural identity formation that enable positive connection between history, heritage and the present day. In later sections, we explore how dance is seen to contribute to quality of life for Indigenous communities; but first we explore conceptions of quality of life in relation to dance more broadly.

Dance and Quality of Life

Scholars have suggested that participation in dance has likely contributed to good quality of life for human beings since pre-historic times (Dissanayake, 2000, Coda, this volume; Nemetz, 2006; Schott-Billman, 1992). Dance is ubiquitous in human societies, and people from most world cultures have expressed themselves by moving together to common rhythms in relation to important events such as harvests, hunts, and wars, and in times of transition such as birth, puberty, courtship, marriage, and death. Feelings and emotions have probably always been shared through co-participation in movement (Schmais & White, 1986).

Karen Bond (2014) offers a comprehensive overview of the relationship between dance and quality of life. She begins by defining complex human practices of dance as "nonverbal behaviour composed of movements that convey a heightened, aesthetic sense of body, rhythm, and space" (p. 1419). She suggests that dance can have multiple meanings for participants and observers, encompassing individual, social, cultural, and spiritual dimensions. These have parallels with domains of wellbeing considered significant for Australian Indigenous people.

Bond (2014) notes that most empirical research on dance and quality of life in both recreation and clinical settings focuses on emotional, mental/cognitive and social outcomes of dance. The contemporary field of dance movement therapy posits that humans have always danced for integrative purposes of health and healing (Quiroga & Kreutz, 2012). Ellen Dissanayake (2000, Coda, this volume) also describes integrative functions of dance, proposing that human beings are potentially designed for dancing and other aesthetic behaviors that help satisfy needs for identity, belonging, meaning and personal competence. Dance participation can lead to increased spontaneity and ability to play, with "a powerful motivation for dancing…the need to express oneself through rhythmic play and exploration of one's bodily powers and physical environment" (Quiroga & Kreutz, 2012, p. 128).

The value of dance participation for people who have a specific cultural identity—beyond the "mainstream"—is affirmed by research from diverse contexts. Engagement in traditional music and dance practices has been reported to facilitate social interaction amongst the cultural in-group, including inter-generational connections, as well as symbolic connection to earlier generations. Performance of these art forms also offers a "public articulation of [that cultural identity]" (Leonard, 2005, p. 516). These phenomena have been documented for groups such as Irish migrants to the UK (Leonard, 2005) and Maori migrants to Australia (Dunphy, 1996).

For Indigenous peoples in countries beyond Australia, there is also evidence of the contribution of dance to quality of life and wellbeing. For example, in Canada, arts are incorporated in holistic models of healing encompassing physical, emotional, intellectual, and spiritual worlds (Aboriginal Healing Foundation, 2012). Traditional healing interventions and ceremonies involving dance indicate positive outcomes for this cultural group (Castellano, 2006; McCormick, 1994; Schiff & Moore, 2006). Jacqueline Shea Murphy (2007) documents how Indigenous peoples of the US and Canada practice dance for a range of integrative purposes, enacting cultural connections to land, ancestors, and animals, as well as spiritual and political concerns through dance (Chaps. 5 and 17, this volume).

The adaptive value of hybrid genres is also documented. Mixing of traditional and modern cultural practices has been discussed as particularly valuable in assisting younger community members to bridge old and new worlds. In periods of rapid change, hybrid arts practices can provide a space where participants make sense of and adapt to the new while maintaining connections with the old order (Ware, 2006). Hickey-Moody's (2013) study with young Sudanese women living in

Melbourne, Australia found that explorations involving traditional and global pop dance provided these newcomers with ways of "writ[ing] themselves into the local community imaginaries" (p. 90) (see Chap. 26, this volume). This opportunity mitigated newcomers' experiences of alienation and increased their sense of belonging in a new culture.

Drawing in part on Bourdieu's (1986) conceptual framework, Laura Moran (2015) suggests that young people, especially those outside dominant ethnic groups, often embrace symbols of "race and ethnicity," such as might be enabled through arts practices, to build social capital. Such capital can then be used to help define their place in society (p. 711). This is important, as cultural identity needs to be generated and replenished continually. As Hall (1990) suggests, cultural identity is 'not a fixed essence at all'... but always in the process of being constructed, 'through memory, fantasy, narrative and myth' (p. 220). At the same time, some are cautious about the value of hybrid performance genres, citing communities' fears that hybridity might threaten the integrity and vitality of their cultural heritage (Dunphy, 2013; Wanyema, 2008).

Quality of Life and Dance in Indigenous Cultures in Australia

The First Nations people of Australia practice the oldest living cultures on the planet, expressed in an unbroken lineage for at least 60,000 years (Al-Yaman, 2016). Prior to colonisation 250 years ago, around 700 Indigenous languages and dialects were spoken amongst 250 Indigenous nations who each had their own territories and systems of law (Cowling & Searle, 2008). Ceremonies involving dance, song and related art forms have been vital aspects of cultural life throughout these millennia (Byard, 1988; Perkins & Langton, 2008). The arts of dance and music were functionally indivisible, music being considered fundamental to the performance of dance and vice versa (Magowan, 2007; Stubbington, 2007). In earlier times, these practices had a range of purposes, including teaching and maintaining cultural knowledge, activating health, wellbeing and community connection (Byard, 1988; Stubbington, 2007), mourning loss through death (Magowan, 2007; Stubbington, 2007), and sustaining relationships with nature and spirituality (Magowan, 2007; Perkins & Langton, 2008; Stubbington, 2007).

Contemporary Indigenous Australians in urban and remote communities continue such cultural practices, including ceremonies with perceived similarities to ancient ones (Al-Yaman, 2016; Phipps & Slater, 2010; Treloyn & Martin, 2014). The "essential" role of song and dance in contemporary Indigenous culture and society is articulated by the General Assembly of the International Council for Traditional Music (ICTM). This significant body reports that through song and dance,

> Indigenous Australians maintain social and personal wellbeing, sustain their cultures, and maintain Law and their own identity. Performance traditions also serve to strengthen Indigenous languages and provide intergenerational links between families and communities. (ICTM-ANZ, 2011)

The functions of ceremonies involving dance are highlighted in Judy Atkinson's (2002, 2012) important work on intergenerational trauma and healing. She articulates the cultural and spiritual powers that are evoked to ensure a continuing relationship between past, present and future: "Song, dance, art and ritual, used in ceremony, remind the ancestral beings to continue to release their powers, to ensure the ongoing reproduction of life cycles" (p. 33).

Ware's (2014) synthesis of research on arts in Indigenous Australian communities indicates multiple avenues for improved quality of life and wellbeing, which include: maintenance and transmission of cultural knowledge, increased sense of agency, resilience and pride in personal or community achievements, and reduced shame (p. 6.). Allain (2011) also notes physical and mental health benefits of arts participation for Australian Indigenous communities, including healing from traumatic life experiences and reduction in self-harm. The wellbeing engendered through maintenance of traditional cultural knowledge provides a potential foil to narrowed identities that Sen (1999) warns can adversely affect wellbeing and quality of life in disadvantaged communities (p. 8).

At the same time, traditional cultural practices and ceremonies are being adapted to include both customary and contemporary elements. These developments might be one way that dance supports the renegotiation and adjustment of identities in new circumstances (Costigan & Neuenfeldt, 2002; Dussart, 2000), including urban life. Art forms such as dance, involving old and new practices, are also being used specifically to promote health and wellbeing. The Djuki Mala (formerly Chooky) dance group from Elcho Island was established by an elder, Frank Djirrimbilpilwuy, around 2007 to assist young men in the community to keep healthy, active and fit in the face of significant stressors including lack of employment, substance misuse, poor schooling, boredom, and depression (Healy, 2013).

This group have attracted international recognition for their unique rendering of traditional Yolngu dance moves with contemporary styles, including their first performance piece, *Zorba the Greek Yolngu Style* (2007) which was accompanied by Mikis Theodorakis's music based on traditional Cretan folk songs. Another initiative undertaken to improve social and emotional wellbeing of young people in remote Indigenous communities incorporated traditional Indigenous culture fused with hip-hop, rap, beat boxing and break dancing. A formal evaluation indicated some success of this project in raising awareness of services, basic principles for preventing depression and anxiety, and supporting those at-risk (Kurongkurl Katitjin Centre for Indigenous Australian Education and Research, 2009).

Western researchers and practitioners are increasingly investigating and drawing on Indigenous knowledge and ways of healing. Evidence from emerging fields of neuroscience and neurobiology suggests that Indigenous dance practices, such as the use of patterned repetitive stimuli of words, dance or song, can promote healing and recovery for traumatized children. In his foreword to Malchiodi (2008/2015), neurodevelopmental researcher Bruce Perry (2015) asserts that this science supports "what the elders and healers, in some ways, have always known" (p. ix). Perry has found that "repetitive, rhythmic, relevant, relational, respectful, and rewarding" movement (p. xi) can alter neural systems involved in the stress response. His research affirms the knowledge that Indigenous people hold of the value of dance participation.

Benefits of arts participation correspond closely with aspects of wellbeing considered important by and for Indigenous people discussed previously: physical, mental, emotional, social, cultural, ecological, and spiritual. Taken together with the fact that cultural participation, including the arts is high— with almost two-thirds (63%) of Aboriginal and Torres Strait Islander people aged 15 years and over, and 75% aged 4–14 years reporting involvement in cultural events, ceremonies or organisations in a year, and even higher participation rates in remote areas (82% of people 15 and over, and 87% of children) (Australian Bureau of Statistics, 2016)— these findings suggest the importance of government and philanthropic support for such participation in Indigenous communities.

Dunphy's (2013) research on arts participation in Timor Leste found that factors supporting positive changes through arts programs include good planning, skilled leadership, emphasis on collaboration, and strong stimulation of creativity. When dance program leaders and participants are from different cultural backgrounds, facilitators' capacity for improvisation and responsiveness in the moment, cultural sensitivity and respect, and appropriate inclusion of cultural elements have been identified as important process factors (Dunphy, Elton, & Jordan, 2014). Dance scholar Judith Lynne Hanna (2006) suggests that dance leaders who disregard cultural elements and values can create stress for participants.

Junba and *Milpirri*

We now offer two examples of cultural activities focused on dance-making and participation that authors documenting them posit as contributing to quality of life in Australian First Nations communities: *Junba*, a ceremonial practice continuing with vital energy, while largely unchanged over centuries, and *Milpirri*, a relatively recent festival involving customary practices combined with new artistic elements and collaborations. Formal "academic" evaluations of these activities were not available for our review, but we include perspectives on the events from senior Indigenous practitioners and their non-Indigenous partners/collaborators. Thus, this discussion reflects narratives of those in leadership positions rather than those of participants or the wider community.

Junba *Dance-Song Tradition, Western Australia*

Junba is the dance-song tradition of the Ngarinyin, Wunambal, and Worrorra peoples of the remote Kimberley region of northwest-Australia. *Junba*, in which the music and accompanying dance are inseparable, is considered one of Australia's oldest and richest song-dance traditions. While it originated thousands of years ago, it remains dynamic. As many as 3000 new dance-songs have been created by 35 composers in more than five languages over the last two centuries (Treloyn & Martin, 2014). Non-Indigenous scholar Sally Treloyn and *Junba* performer Matthew "Scotty" Martin describe *Junba* as an open or "public" genre performed at private, community, and public events, including festivals. Male and female performers are directed by a leader/composer, and community members contribute as dancers, singers, onlookers, helpers, or patrons. Elders explain performances to audiences, providing details about stories presented and issues affecting their communities (Treloyn & Martin, 2014).

Junba is now performed for advocacy purposes—to raise concerns about the health and wellbeing of communities and young people. This function is considered particularly salient due to the loss of elders and high rates of youth suicide. *Junba* is also seen as a key resource for Indigenous peoples of the region to adapt to changing social, economic, and cultural conditions in the Kimberleys since colonization began in the mid-to-late 1800s (Redmond, 2001; Treloyn, 2006).

Treloyn and Martin (2014) explore Junba's relationship with diverse aspects of wellbeing in careful detail. The analysis of Junba offered here derives from Treloyn's extended fieldwork in Junba-performing communities in the Kimberley region and later transcription, analysis, and integration of this information with research. The authors employ both Indigenous and formal academic, or "scientific," ways of knowing in this process. As a *Junba* cultural proponent, Martin brings skills in "traditions of intercultural teaching, learning, and collaborative research" (p. 1) as fostered by senior Indigenous cultural knowledge holders, while Treloyn brings analytic approaches from her discipline of ethnomusicology. They apply both types of knowledge to draw out the interrelated aesthetic elements of *Junba* that its proponents consider instrumental in positive change. Notably, the holistic indicators of health and wellbeing they identify correspond with the seven domains of Indigenous wellbeing discussed earlier (Gee et al., 2014). Specifically, Treloyn and Martin see a causal association between *Junba* cultural practice and the social and emotional wellbeing of *Junba*-performing communities.

First, there is "connection between people and moieties" (Treloyn & Martin, 2014, p. 6) or clans, which can be considered as social wellbeing; then there is "connection between people and spirits" (p. 7), related most closely to spiritual wellbeing; and "connection between people and country" (p. 9) or land, which can be considered ecological wellbeing. The entire creative process of *Junba*, from composition and design to choreography, costuming, props and musical accompaniment, works in integrated ways, as examined in detail in the next paragraphs.

Social Wellbeing A significant aspect of social wellbeing is relationships between people, which we view here through a lens of contemporary social capital (CDN, 2017; Halpern, 2005; Putnam, 2000). While not unproblematic (Haynes, 2009; Warr, 2006), this concept can be useful in understanding the impacts of the Junba case study. In this case, it is possible to see that both *bonding* and *bridging* social capital (Putnam, 2000) are engendered. Bonding capital—connections between people who know each other already, such as members of the same family group/community—are fostered through sharing of dances and songs in public performances. Dance elements are passed across generations, from spirits to adult performers and on to younger generations who are either participants or audience members. Thus, participation in this cultural practice is highly significant for intergenerational connection, in tying living dancers to "the family that came before him, …that surrounds him, and… that will follow him" (Treloyn & Martin, 2014, p. 7).

Connections between individuals and wider communities, or moieties, are embodied in choreography. Dance steps require performers to move together, then split, then come back together and dance in each other's tracks. Thus, performers literally dance the links between themselves into existence, both collectivizing and differentiating themselves from others through shared and separate movements.

A different type of social capital, bridging capital—building relationships between people who are not alike or not already connected (Putnam, 2000)—is also generated through *Junba*. These dance-songs serve to manage relationships between proponents and Indigenous people from other communities, with whom different and more frequent types of contact has been catalysed by changed socioeconomic forces, such as the growing pastoral industry in that area.

Spiritual Wellbeing *Junba*'s spiritual dimension of wellbeing is afforded through the fostering of relationships between people and their deceased kin—ancestors and spirits, as highlighted earlier by Atkinson (2002). This spiritual connection happens through many aspects of *Junba*. In composition, the performer receives the dance-songs in dreams from spirits of deceased family members or other song men and women (Treloyn 2006), rather than creating them from their imagination, as can often occur in cultural creative processes.

All aspects of *Junba* performance design, from stage sets and lighting to costuming and make-up, are considered to enhance spiritual connection and wellbeing. Ceremonies are staged as darkness falls, with firelight, bough screens used as stage "sets," and dancers' ochre face painting obscuring visibility of them. These devices enable performers to first appear as ghosts, who gradually become more human-like as they move forward into the light. "Thus, a line of descent from deceased to living relatives is marked and enacted on the dance ground" (Treloyn & Martin, 2014, p. 8). Connection to the spirit world is augmented further by costuming: for example, the paperbark used for headpieces is the same as that employed to wrap the bones of deceased people for interment (Redmond, 2012).

Ecological Wellbeing *Junba* participation also enhances a third type of wellbeing—ecological—in its fostering of relationships between people and country. Dance is seen to be causal in wellbeing of the land, as when people dance *Junba*, "Country becomes healthy" (Treloyn & Martin, 2014, p. 9). The performance renews and asserts participants' connections with their ancestral homes. This connection is enhanced by props used in performance, with totems enabling people to invoke an identity attached to their ancestral country. This link is able to be engendered through *Junba* even when proponents are in new physical locations.

Health of country is interconnected, again, to physical wellbeing of inhabitants. When country is made healthy through people dancing on it, in turn they are made healthier by the food and resources the land provides. Physical health is stimulated further by *Junba*'s accompanying music, with beating of clapsticks seen to strengthen young peoples' bones. In a public lecture in Melbourne, Scotty Martin described:

> That's why you see them kids real happy and thing. They're not looking sad, they're looking forward for dancing or anything, they'll do anything. Now the bone, that *ornorr*, is strong to do anything, dance. They can run all day too if they want to. … They have the Country and for themselves they feel strong, they not weak. … The spirit, the singing, the dancing, that makes them healthy. It's always been there. (Treloyn & Martin 2012).

In sum, *Junba* participation can potentially contribute to wellbeing across all domains identified by Gee et al. (2014): connection to body (physical wellbeing), to mind and emotions, family and kinship, community, culture, land or country, and spirituality and ancestors. Additionally, it addresses specific aspects of the cultural domain identified by CDN (2017), in stimulating creativity and aesthetic enrichment of participants and wider communities. Such affordances are supported by many aesthetic elements: composition-choreography, design and staging, costuming, props, musical accompaniment, and environmental elements of location on country.

Milpirri *Festival, Lajumanu, Northern Territory*

Our second example is *Milpirri*, a bi-annual festival of the *Warlpiri* people from the remote Lajumanu community in Northern Territory. *Milpirri* is like *Junba* in involving some elements of traditional cultural practices, for example, being held regularly at the traditional time for *Warlpiri* ceremonies, just before replenishing annual rains (Patrick, 2015). Festival creative director *Warlpiri* man Steve Jampijinpa Patrick considers *Milpirri* to have several functions that can also be seen to match the domains of wellbeing discussed earlier (Gee et al., 2014).

Milpirri is intended to teach the community's children about *ngurra-kurlu,* the Warlpiri people's sense of place and home, which consists of five pillars of family, law, land, language and ceremony (Patrick, Holmes, & Box, 2008). *Milpirri* is like *Junba* in responding to challenges facing young people, as it seeks to provide a sense of belonging in times of rapid change (Tracks Dance, 2017). In intending to make people feel good about who they are and where they live, the festival also has mental and physical health goals. One recent event themed around the wind songline *Pulya-ranyi* addressed community members' potentials and how they can be realised, controlled, taught and passed on.

Like *Junba, Milpirri* activities are intended to enhance bonding social capital by bringing together people of different generations. Elders and younger people contribute to the festival according to skills and interest, with youth energy linked to the wisdom of the old. The festival also serves a bridging capital function to increase understanding between *Yapa* (Warlpiri, Aboriginal people) and *Kardiya* (non-Warlpiri, non-Aboriginal people). Patrick (2015) considers this "the beginning of a revisioning of the way that both Western and Warlpiri values could work together" (p. 4).

Dissimilar to *Junba*, *Milpirri* is not an ancient tradition but a recent initiative, first run in 2005. *Milpirri* was inspired by the *Garma* Festival of east Arnhem Land, a partnership between the *Yolngu* people and multiple non-Indigenous contributors, developed to advance interactions between *Yolngu*, other Indigenous people, and people of other cultures (Garma Forum on Indigenous Performance Research, 2002). Like *Garma*, *Milpirri* involves collaboration between Indigenous people—the Warlpiri community and the Lajamanu School, as well as non-Indigenous people and Darwin's contemporary dance company, Tracks Dance (see Chap. 30, this volume). While the *Milpirri* project began just over ten years ago, it is based upon a relationship between Tracks Dance and the Lajamanu community established three decades earlier. Community members write music compositions in Warlpiri and English and Tracks support this creativity including provision of digital recording equipment.

Milpirri is also different from *Junba* in that it reinterprets traditional cultural practices in new ways. Its cultural functions include the intention to "enliven tradition for an intercultural twenty-first-century future" (Tracks Dance 2017, p. 1). This does not mean returning to historical times, but maintaining core Warlpiri values alongside mainstream Australian culture. *Milpirri's* model of "aesthetic innovation" developed by Patrick (2015) promotes the five pillars of *ngurra-kurlu*. The festival includes experimental practices, with older people dancing to "express the meaning of the story" in traditional *ngurra-kurlu*, while younger members interpret the same stories using hip hop (p. 1).

As noted above, we found no formal evaluation of the festival as we wrote this article, but stakeholders have reflected on its contributions to quality of community life. Patrick et al. (2008) reported "an enormous effect on the community" in educational, employment, health and wellbeing enhancements (p. 7), and Tracks Dance (2017) notes higher educational engagement and general fitness improvements (Tracks Dance, 2017). In 2015, the festival was recognised with the Australian Dance Award for Outstanding Achievement in Community Dance.

Patrick (2015) attributes the festival's success to participants' enjoyment of connection and reconnection with culture—how this stimulates a common sense of belonging. Through *Milpirri*, he suggests, people feel "human again and not a shadow, … like we have a voice and are not just a background people" (p. 8). This perspective aligns with Sen's (1999) emphasis on the importance, for quality of life, of a positive and unrestricted sense of identity. Tracks members perceive that *Milpirri* is successful in its maintenance of traditional cultural knowledge, and identify its ever-evolving contemporary interpretation and presentation as the causal factor in achieving this (Newth, McMicken, & Biddle, 2015).

Thus, while both events involved creative stimulation and enactment, the processes utilised in *Milpirri* are different than those of *Junba*, with inspiration for performance not coming primarily from ancestors in dreams, but through collaboration between Warlpiri people and the non-Indigenous professional dance artists of Tracks Dance Company. These artists' long term relationship with the community offers new possibilities for learning, skill development and creative expression. *Milpirri* exemplifies how long-term relationships are vital to creative, collaborative, heritage-making. Notably, these practices can also contribute in integrated ways to Indigenous quality of life.

Conclusion

This study examines existing literature to explore the relationship between dance and quality of life for Aboriginal and Torres Strait Islander Australians, as considered meaningful in Indigenous terms. We discuss quality of life broadly and in the Indigenous context, highlighting the holistic approaches to health and wellbeing recommended by and for First Nations communities. This leads to a proposal that dance participation can support Indigenous quality of life across the seven domains of social and emotional wellbeing identified by Gee et al. (2014)—physical (body), mental, family and kinship, community, culture, land, and spirituality, as well as the CDN's (2017) measures of cultural engagement—creative stimulation, aesthetic enrichment, new knowledge and insight, and sense of belonging.

The two examples offered of lively cultural practices that prioritise dance illustrate significant quality of life enhancements for both communities. Spiritual, social, and individual emotional wellbeing are engendered in the ancient and still vital *Junba* dance-song tradition from remote north western Australia—through rehearsing relational connections across the community (between the living, and between the living and those who have passed on). As it did for the ancestors, ecological wellbeing is fostered through connection to country in the process of dancing on it. The contemporary *Milpirri* festival collaboration between Indigenous cultural members and non-Indigenous dancers also engenders quality of life enhancements for participants, including activation of intergenerational relationships, increased understanding between Indigenous and non-Indigenous communities, and a space for adaptation of traditional practices in the context of the dominant settler-society.

Given indications of the contribution of dance to quality of life across salient domains and selected sites found in the highlighted literature, we conclude that further research is clearly important. By growing understanding of dance and its relation to Indigenous quality of life, the potential for benefits accruing through dance participation can be maximised, in turn contributing to knowledge about how services for Aboriginal and Torres Strait Islander Australians might be improved.

Acknowledgements We thank editors and anonymous reviewers for their contributions to the current version.

References

Aboriginal Healing Foundation. (2012). *Dancing, singing, painting, and speaking the healing story: Healing through creative arts*. Ottawa, Ontario: Aboriginal Healing Foundation. Retrieved from http://www.ahf.ca/downloads/healing-through-creative-arts.pdf

Aboriginal Health and Medical Research Council of New South Wales. (1989). *National aboriginal health strategy*. Sydney, NSW: Aboriginal health and Medical Research Council of New South Wales.

Allain, G. (2011). An art-based healing process: The Aurukun Creative Livelihoods Project at the Wik and Kugu Arts and Craft Centre. *Australasian Psychiatry, 19*(S1), S42–S44.

Al-Yaman, F. (2016). Australia: Aboriginal and Torres Strait Islander peoples. In K. Silburn, H. Reich, & I. Anderson (Eds.), *A global snapshot of Indigenous and tribal peoples' health* (pp. 6–7). Melbourne, VIC: The Lowitja Institute.

Atkinson, J. (2002). *Trauma trails, recreating song lines: The transgenerational effects of trauma in Indigenous Australia*. North Melbourne, VIC: Spinifex.

Atkinson, J. (2012). *Educaring: A trauma informed approach to healing generational trauma for aboriginal Australians*. South Goolmangar, NSW: We Al-li. Retrieved from http://www.wealli.com.au.

Australian Bureau of Statistics. (2015). *Aboriginal and Torres Strait islander prisoner characteristics*. Canberra: ACT: Australian Bureau of Statistics.

Australian Bureau of Statistics. (2016). *National Aboriginal and Torres Strait islander social survey, 2014–15*. Canberra, ACT: Australian Bureau of Statistics.

Australian Indigenous Health Infonet. (2015). *What is closing the gap?* Retrieved from http://healthinfonet.ecu.edu.au/closing-the-gap/key-facts/what-is-closing-the-gap.

Australian Institute of Aboriginal and Torres Strait Islander Studies [AIATSIS] (2015). *Mabo case*. Retrieved from https://aiatsis.gov.au/explore/articles/mabo-case.

Bergland, A., & Narum, I. (2007). Quality of life: Diversity in content and meaning. *Critical Review of Physical Rehabilitation Medicine, 19*, 115–139.

Bond, K. E. (2014). Dance and quality of life. In A. C. Michalos (Ed.), *Encyclopedia of quality of life and Well-being research* (pp. 1419–1424). Dordrecht, NL: Springer.

Byard, R. (1988). Traditional medicine of aboriginal Australia. *CMAJ, 139*(8), 792–794.

Calma, T. (2008). *Social justice report*. Sydney, NSW: Australian Human Rights Commission.

Castellano, M. B. (2006). *Final report of the aboriginal Healing Foundation, volume 1: A healing journey: Reclaiming wellness*. Ottawa, ONT: Aboriginal Healing Foundation.

Clark, I. (1995). *Scars on the landscape. A register of massacre sites in Western Victoria 1803–1859*. Canberra, ACT: Aboriginal Studies Press.

Commonwealth of Australia. (1997). *Bringing them home: National inquiry into the separation of aboriginal and Torres Strait islander children from their families*. Sydney, NSW: Human Rights and Equal Opportunity Commission.

Costigan, L., & Neuenfeldt, K. (2002). Torres Strait Islander music and dance in informal and formal educational contexts in Australia. *Research Studies in Music Education, 19*(1), 46–55.

Cowling, V., & Searle, S. (2008). *Wiyiliin ta nubaliin ta – Awabakal language for talking, learning. Working with aboriginal families and communities. The clinician, Vol 4 – Vulnerable families: Children of parents with mental illness (pp. 135–141)*. Sydney, NSW: MH-Kids/NSW Health.

Cultural Development Network (CDN). (2017). *A schema of measurable outcomes for cultural engagement*. Melbourne, VIC: Cultural Development Network. Retrieved from http://www.culturaldevelopment.net.au/outcomes/.

Dissanayake, E. (2000). *Art and intimacy: How the arts began*. Seattle, WA: University of Washington Press.

Dudgeon, P., Milroy, H., & Walker, R. (Eds.). (2014). *Working together: Aboriginal and Torres Strait islander health and wellbeing principles and practice*. Canberra, ACT: Department of the Prime Minister and Cabinet and the University of Western Australia Press.

Dunphy, K. (1996). *The cultural arts experience of Maori migrants in Melbourne* (Master's thesis). Melbourne, VIC: University of Melbourne. Retrieved from http://repository.unimelb.edu.au/10187/11603

Dunphy, K. (2013). *The role of participatory arts in social change in Timor-Leste* (Doctoral thesis). Melbourne, VIC: Deakin University. Retrieved from www.manyhands.org.au/resources

Dunphy, K., Elton, M., & Jordan, A. (2014). Exploring dance-movement therapy in post-conflict Timor-Leste. *American Journal of Dance Therapy, 36*(2), 189–208.

Dussart, F. (2000). *The politics of ritual in an Aboriginal settlement: Kinship, gender and the currency of knowledge*. Washington, DC: Smithsonian Institution.

Elder, B. (2003). *Blood on the wattle: Massacres and maltreatment of Aboriginal Australians since 1788* (3rd ed.). Chatswood, NSW: New Holland.

Galloway, S. (2006). Cultural participation and individual quality of life: A review of research findings. *Applied Research on Quality of Life, 1*, 323–342.

Garma Forum on Indigenous Performance Research. (2002). *Garma statement on Indigenous music and dance*. National Recording Project for Indigenous Performance in Australia. Retrieved from www.aboriginalartists.com.au?NRP_statements.htm.

Garvey, D. (2008). A review of the social and emotional wellbeing of Indigenous Australian peoples. Australian Indigenous Health*InfoNet*. Retrieved from http://www.healthinfonet.ecu.edu.au/other-health-conditions/mental-health/reviews/our-review

Gee, G., Dudgeon, P., Schultz, C., Hart, A., & Kelly, K. (2014). Understanding social and emotional wellbeing and mental health from an Aboriginal and Torrres Strait Islander perspective. In P. Dudgeon, H. Milroy, & R. Walker (Eds.), *Working together: Aboriginal and Torres Strait islander health and wellbeing principles and practice* (2nd ed., pp. 55–68). Canberra, ACT: Department of the Prime Minister and Cabinet.

Hall, S. (1990). Cultural identity and diaspora. In J. Rutherford (Ed.), *Identity: Community, culture, difference* (pp. 222–237). London: Lawrence and Wishart.

Halpern, D. (2005). *Social capital*. Cambridge, UK: Polity.

Hanna, J. L. (2006). *Dancing for health: Conquering and preventing stress*. Lanham, MD: AltaMira Press.

Haynes, P. (2009). *Before going any further with social capital: Eight key criticisms to address*. INGENIO (CSIC-UPV) Working Paper Series 02. Valencia: Instituto de Gestion de la Innovacion y del Conococimiento. Retrieved from http://www.ingenio.upv.es/en/going-any-further-social-capital-eight-key-criticisms-address#.WoY3phNuauN

Healy, J. de L. (2013). Yolngu Zorba meets Superman. *Anthrovision, 1*(1). Retrieved from http://anthrovision.revues.org/362

Hickey-Moody, A. (2013). *Youth, arts and education: Reassembling subjectivity through affect*. Abingdon, Oxfordshire: Routledge.

International Council for Traditional Music – Australia/New Zealand Regional Committee. (2011). *Statement on Indigenous Australian music and dance*. Retrieved from http://www.ictmusic.org/sites/default/files/documents/IAMD_statement.pdf.

Kiernan, B. (2007). *Blood and soil: A world history of genocide and extermination from Sparta to Darfur*. New Haven, CT: Yale University Press.

Kite, E., & Davy, C. (2015). Using indigenist and indigenous methodologies to connect to deeper understandings of Aboriginal and Torres Strait Islander people's quality of life. *Health Promotion Journal of Australia, 26*, 191–194.

Krakoeur, J. (2015). *Literature review relating to the current context and discourse on Indigenous cultural awareness in the teaching space: Critical pedagogies and improving Indigenous learning outcomes through cultural responsiveness*. Melbourne, VIC: ACER.

Kurongkurl Katitjin Centre for Indigenous Australian Education and Research. (2009). *Evaluation of indigenous hip-hop projects*. Perth, WA: Edith Cowan University Press.

LaMothe, K. L. (2015). *Why we dance: A philosophy of bodily becoming*. New York: Columbia University Press.

Leonard, M. (2005). Performing identities: Music and dance in the Irish communities of Coventry and Liverpool. *Social & Cultural Geography, 6*(4), 515–529.
Maddison, S. (2013). Indigenous identity, "authenticity" and the structural violence of settler colonialism. *Identities, 20*(3), 288–303.
Magowan, F. (2007). *Melodies of mourning: Music and emotion in Northern Australia.* Crawley, UK: University of Western Australia Press.
Malchiodi, C. (Ed.). (2015). *Creative interventions with traumatized children* (2nd ed.). New York: Guilford Press.
McCormick, R. (1994). *The facilitation of healing for the First Nations people of British Columbia* (Doctoral dissertation). Retrieved from https://open.library.ubc.ca/cIRcle/collections/ubctheses/831/items/1.0053949
McKevitt, C., Redfern, J., La-Placa, V., & Wolfe, C. (2003). Defining and using quality of life: A survey of health care professionals. *Clinical Rehabilitation, 17*(8), 865–870. https://doi.org/10.1191/0269215503cr690oa.
Møller, V. (Ed.) (1997). *Quality of life in South Africa* (Social Indicators Research Series, Vol. 1). Dordrecht: Kluwer.
Moran, L. (2015). Constructions of race: Symbolic ethnic capital and the performance of youth identity in multicultural Australia. *Ethnic & Racial Studies, 39*(4), 708–726.
Murphy, J. S. (2007). *The people have never stopped dancing: Native American modern dance histories.* Minneapolis, MN: University of Minnesota Press.
National Aboriginal Community Controlled Health Organisation. (2014, February). Aboriginal health and racism: What are the impacts of racism on Aboriginal health? *NACCHO Aboriginal health news alerts.* Retrieved from https://nacchocommunique.com/2014/02/28/
Nemetz, L. D. (2006). Moving with meaning: The historical progression of dance/movement therapy. In S. L. Brooke (Ed.), *Creative arts therapies manual: A guide to the history, theoretical approaches, assessment, and work with special populations of art, play, dance, music, drama, and poetry therapies* (pp. 95–108). Springfield, IL: Charles C. Thomas.
Newth, T., McMicken, D., & Biddle, J. (2015). Milpirri: Jennifer Biddle in discussion with Tracks Dance Company. *Cultural Studies Review, 21*(1), 132–148.
Patrick, S., Holmes, M., & Box, A. (2008). *Ngurra-kurlu: A way of working with Warlpiri people.* Alice Springs, NT: Desert Knowledge Cooperative Research Centre.
Patrick, W. S. J. (2015). Pulya-ranyi: Winds of change. *Cultural Studies Review, 21*(1), 121–131.
Perkins, R., & Langton, M. (2008). *First Australians: An illustrated history.* Carlton, VIC: Miegunyah.
Perry, B. (2015). Foreword. In C. Malchiodi (Ed.), *Creative interventions with traumatized children* (pp. ix–xii). New York: Guilford Press. (Original work published 2008).
Phipps, P., & Slater, L. (2010). *Indigenous cultural festivals: Evaluating impact on community health and wellbeing: Report to the Telstra Foundation.* Melbourne, VIC: RMIT Globalism Centre.
Putnam, R. (2000). *Bowling alone: The collapse and revival of American community.* New York: Simon & Schuster.
Quiroga, M. C., & Kreutz, G. (2012). Dance and health: Exploring interactions and implications. In R. Macdonald, G. Kreutz, & L. Mitchell (Eds.), *Music, health, and wellbeing* (pp. 125–133). Oxford: Oxford University Press.
Redmond, A. (2001). *Rulug Wayirri: Moving kin and country in the Northern Kimberley* (Doctoral dissertation). Sydney, NSW: The University of Sydney.
Redmond, A. (2012). Tracking Wurnan: Transformations in the trade and exchange of resources in the northern Kimberley. In N. Fijn, I. Keen, C. Lloyd, & M. Pickering (Eds.), *Indigenous participation in Australian economies II: Historical engagements and current enterprises* (pp. 57–72). Canberra, ACT: Australian National University E Press.
Ruta, D., Camfield, L., & Donaldson, C. (2007). Sen and the art of quality of life maintenance: Towards a general theory of quality of life and its causation. *Journal of Socio Economics, 36,* 397–423.

Ryan, F. (2011). Kanyininpa (holding): A way of nurturing children in Aboriginal Australia. *Australian Social Work, 64*(2), 183–197.
Schiff, J. W., & Moore, K. (2006). The impact of the sweat lodge ceremony on dimensions of well-being. *American Indian and Alaska Native Mental Health Research, 13*(3), 48–69.
Schmais, C., & White, E. (1986). Introduction to dance therapy. *American Journal of Dance Therapy, 9*(1), 23–30.
Schott-Billman, F. (1992). Primitive expression: An anthropological dance therapy method. *The Arts in Psychotherapy, 19*(2), 105–109.
Scott, R., & Heiss, A. (Eds.). (2016). *The intervention: An anthology*. Sydney, NSW: NewSouth.
Secretariat of National Aboriginal and Islander Child Care. (2011). *Growing up our way: Aboriginal and Torres Strait islander child rearing practices matrix*. Melbourne, VIC: SNAICC. Retrieved from https://www.health.act.gov.au/sites/default/files/SNAICC%20Growing%20up%20our%20way%20Aboriginal%20and%20Torres%20Strait%20Islander%20Child%20Rearing%20Practices%20Matrix.pdf.
Sen, A. (1999). *Development as freedom*. Oxford, UK: Oxford University Press.
Stubbington, J. (2007). *Singing the land: The power of performance in aboriginal life*. Sydney, NSW: Currency House.
Tracks Dance. (2017). *The story behind Milpirri festival*. Retrieved from http://www.tracksdance.com.au/story-behind-milpirri-festival.
Treloyn, S. (2006). *Songs that pull: Jadmi Junba from the Kimberley region of northwest Australia* (Doctoral dissertation). Sydney, NSW: The University of Sydney.
Treloyn, S., & Martin, M. D. (2012, July 24). *Australia's endangered song traditions*. Music on the Mind Public Lecture Series. Melbourne, VIC: Melbourne Recital Centre.
Treloyn, S., & Martin, M. D. (2014). Perspectives on dancing, singing and well-being from the Kimberley, Northwest Australia. *Journal for the Anthropological Study of Human Movement, 21*(1), 1–13.
Valenkamp, M., & van der Walt, J. L. (2009). The spiritual dimension of quality of life. In V. Moller & D. Huschka (Eds.), *Quality of life and the millennium challenge* (Social indicators research series) (Vol. 35, pp. 81–97). Dordrecht, Eastern Cape: Springer.
Wanyema, M. N. (2008). Dance as a means of cultural identity: A case of the Bukusu Kamabeka dance. *Muziki, 5*(2), 213–222.
Ware, V. (2006). *Stylistic and cultural transformations in Bangkok fusion music from 1850 to the present day, leading to the development of Dontri Thai Prayuk* (Doctoral thesis). Melbourne, VIC: Monash University.
Ware, V. (2012). *Improving access to urban and regional early childhood services: Resource sheet no. 17*. Canberra, ACT/Melbourne, VIC: Australian Institute of Health and Welfare/Australian Institute of Family Studies.
Ware, V. A. (2014). *Supporting healthy communities through arts programs* (Resource sheet no. 28). Canberra, ACT: Australian Institute of Health and Welfare.
Warr, D. (2006). Gender, class and the art and craft of social capital. *The Sociological Quarterly, 47*(2006), 497–520.
World Health Organization. (1995). Quality of life assessment (WHOQOL): Position paper from the World Health Organization. *Social Science Medicine, 41*, 1403–1409.

Part VIII
Dancing the Lifespan

Chapter 29
Memoir of a Dancing Life

Teresa Benzwie

Have you ever seen a blade of grass growing up through a crack in concrete? When I look back over my life, this seems the perfect metaphor, as dance infused my being and wouldn't be ignored no matter what the challenges—like a dandelion, once freed, spreading its seedlings into the wind, each finding its own place in my world. Dance has defined and sustained me throughout my life. As a young child, I put music on the radio, shut the door, and danced to blot out my parents yelling. It was a safe way to keep out the craziness and make beautiful worlds of my own. My mother sent me to dancing school at about age seven to "help heal my rickets" (I didn't have rickets but who cares—this put me into the world of dance). Ever since then, dance has been a crucial part of my life.

Today I continue, persistently and tirelessly, to put my energy, heart and soul into promoting dance in the early childhood curriculum. My vision is for all children to have the opportunity to fully express their individuality through dancing while working together cooperatively as they learn. I know how important this was for me—perhaps for all beings, to be able to release and escape into beautiful worlds, worlds of our own making that dance can give us.

As a child, I wanted to become a professional ballerina or modern dancer but my mother didn't think I had the stamina for what she called a "nightlife." Nevertheless, I often danced in the privacy of my own living room for imaginary audiences and continued to take classes throughout my teen years at the New Dance Group in New York City. I danced spontaneously at every opportunity, sometimes winning Charleston dance contests. Having difficulty expressing myself with words, I began to claim English as a second language and dance as my first language. I still like to say dance is my first language as it does feel like a primary mode of expression and the passion in my work.

I also had a great love of children, so when it came time to decide on a college major I chose early childhood education. It was 1953 and I commuted every day on

T. Benzwie (✉)
Center for Creative Change, Cherry Hill, NJ, USA

K. Bond (ed.), *Dance and the Quality of Life*, Social Indicators Research Series 73,
https://doi.org/10.1007/978-3-319-95699-2_29

the "D" train from the Bronx to New York University in Greenwich Village. The 30 other young women in my program were dressed impeccably with their gloves and smart shoes. I, on the other hand, not having any sense of style, might show up with a stripes and polka dots combination. Also, having alopecia (hair loss) since age 13, I wore a wig. I didn't fit the NYU image of an early childhood teacher and was excluded from my peers' social activities. My supervisors suggested I transfer to physical education. I was strong enough to resist (I thank my father for this capability), and with parental support completed a master's in early childhood education. A fulfilling experience during my time at NYU was participation in the Boaz Arts performing arts festivals where I had the dance lead for all performances.

Fast forward ten or so years, to the late sixties. I am married with three sons, and after my youngest entered first grade, I began teaching kindergarten full time in Camden, New Jersey. I believed it was important for children to express themselves freely and have an outlet for their abundant energies. These children were quick to fight, as well as affectionate and excited by the learning experience. Being high energy myself and with a background of getting into trouble in elementary school for not paying attention, I understood these children.

Since movement felt so natural to me, I taught through engaging bodies and the space around us. I moved all the desks and chairs to one end of the room to create a large open space to dance, explore and learn. Children were able to apply their energy to create and problem-solve. Instead of getting into trouble, they were actively involved in the learning process. Instead of fighting, creative movement helped us to cooperate and get along with each other. At this time, I didn't know if there was anyone else combining dance with academics or if there were books on the subject or anything called "dance education." I was in my own little world doing what I loved.

During this period, an acquaintance suggested I look into a program at Temple University in Philadelphia, PA that was similar to how I was teaching. I was 34 years old and at a crossroads, having just become a single parent of three pre-teen sons. I followed through, not fully knowing why, but intuitively feeling there was something more for me. First I called the elementary education department, but was directed to the physical education department, who suggested I contact Edrie Ferdun in the dance program. *Finally, I landed where I belonged.* I met with Edrie (then in charge of the dance program in the College of Health, Physical Education, and Recreation, or HPER) in September of 1971. This was a momentous meeting that changed my life. I told Edrie about how I taught and she said, "What you do, we teach, and why don't you start your doctorate with us?" I entered the dance doctoral program in 1972 and for the first time received full support and acknowledgement for how I worked with children through movement.

Another life transformation happened in 1971 when I stopped wearing wigs, no longer wanting to hide my baldness. Being publicly without hair, artists stopped me in the street, asking to photograph, paint or sculpt me, and I was asked by choreographers who knew I was interested in dance to join their companies (Fig. 29.1). I performed in Philadelphia with South Street Dance Company at the Painted Bride, the Rita Jones Company at the Wilma Theater, and Plays and Players, as well as with

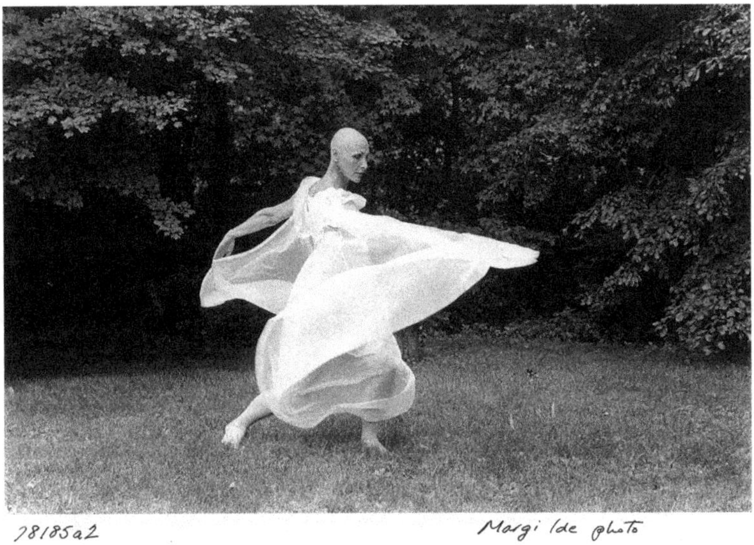

Fig. 29.1 Teresa Benzwie, early 1970s

the Manning-Fried Dance Company at the McCarter Theater in Princeton, New Jersey and Black Box in New York City. This was so exciting! At age 35, I was performing and realizing my childhood dream. I loved the camaraderie of being with dancers in rehearsal, however, actually performing made me extremely anxious.

One might assume I would have started studying more rigorously at this time to excel at being a "dancer," but I didn't. I realized I was no longer serious about performing, but found it interesting that becoming more myself, that is, getting rid of my wigs, gave me entry to the world of performance. My dancing career ended abruptly at age 40 when I fractured my hip. Some thought this was caused by too much stress: studying for doctoral comprehensive exams, teaching part time in the dance department at Temple, teaching kindergarten, and all the while being a single mom of three pre-teen sons. I guess I needed a "break," but not the one I got.

A few years later my oldest son Lawrence completely surprised me. In 1976, while studying civil engineering at the University of Maine, he telephoned to report that his girlfriend had invited him to take an African dance workshop with a visiting artist, Arthur Hall. I knew Arthur from Philadelphia and thought it fascinating that Lawrence met a dancer from "our own back yard." Furthermore, never having been interested in dance before, he now wanted a career as a modern dancer. He continued to study dance after graduation with Maggie Black and gained a scholarship to study with Luis Falco in New York City. Although he began late, Lawrence received a lot of support to become a professional dancer.

I saw a transformation in my son's body and his being. He stood taller and his face was more gentle and open. He was happier than I had ever experienced him, and we seemed to understand each other in a deeper way. Eventually, knee and back injuries stopped Lawrence from continuing. It was very sad to see that passion

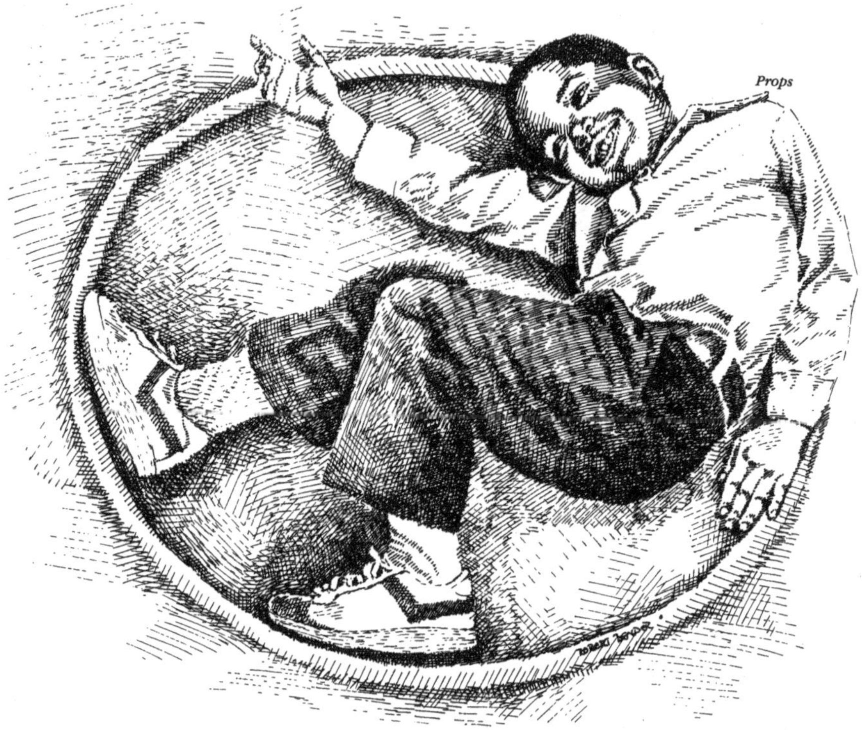

Fig. 29.2 Can you shape your body into something round? Feel your body soft and round. (Illustration: Robert Bender)

stamped out, but the affective changes remained. Years later, he named his son Misha after Mikhail Baryshnikov. Dance had reached his core. This is, I believe, what dance can do. It can change you physically and emotionally into a more creative, appreciative, spiritual being.

While Lawrence became passionate about dance, my youngest son Robert fell in love with drawing and later offered to illustrate my books, making my kindergarten children dance off the pages as in the images below (from Benzwie, 1987) (Figs. 29.2 and 29.3). My son Craig, having had piano lessons in both youth and adulthood, became an advocate for music. He was well into his career with IBM when he began to hold professional music concerts in his home to raise money to buy musical instruments for the local elementary school. He named this effort, "Kids need Music." It is deeply gratifying as a parent to know that my children "caught" my love of the arts and are passing it into the future.

As introduced above, I entered doctoral coursework at Temple in 1972, where I began to develop a language to describe and explain my teaching methods and gain confidence to share my work with administrators in the Camden, New Jersey school district. Prior to that I was a "closet" dance teacher. I would switch to a more traditional way of teaching when any supervisors came into my classroom. I did however, choreograph dances for special holidays and my students performed in the

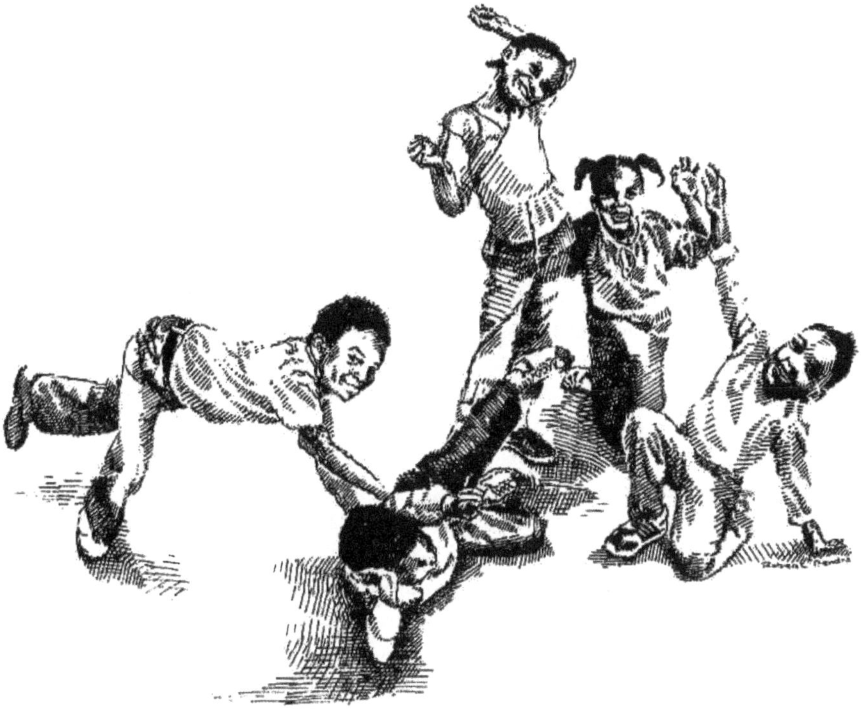

Fig. 29.3 Creating real, fantasy or current events stories with different levels, directions and group cooperation. (Illustration: Robert Bender)

auditorium for the whole school. For example, on Arbor Day the children danced as trees burning to Wagner's (1856) *Die Walküre* and then grew into new beautiful trees to "Morning" from Edvard Grieg's (1875) *Peer Gynt Suite*.

On Martin Luther King Day, we danced to his famous speech, "I have a dream" (King Jr., 1963). We began our performance by marching from the back of the auditorium onto the stage carrying peace and civil rights signs and singing, "We shall overcome…" Children's dances showed how we could get along together. My kindergarteners also performed at Temple University for my choreography class. It was the early 70s and I was an activist. I marched on Washington for the civil rights and peace movement with my three sons and held fund raising parties in my home. Activism stimulated my educational philosophy in which dance was a way to help children cooperate and get along as well as appreciate themselves and each other's differences. This evolved into appreciation for nature and our world. Our performances and learnings highlighted respect and care for all life. Philosophical influences also included the pioneers of humanistic psychology: Abraham Maslow's (1962/1999) theory of self-actualization (see Chap. 30, this volume), Carl Rogers' (1961/1995) "person-centered approach," and Fritz Perls' (1969/1992) *Gestalt Therapy Verbatim*. These psychology giants founded the Association for Humanistic Psychology, where I took many workshops as well as presenting my work on creative movement. Presenters I remember best who added to my teaching repertoire were psychologist and author Jean Houston, and dance therapist Poldi Orlando.

During the 15 years I taught in Camden, I tried different ways to persuade the administration to incorporate dance in the academic programs. One year I joined the Curriculum Steering Committee and another year wrote a paper about learning through movement. Yet another year I researched how movement helps learning and the next year gave the teachers in my school 20-minute workshops every morning before the children arrived. I went into other schools on my lunch hour to give movement workshops. Teachers showed up and seemed to enjoy the movement experiences, but no one that I knew of made practical use of it with their own students. Each year I looked for another way to stimulate interest in learning through creative movement. Nothing seemed to work. I began to have a reputation for being creative but it felt more like I was being patted on the head condescendingly, like a pet dog.

As part of my doctoral dissertation Edrie suggested I make a film showing my kindergarten children learning through dance. I found a filmmaker, Richard Gaughan, who wanted to make a 16 mm color and sound film without being paid. I only had to fund materials and printing. A close friend, Sheila Greenberg, narrated and edited, while another friend, Aida Epstein, a professional pianist, played classical music as background. My students' parents gave permission for their children to participate. The result, *Math: A Moving Experience* shows children exploring creative movement, imagination, and props to learn mathematical concepts such as numbers, counting, shapes and vocabulary (Benzwie & Gaughan, 1981).

The film depicts a holistic environment where children and teacher are free to cooperate, laugh, touch, and dance together. It demonstrates a child-centered and process-oriented approach that emphasizes creative problem solving and positive reinforcement. It highlights children as individuals and in interactive relationships. Making the film was a fun and loving experience. I was excited to see the children take leadership spontaneously and come up with ideas of their own. During the making process, I often played the film back in my mind reconfiguring its parts. Then I would splice these different scenes together, which felt like magic. Even now in 2017, when I look at the film I smile and feel proud of the children, knowing how important it was for them to have had the opportunity to dance to learn.

One year, a professional dance company came into our school for 2 weeks for an "Arts in Education" residency. I remember that day they arrived very clearly. The dancers came down the school hallway dressed in leotards and ballet slippers. I recall one teacher's negative reaction. In an annoyed voice, she said, "Are we here to teach reading or dance?" Her arms gestured strongly and quickly to the right and then to the left to accentuate her "either-or" question. I kept her in mind when creating the film, as my philosophy was to incorporate movement as another teaching modality for all subjects.

As the years went on, I continued being committed to this work by writing books (Benzwie, 1987, 1996, 2002, 2011; Benzwie & Scott, n.d.) and giving workshops. More and more children were being diagnosed with attention-deficit/hyperactivity disorder (ADHD). I didn't understand why teachers were insisting on seeing children as dysfunctional and badly behaved when I felt many just loved being physically engaged in the learning process. Why not use children's energies constructively to learn and enjoy school? Instead many children were being given medication. I was only half-joking when I said it would be better to put teachers on medication to help them be with children with bodily enthusiasm.

Sometimes I was asked what I wanted to do after completing the doctorate. I always answered: "I might become the only kindergarten teacher in the world who has a doctorate in dance." I loved what I was doing and had no intention of changing my work. I gained permission to work only a half-day with the morning kindergarten class, as I wanted to have time to give workshops outside the Camden, New Jersey school district. I was then moved from one school to another depending on which had a half-day kindergarten.

After 15 years of teaching, giving professional development workshops, and showing my film, I realized that I wasn't going to fulfill my dream in Camden. During my final year, my students and I shared space in an extra-large room divided by a barrier with the reading teacher on the other side. She was the wife of an assistant superintendent and complained to my supervisor that there was too much noise coming from my space. We often accompanied our dancing with music and the children's self-expression created an "enthusiastic environment." My supervisor paid me a visit. She asked if I could take my children into the gym for the movement lesson so there wouldn't be so much noise for the other teacher. I remember saying, "Yes ma'am" (I don't usually use the term "ma'am") and "knew" in that moment they were never going to understand my work. Although I loved working with the children, who I continued to experience as sweet, loving, accepting, and committed to learning and being together, I no longer wanted to put energy into fighting the system. As for the "gym," which was dirty and smelly, it was also the cafeteria and a walk-through to other areas of the school.

The philosophy of my work is to incorporate creative movement throughout the day in the classroom rather than as a different subject in a gym. For example, movement can be offered for a few moments, with one child sitting at their desk attempting to write the letter B and needing help to make the round parts go to the right. I would take the child's hand and arm, assisting her to move to the right, saying, "The B goes this way to the right," helping the child experience the direction of the B in their body. Or, I would work with the whole class for 20 min using the entire space, with music to introduce or culminate a lesson. I integrated dance into all subjects throughout the day. While I wanted to think that teachers and administrators in the Camden school district were "getting it," I finally concluded that no matter what I might do, it wasn't going to make a difference to how the system thought about working through the arts. I left at the end of that school year, 1986, 5 years after completing the EdD in Dance degree at Temple.

I continued writing and giving workshops around the country and abroad, promoting and encouraging others to include creative movement in the classroom. It was an exciting time and I met many who believed in this way of working. My books were selling and participants in my workshops appreciated creative arts methods. However, I didn't see any systemic changes in how children were being taught in public schools. More and more, standardized tests were being used to assess children's learning. Teachers began teaching to these tests, as there was a lot of pressure for children to achieve. It seemed a vicious circle, as children became stressed in the face of a very difficult and arguably boring way of learning. I trudged along teaching and writing, never giving up. During my doctoral work, I was asked to teach "Dance Experiences for Children" in Temple University's dance department. I had never taught college before and came across Barbara Mettler's self-published books, *Basic Dance on a College Level* (Mettler & Warner, 1954) and *Materials of Dance as a Creative Art Activity* (Mettler, 1960/1979), which were aligned with my humanistic philosophy.

Opportunities present themselves from seemingly nowhere. At one particular time, I was asked to present to a group of psychology professors at the University of Copenhagen. I was nervous about this, as I was not used to standing on a stage lecturing. Normally I have my group actively participating with me. So I asked a child psychiatrist, Edwin Castillo, MD, whom I knew casually, to review my slide presentation. Afterwards, he invited me to work with him in his psychiatric practice with pre-teen boys. We connected and developed an ongoing professional relationship that included his mentoring and supervising my therapeutic practice with other clients. I loved this new venture and decided to go back to school one more time to get a master's in clinical social work. After graduation, I opened my own office/studio/space (I didn't know how to refer to this "alternative" kind of work space). It was full of expressive materials, art supplies, toys, and plenty of room to dance. I had my perfect place to do all the things I loved, connecting education with feelings and the arts.

My work in dance took me to new places where I felt at peace and the world seemed welcoming. In 1982 the International Conference on Universal Education invited me to offer a workshop in dance education in Pomona, Italy at a monks' sanctuary. The monks participated with their robes flying in the wind and faces filled with smiles. Surrounded by gentle rolling hills, it was so peaceful that butterflies would light on my shoulder or arms and remain there. One evening a group of us decided to go to a local pub, and it was suggested I bring my records. Yes, I lugged about 40 long playing records with me across the Atlantic along with my many colorful scarves.

We entered the pub and found a group of middle-aged men sitting in a row with serious expressions on their faces. None were interacting in any way. In another corner of the room I observed a group of young men and women in their early twenties, also not interacting. I played my records and threw about 100 scarves up in the air. My conference friends immediately caught the scarves and began to dance. The young group followed suit and also began to dance with each other, wearing and using the scarves to create choreography and costumes. Finally, the older men each took a scarf and waved it from their seats, smiling. The pub was transformed into a good humored, energetic, intermingling group.

Another strong dance memory is from 1995 when I took a photographic safari to Tanzania with a museum group. One day we visited a Masai Village. About 25 of us arrived to find some 40 Masai men, women and children of all ages lined up waiting. We stood this way for a while, looking at each other, neither group crossing over to connect with the other. Eventually, I walked over to say hello to a baby held by their mother. Then some of the Masai began to drum and I started moving to the rhythm. Some of the women began laughing and I felt encouraged to move more.

Eventually a Masai woman who was laughing more than the others came into the center and began dancing. I moved toward her and joined in her dance as she continued to smile. I followed her lead and mirrored her as much as possible. Two decades later, I still remember how we ended our dance. Kneeling down on one knee and facing a little to the left and right of one other, we each rested a hand on the other's shoulder, still smiling. It felt so good to be in communication this way as we didn't know each other's language. We eventually stood up and separated. My group then began to approach the Masai people, who were also moving toward their visitors. We began to intermingle. Dance was the connector. While dance scholars have debated whether dance can be called a universal language, my experience is that dance can be a mutual language across cultures—it is my first language.

I was getting older—70 years old to be exact, and it was becoming more difficult to get up from the floor and run around doing workshops to promote dance in education. In 2005, I decided it was time to start an award program to stimulate young dance majors to do this work. I felt Temple University's Department of Dance, specifically Edrie Ferdun, had done so much for me that I wanted to give back. I created the Teresa Benzwie Dance in Education Award to be granted annually to a dance major interested in promoting "dancing to learn." After a few years, dance faculty Karen Bond suggested that I mentor dance majors who received the award, and a new phase of professional advocacy began. Our first program was at Meade Elementary School, a local school near the Temple campus. The following year, a change in school administration at Meade necessitated a shift of venue, which ended up being the Barclay Early Childhood Center in Cherry Hill, New Jersey. Two years later, the BFA in Dance coordinator, Jillian Harris, developed the program into a credit-bearing fieldwork elective, which enables more students to participate.

Since 2009, I have been bringing groups of dance majors into classrooms at the Barclay Early Childhood Center where William Marble, then principal, was excited to have us and completely supported the program. We develop dance experiences from the classroom teacher's lesson plans. The children, ages three to five, some with special needs, are learning academics through creative movement. Many of the classroom teachers continue to use our dance lessons afterwards. It is fulfilling and heartwarming to finally have this program accepted, supported, and consistently sought after.

In 2014, with a new principal, Karen Rockhill, environmental studies became a focus at the Barclay school. Coincidentally, I had become more involved in global warming issues. I began to include environmental topics in our creative movement lessons such as: the cycle of apples, weather, trees, and recycling. Karen invited me to join the school's "Green Team," a group of teachers who were developing an environmental program to fulfill the requirements of a small grant. To this end I expanded the lesson plans my students and I developed about environmental issues into a creative movement curriculum called *Have Apples - Will Move* (Benzwie 2016). The principal offered to share this work with all her teachers.

After many years of trying to establish creative movement as part of the curriculum—with all the degrees, books, workshops and energy put toward this effort—the dots were starting to connect. In 2016, the Cherry Hill, New Jersey school superintendent disseminated *Have Apples - Will Move* to early childhood classrooms throughout the district. At the Barclay Early Childhood Center, Karen Rockhill now asks all teachers to integrate movement into their lesson plans and is hoping to create a part-time position in the school for a graduate of my program. I often say (tongue in cheek), you just have to live long enough to see your dreams fulfilled. This is an exciting time, as life can begin again at 80.

Through my experience with alopecia, I learned to appreciate difference and that differences can be celebrated and cherished. Creative movement emphasizes that all individuals have a unique way of moving, that there is more than one answer to a problem, and all interpretations can be valid. How many ways can we make the letter B with our body? We can use our fingers or our whole body; we can do it standing or lying down, by ourselves or with a partner or a whole group. These are just a few of the many ways children can discover. Dance can promote individuality, laughter, learning, and self-awareness, no matter who "the self" might be on a given day. Dance can make things right, with no need to bully or harm others.

What makes one so passionate about something to make it a life-long adventure? Possibly some of this is inherited and some modeled. My mother told me stories of her childhood—such as dancing in the street to the tune of the organ grinder with his little monkey holding a tin cup for donations, and also shared her love of children and the arts. My father had a beautiful singing voice and sometimes I accompanied him on the piano. Whatever I was doing, becoming, professionally interested in, or emotionally growing into, dance was my entrance—the place I could be myself, develop, and share my passions.

Dance has been my way of surviving through trauma and celebrating important events. Dance has given me opportunities to create special worlds, a home that I could count on, a space of worship I could go to, where the world became the perfect place to be. Dance was transformative, permeating the different phases of my life. I'm still teaching, writing, and especially daydreaming about a world where all children feel loved and appreciated while they learn through creative movement to be all they can be.

In 2015, I turned 80 and threw myself a big outdoor celebration. Dance was the main attraction. I began a performance dancing to Debussy's (1905) *Clair de Lune*, with my Temple dance students joining in. A DJ played throughout the day. It was a great party with close to a hundred family, friends and colleagues involved, feeling good, and dancing. My nine-year-old grandson, Ellis, surprised me by breaking out into spontaneous performance. I was ecstatic throughout the day as most of those I cared about were dancing with me. With dance my life took flight and still does.

Did I say life begins at 80? Little did I realize what else was in my future. In July 2017 at age 82, I happened to meet Carrie Christiansen, a teacher of horsemanship. I began learning how to communicate with, ride, and dance with a horse named

Pegasa—17.1 hands high—a very big and beautiful horse. She was gentle and patient with me as I learned how to use my energy and intention to let her know what I would like from her. I am sharing Dancing with Horses with my Temple dance students and the teenage students at the horse barn. It's a whole new non-judgmental world where I am also learning more about myself. There doesn't seem to be any end to the ways I can find love and happiness, and create beautiful worlds through dance.

Acknowledgment I am grateful to Jane Bonbright and Rima Faber of the National Dance Education Organization (NDEO) for their support in publishing my 2002 book, *Alphabet Movers*.

References

Benzwie, T. (1987). *A moving experience: Dance for lovers of children and the child within*. Tucson, AZ: Zephyr.
Benzwie, T. (1996). *More moving experiences: Connecting the arts, feelings and imagination*. Bethesda, MD: National Dance Education Organization.
Benzwie, T. (2002). *Alphabet movers*. Bethesda, MD: National Dance Education Organization.
Benzwie, T. (2011). *Numbers on the move*. Philadelphia, PA: Temple University Press.
Benzwie, T. (2016). Have apples – Will move. Complimentary copies available from Teresa Benzwie: benzwie@aol.com.
Benzwie, T. (Producer), & Gaughan, R. (Director). (1981). Math: A moving experience (16 mm film). Cherry Hill, NJ: T. Benzwie.
Benzwie, T., & Scott, D. Write dance draw: Creating peace and health for self and our world. (Unpublished monograph).
King, M. L., Jr. (1963). I have a dream… Retrieved from https://www.archives.gov/files/press/exhibits/dream-speech.pdf
Maslow, A. (1999). *Toward a psychology of being* (3rd ed.). New York: Wiley (Original work published 1962).
Mettler, B. (1979). *Materials of dance as a creative art activity*. Tucson, AZ: Mettler Studios (Original work published 1960).
Mettler, B., & Warner, J. (1954). *Basic dance on a college level*. Tucson, AZ: Mettler Studios.
Perls, F. H. (1992). *Gestalt therapy verbatim*. Gouldsboro, ME: The Gestalt Journal Press (Original work published 1969).
Rogers, C. (1995). *On becoming a person*. New York: Houghton Mifflin (Original work published 1961).

Chapter 30
Dancing in the Setting Sun: Performance, Self-Actualization and the Elderly

Nicholas Rowe, David McMicken, and Tim Newth

The Dancing Elderly

> I thought how little we know about the feelings of old people. Children we understand, their fears and hopes and make-believe. (Du Maurier, 1938, p. 43)

It was once presumed that the human inclination to shift between reality and make-believe diminishes with our exit from childhood (Piaget, 1929). An interest in imaginary realms however, can continue throughout life; perhaps this is part of our human bio-cultural endowment, what Ellen Dissanayake calls "aesthetic imagination" (Dissanayake, 2001). While age brings increasing physical challenges, dancing can remain a vehicle for elderly individuals to navigate fear, to realize hope, and to become immersed in make-believe. Dancing, as an embodied way to re-imagine the past, present and future, provides a life-long doorway to experiences of fantasy (Stinson, 1985, 1997; Chap. 29, this volume).

The feelings of children and the elderly have received much scholarly attention in the eight decades since Daphne Du Maurier wrote the above lines, yet the uncertainty expressed by them continues to resonate. While research into young people has contributed to the advancement of dance in formal education, academic attention to elderly people has tended to focus on the remedial functions of dance and creativity in affording mental and physical wellbeing. There has been scant consideration of how dance performance can enhance the personal and creative development of older participants.

N. Rowe (✉)
University of Auckland, Auckland, New Zealand
e-mail: n.rowe@auckland.ac.nz

D. McMicken · T. Newth
Tracks Dance Company, Darwin, Australia
e-mail: david@tracksdance.com.au

K. Bond (ed.), *Dance and the Quality of Life*, Social Indicators Research Series 73,
https://doi.org/10.1007/978-3-319-95699-2_30

What are our ongoing assumptions about the creative concerns and aspirations of elderly people? As community dance practitioners, the authors of this chapter acknowledge the importance of such reflective exploration. Two of the authors (David and Tim) are directors of Tracks Dance Company, based in the city of Darwin in northern Australia, sometimes known at The Top End. Tracks Dance Company administers the Grey Panthers, a volunteer-based dance organization that has sustained an active community-of-practice amongst elderly dancers for three decades. The third author (Nicholas) designs and researches undergraduate and postgraduate dance programs, and has worked with the Grey Panthers as a guest choreographer and teacher. During a post-workshop discussion, Nicholas commented on the remarkable commitment that the Grey Panthers show towards their art, and we began to reflect on the performance aspirations of older dancers. We sought to understand more fully elderly individuals' experiences of learning, creating and especially performing dance, and to begin to consider how particular pedagogic and choreographic practices might support or inhibit their engagement.

The dancers in this group generally start to perform dance after middle age, and so their transition into dance performance as elderly people opens further queries as to what motivates such a deliberate engagement. Their needs and aspirations as "the dancing elderly" can be seen as distinct from those of "elderly dancers," that is, aging professional dance artists who continue to explore their art later in life, notably Dame Margaret Scott (Potter, 2014) and Sir Robert Helpman (Salter, 1978) in Australia and Anna Halprin (Ross, 2007b) and Liz Lerman (2011) in the United States. We have sought to understand why dancers in the Grey Panthers chose to start performing, what they value about performing dance, and how performing might affect their sense of belonging, visibility and distinction within their local community.

This research extends the literature on associations between quality of life, dancing, and the elderly (Bolwell, 2017; Centre for Policy on Ageing, 2011; Connolly & Redding, 2010; Cooper & Thomas, 2002; Hanna & Perlstein, 2008; Houston, 2005; Keogh, Kilding, Pidgeon, Ashley & Gills, 2009; Thomas & Cooper, 2003). Within this field of inquiry, three broad associations with quality of life recur: dance and physical health, dance and mental health, and dance and social inclusion. Existing literature generally focuses on exercise and socializing aspects of participating in dance, as distinct from performing dance (Nahachewsky, 1995). This study's additional interest in dance performance by the elderly allows us to expand the discourse on dance and the elderly into relatively uncharted terrain. Through a grounded theory approach (Bryant & Charmaz, 2007), the study elucidates participating Grey Panthers' motivations for dancing and performing through humanistic psychologist Abraham Maslow's (1943, 1970) hierarchy of human needs.

Darwin, Northern Territory and the Grey Panthers: "You lot are making the oldies invisible!"

Darwin is the administrative capital of the sparsely populated Northern Territory of Australia. It was established as a colonial port in 1869 on land inhabited by the indigenous Larrakia people, and has been completely destroyed four times, by war and weather events. The population is predominantly young, with a median age 33 (the youngest of Australian capital cities), and descended from Northern Europe, with substantial minorities identifying as indigenous Australian, Pacific, South and East Asian, and Southern European. A significant proportion of the population is employed in the public sector and the military, many of whom are from other Australian cities completing temporary postings in Darwin. This, along with Darwin's remoteness (more than 3,000 kilometres distant from other Australian cities), contributes to a relatively transient population. The hot, wet, and dry tropical weather and distance from family members in the more populous south and east of Australia also result in relatively few people choosing to spend their retirement in Darwin (Australian Bureau of Statistics, 2016). These factors all contribute to invisibility of the elderly population and of the ways that a sense of intergenerational and intercultural community might be constructed and sustained.

The Grey Panthers emerged out of the *Dance on Darwin* community arts project in 1988, which sought to showcase the variety of local community dance organizations within an open-air festival. Community artist Beth Shelton was visiting Darwin, co-directing the project with Darwin Dance Mob, a local modern dance group, and Brown's Mart Community Arts, Darwin's longstanding community arts hub (Tracks Dance Company, 2015a). Tim recalls that Shelton commended the inclusion of various types of cultural dancers from the local community, but she noted the absence of anyone over the age of 40, exclaiming, "Where's the rest of the community? Where are the oldies? You lot are making the oldies invisible!"

This prompted Shelton to initiate the Senior Adult Darwin Dance Mob, which, according to Tim, she announced by standing on a table in the bar at the local Returned Services League (RSL) Club. In a venue and a city that exemplifies Australia's veneration of youth and masculinity (Mewett, 1988), this declaration that the elderly—particularly elderly women—should be seen and valued, established the loud-and-proud tone of what would become the Grey Panthers. Tim recounts that from its inception, the group aimed to be a performance troupe and not simply a participatory social dance group.

Grey Panthers' productions have included small-scale performances in theatres, retirement homes, and social clubs, for community events and television advertisements, and for large scale, evening length, site-specific productions such as Old Spice Club Cabaret (1992), Healthy Wealthy and Wise (1995), Reluctant Retirees

(1999), Dear Auntie (2001), A Bowls Club Wedding (2003, 2006), Lipstick and Ochre (2008), and Future Age (2013). The Grey Panthers have also collaborated inter-generationally as guest performers within Tracks Dance's major performances 4WD Sweat Dust and Romance (1997), Bodies of Light (1997), Love Versus Gravity (2000), Fierce, the Story of Olive Pink (2001), Allure of Paradise (2010), and Last Light (2015) (Tracks Dance Company, 2015b).

As David recalls, establishment of the Senior Adult Darwin Dance Mob coincided with Tracks Dance's initiation of an annual dance residency in Lajamanu (a remote town in Northern Australia) with Indigenous elders through Yawulyu Senior Women's Traditional Dance Group. The idea of maintaining the cultural relevance and visibility of elderly people underpinned Track's engagement with elders as dancers in both multicultural Darwin and indigenous Lajamanu. The relationship between the two groups was further extended through creative and performance collaborations in the productions Fierce, the Story of Olive Pink (2001) and Lipstick and Ochre (2008).

Maintaining a regular weekly class throughout the year, the Darwin-based dancers' commitments to the group escalate during performance seasons, to daily rehearsals and performances. While the age of the dancers was originally stipulated as 50 and above, by 2010 the Grey Panthers had grown to over 30 active members, so the group established a minimum entry age of 60. As a result, the group became predominantly one of retirees, who could commit the time to regular classes, rehearsals and performances. Social inclusion otherwise remained central to the group's values, the only requirement of those wishing to join being a willingness to move and a commitment to attend classes and rehearsals.

The longevity and reputation of the group allowed the idea to crystalize in the local psyche, so that people who were in their twenties and thirties when the group first began are becoming eligible to join. As dancer Val Hristova shared, "My daughter can't wait to become a Grey Panther!" Janine Sutter explained how the idea of joining developed for her:

> I'd seen Tracks perform and knew a couple of the ladies that do it…I was having a chat with them and they said "come along, come along, it's good fun!" so I thought when I retire that's something I'd like to do.

In some cases, joining meant dancing and performing for the first time. For others, it's a return to a practice they had engaged in in their youth.

The tropical environment of Darwin has been central to the group's major productions, which are created and performed in local sites such as bowling clubs and public gardens. These site-responsive productions explore local cross-cultural histories and themes of multicultural isolation, reflecting a distinct Indigenous/Asian/European/Pacific cultural ambience in the Top End, and the performers in the group at any one time usually represent Darwin's multi-ethnic diversity. Dance pieces ultilizing local props and sets, such as washing lines and Banyan trees, further locate the choreographed works within contexts that are familiar to the performers. These works have been created collaboratively through commissions with local and international dance artists and teachers (Tracks Dance Company, 2015b).

As of 2017, more than 103 dancers, mostly women, have at one period or another considered themselves members of the Grey Panthers, participating in weekly classes, daily rehearsals, and seasons of performance. The majority have remained members of the group for more than five years. This involves a significant investment of time and energy, raising the question of what attracts them to the group and retains their commitment, year after year, especially since many do not seem to lack a satisfying social life. Resident director and teacher David observes that when he attends funerals for Grey Panther members, he is "continually amazed to hear stories about the rich and diverse lives these women have led. They are all so different, and have so much else going on in their lives and with their families."

Grounded Theory to Hierarchy of Needs: "There's no forced performance"

Following University of Auckland Human Participant Ethics protocols, dancers of the Grey Panthers were offered the opportunity to be interviewed for this study. Twelve dancers volunteered to participate and gave their informed consent to be identified by their real names. Interviewees include Judith Allen, Toni Vine Bromley, Darryl Butler, Jan Hastings, Val Hrstova, Marg Lee, Lillian Mann, Judy McKerr, Glad Morris, Shirley Somers, Janine Sutter, and Maria Vlastuin. All are over 65 years of age and had been with the group for at least five years.

Our orienting research question concerned why Grey Panther members make time for this activity and how they derive value from it. As educator-artists aspiring to dialogic (Freire, 1972) and humanizing (Salazar, 2013) approaches to community development, our research practices began through discussion with the dancers—listening to their viewpoints and prompting their reflections. We were concerned to avoid the common situation where voices of dancers themselves are not present within scholarly research and where there are too many assumptions and stereotypes regarding their interests (Bond & Stinson, 2000/2001; Risner, 1995; Stinson, Blumenfeld-Jones, & Van Dyke, 1990).

Through semi-structured, qualitative interviews (Denzin & Lincoln, 1998), we invited participants to consider the various learning, choreographic, rehearsal and performance experiences they had had with the group, to identify what they valued and found problematic, and to reflect on meanings they made from these experiences. Our mix of insider (David and Tim) and outsider (Nicholas) roles, present in both interviews and subsequent analysis, helped initiate fresh dialogues with the research participants and prompt them to contextualize their perspectives, while confronting assumptions that can become established through day-to-day practices and relationships (Fine, 1994). Participants were offered the opportunity to withdraw, pause or revisit their reflections throughout the interviews. The research process involved five individual interviews, allowing singular personal narratives to be extended, and two focus group discussions in which group members prompted each other's reflections.

While the number of research participants is limited, the diversity of their perspectives reveals that aspirations of elderly dancers are varied. This aligned with our research aim, which was to avoid reductive analysis and instead to reveal differences and complexity within the phenomenon of dance, performance and the elderly. Following a grounded theory approach (Bryant & Charmaz, 2007), we allowed the responses from the initial interviews to give rise to salient themes. These themes were coded, which prompted realizations associated with psychologist Abraham Maslow's (1970) "hierarchy of needs" and a return to subsequent interviews to further explore these emergent themes (Boyatzis, 1998). Both distinct and overlapping concepts elucidated the dancers' valuing of dancing and performance.

Our interest in performance as a *sustained* community-building activity, within an organization that retains membership over several years, brings a depth perspective to questions of dance, performance and the elderly. Our premise was that a sense of community can be constructed by the significance and solidarity felt by long-term members of Grey Panthers (Clarke, 1973), and that performing dance can support this community-building process (Rowe, Buck & Martin, 2015). We wanted to discover whether a sustained practice of performing within a localized repertory company could benefit elderly dancers' holistic quality of life (physical, social, cognitive and emotional), both within the Grey Panthers and within the culturally diverse but youth oriented and somewhat isolated society of Darwin.

While the Grey Panthers have a public profile as a performance troupe, the group does not require its members to perform. Sometimes the dancers participate in class and rehearsal for several years before they join performances. Experienced members may break from performing in response to personal issues or health concerns. Janine Sutter explains, "There's no forced performance. Whoever was teaching us always said, 'If you don't want to do a performance you don't have to.'" According to Jan, most Grey Panthers do choose to perform; we view such agency as an indicator of self-actualization.

Each Grey Panthers production has involved a devising process to prepare the dancers to perform through helping to create original productions. This approach contrasts with performance contexts where dancers present traditional dance steps or sequences of choreography that have been created elsewhere (Silvester & Frampton, 2014) and, further, allows experiences of exploring and exercising one's imagination (Craft, 2005). Research has indicated that performing dance can be valued by the elderly, although such studies have focused on more transient gatherings of elderly individuals within specific dance performance projects (Barr, 2013; Eisner, 2010; Lerman, 2011; Lomas, 2007; Ross, 2007a).

Research Findings: From Physiology to Self-Actualization

As introduced earlier, grounded theory analysis of dancers' interviews led us to frame the research findings in Abraham Maslow's (1943, 1970, 1976) theory of motivation as articulated in a tiered hierarchy of human needs, often depicted as a

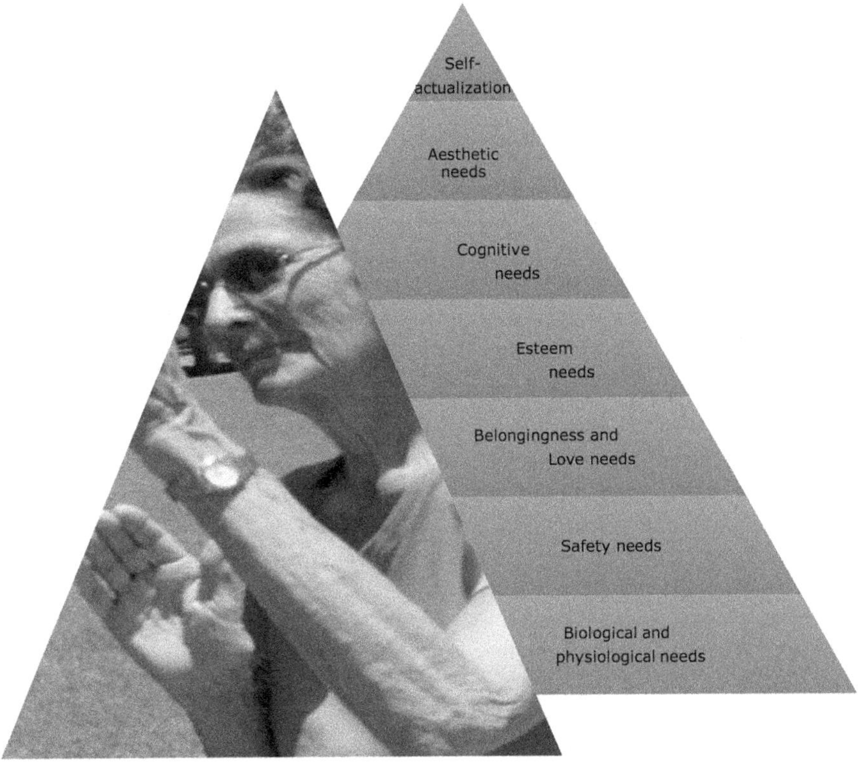

Fig. 30.1 Maslow's hierarchy

pyramid (Fig. 30.1). Maslow originally identified five needs—physiological, safety, belonging, esteem and self-actualization, and by the 1970s two others were elaborated that are salient to the present study: cognitive and aesthetic.

Physiological and Safety Needs: "Its better than taking a pill!"

The base of Maslow's hierarchy is the composite of bio-physiological needs that are fundamental to life, often listed as air, water, food, sleep and sex. For purposes of this chapter, we highlight moving as a human need, arguing that all other physiological needs support fulfillment of animate life's primary process: productive, and for humans, meaningful movement (Sheets-Johnstone, 1999/2011). In interviews, dancers talked about the importance of moving for the aged and its centrality in motivating them to join and stay with the group. As Glad Morris noted when the Grey Panthers started, "It is better than taking a pill!" (Tracks Dance Company, 2015b). Val Hristova sums up, "I came for all the usual reasons—to keep weight down, keep fit, keep flexible." Maintaining their dance practice has been a way to navigate the physiological challenges that older age brings, and for recovering from illness or injury. Marg Lee reflects, "Since the cancer I don't have the flexibility I used to have. One of the side effects is stiffening of the joints. So the exercise is good. I want to get my stamina back." Instead of being a reason to stop dancing, age becomes a reason to start or *keep* dancing.

Touch and Sensuality Physical interactions between the Grey Panthers provide moments during the week when the dancers can safely touch other human beings. Tactility threads throughout classes and rehearsals. Dancers engage in non-weight bearing physical connection within improvisational tasks and choreographed moves; during rehearsals, they hold hands and share hugs in response to dance sequences working or moves being forgotten.

The Grey Panthers are mostly women, which within the 'frontier masculinity' of Darwin (Mewett, 1988), provides a safe space for frank expression of sensuality and sexual desire. One of the 'Broadway numbers' the Grey Panthers dance within the social club circuit is performed to the Tom Jones song, *It's not Unusual*. At a particular point, the dancers sing over the lyrics with a new line, "It's not unusual to want sex at sixty-five!" David remarked that the shimmies and wiggles within some of the choreography allow the dancers to express themselves as sensual and sexual beings. While this theme does not pervade the Panthers' creative work, opportunities for sexual expression allow dancers to challenge age-norms regarding sexual presence.

One of Maslow's (1943) early premises was that human motivation transcends any distinct categorical criteria: "The integrated wholeness of the organism must be one of the foundation stones of motivation theory" (p. 370). Over 50 years later, advances in neuroscience validate a more holistic perspective on 'the physiological' (Lane & Nadel, 2001; Simonov, 2013) and we elaborate Maslow's physiological needs criteria to include dancers' psycho-physical descriptions. For example, emotional experience requires arousal of the nervous system, as affirmed by Judy McKerr's comment about how quickly the mood changes "as soon as the music is on." Val shared, "I've always loved dance and loved moving." From the laughter and smiles authors have observed permeating classes and rehearsals, it seems apparent that dancing provides these dancers an emotional high, or physiologically, a boost in endorphins.

Perhaps for the elderly dancer in particular, safety needs are closely related to the physiological, including the emotional. Some dancers expressed concerns over fears of injury in some structured exercise classes, such as aerobics. Several identified how much they value the Panther dance classes being tailored for them. Janine Sutter noted, "Whoever has been teaching the class has been very aware of the limitations of the people, but trying to extend them as far as they could."

Jan Hastings talked about her sense of emotional safety being part of the group:

> I'm shy, but since being at Panthers I can cope with a lot more things. When we did one of the shows where you had to mix with the audience, I was terrified at first…, meeting strangers, talking, dancing around them. I was a lot more confident doing the show the second time. The fact that you're doing this with your friends, the Panthers, that you are all doing the same thing, that nobody is being visibly attacked or anything!

Love and Belonging: "You know, I'm with friends!"

Many Grey Panthers' disclosures about reasons for participating in dance and performance highlight the fulfillment of social needs. Janine explained, "It wasn't the performances, it was the coming every week." Many identified themselves as widows, and expressed that the obligation to attend regular dance classes and rehearsals provided a sense of belonging that helped them recover from the loss of a partner. Marg reflects on her time with the Grey Panthers, "It's been eleven years, because it's eleven years today that I lost my husband."

Participants value dancing and performing as a way of creating community, providing a focal point for friendships to be sustained and new relationships to form. Janine explains,

> I wouldn't be doing it if I didn't think I could be part of a team. We've got lovely relationships amongst the ladies. We get to know each other and share our lives – it's nice to be able to do that at our stage of life… All of us come from different backgrounds and yet we are on a level playing field when it comes to dance.

Shirley Somers emphasized how her sense of belonging within the group enhances her confidence on stage:

> The first time one of the ladies here said to me, "Are you nervous?" I hadn't thought about that. You know, I'm with friends! They've all been practicing with me. I'm quite comfortable.

Describing the process of *Swings and Flings* (2013), Lillian Mann reflected on how the dancers' social bond was enhanced through their shared contributions to the conception of a choreographic work:

> That rural one was really excellent … it really showed the other side of how people lived. We all bonded together very well... When waving goodbye, I can always remember people saying, "Stay there until your visitors go." And in that scene, when we were waving goodbye, we all had tears in our eyes. And here was dance, mixing with everyday life, making it so beautiful.

The above narratives depict a sense of belonging as dancers among other dancers—the Panthers form a community of practitioners. Lillian suggests this community is privy to particular segments of the wider Darwin population, with the "other side of how people lived' suggesting insights into the isolated life of rural women in past eras, with lost cultural practices such as waving to departing visitors until they are out of sight. This aligns with research investigating the impact of intergenerational dance performance practices (Borstel, 2006; Lerman, 2011).

Belonging Within the Local Community The Grey Panthers was established to make Darwin's elderly more visible and reveal their creative potential. Regard for the Grey Panthers is shown by a strong and loyal audience base, and affirmed by fellow performers within the intergenerational productions that they join, such as the Tracks Dance Company's 2015 outdoor production of *Last Light*. Such performative engagement with audiences can support the creation of community within the wider context of Darwin. Shirley described her sense of belonging in the wider community this way: "I don't worry too much because I know the audience are always very kind to us." Janine elaborated on how presenting a work that clearly engages an audience contributes to her perception that the Panthers are valued in the wider community.

> *Bowl's Club Wedding* was the favourite show I have done. The script was funny. We had young people working with us. We dressed up and we bowled on the lawn. So it was bowling, dancing, acting. The location in the bowl's club was really good. Everyone who came along, you could see they were really looking for a fun time. It involved the audience. People quite enjoy that.

According to our interviews, performing dance as a community-building activity within Darwin was not a reason for joining the group. Through reflection, however, dancers acknowledged this as a valued aspect. Val described,

> On the census they asked, "What do you do to help out in the community?" and someone said to me, "Well, you do plenty! You sing with the Chorale. You dance with Grey Panthers!" I'd never thought of it as giving to the community...I felt pretty great.

While the dancers did not identify performing in order to "help out" in the community as a reason for starting to dance, actual experiences of performance gave the dancers opportunities to realize how their creative contributions are valued by the wider community. Providing a segue to the next motivator in Maslow's hierarchy of needs, that of "esteem," Jan said, "After you've done a show, people in the street recognize you, and come up and compliment you!"

Esteem: "They thought my dancing was pretty cool"

According to Maslow (1943, 1970), the "pre-potent" needs of physiology, safety and belonging enable the individual to grow confidence and self-esteem. Maslow's concept of esteem encompasses achievement, mastery, independence, status, dominance, prestige, self-respect, and respect from others. Transitioning into dance performance later in life can be a deeply emancipatory experience. Shirley describes, "I like having an audience. I'm really in the moment when I'm out onstage. … I'm relaxed because I know what I'm doing." Her sense of being "in the moment" can be considered a *peak experience* across the lifespan (Bond & Stinson, 2000/2001; Maslow, 1962). Jan described audience feedback as a confidence-boosting motivator: "That helps too. It must have looked alright. It gives you confidence to continue...to move forward."

Some Panthers experience the inter-generational productions with Tracks Dance Company as confidence building. Val recalled, "We did *Last Light*. I really, really enjoyed that, and dancing with the young group as well. These young girls were fit and great, and they appreciated *us*!" Marg shared another example of inter-generational regard: "My granddaughters are dancers. They thought [me dancing] was pretty cool." Esteem in the form of personal power can be enhanced when a performer challenges social boundaries and connects with others imaginatively. Darryl Butler reflected,

> The nervousness disappeared when I could see the audience. If I look at someone in the audience and they look back at me, there's something going on there. It's a connection. You have some power, you are setting the agenda. In *Eight to Eighty*, in the mall, I caught someone's eye and played to that person.

Cognition and Aesthetics: "You get a little bit of a rev!"

By the 1970s Maslow had added two further "growth needs" to his theory of motivation: cognitive and aesthetic, the first related to the human quest to keep growing "intelligence" and the other related to the classical notion of aesthetics as the need for beauty, harmony, and balance, especially in relation to nature (Maslow, 1970, 1976). Twenty-first century definitions of intelligence and aesthetics have grown to accommodate multiple forms of sensory and embodied knowledge, extending beyond the mental and abstract orientation of earlier universal definitions (Gardner, 1983). Human beings demonstrate sensory-aesthetic preferences from a young age (Bond, 2001, 2018) and the need to play and be creative continues throughout life.

Cognitive Needs Dancers appreciate the didactic content of Grey Panther classes, as illustrated by Janine: "I love the ways it's explained: 'We are doing this for the core… We are doing this for the 26 bones in the foot.' It's satisfying to know." Cognitive motivation can extend beyond class contact time, as Judith Allen noted: "When we are learning a new dance, I go and write it down. This helps me to learn, and I continue thinking about it through the week." Toni Vine Bromley added, "I always feel that once I've learnt the dance, I've grown." Maria Vlastuin corroborated, "It's like always growing up." A number of dancers noted cognitive gains from performance. Val explained,

> You get a little bit of a rev! You're lifted to the next height, and then you are comfortable at that level… I always perform much more onstage than in rehearsal. It brings it out. … I think the performance pushes us just that little bit further, because there is an audience.

Val's state of mental charge emerges in the performance moment, yet performing could as easily occasion unwanted stress. Maintaining "rev" within dance performance can require activities that are challenging enough to motivate, but not so challenging that they create overwhelming anxiety (Bond & Stinson, 2007/2016).

Achieving cognitive balance between the familiar and the novel can allow an individual to achieve a sense of flow, which, according to performance psychologist Mikhail Csikszentmihalyi (1996), supports self-actualization. Jan describes how she achieves a sense of flow, alluding to both psycho-physiological requisites and aesthetic needs:

> I still get nervous, but when doing shows, I relax and remember everything. It all comes back, what I have done in class. Memory is very important, at this stage in life especially… It has built up to such a stage that I am comfortable. It seems to come to me, because I need to put my best effort into it, as people are watching. It's important to get it right, for my own

> peace of mind. I guess it is a bit like autopilot, after all the rehearsals, and once you have costuming on, which seems to be something else that adds to it. You have the full thing going. It's a wonderful experience.

Like experienced dancers across the lifespan, when on "autopilot," Jan trusts her body to think and complete tasks without conscious effort and deliberation. For Val, too, having dance knowledge well-embodied by the time of performance allows mental alertness within a state of relaxation:

> Near the beginning, we are trying to figure out the steps. Our muscle memory hasn't worked in. But by the time we perform, all of that has come together and that's how I can relax. By that stage we are not stressed, because we've practiced the routines.

She adds, "I don't perform if I have been away for a while. I don't do it if I don't feel comfortable." Lillian describes also how the process of retaining, repeating, and refining the performance of dances builds confidence in her memory:

> Routine gives me a lot of confidence. It's like a little child. You give them the same routine, they become very confident. It's the same with us. With the constant routine, I begin to know exactly where I stand and what I can do.

The dancers' reflections align with previous research supporting associations between dance, the elderly and mental health (Hill, 2015; Ray, 2016).

Aesthetic Needs According to Maslow's hierarchy of needs, humans require novelty and aesthetic pleasures of, for example, balance and harmony to achieve self-actualization. As introduced above, in this chapter we elaborate Maslow's (1970) emphasis on beauty and intimacy with nature to include the bio-aesthetic—our human multi-sensory capacity to appreciate and create holistic forms and felt, rhythmic connections to self, others and place, a capacity we may be born with (Bond, 2008, 2018; Dissanayake, 2001; Coda, this volume). As Marg commented, "I'd always been involved in musicals … I'd always wanted to dance. And then I came back to it, when I retired."

Where aesthetic needs are concerned, "one size does not fit all." Grey Panther works are made to fit the dancers. David explains how the choreographic process involves an "unspoken constant negotiation" in which performers' talents, capabilities, and limitations are explored as a central part of the creative practice. Janine described,

> I've just loved the way that, when learning a dance, if you can't do this step, if you can't turn around, if you get dizzy, they say, "just do this step instead." It's just lovely that it encompasses everybody. I really like that feeling. At our age, it is something that's really nice. All the people, who come from all the different sorts of backgrounds…we are on a level field when it comes to dance.

Creativity is central to all Grey Panther activities. Janine provides a holistic description:

> What I find with dance is that every week it's a little bit different. You're learning something, you are revising something. It makes you think. There is a combination of exercise with creativity.

Jan expressed her pleasure in "presenting work of high quality." All the preceding comments reference the satisfaction of aesthetic needs, as conceptualized above, pointing to self-actualization.

Choreographic approaches within the Grey Panthers vary along the didactic-to-democratic spectrum (Butterworth, 2004), offering the dancers a great variety of experiences. Sometimes the work involves an evolving, collaborative process with the dancers contributing movement material and creative ideas. Tim explained that other times the process is predetermined by the choreographer, and the final dance movements are presented (or adapted) to the group and each dancer. Dancers spoke of enjoying opportunities to create as well as the freedom to simply perform someone else's steps, or as Janine described, "…adding the finesse to the dance."

The Grey Panther repertoire is created with and for local performers in response to local sites and cultural issues, and maintained locally as repertoire. All works performed are created for and mostly with the dancers, so there is no sense of replicating movements out of a book. Choreographic methods include varying degrees of collaboration, depending on who is working with the dancers, and so the creative process may involve shared conceptualization of the dance, movement generation, composition, or improvisation during performance. Dancers' creative potentials often extend to performances where they are asked to behave spontaneously with an audience. Lillian recalled,

> One time, we had to walk amongst the audience and ask people if they would give us a hand. I went over to this chap and said, "Would you mind giving me a hand to hang out the washing?" and he immediately said, "Yes! I'll be there!" and his wife said, "Yeah, he'll come and give you a hand!" …The reaction of this guy! I can still see him now.

Creative exploration can afford aesthetic satisfaction when personal and local histories gain artistic quality. Marg described,

> *Swings and Flings* reduced me to tears at the end. Every time. It was a journey. It was set in a rural area, and quite a few of us had lived that life. When I first came up here teaching back in the sixties, I was out in the settlements. Then I went out on the cattle stations, teaching out there. I just identified with all of that. And there were some great scenes in it, and right at the end the audience would be in tears.

Here, meanings extend beyond the stage, emphasizing the significance of a dancer's life "journey" and sense of place. While some of the cabaret-style works adapt to fit into different performing contexts of social halls and small theatres, all major evening-length festival works are purposely created in local sites, responding to the architecture, nature, and cultural histories of the site. *A Bowl's Club Wedding* (2003, 2006) was situated within a local bowls club and its greens. For 2015's *Last Light*, a clifftop venue was chosen to explore the phases of Darwin's renowned sunset over the water.

Local issues also pervade Grey Panthers' repertoire. For example, *The Story of Olive Pink* (2001) explored local historical figures, while *Lipstick and Ochre* (2008) presented intercultural dialogues. Local issues have been set within global paradigms: drawing on Romeo and Juliet, *A Bowl's Club Wedding* explores the local rivalry of competing bowling clubs, within the fractious "you're with us or against us" political context of post-9/11 global conflicts. Further, these works are not lost within a season, but maintained as repertoire, passed (with adaptations) from generation to generation of performers. This continuity keeps each work tangible and strengthens the vision that art created locally *remains* local.

Self-Actualization: "It brings me out of myself"

Maslow did not coin the term "self-actualization," but gave it popular currency as a guiding beacon of the 1960 and 70s' human potential movement in the United States. Drawing the concept from German neurologist Kurt Goldstein's (1936/1995) holistic "theory of the organism," Maslow (1943) viewed self-actualization as the fulfillment of an instinctual desire to make the most of one's abilities and become all that one is "fitted for." He wrote, "A musician must make music, an artist must paint, a poet must write…" for ultimate happiness (p. 383). As noted in the introduction to this chapter, we view the elderly dancers of the Grey Panthers' *choice to perform* as an indicator of self-actualization.

The process of retirement allows for reflections, renewed directions and personal goal-setting, and the Grey Panthers therefore seems an exemplary context to theorize self-actualization in dance. Lillian's comment is illuminating in this regard:

> I can remember when I was very young and learning dance, and the nuns saying, "if you keep up that dance, we will excommunicate you!" All because I was doing dance! All that time, from when I was nine until now, I never got back into something where I could really express myself and enjoy. It's just been so great.

Val shared,

> I'd retired, I was 65 and looking round for things to do, a friend of mine was coming then, and she said, "you like dance and movement and singing and carrying on." I came along.

Dancers emphasized in particular the power of performance to generate the kinds of cognitive and aesthetic growth that support self-actualization for participating dancers, including what Maslow called "peak experiences" (Bond & Stinson, 2000/2001; Privett, 2001), in which dancers explore heightened emotions and new ways of being. Shirley reflected that performing transforms her from a more introverted to a more extroverted state: "I'm a show off! Actually, I'm very shy, but not on stage. I'm quite different at that time. I've never been worried by being nervous or anything like that." Some Grey Panthers view the experience of becoming a more extroverted person on stage as a product of social combustion. Val described how a desire for visibility is generated within the group: "I get those feelings when I get on stage. Like everyone else. We always fight for the front of the stage! We don't start off as show offs."

Dancers' transformations through performance are observable in both the emergence of alternate and seemingly contradictory aspects of their "normal" personalities, and through sheer playfulness and imagination. Jan reflected on her transformation:

> It makes me feel more feminine. I'm not a feminine person, I'm more mannish in my ways, but I enjoy the excitement of dressing up, even though I hate dresses! I enjoy the chance to be feminine. I've been a tomboy most of my life, but performance gives me a chance for that sort of thing. It brings me out of myself.

Janine described how the sensation of transforming during a performance involved a clear shift from the experience of rehearsal—that entering a performance persona allows her greater ownership of the choreography.

> In *Last Light*, we didn't have a whole audience in front of us. You could dance more one-to-one, do whatever you liked. That was rather fun. It's nice to be able to just jump outside of yourself and away you go. I could do this or do that (performing arm movements) and nobody is going to say you are right or wrong.

Reaching this point of confidence in creative improvisation on stage seems noteworthy in terms of self-fulfillment. Such experiences suggest how performance allows for personal transformation and make-believe, prompting individuals to momentarily redesign the world, and through that experience, realize their potential and 'self-actualization' within it from a new perspective.

Conclusion: Dancing in the Sunset

Performing dance can be a means of personal discovery and creative expression, generating enhanced feelings of having and using imagination, creativity, skill and other positive and valued attributes amongst the elderly. The dancers of the Grey Panthers have shared their understandings of how dancing and performing dance fulfill motivational needs across a holistic spectrum – physical, social, emotional, cognitive and aesthetic. Central to dancers' needs fulfillment has been their developing confidence that their dance work is valued—by each other and by the local community, meeting growth needs of esteem, aesthetics, and self-actualization (Maslow, 1970).

Community artists have observed that amongst the elderly, expectations of movement improvisation and innovation can lead to feelings of dissatisfaction and anxiety (Barr, 2013; Davidson, 2002). This suggests that the creation and rehearsal processes of the Grey Panthers deserves further research to illuminate pedagogic and choreographic practices that allow such performances to be achieved, and how elderly dancers can continue to be represented as performers in the literature on dance and the quality of life.

A recent performance of the Grey Panthers, *Last Light* (2015), presents a strong visual metaphor for elderly performers, evidencing their artistic distinction and emphasizing the need for more scholarship in the zone of dance, performance and the elderly. Set atop a cliff-bound coastline amidst the tropical sunset, the dancers move against the skyline. Just as the sunset demonstrates that its later hues can be the most vibrant, the dancers illustrate that some of the most poignant and surprising physical expressions can emerge later in life.

References

Australian Bureau of Statistics. (2016). *Darwin.* Retrieved from http://www.censusdata.abs.gov.au/census_services/getproduct/census/2006/quickstat/705

Barr, S. (2013). Learning to learn: A hidden dimension within community dance practice. *Journal of Dance Education, 13*(4), 115–121.

Bond, K. (2008). The human nature of dance: Towards a theory of aesthetic community. In S. Malloch & C. Trevarthen (Eds.), *Communicative musicality: Exploring the basis of human companionship* (pp. 401–422). Oxford: Oxford University Press.

Bond, K. (2018). "Me, a tree": Young children as natural phenomenologists. In S. Fraleigh (Ed.), *Back to the dance itself: Phenomenologies of the body in performance* (pp. 205–232). Urbana: University of Illinois Press.

Bond, K. E. (2001). "I'm not an eagle, I'm a chicken!" Young children's perceptions of creative dance. *Early Childhood Connections, 7*(4), 41–51.

Bond, K. E., and Stinson, S. W. (2000/2001). "I feel like I'm going to take off!": Young people's experiences of the superordinary in dance. *Dance Research Journal, 32*(2), 52-87.

Bond, K. E., & Stinson, S. W. (2016). "It's work, work, work, work:" young people's experiences of effort and engagement in dance. In S. W. Stinson (Ed.), *Embodied curriculum theory and research in arts education: A dance scholar's search for meaning* (pp. 269–295). Dordrecht, Eastern Cape: Springer (Original work published 2007).

Bolwell, J. (2017). Wellbeing and the ageing dancer. In V. Karkou, S. Oliver, & S. Lycouris (Eds.), *Oxford handbook of dance and wellbeing* (pp. 311–328). Oxford: Oxford University Press.

Borstel, J. (2006). Liz Lerman dance exchange: Superheroes and everyday dancers, old and young. *Generations, 1*(3), 65–67.

Boyatzis, R. E. (1998). *Transforming qualitative information.* Thousand Oaks, CA: Sage.

Bryant, A., & Charmaz, K. (2007). *The sage handbook of grounded theory.* Thousand Oaks, CA: Sage.

Butterworth, J. (2004). Teaching choreography in higher education: A process continuum model. *Research in Dance Education, 5*(1), 45–67.

Centre for Policy on Ageing. (2011). *Keep dancing: The health and wellbeing benefits of dance for older people.* Retrieved from http://www.cpa.org.uk/information/reviews/shall-we-dance-report.pdf

Clarke, D. B. (1973). The concept of community: A re-examination. *Sociological Review, 21*(3), 32–37.

Connolly, K., & Redding, E. (2010). *Dancing towards wellbeing in the third age: Literature review on the impact of dance on health and wellbeing of older people.* Retrieved from https://www.trinitylaban.ac.uk/media/315435/literature%20review%20impact%20of%20dance%20elderly%20populations%20final%20draft%20with%20logos.pdf

Cooper, L., & Thomas, H. (2002). Growing old gracefully: Social dance in the third age. *Ageing & Society, 22*(6), 689–708.

Craft, A. (2005). *Creativity in schools: Tensions and dilemmas.* Oxon, UK: Routledge.

Csikszentmihalyi, M. (1996). *Creativity: Flow and the psychology of discovery and invention.* New York: Harper Collins.

Davidson, P. (2002). *Evaluation of Gener8: A dance group for the over-sixties run by Scottish ballet.* Edinburgh, UK: SCRE Centre.

Denzin, N. K., & Lincoln, Y. S. (1998). *Strategies of qualitative inquiry.* Thousand Oaks, CA: Sage.

Dissanayake, E. (2001). Becoming homo aestheticus: Sources of aesthetic imagination in mother-infant interactions. In H. P. Abbott (Ed.), *On the origin of fictions: Interdisciplinary perspectives* (pp. 85–103). Madison, WI: University of Wisconsin Press.

Du Maurier, D. (1938). *Rebecca.* London: Pan.

Eisner, R. S. (2010). 'I am cultures': Ea Sola's transnational, transcultural arts and answerability. In L. Noszklopy & M. Cohen (Eds.), *Contemporary southeast Asian performance: Transnational perspectives* (pp. 133–163). Newcastle, UK: Cambridge Scholars.

Fine, M. (1994). Working the hyphens: Reinventing self and other in qualitative research. In N. K. Denzin & Y. S. Lincoln (Eds.), *Handbook of qualitative research* (pp. 70–82). Thousand Oaks, CA: Sage.

Freire, P. (1972). *Pedagogy of the oppressed.* Harmondsworth, England: Penguin.

Gardner, H. (1983). *Frames of mind: The theory of multiple intelligences.* New York: Basic Books.

Goldstein, K. (1995). *The organism.* New York: Urzone (Original work published 1936).

Hanna, G., & Perlstein, S. (2008). *Creativity matters: Arts and aging in America.* Washington, DC: Americans for the Arts Monograph.

Hill, H. (2015). Dancing with hope: Dance therapy for people with dementia. In S. Chaiklin & H. Wengrower (Eds.), *The art and science of dance/movement therapy: Life is dance* (2nd ed., pp. 219–232). New York: Routledge.

Houston, S. (2005). Dance for older people. *Primary Health Care, 15*(8), 18–19.

Keogh, J., Kilding, A., Pidgeon, P., Ashley, L., & Gills, D. (2009). Physical benefits of dancing for healthy older adults: A review. *Journal of Ageing and Physical Activity, 17*, 1–23.

Lane, R. D., & Nadel, L. (Eds.). (2001). *Cognitive neuroscience of emotion.* Oxford: Oxford University Press.

Lerman, L. (2011). *Hiking the horizontal.* Middletown, CT: Wesleyan University Press.

Lomas, C. (2007). Culture constructs, community and celebration. In P. Kuppers & G. Robertson (Eds.), *The community performance reader* (pp. 213–216). New York: Routledge.

Maslow, A. (1943). A theory of human motivation. *Psychological Review, 50*(4), 370–396.

Maslow, A. (1962). *Toward a psychology of being.* New York: Van Nostrand Reinhold.

Maslow, A. (1970). *Motivation and personality.* New York: Harper & Row.

Maslow, A. (1976). *The farther reaches of human nature.* New York: Penguin.

Mewett, P. (1988). Darwin's Beer Can Regatta: Masculinity, frontier and festival in Northern Australia. *Social Analysis: The International Journal of Social and Cultural Practice, 23*, 3–37.

Nahachewsky, A. (1995). Participatory and presentational dance as ethnochoreological categories. *Dance Research Journal, 27*(1), 1–15.

Piaget, J. (1929). *The child's conception of the world* (J. & A. Tomlinson, Trans.). New York: Harcourt Brace.

Potter, M. (2014). *Dame Maggie Scott: A life in dance.* Melbourne, VIC: Text Publishing.

Privette, G. (2001). Defining moments of self-actualization: Peak performance and peak experience. In K. J. Schneider, J. F. T. Bugental, & J. F. Pierson (Eds.), *The handbook of humanistic psychology* (pp. 161–180). Thousand Oaks, CA: Sage.

Ray, M. (2016). Creativity and the arts for older people living with depression. In C. A. Chew-Graham & M. Ray (Eds.), *Mental health and older people: A guide for primary care practitioners* (pp. 133–144). Dordrecht, The Netherlands: Springer.

Risner, D. (1995). Voices seldom heard: The dancers' experience of the choreographic process. *Impulse, 3*(2), 76–85.

Ross, F. (2007a). Company of elders. *Working with Older People, 11*(4), 37–40.

Ross, J. (2007b). *Anna Halprin: Experience as dance.* Berkeley: University of California Press.

Rowe, N., Buck, R., & Martin, R. (2015). The gaze or the groove? Emerging themes from the New meanings and pathways: Community dance and dance education symposium. *Research in Dance Education, 16*(2), 184–197.

Salazar, C. (2013). A humanizing pedagogy: Reinventing the principles and practice of education as a journey toward liberation. *Review of Research in Education, 37*, 121–148.

Salter, E. (1978). *Helpmann: The authorized biography of sir Robert Helpmann.* Melbourne, VIC: Angus and Robertson.

Sheets-Johnstone, M. (2011). *The primacy of movement* (expanded 2nd ed.). Amsterdam: John Benjamins. (Original work published 1999)

Silvester, D., & Frampton, S. (2014). *Dance and movement sessions for older people: A handbook for activity coordinators and carers*. London: Jessica Kingsley.

Simonov, P. V. (2013). *The emotional brain: Physiology, neuroanatomy, psychology, and emotion* (M. J. Hall, Trans.). New York: Springer. (Original work published 1986)

Stinson, S. W. (1985). Piaget for dance educators: A theoretical study. *Dance Research Journal, 17*(1), 9–16.

Stinson, S. W. (1997). A question of fun: Adolescent engagement in dance education. *Dance Research Journal, 29*(2), 49–69.

Stinson, S. W., Blumenfeld-Jones, D., & Van Dyke, J. (1990). Voices of young women dance students: An interpretive study of meaning in dance. *Dance Research Journal, 22*(2), 13–22.

Thomas, H., & Cooper, L. (2003). *Dancing into the third age: Social dance as cultural text: A research report*. London: Goldsmiths College.

Tracks Dance Company. (2015a). *Dance on Darwin*. Retrieved from http://tracksdance.com.au/dance-darwin

Tracks Dance Company. (2015b). *The Grey panthers*. Retrieved from http://tracksdance.com.au/grey-panthers-13

Chapter 31
Babies and Dance: Questions of Origin

Karen Bond and Kirsten Kaschock

Part I

Babies and Dance – Karen Bond

I was fortunate to study modern dance in high school physical education. I remember being fascinated by how it felt to sit on the gym floor—knees bent with soles of feet together, practicing Martha Graham's contraction and release to the beats of a hand drum. This bodily "re-cognition" was different from "real life" and from the ballet classes I had taken from a young age. I continued to study modern dance in college and wrote my first essay in freshman English on the subject, incorporating Martha Graham's (1952/1998) well-known quote: "dance is a symbol of the performance of living" (p. 66). Philosopher Zachary Simpson (2012) interprets Graham's meaning dynamically, suggesting that for her dance was an "opening to life through movement and embodiment" (p. 160).

As a novice dance tutor in an Australian early childhood teacher's college, I gained further ideas from Graham's (1952/1998) "I am a Dancer," which was originally a radio talk for Edward R. Murrow's program, *This I Believe,* on National Public Radio. Along with embodied research on various somatic methods that involved spending a lot of time "in the floor": spiraling, pushing, pulling, expanding, condensing, reaching, gesturing, balancing, listening, gazing, flowing, Graham supported my growing sense that babies and young children are essential sources of dance knowledge—teaching us "the miracle of small beautiful bones and their

K. Bond (✉)
Department of Dance, Temple University, Philadelphia, PA, USA
e-mail: kbond003@temple.edu

K. Kaschock
Drexel University, Philadelphia, PA, USA
e-mail: kjk42@drexel.edu

K. Bond (ed.), *Dance and the Quality of Life*, Social Indicators Research Series 73,
https://doi.org/10.1007/978-3-319-95699-2_31

delicate strength" (p. 67). Further, infants are exemplars of the human potential for learning through experience and practice (Bond, 2018).

In the early 1980s, I picked up a notion (source lost) that Graham developed her method of contraction and release in part through observation of infants breathing. I started collecting empirical evidence towards the possibility of making a case for infants as pioneers of modern dance; clearly, they—along with dancers—represent the gold standard of observable "whole body breathing." I began assigning baby observations in dance practicum classes, a practice that continued intermittently over decades (1985–2011):

> *Do babies dance?*
>
> Spend time in the next week observing, playing with, and/or dancing with a baby (a pre-walker). In your class journal, describe the baby's dance or discuss your reasons why babies *don't* dance. If you do not have access to a live baby, video observation will suffice. (Bond, Practice and Theory of Movement archive, 1985)

Early this year, research assistant Kakali Paramguru and I performed preliminary descriptive coding of my treasure trove of student papers, creating a baby dance profile of approximately 1,000 codes (6,000 words total). Perhaps unsurprisingly, we found an overall affirmative response to the question, *Do babies dance*? (approximately six per cent said no). While one might see this as a predictable outcome for a population of dance teaching artists, I concur with van der Leeuw (1932/2006) that of all the arts, dance *requires participation* to be understood. I propose, therefore, that the two groups—dance specialists and infants—are expert and reliable informants. Metaphorical support for the value of infant dance (and dance, the phenomenon) comes from countless literary sources, for example Henry David Thoreau (1854) who suggested in *Walden*, "To affect the quality of the day, that is the highest of arts" (as cited in Berleant, 2016, n.p.). Multiple observations over an extended period suggest that for both sets of participant observers (babies and professionals), "quality of the day" was heightened during these quality moments captured over 25 years. In Part II of this final chapter, dancer, poet, and novelist Kirsten Kaschock presents a poetic interpretation of both the historical sketch and the distilled data.

Part II

Questions of Origin - Kirsten Kaschock

1. Did Martha watch the small ribcages / expand? Did she find

   : smile wiggle move a dance to music special love a twitching her biggest love dancing—it's second nature songs sung at church rock&dance sounds they make bang toot stomp that off-on key duet wiggledance & happysmile

2. in their breathing the spine / of her practice?

   : jiggle try to keep rhythm sing along with all sorts Baby Loves to Dance to her own beat bangs on a toy chest shakes back&forth most love to happytime kicks in the car her little heart out jiggle wiggle a little boogie

3. And if she did—are they then our ancestors / unsung-but-ever-singing?

   : bob of head back&forth beat-bounce up&down rhythm bottom-shakes bobs&grooves side-to-side singing singing singing&dancing bobs head—now—stomps feet tries to sing along certain songs sounding nothing-like

4. Can Wordsworth's conundrum / maintain—

   : the song dances allllllllllll the time slow to slower songs on tempo to everything to the music to dance drops it like it's hot bouncing little bum-bum whenever music moving&grooving makes his own by banging shaking&bouncing

5. that the child is father of the man? / And then, what of woman

   : shaking&bouncing fast babble—constantly walking climbing walking backwards almost-running grooving saying "bubble&puppy" up&down then she throws head down between her knees this—for over an hour

6. —can an infant(s) mother our movement?

   : a long time now they hone in kick legs move arms shake heads into different parts of the body they can sink have great release how weighted into the floor their torso grounded in the floor so limbs are free arms to articulate

7. I have had and held them, felt / them bob and rock, coo and curl, contract / and crawl—and the words of their parents / echo. Is it echoing them?

   : legs free to explore relying on the floor released weight into the floor the weight of the head or standing using chair for balance chair with one hand tapping&waving the other correspondence a sense of awe enthusiasm

8. The root of language, does it / babble as it reaches towards some / deeper stream?

   : celebratory laughter not spinning moving in all directions clapping her hands spontaneous joying pelvic rock hand-tapping all rhythmical dancing internally repetitively social interaction mother&child facial gestures mirroring

9. When we enter the dance, tell me, is it / something *other* than a reclamation?

   : a subtle form spontaneous play delight impulse to move reaction&interaction of sorts any&every muscle or bone finds a way to move constant motion crawling attempting to gain the alignment to walk falling over&over again matching song

10. If it is, I don't know what / it is—other than this

: worth / our words. Our study. Yes?yes.

References

Berleant, A. (2016). The art in knowing a landscape. In *Aesthetics beyond the arts* (pp. 67–80). New York: Routledge.

Bond, K. (2018). "Me, a tree": Young children as natural phenomenologists. In S. Fraleigh (Ed.), *Back to the dance itself: Phenomenologies of the body in performance* (pp. 205–232). Urbana: University of Illinois Press.

Graham, M. (1998). I am a dancer. In A. Carter & J. O'Shea (Eds.), *The Routledge dance studies reader* (pp. 66–71). New York: Routledge (Original work published 1952).

Simpson, Z. (2012). *Merleau-Ponty and Marion on the thought of being. Life as art: Aesthetics and the creation of self* (pp. 159–204). Lanham, MD: Lexington Books.

van der Leeuw, G. (2006). *Sacred and profane beauty: The holy in art* (D. E. Green, Trans.). D. Apostolos-Cappadona (Ed.). Oxford: Oxford University Press. (Original work published 1932).

Coda

Ellen Dissanayake

Days before I started to write this essay, ethnolinguist Ekkehart Malotki and I completed a book that we've been working on for more than five years. It is a study of petroglyphs and pictographs that our human ancestors and relatives have left behind on stone surfaces all over the world. The book is concerned entirely with geometric or abstract markings, rather than the better-known pictorial representations of animals and people that include depictions of dance or "dance-like" behavior worldwide (Gillette, Greer, Hayward, & Murray, 2014). Its subtitle, *The Geometric Enigma*, is derived from the puzzling fact that abstract geometric marks are the oldest and most numerous rock markings everywhere they are found (Malotki & Dissanayake, 2018). A study of abstract petroglyphs might seem remote from the topic of dance and even more so from dance and the quality of life. Yet as I thought more, I realized there are connections after all. In this coda, I point not only to what the two art forms have in common, but propose a common denominator of all the arts.

"Making Special"

My work over four decades has focused on the biological and evolutionary basis of the arts. Almost from the beginning, I have thought of art not as a thing—a choreography or sonata, a quality like beauty or skill, or a label assigned by an "artworld" of critics and historians. Instead, I think of art as something people *do*, a *behavior* of art. It remains to be understood fully what people do when they behave "artfully," but this perspective allows me to treat art(s) as a characteristic of our species, from earliest times, that can be found in every known human society. Art as behavior characterizes everyone.

E. Dissanayake (✉)
University of Washington, Seattle, Washington, USA
e-mail: ed3@u.washington.edu

K. Bond (ed.), *Dance and the Quality of Life*, Social Indicators Research Series 73,
https://doi.org/10.1007/978-3-319-95699-2

It is easy to appreciate art as behavior when considering dance. Dancing unfolds in time and when it ends, exists only in memory—at least this was so until the invention of film and more recent visual technologies. The first line of Erin Brannigan's (2011) monograph on "dancefilm" reads, "The nature of dance performance has been irrevocably altered by the cinema" (p. 3), although screen dance is not usually considered equivalent to live dancing for participants or viewers (Dodds, 2004; Mitoma, Zimmer, & Stieber, 2002). In terms of evolutionary history, dance is dancing, and more broadly, song is singing, performance is performing—all "things that people do." Visual art, like a petroglyph or statue, would seem to be different; but, although it is a thing or a work, it is possible to think of visual art as the result of behavior. A petroglyph during its making can be considered an instance of a behavior of gestural or whole body mark making—a kind of dance perhaps, and we can ask what characterizes *that*.

In my early work on the arts as behavior, I called the doing of art "making special" (see Dissanayake, 1992), which I eventually made more academically acceptable with a verb, "artify," as an ethological construct denoting our human adaptive predisposition to "make special." As such, artifying is not confined to the highly-skilled specialist; nor is it "disinterested" or separate from biological function (Dissanayake, 2014, p. 57). Archaeological evidence indicates that from very early times humans were able to distinguish between the ordinary and the extra-ordinary, and to artify or make the ordinary "special." At Gönnerdorf, an open-air site near Koblenz, Germany, for example, excavators have found stone plaques engraved with groups of female figures in rows (from 14-12 millennia BCE). Some figures are facing right in half-crouching positions with arms raised in "dynamic body gestures" (Garfinkel, 2014, p. 6), special movements outside of the everyday that certainly suggest dance.

The Austrian pioneer human ethologist, Irenäus Eibl-Eibesfeldt (1988), proposed that aesthetic perception is grounded in physiological biases that humans share with higher vertebrates (for example, birds and monkeys), and that these evolved for pattern recognition, perceptual constancy, and spatial orientation. He notes, "Our perception seeks and enjoys order" (p. 30). Through this lens, perhaps early humans' appreciation of the moon's passage across the sky—its regularity, its shininess and changing shapes—inspired an extra-ordinary response of expressive reaching and whole body circling movements, a solo for—or a duet with—the celestial body.

Although dance can certainly produce or display order, my view is that it is most importantly a mode of social communication, as a number of chapters in this volume illustrate. Biologist E. O. Wilson saw parallels between chimpanzees' carnival behavior and human dancing and singing, suggesting that both species dance to reinforce group identity (Rampley, 2017). My own evolutionary perspective is that the behaviors of making special arise from the earliest communication between mother and infant, where mutual coordination is first experienced and practiced in time and space. I was interested to encounter developmental theorist Daniel Stern's (1977, 2010) use of the metaphors "dance," "performance," and "duet" to describe mother-infant interaction, and subsequently further explored the relationship between art and intimacy in my own work (for example, Dissanayake, 2000, 2014).

Origins of Artistic Practice

Ethological descriptions of "ritualized" super-ordinary behaviors in animals eventually led me to propose that human arts began when our Pleistocene ancestors (2.6 million to 11,700 years ago) deliberately began to use aesthetic strategies (initially untaught and then learned) to transform ordinary objects and behavior so that they were then experienced as extra-ordinary, or special. Ritualized behaviors occur spectacularly in birds, and it was not lost on evolutionary theorist Charles Darwin (1874) and others that the lavish products of human artists can resemble the courtship displays of birds. Some even attribute the origin and function of human art-making to sexual selection (Dutton, 2009; Miller, 2000), a hypothesis that continues to be contested or qualified (see Dennett, 1995/2014; Dissanayake, 2000).

Dance and Dancing

It is not known when dance began. It leaves few or no traces in the sites where ancestral humans once lived, although existing traces suggestive of dance are spread widely in the world (Garfinkel, 2014). My own belief is that dance and song, along with body decoration, probably preceded or at least accompanied the invention of mark making, of which we have evidence in *Homo sapiens* as early as 200 thousand years ago (Van Peer et al., 2003). Ancestral environments required biologically relevant physical abilities such as toolmaking, tracking or navigating, using one's body for work, play, and locomotion. Dance is made of these movements and others, first perhaps through imitation of natural forms and occurrences and eventually transforming them with aesthetic sensibilities (Dissanayake, 1979) or "operations," such as composing, formalization (organizing, composing), repetition, exaggeration, elaboration, and the manipulation of expectation (Dissanayake, 2014). These all make something special and *noticeable*. Prominence or emphasis of any sort is potentially *emotional*. In dance, ordinary body movements are shaped, patterned, and made vivid through the above innate aesthetic operations.

Infants are born prepared to engage in rhythmic, coordinated interactions with their caretakers (Dissanayake, 2000; Stern, 1977, 2010; Trevarthen, 1999). The facial, vocal, and gestural expressions and responses used and developed in these early interactions are composed of behaviors that resemble the methods and effects in two other behavioral contexts: ritualization in other-than-human animals and in the temporal arts, such as dance, song, and instrumental music (Dissanayake, 2001), thus spanning the biology and evolution of our prehuman relatives, our ancient human ancestors and infants, as well as into our own adult lives.

Being a baby means desiring to participate in patterned, multimodal, emotionally communicative improvisations with caretakers and others, to imitate their movements and sounds, move rhythmically to music, and play with words and other vocal sounds (see Chap. 31, this volume). Babies do not have to be trained to learn these things in the way that lions must be trained to jump through hoops. Patterning and elaborating, recurrence and variation begin to occur in all modalities of movement, including vocalization, as precursors of what will become dance, song, and poetry. All children are predisposed to play and dance—that is, to notice, participate in, and create a special, extra-ordinary dimension of experience. These universal actions feel good and are actively sought out, a sure sign for an ethologist that they are critical to a child's ongoing development.

Having all been babies, early humans, too, possessed an innate susceptibility to elements of repetition, emphasis, and extravagance in kinesthetic, vocal, and visual modalities. In this way, components of mother-infant interaction became transmuted into the first arts, developed in ritual ceremonies as what we now call song, dance, dramatic performance, poetic language, and visual display. As with mothers and infants, ceremonial arts generally occur all together as *bodily-based* "multimedia," and they have multimodal, interpenetrating sensory and emotional effects. At the same time, one could say that all the arts are "dance-based"; there are no arts without aesthetic embodiment.

The Dancing Brain Elements of dance are born through the perceptual and organizational properties of the human brain (Bläsing et al., 2012; Brown, Martinez, & Parsons, 2006), neurophysiological features essential for ordinary life in the world. Our inborn receptivity to elements such as rhythm, balance, symmetry, proportion, perspective—and deviations from these—makes them good candidates for elaborations that attract attention, sustain interest, and arouse and shape emotions. Neurophysiological studies have shown that activities such as group dancing, rhythmic clapping, and chanting promote affiliative emotions and brain states conducive to accepting and incorporating collective values (Ehrenreich, 2007; Freeman, 1995; McNeill, 1995; Sheets-Johnstone, 2017). Further, rhythmic sequential organization of movements and sounds, in both synchrony and antiphony, together build community (Malloch & Trevarthen, 2008). Participating with others in coordinated movements and sounds is a sign of good working order, which feels good (Bond, 2008).

Conclusion

From an evolutionary perspective, I align with the view that dance (or any other performative or processual arts) need not show or tell a story "about" anything (see Daly, 2002). Similarly, not all geometric abstract marks on stone surfaces "mean" something other than themselves, but are made with the intention that the act of making will have an effect on the world—on quality of life (Malinowski, 1925/1954; Malotki & Dissanayake, 2018). Dancing is behavior with noticeable changing characteristics and effects as it occurs in time and space. Its effects can be felt through expressive and formal properties as much as through subject matter (Sheets-Johnstone, 1966/2015). As proposed by Jane Austen (1815/2016) through the character Mr. Knightley in her novel *Emma,* "Fine dancing…like virtue, must be its own reward" (p. 310).

Dancing, along with vocalizing, might be called the earliest form of human "making special." As illustrated in the final chapter of this volume, even very young babies will bounce, jiggle, and sway to sequential rhythmic sounds that they hear, well before they have the physical strength and coordination to create patterned locomotor movements in space and time, and they often vocalize to accompany themselves moving. In the second year, as soon as they can hold a drawing instrument, infants will make marks using their whole arm, and as they start to imitate speech, they will play with sounds and eventually words. The precursors to artful behavior and appreciation are there, "ready to go."

It makes sense that our remote human ancestors would have first transformed their movements and vocal sounds in elementary ways before gradually coming to use aesthetic strategies (both untaught and learned) to create dance and song in space and time. Similarly, they would have made marks on soft surfaces, including their bodies, also occurring in space and time. Although dance today might be relegated by some to the province of virtuosic specialization and by others to the realm of evil and sin, what brings the *aesthetic behavior* of dance into being is an inborn capacity in all human beings everywhere. In the most fundamental sense, humans are "born to dance," and dancing is intrinsic to the vitality and quality of life.

References

Austen, J. (2016). *Emma*. London: Macmillan Collectors Library (Original work published 1815).

Bläsing, B., Calvino-Merino, B., Cross, E. S., Jola, C., Honisch, J., & Stevens, C. J. (2012). Neurocognitive control in dance perception and performance. *Acta Psychologia, 139*, 300–308.

Bond, K. E. (2008). The human nature of dance: Towards a theory of aesthetic community. In S. Malloch & C. Trevarthen (Eds.), *Communicative musicality: Exploring the basis of human companionship* (pp. 401–422). Oxford: Oxford University Press.

Brannigan, E. (2011). *Dancefilm: Choreography and the moving image*. Oxford: Oxford University Press.

Brown, S., Martinez, M. J., & Parsons, L. M. (2006). The neural basis of human dance. *Cerebral Cortex, 16*, 1157–1167.

Daly, A. (2002). *Critical gestures: Writings on dance and culture*. Middletown, CT: Wesleyan University Press.

Darwin, C. (1874). *The descent of man and selection in relation to sex* (2nd ed.). New York: A. L. Burt.

Dennett, D. C. (2014). *Darwin's dangerous idea: Evolution and the meanings of life*. New York: Simon & Schuster (Original work published 1995).

Dissanayake, E. (1979). An ethological view of ritual and art in human evolutionary history. *Leonardo, 12*(1), 27–31.

Dissanayake, E. (1992). *Homo aestheticus: Where art comes from and why*. Seattle: University of Washington Press.

Dissanayake, E. (2000). *Art and intimacy: How the arts began*. Seattle: University of Washington Press.

Dissanayake, E. (2001). Becoming *Homo aestheticus*: Sources of aesthetic imagination in mother-infant interactions. *SubStance, 30*(1/2), 85–103.

Dissanayake, E. (2014). A bona fide ethological view of art: The artification hypothesis. In C. Sütterlin, W. Schiefenhövel, C. Lehmann, J. Forster, & G. Apfelauer (Eds.), *Art as behavior: An ethological approach to visual and verbal art, music and architecture* (pp. 43–62). Oldenburg, Germany: Carl von Ossietzky University of Oldenburg Press.

Dodds, S. (2004). *Dance on screen: Genres and media from Hollywood to experimental art*. Basingstoke, UK: Palgrave Macmillan.

Dutton, D. (2009). *The art instinct: Beauty, pleasure and human evolution*. New York: Bloomsbury.

Ehrenreich, B. (2007). *Dancing in the streets: A history of collective joy*. New York: Henry Holt.

Eibl-Eibesfeldt, I. (1988). The biological foundation of aesthetics. In I. Rentschler, B. Herzberger, & D. Epstein (Eds.), *Beauty and the brain: Biological aspects of aesthetics* (pp. 29–70). Basel, Switzerland: Berkhauser Verlag.

Freeman, W. J. (1995). *Societies of brains*. Hillsdale, NJ: Erlbaum.

Garfinkel, Y. (2014). Archaeology of dance. In K. Soar & C. Aamodt (Eds.), *Archaeological approaches to dance performance* (pp. 5–14). Oxford, England: Archaeopress.

Gillette, D. L., Greer, M., Hayward, M. H., & Murray, W. B. (Eds.). (2014). *Rock art and sacred landscapes*. New York: Springer.

Malinowski, B. (1954). *Magic, science, and religion*. Garden City, NY: Doubleday Anchor. (Original work published 1925).

Malloch, S., & Trevarthen, C. (Eds.). (2008). *Communicative musicality: Exploring the basis of human companionship*. Oxford: Oxford University Press.

Malotki, E., & Dissanayake, E. (2018). *Early rock art in the American West: The geometric enigma*. Seattle: University of Washington Press.

McNeill, W. H. (1995). *Keeping together in time: Dance and drill in human history*. Cambridge, MA: Harvard University Press.

Miller, G. F. (2000). *The mating mind: How sexual choice shaped the evolution of human nature*. New York: Doubleday.

Mitoma, J., Zimmer, E., & Stieber, D. A. (Eds.). (2002). *Envisioning dance on film and video*. New York: Routledge.

Rampley, M. (2017). *The seductions of Darwin: Art, evolution, neuroscience*. University Park: Pennsylvania State University Press.

Sheets-Johnstone, M. (2015). *The phenomenology of dance* (50th anniversary edition). Philadelphia: Temple University Press. (Original work published 1966).

Sheets-Johnstone, M. (2017). Moving in concert. *Choros International Dance Journal, 6*, 1–19.

Stern, D. (1977). *The first relationship*. Cambridge, MA: Harvard University Press.

Stern, D. (2010). *Forms of vitality: Exploring dynamic experience in psychology, the arts, psychotherapy and development*. Oxford: Oxford University Press.

Trevarthen, C. (1999). Musicality and the intrinsic motive pulse: Evidence from human psychobiology and infant communication. *Musicæ Scientiæ, 3*(1), 155–215.

Van Peer, P., Fullagar, R., Stokes, S., Bailey, R. M., Moeyersons, J., Steenhoudt, F., et al. (2003). The early to middle stone age transition and the emergence of modern human behaviour at site 8-B-11, Sai Island, Sudan. *Journal of Human Evolution, 45*(2), 187–193.

Index

K. Bond (ed.), *Dance and the Quality of Life*, Social Indicators Research Series 73,
https://doi.org/10.1007/978-3-319-95699-2

D

G

H

I

Q

CPSIA information can be obtained
at www.ICGtesting.com
Printed in the USA
BVHW041257070319
542048BV00004B/11/P

9 783319 956985